DATE DUE

APR 17 2003			

FOOD FOR HEALTH IN THE PACIFIC RIM

3rd International Conference of Food Science and Technology

F N P PUBLICATIONS IN FOOD SCIENCE AND NUTRITION

Books

DICTIONARY OF FLAVORS, D.A. DeRovira
FOOD FOR HEALTH IN THE PACIFIC RIM, J.R. Whitaker *et al.*
DAIRY FOODS SAFETY: 1995–1996, A COMPENDIUM, E.H. Marth
OLIVE OIL, SECOND EDITION, A.K. Kiritsakis
MULTIVARIATE DATA ANALYSIS, G.B. Dijksterhuis
NUTRACEUTICALS: DESIGNER FOODS III, P.A. Lachance
DESCRIPTIVE SENSORY ANALYSIS IN PRACTICE, M.C. Gacula, Jr.
APPETITE FOR LIFE: AN AUTOBIOGRAPHY, S.A. Goldblith
HACCP: MICROBIOLOGICAL SAFETY OF MEAT, J.J. Sheridan *et al.*
OF MICROBES AND MOLECULES: FOOD TECHNOLOGY AT M.I.T., S.A. Goldblith
MEAT PRESERVATION, R.G. Cassens
S.C. PRESCOTT, PIONEER FOOD TECHNOLOGIST, S.A. Goldblith
FOOD CONCEPTS AND PRODUCTS: JUST-IN-TIME DEVELOPMENT, H.R. Moskowitz
MICROWAVE FOODS: NEW PRODUCT DEVELOPMENT, R.V. Decareau
DESIGN AND ANALYSIS OF SENSORY OPTIMIZATION, M.C. Gacula, Jr.
NUTRIENT ADDITIONS TO FOOD, J.C. Bauernfeind and P.A. Lachance
NITRITE-CURED MEAT, R.G. Cassens
POTENTIAL FOR NUTRITIONAL MODULATION OF AGING, D.K. Ingram *et al.*
CONTROLLED/MODIFIED ATMOSPHERE/VACUUM PACKAGING, A.L. Brody
NUTRITIONAL STATUS ASSESSMENT OF THE INDIVIDUAL, G.E. Livingston
QUALITY ASSURANCE OF FOODS, J.E. Stauffer
SCIENCE OF MEAT & MEAT PRODUCTS, 3RD ED., J.F. Price and B.S. Schweigert
HANDBOOK OF FOOD COLORANT PATENTS, F.J. Francis
ROLE OF CHEMISTRY IN PROCESSED FOODS, O.R. Fennema *et al.*
NEW DIRECTIONS FOR PRODUCT TESTING OF FOODS, H.R. Moskowitz
PRODUCT DEVELOPMENT & DIETARY GUIDELINES, G.E. Livingston, *et al.*
SHELF-LIFE DATING OF FOODS, T.P. Labuza
ANTINUTRIENTS AND NATURAL TOXICANTS IN FOOD, R.L. Ory
POSTHARVEST BIOLOGY AND BIOTECHNOLOGY, H.O. Hultin and M. Milner

Journals

JOURNAL OF FOOD LIPIDS, F. Shahidi
JOURNAL OF RAPID METHODS AND AUTOMATION IN MICROBIOLOGY, D.Y.C. Fung and M.C. Goldschmidt
JOURNAL OF MUSCLE FOODS, N.G. Marriott, G.J. Flick, Jr. and J.R. Claus
JOURNAL OF SENSORY STUDIES, M.C. Gacula, Jr.
JOURNAL OF FOODSERVICE SYSTEMS, C.A. Sawyer
JOURNAL OF FOOD BIOCHEMISTRY, N.F. Haard and H. Swaisgood
JOURNAL OF FOOD PROCESS ENGINEERING, D.R. Heldman and R.P. Singh
JOURNAL OF FOOD PROCESSING AND PRESERVATION, D.B. Lund
JOURNAL OF FOOD QUALITY, J.J. Powers
JOURNAL OF FOOD SAFETY, T.J. Montville and D.G. Hoover
JOURNAL OF TEXTURE STUDIES, M.C. Bourne and M.A. Rao

Newsletters

MICROWAVES AND FOOD, R.V. Decareau
FOOD INDUSTRY REPORT, G.C. Melson
FOOD, NUTRACEUTICALS AND NUTRITION, P.A. Lachance and M.C. Fisher

FOOD FOR HEALTH IN THE PACIFIC RIM

3rd International Conference of Food Science and Technology

Edited by

JOHN R. WHITAKER, Ph.D.
Professor Emeritus
University of California, Davis
Department of Food Science and Technology
Davis, California

NORMAN F. HAARD, Ph.D.
Professor
University of California, Davis
Department of Food Science and Technology
Davis, California

CHARLES F. SHOEMAKER
Professor
University of California, Davis
Department of Food Science and Technology
Davis, California

R. PAUL SINGH, Ph.D.
Professor
University of California, Davis
Department of Biological and Agricultural Engineering
Davis, California

FOOD & NUTRITION PRESS, INC.
TRUMBULL, CONNECTICUT 06611 USA

FOOD & NUTRITION PRESS, INC.
Trumbull, Connecticut 06611 USA

Library of Congress Catalog Card Number: 98-073839
ISBN: 0-917678-46-X

Printed in the United States of America

CONTRIBUTORS

FIKRAT ABDULLAEV, Department of Food Research and Postgraduate Studies, Autonomous University of Queretaro, Mexico, Cerro de las Campanas, Queretaro, Qro 76010, Mexico.

YOICHI ABE, Rakuno Gakuen University, Ebetsu, Hokkaido 069, Japan.

H. AKO, Department of Environmental Biochemistry, University of Hawaii at Manoa, Honolulu, HI 96822.

S. ALCOCK, British Sugar Technical Centre, Norwich NR4 7UB, England.

RASHDA ALI, Department of Food Science and Technology, University of Karachi, Karachi-75270, Pakistan.

KEN-ICHI ARAI, Rakuno Gakuen University, Ebetsu, Hokkaido 069, Japan.

TOYOHIKO ARIGA, Department of Nutrition and Physiology, School of Agriculture and Veterinary Medicine, Nihon University, Setagaya, Tokyo 154, Japan.

OFELIA PÉREZ ARVIZU, Dept. of Food Research and Postgraduate Studies, Universidad Autónoma de Querétaro, Querétaro, 76010 Qro., México.

DIANE M. BARRETT, Department of Food Science and Technology, University of California, Davis, CA 95616.

FELICIANO P. BEJOSANO, Cereal Science Laboratory, Department of Botany, University of Hong Kong, Pokfulam Road, Hong Kong.

CHRISTINE M. BRUHN, University of California, Davis, One Shields Ave., Davis, CA 95616.

E. CARSTENS, Section of Neurobiology, Physiology and Behavior, University of California, Davis, CA 95616.

CHI-FAI CHAU, Department of Biology, The Chinese University of Hong Kong, Shatin, New Territories, Hong Kong.

FENG CHEN, Department of Botany, The University of Hong Kong, Pokfulam Road, Hong Kong.

GONG-RUI CHEN, Institute of Biotechnology, Fuzhou University, Fuzhou, Fujian, 350002, P.R. China.

HUA-MING CHEN, Marine Food Science Department, National Taiwan Ocean University, 2 Pei-Ning Rd., Keelung, Taiwan, R.O.C.

J.M. CHEN, Science Association at Liyuan Township of Wuxi City, Wuxi 214074, China.

RU-MING CHEN, Institute of Biotechnology, Fuzhou University, Fuzhou, Fujian, 350002, P.R. China.

SUSAN CHEN, Marine Food Science Department, National Taiwan Ocean University, 2 Pei-Ning Rd., Keelung, Taiwan, R.O.C.

TIAN-BAO CHEN, Institute of Biotechnology, Fuzhou University, 523 Gong-ye Road, 350002, Fuzhou, Fujian, P.R. China 350002.

M.K. CHENG, Department of Biology, The Chinese University of Hong Kong, Shatin, NT, Hong Kong.

PETER C.K. CHEUNG, Department of Biology, The Chinese University of Hong Kong, Shatin, Hong Kong.
DEAN O. CLIVER, W.H.O. Collaborating Center on Food Virology, School of Veterinary Medicine, University of California, Davis, CA 95616.
B. CLOUGH, British Sugar Technical Centre, Norwich NR4 7UB, England.
LILIA S. COLLADO, Cereal Science Laboratory, Department of Botany, University of Hong Kong, Pokfulam Road, Hong Kong.
HAROLD CORKE, Cereal Science Laboratory, Department of Botany, University of Hong Kong, Pokfulam Road, Hong Kong.
ELBA CUBERO, Department of Food Science and Technology, University of California, Davis, 95616.
GLORIA S. DÁVILA-ORTÍZ, Departamento de Biotecnología, Centro de Desarrollo de Productos Bióticos, del Instituto Politécnico Nacional, Apartado Postal 24, 62730 Yautepec, Mor., Mexico.
BENITO O. DE LUMEN, Division of Nutritional Sciences and Toxicology, University of California, Berkeley, CA 94720.
HANSHU DING, Department of Food Science and Technology, University of California, Davis, and California Institute of Food and Agricultural Research, Davis, CA 95616.
XIAO LIN DING, School of Food Science and Technology, Wuxi University of Light Industry, Wuxi, 214036, P.R. China.
JINGLIE DOU, Department of Food Science, The University of British Columbia, 6650 NW Marine Drive, Vancouver, B.C., Canada V6T 1Z4.
D. ENG, Pokka Ace (M) SDN BHD; Lot 39, 41050 Klang, Selangor, Darul Ehsan, Malaysia.
CHANG-TENG FAN, Department of Food Science, Tunghai University, Taichung, Taiwan 407, R.O.C.
FANG FAN, Institute of Biotechnology, Fuzhou University, Fuzhou, Fujian, 350002, P.R. China.
LIR-WAN FAN, Graduate Institute of Food Science, Tunghai University, Taichung, Taiwan, R.O.C.
DANIEL F. FARKAS, Department of Food Science and Technology, Oregon State University, Corvallis, OR 97331.
HONG FU, Institute of Biotechnology, Fuzhou University, 523 Gong-ye Road, Fuzhou, Fujian, 350002 P.R. China.
G.K. FUKUMOTO, Cooperative Extension Service, Kealakekua, HI 96750.
A. FULLER, British Sugar Technical Centre, Norwich NR4 7UB, England.
YASUHIRO FUNATSU, Toyama Prefectural Food Research Institute, 360 Yoshioka, Toyama 939, Japan.
ALFREDO F. GALVEZ, Division of Nutritional Sciences and Toxicology, University of California, Berkeley, CA 94720.
WEN-HONG GAO, Institute of Biotechnology, Fuzhou University, Fuzhou, Fujian, 350002, P.R. China.

BLANCA E. GARCÍA, Dept. of Food Research and Postgraduate Studies, Universidad Autónoma de Querétaro, Querétaro, 76010 Qro., México.

S. GOHTANI, Department of Bioresource Science, Kagawa University, Miki, Kagawa 761-07, Japan.

WENYING GU, Food College, Wuxi University of Light Industry, Wuxi, Jiangsu, 214036, P.R. China.

ZHENGBIAO GU, School of Food Science and Technology, Wuxi University of Light Industry, Wuxi 214036, P.R. China.

JEAN-XAVIER GUINARD, Department of Food Science and Technology, University of California, Davis, Davis, CA 95616.

JIN-MING GUO, Institute of Biotechnology, Fuzhou University, Fuzhou, Fujian, 350002, P.R. China.

HIROSHI HARA, Laboratory of Foods and Nutrition, Faculty of Agriculture, Hokkaido University, Hokkaido, Japan.

GRUO BEN HENG, Shang Hai Dairy Training and Research Center, 101 Peng Lian Road, Shanghai, China 200072.

TIEN-KEN HSU, Graduate Institute of Food Science, Tunghai University, Taichung, Taiwan, R.O.C.

HSIU-HUA HSU, Marine Food Science Department, National Taiwan Ocean University, 2 Pei-Ning Rd., Keelung, Taiwan, R.O.C.

CHUN HU, Department of Food Science, University of British Columbia, Vancouver, B.C., Canada, V6T-1Z4.

CHUN-JIAN HUANG, Institute of Biotechnology, Fuzhou University, 523 Gong-ye Road, Fuzhou, Fujian, 350002 P.R. China.

JIANZHONG HUANG, Biological Engineering College, Fujian Normal University, Fujian, Fuzhou, 350007, P.R. China.

W. HUANG, 215/F 66A Broadway St. Mei Foo, Kowloon, Hong Kong.

Z.Y. JIN, School of Food Science and Technology, Wuxi University of Light Industry, Wuxi 214036, China.

TAKANORI KASAI, Laboratory of Foods and Nutrition, Faculty of Agriculture, Hokkaido University, Hokkaido, Japan.

S. KAWAKISHI, Laboratory of Food and Biodynamics, Nagoya University School of Agricultural Sciences, Nagoya 464-01, Japan.

KEN-ICHI KAWASAKI, Toyama Prefectural Food Research Institute, 360 Yoshioka, Toyama 939, Japan.

CHANG KECHANG, School of Biotechnology, University of Light Industry, Wuxi 214036, P.R.China.

K.H. KIM, Department of Bioresource Science, Kagawa University, Miki, Kagawa 761-07, Japan.

K.H. KIM, Department of Animal Sciences, University of Hawaii at Manoa, Honolulu, HI 96822

Y.S. KIM, Department of Animal Sciences, University of Hawaii at Manoa, Honolulu, HI 96822.

JANET C. KING, Western Human Nutrition Research Center, USDA/ARS, P.O. Box 29997, Presidio of San Francisco, CA 94129.

DAVID D. KITTS, Department of Food Science, University of British Columbia, Vancouver, B.C., Canada V6T-1Z4.

KOICHI KOSHIMIZU, Department of Biotechnological Science, Faculty of Biology-Oriented Science and Technology, Kinki University, Iwade-Uchita, Wakayama 649-64, Japan.

DEANNE C. KRENZ, Division of Nutritional Sciences and Toxicology, University of California, Berkeley, CA 94720-3104.

H.S. KWAN, Department of Biology, The Chinese University of Hong Kong, Shatin, N.T., Hong Kong.

G.S.W. LEUNG, Department of Biology, The Chinese University of Hong Kong, Shatin, N.T., Hong Kong.

CHUNLI LI, School of Food Science and Technology, Wuxi University of Light Industry, Wuxi 214036, P.R. China.

JIAN-CAI LI, Institute of Biotechnology, Fuzhou University, 523 Gong-Ye Road, Fuzhou, Fujian, 350002, P.R. China.

LONG LI, Institute of Biotechnology, Fuzhou University, 523, Gong-Ye Road, Fuzhou, Fujian, 350002, P.R. China.

PINGZUO LI, School of Biotechnology, Wuxi University of Light Industry, Wuxi, 214036, P.R China.

YANQUN LI, Food Engineering Department of Sino-German Joint Institute (Jiangxi-OAI), No.17 Nanjingdong Road, Nanchang 330047, P.R. China.

YAO-XIN LIN, Biological Engineering College, Fujian Normal University, Fujian, Fuzhou, 350007, P.R. China.

SHU-TAO LIU, Institute of Biotechnology, Fuzhou University, 523, Gong-ye Road, Fuzhou, Fujian, P.R. China 350002.

P.H. LU, Science Association at Liyuan Township of Wuxi City, Wuxi 214074, P.R. China.

B.S. LUH, Department of Food Science and Technology, University of California, Davis, CA 95616.

IRENE LUNA-GUZMAN, Department of Food Science and Technology, University of California, Davis, CA 95616.

HIROKI MAKITA, First Department of Pathology, Gifu University School of Medicine, 40 Tsukasa-machi, Gifu 500, Japan.

ALMA L. MARTÍNEZ-AYALA, Departamento de Biotecnología, Centro de Desarrollo de Productos Bióticos, del Instituto Politécnico Nacional, Apartado Postal 24, 62730 Yautepec, Mor., Mexico.

ALEXANDER McPHERSON, University of California, Riverside, Department of Biochemistry, Riverside, CA 92521.

ELVIRA GONZALEZ de MEJIA, Department of Food Research and Postgraduate Studies, Autonomous University of Queretaro, Mexico, Cerro de las Campanas, Queretaro, Qro 76010, Mexico.

TERUO MIYAZAWA, Food Chemistry Laboratory, Department of Applied Biological Chemistry, Tohoku University, Sendai 981, Japan.

YASUJIRO MORIMITSU, Laboratory of Food and Biodynamics, Nagoya University School of Agricultural Sciences, Nagoya 464-01, Japan.

AKIRA MURAKAMI, Department of Biotechnological Science, Faculty of Biology-Oriented Science and Technology, Kinki University, Iwade-Uchita, Wakayama 649-64, Japan.

YUKAKO NABESHIMA-ITO, Toyama Prefectural Food Research Institute, 360 Yoshioka, Toyama 939, Japan.

KIYOTAKA NAKAGAWA, Food Chemistry Laboratory, Department of Applied Biological Chemistry, Tohoku University, Sendai 981, Japan.

SHURYO NAKAI, Department of Food Science, The University of British Columbia, 6650 NW Marine Drive, Vancouver, B.C., Canada V6T 1Z4.

SOICHIRO NAKAMURA, Department of Food Science, The University of British Columbia, 6650 NW Marine Drive, Vancouver, B.C., Canada V6T 1Z4.

YOSHIMASA NAKAMURA, Division of Applied Life Sciences, Graduate School of Agriculture, Kyoto University, Kyoto 606-01, Japan.

SHAHINA NAZ, Department of Food Science and Technology, University of Karachi, Karachi-75270, Pakistan.

LI NI, Institute of Biotechnology, Fuzhou University, 523 Gong-Ye Road, Fuzhou, Fujian, 350002, P.R. China.

HIROYUKI NISHIMURA, Department of Bioscience and Technology, School of Engineering, Hokkaido Tokai University, Sapporo 005, Japan.

ELISA GIRARDELLI PINTO NOVAIS, Department of Food Science, University of British Columbia, Vancouver, B.C. Canada V6T-1Z4.

HAJIME OHIGASHI, Division of Applied Life Sciences, Graduate School of Agriculture, Kyoto University, Kyoto 606-01, Japan.

YOSHIMI OHTO, Division of Applied Life Sciences, Graduate School of Agriculture, Kyoto University, Kyoto 606-01, Japan.

TOORU OOIZUMI, Department of Marine Bioscience, Fukui Prefectural University, Obama, Fukui, 917 Japan.

T. OSAWA, Laboratory of Food and Biodynamics, Nagoya University School of Agricultural Sciences, Nagoya 464-01, Japan.

BONNIE SUN PAN, Marine Food Science Department, National Taiwan Ocean University, 2 Pei-Ning Rd., Keelung, Taiwan, R.O.C.

M. PANTELLA, Department of Food Science, RMIT University, 124 Latrobe Street, Melbourne 3001, Australia.

OCTAVIO PAREDES-LÓPEZ, Departamento de Biotecnología y Bioquímica, Centro de Investigación y de Estudios Avanzados del Instituto Politécnico Nacional, Apartado Postal 629, 36500 Irapuato, Gto., Mexico.

XIUPING QIAN, Laboratory of Natural Product Research, Department of Tea Science, Zhejiang Agriculture University, Hangzhou 310029, P.R. China.

PING-FAN RAO, Institute of Biotechnology, Fuzhou University, Fuzhou, Fujian, 350002, P.R. China.
CARLOS REGALADO, Dept. of Food Research and Postgraduate Studies, Universidad Autónoma de Querétaro, Querétaro, 76010 Qro., México.
M. JAMELA REVILLEZA, Division of Nutritional Sciences and Toxicology, University of California, Berkeley, CA 94720.
NURIA ROCHA, Department of Food Research and Postgraduate Studies, Autonomous University of Queretaro, Mexico, Cerro de las Campanas, Queretaro, Qro 76010, Mexico.
KANZO SAKATA, Faculty of Agriculture, Shizuoka University, 836 Ohya, Shizuoka 422, Japan.
LUIS A. SALAZAR-OLIVO, Department of Food Research and Postgraduate Studies, Autonomous University of Queretaro, Mexico, Cerro de las Campanas, Queretaro, Qro 76010, Mexico.
KUNIHIKO SAMEJIMA, Rakuno Gakuen University, 582 Midori-cho, Bunkyodai, Ebetsu, Hokkaido 069, Japan.
ATSUSHI SATOH, Department of Bioscience and Technology, School of Engineering, Hokkaido Tokai University, Sapporo 005, JAPAN.
KOUJI SAYAMA, Research Laboratories, Nitten Co., Ltd., Hokkaido Japan
HOWARD G. SCHUTZ, Tragon Corporation, 365 Convention Way, Redwood City, CA 94063.
VALDEMIRO C. SGARBIERI, Centro de Química de Alimentos e Nutrição Aplicada, Instituto de Tecnologia de Alimentos, C.P. 139, Campinas, São Paulo, Brasil.
SHIWANG SHE, Food Engineering Department of Sino-German Joint Institute (Jiangxi-OAI), No.17 Nanjingdong Road, Nanchang 330047, P.R. China.
F. SHERKAT, Department of Food Science, RMIT University, 124 Latrobe Street, Melbourne 3001, Australia.
FUU SHEU, Department of Horticulture, National Taiwan University, Taipei, Taiwan R.O.C.
BI-HONG SHI, Institute of Biotechnology, Fuzhou University, Fuzhou, Fujian, 350002, P.R. China.
GUIYANG SHI, School of Biotechnology, Wuxi University of Light Industry, Wuxi, Jiangsu 214036, P.R. China.
QIAO-QIN SHI, Biological Engineering College, Fujian Normal University, Fujian, Fuzhou, 350007, P.R. China.
CHARLES SHOEMAKER, Department of Food Science and Technology, University of California, Davis, and California Institute of Food and Agricultural Research, Davis, CA 95616.
SHARON SHOEMAKER, Department of Food Science and Technology, University of California, Davis, and California Institute of Food and Agricultural Research, Davis, CA 95616.

YUAN-TAY SHYU, Department of Horticulture, National Taiwan University, Taipei, Taiwan R.O.C.

JOEL L. SIDEL, Tragon Corporation, 365 Convention Way, Redwood City, CA 94063.

HERBERT STONE, Tragon Corporation, 365 Convention Way, Redwood City, CA 94063.

JENG-DE SU, Department of Food Science, Tunghai University, Taichung, Taiwan 407, R.O.C.

SAMUEL S.M. SUN, Department of Biology, The Chinese University of Hong Kong, Shatin, NT, Hong Kong and Department of Plant Molecular Physiology, University of Hawaii, Honolulu, Hawaii.

TAKUJI TANAKA, First Department of Pathology, Gifu University School of Medicine, 40 Tsukasa-machi, Gifu 500, Japan.

AL TAPPEL, Dept. of Food Science and Technology, University of California, Davis, California 95616.

HEATHER THOMAS, Tragon Corporation, 365 Convention Way, Redwood City, CA 94063.

FUSAO TOMITA, Laboratory of Applied Microbiology, Faculty of Agriculture, Hokkaido University, Hokkaido, Japan.

HAU-YANG TSEN, Department of Food Science, National Chung-Hsing University, Taichung, Taiwan, ROC.

HELEN M. TU, Department of Plant Molecular Physiology, University of Hawaii, Honolulu, Hawaii.

TAIICHI USUI, Faculty of Agriculture, Shizuoka University, 836 Ohya, Shizuoka 422, Japan.

ELENA VLASENKO, Department of Food Science and Technology, University of California, Davis, and California Institute of Food and Agricultural Research, Davis, CA 95616.

MARY Y. WANG, California Department of Health Services, Sacramento, CA.

MING-LI WANG, Department of Plant Molecular Physiology, University of Hawaii, Honolulu, Hawaii.

WEN WANG, Institute of Biotechnology, Fuzhou University, 523 Gong-Ye Road, Fuzhou, Fujian, 350002, P.R. China.

HONG JIANG WANG, Laboratory of Natural Product Research, Department of Tea Science, Zhejiang Agriculture University, Hangzhou 310029, P.R. China.

MEI WANG, Food College, Wuxi University of Light Industry, Wuxi, Jiangsu, 214036, P.R. China.

SHAO-YUN WANG, Institute of Biotechnology, Fuzhou University, 523 Gong-ye Road, Fuzhou, Fujian, 350002 P.R. China.

MIAO WANG, School of Food Science and Technology, Wuxi University of Light Industry, Wuxi, China.

NAOHARU WATANABE, Faculty of Agriculture, Shizuoka University, 836 Ohya, Shizuoka 422, Japan.

CHARLENE WEE, Department of Food Science and Technology, University of California, Davis, CA 95616.

MING C. WEN, Graduate Institute of Food Science, Tunghai University, Taichung, Taiwan, R.O.C.

C. HANNY WIJAYA, Faculty of Agricultural Technology, Bogor Agricultural University, P.O. Box 122, Bogor, Indonesia.

AROSHA N. WIJEWICKREME, Department of Food Science, University of British Columbia, Vancouver, B.C., Canada V6T-1Z4.

J. WILSON, Simplot Foods, PO Box 177, Southland Centre, Cheltenham, 3192, Melbourne, Australia.

SONG-GANG WU, Biological Engineering College, Fujian Normal University, Fujian, Fuzhou, 350007, P.R. China.

BI-FENG XIE, Biological Engineering College, Fujian Normal University, Fujian, Fuzhou, 350007, P.R. China.

W.J. XIE, Department of Biology, The Chinese University of Hong Kong, Shatin, N.T., Hong Kong.

LIWEN XIONG, Department of Plant Molecular Physiology, University of Hawaii, Honolulu, Hawaii.

ROU XU, School of Biotechnology, Wuxi University of Light Industry, Wuxi, 214036, P.R China.

RUO-JUN XU, Department of Zoology, The University of Hong Kong, Hong Kong.

X.M. XU, School of Food Science and Technology, Wuxi University of Light Industry, Wuxi 214036, P.R. China.

Y. YAMANO, Department of Bioresource Science, Kagawa University, Miki, Kagawa 761-07, Japan.

MASAKATSU YAMAZAWA, National Research Institute of Fisheries Science of Japan, Fukuura 2-12-4, Kanazawa, Yokohama 236, Japan.

M.T. YAN, Department of Food Science and Technology, University of California, Davis, CA 95616.

XU YAN, School of Biotechnology, University of Light Industry, Wuxi 214036, P.R. China.

KOSAKU YASUNAGA, National Research Institute of Fisheries Science of Japan, Fukuura 2-12-4, Kanazawa, Yokohama 236.

ATSUSHI YOKOTA, Laboratory of Applied Microbiology, Faculty of Agriculture, Hokkaido University, Hokkaido, Japan.

XINGHUA YUAN, Wuxi University of Light Industry, Wuxi 214036, Jiangsu, P.R. China.

KECHANG ZHANG, School of Biotechnology, Wuxi University of Light Industry, Wuxi, Jiangsu 214036, P.R. China.

LIXIN ZHANG, School of Biotechnology, Wuxi University of Light Industry, Wuxi, Jiangsu 214036, P.R. China.

M. ZHANG, Department of Biology, The Chinese University of Hong Kong, Shatin, N.T., Hong Kong.

MIN ZHANG, School of Food Science and Technology, Wuxi University of Light Industry, Wuxi 214036, P.R. China.

RONG-ZHEN ZHANG, Institute of Biotechnology, Fuzhou University, Fuzhou, Fujian, 350002, P.R. China.

XIAOMING ZHANG, Wuxi University of Light Industry, Wuxi 214036, Jiangsu, China.

YING ZHANG, Department of Food Science and Technology, Zhejiang Agricultural University, Hangzhou 310029, P.R. China.

ZHENG HUI ZHAO, Laboratory of Natural Product Research, Department of Tea Science, Zhejiang Agriculture University, Hangzhou 310029, P.R. China.

JIANXIAN ZHENG, South China University of Technology, Wuxi, Jiangsu, 214036 P.R. China.

YI ZHENG, Biological Engineering College, Fujian Normal University, Fujian, Fuzhou, 350007, P.R. China.

YU-QIANG ZHENG, Institute of Biotechnology, Fuzhou University, Fuzhou, Fujian, 350002, P.R. China.

XIAO-LAN ZHOU, Biological Engineering College, Fujian Normal University, Fujian, Fuzhou, 350007, P.R. China.

H.K. ZHU, Science Association at Liyuan Township of Wuxi City, Wuxi 214074, P.R. China.

WEI-NENG ZUO, Department of Plant Molecular Physiology, University of Hawaii, Honolulu, Hawaii.

PREFACE

Food for Health in the Pacific Rim includes most of the papers presented at the Conference of the same title held at the University of California, Davis on October 19-23, 1997, jointly sponsored by the University of California, Davis and the Wuxi University of Light Industry of Wuxi, China. This Conference was the third in the series of International Conferences on Food Science and Technology, sponsored by the two Universities as a result of their formalized relationships. The First and Second International Conferences were held at the Wuxi University of Light Industry in October, 1991 and October, 1994. There were more than 120 participants at the Third International Conference, with 105 papers and posters presented.

More than 170 authors are represented by the 71 chapters in the Proceedings *Food for Health in the Pacific Rim*. These include authors from Australia, Brazil, Canada, China, Hong Kong, Japan, Mexico, Taiwan and the United States.

The theme title "Food for Health in the Pacific Rim" was chosen carefully after considerable discussion by the Planning Committee. Other possible titles considered included "Nutraceutical Foods," Healthy Foods" and "Functional Foods," among others. The Committee concluded that these latter titles make more judgmental statements about food than it wished to endorse.

The chapters of the book are arranged under the seven broad titles of "General Topics in Food Science and Technology," "Food Processing and Engineering," "Antioxidants in Foods," "Nutrition and Food Science," "Food Safety," "Sensory Science of Foods" and "Food Biotechnology" as a means of providing some structure to the Book. Obviously, there are overlaps in chapter contents among sections and in the number of chapters in each section. Hopefully, the chapter titles in the Table of Contents and the Subject Index will guide the reader to all contributions on a subject of interest.

The overall quality of the chapters are generally very good. Many of the papers are exceptional in the quality and depth of science and the modern instrumentation and techniques used in the experimentation. Overall, the chapters demonstrated appropriate experimental approaches, interpretation and objectivity in discussing the results. The conclusions are supported by the data. There was none of the hype and salesmanship that have detracted from some other conferences based around the titles discussed in paragraph three above. The Chinese and Japanese scientists demonstrated well their leadership in the science of foods for health.

The Co-Editors owe much to the organizers and management of the Conference. First there were the coordinators in several of the countries that helped in selection of topics, scientists, abstracts, and manuscripts and above all in communication. Professor Ding Xiao Lin, President of the Conference, and Former President of the Wuxi University of Light Industry, coordinated the Chinese delegation. Professor Lucy Sun Huang, National Taiwan University, guided the delegation from Taiwan. Professor Shoichi Takao, Rakuno Gakuen University, along with Professor Hiroyuki Nishamura, Hokkaido Tokai University, guided the Japanese delegation. Professor Harold Corke. University of Hong Kong, guided the Hong Kong delegation.

The Planning Committee included: Professor Emeritus John R. Whitaker, Chair, Professor Emeritus Charles E. Hess, Professor Norman F. Haard, Dr. Emeritus Bor S. Luh and Professor Charles F. Shoemaker, all of UC Davis, who worked for almost two years on the Conference. They were joined near the end by the UC Davis chairs of each of the seven topics. Each of the seven topical sessions had a keynote speaker (listed as the first speaker under each subject title).

President Ding Xiao Lin and Chancellor Larry Vanderhoef served as Co-Presidents of the Conference. The Scientific Committee included: Professor Charles Shoemaker, Professor Ding Xiao Lin, Professor Lucy Sun Huang, Professor Harold Corke and Professor Shoichi Takao. Ms. Judy DeStefano, who served as Secretary to the Chair of the Planning Committee, was undoubtedly the hardest working member of the organization. Our thanks to all the speakers for their presentations and for their manuscripts that permitted these Proceedings and to others who contributed to the success of the Conference and the Proceedings.

We thank John O'Neil, Publisher, Food and Nutrition Press, Inc. and his staff, especially Mrs. Maureen P. Yash, for bringing this book to fruition.

Co-Editors of the book
John R. Whitaker
Norman F. Haard
Charles F. Shoemaker
R. Paul Singh

CONTENTS

CHAPTER **PAGE**

SESSION I. GENERAL FOOD SCIENCE AND TECHNOLOGY

SESSION II. FOOD ENGINEERING AND PROCESSING

SESSION III. ANTIOXIDANTS IN FOODS

SESSION IV. NUTRITION AND FOOD SCIENCE

SESSION V. FOOD SAFETY

SESSION VI. SENSORY SCIENCE AND ACCEPTABILITY

SESSION VII. BIOTECHNOLOGY OF FOODS

APPLICATION OF A GRAPHIC GLOBAL OPTIMIZATION FOR PROTEIN MODIFICATION

SHURYO NAKAI, JINGLIE DOU and SOICHIRO NAKAMURA

Department of Food Science
The University of British Columbia
6650 NW Marine Drive
Vancouver, B.C., Canada V6T 1Z4

ABSTRACT

The Random-Centroid Optimization (RCO) is a sequential optimization technology by repeating a search cycle consisting of random search, centroid search and mapping. A Visual Basic program of RCO was written for Windows 95. The program was applied to five multimodal functions with up to 6 factors after randomizing the locations of the global optima of the model functions. Mapping that was a graphic approximation of the response surfaces was a powerful tool for narrowing the search spaces for the subsequent search cycle. The global optima were mostly found in less than 50 experiments that were substantially less than those of many computational global optimization algorithms. For protein engineering, site numbers in the sequence and amino acid residues to substitute the original residues at the sites are optimized. To select amino acids to substitute, a hydrophobicity scale, propensities of secondary structures or bulkiness are used. RCO thus modified was successfully applied for maximizing the thermostability of B. stearothermophilus *neutral protease by one-site directed mutagenesis of its active-site helix with 16 amino acid residues.*

INTRODUCTION

This paper consists of two parts, namely establishing an experimental global optimization technique and optimization of one-site directed mutagenesis of the active site helix of *B. stearothermophilus* neutral protease.

Experimental Global Optimization

Biological phenomena are unpredictable due to nonlinear and multimodal properties. Therefore, finding the global optimum is extremely difficult but important in biological research and development. The number of papers published on global optimization in chemistry has dramatically increased since 1990. This increase is probably due to the recent introduction of a new technique of Genetic Algorithm (GA). GA is a general methodology for searching for a solution space analogous to the natural selection procedure in biological evolution (Holland 1975). Many other global algorithms, e.g., Lipschiz optimization, Level-Set Program and Simulated Annealing, have also been used (Horst *et al.* 1995). A great majority of the algorithms are used for computational optimization by consuming CPU times in search of the global optima. Therefore, these optimization techniques are inappropriate to apply to slow, expensive biological experiments, especially genetic engineering.

Schwefel (1981) stated that the most reliable global search method is the grid method, which also is time consuming and, thus, most expensive. As an alternative, random strategies received attention due to their simplicity, flexibility and resistance to perturbations. After investigating the feasibility of applying sequential or iterative optimization techniques to food research and processing (Nakai 1982; Nakai *et al.* 1984; Aishima and Nakai 1986), we proposed a new algorithm, namely Random-Centroid Optimization (RCO). RCO is composed of random search, centroid search, and mapping which formulate a search cycle (Nakai 1990; Dou *et al.* 1993). Mapping as an approximation of the response surfaces was first introduced into the super simplex optimization (Nakai *et al.* 1984). Visualization of the optimization progress in a form of maps by approximating the response surfaces greatly improves the optimization efficiency.

Visual Basic is a remarkable improvement from Quick Basic by combining text language with graphic language. It is, therefore, possible to facilitate the mapping process by simplifying the complicated process, thereby enhancing objectivity and reliability in predicting the locations of the global optima. The approach taken in this study is, therefore, a practical solution of the global optimization, rather than purely mathematical solutions. This is an advantage of RCO, because even non-mathematicians can readily manipulate the optimization technique due to the simplicity in algorithm as well as computer operation.

Optimization of Site-Directed Mutagenesis

Rational design of protein engineering was discussed by Blundell (1994). Most efforts have been expended in modeling mutant proteins from their sequences. However, the difficulty in 100% accurate prediction of molecular structure is interfering with obtaining a rational design. Furthermore, the fact that no reliable relationships of the molecular structure with functions of mutant proteins are currently available is making the situation even more difficult. Due to a lack of appropriate working equations, in this case the structure-function relationships, the computational optimization is hard to apply to protein engineering.

Most of the optimization strategy so far published is *in vitro* random selection by mimicking Darwinian evolution of organisms in nature (Breaker and Joyce 1994). A more systematic approach of the design cycle was carried out by the recursive ensemble mutagenesis (REM) of Delagrave *et al.* (1993). REM involves the recursive use of combinatorial cassette mutagenesis (CCM). It is an iterative strategy to continually improve the CCM library. Fuellen and Youvan (1994) applied the genetic algorithm to REM. Delagrave *et al.* (1993) stated that the generation of new and informative mutant protein is necessary to our understanding of protein structure-function relationships.

Unlike REM, we intended to optimize mutation using RCO by selecting site location to be mutated and amino acid residues to replace the ones on the sites selected. Therefore, two factors are needed for altering a site in the sequences of protein molecules. Sander (1994) has suggested that the basic idea is to use our knowledge of protein structure to select a few residue positions, in which mutations may have a functionally beneficial effect. Such an example is provided by the residues lining the active site of an enzyme. These positions are then randomized in a vector carrying the original sequence by using suitably synthesized oligonucleotides. He also recommended that the number of residue positions chosen for randomization must be kept reasonably small to achieve good coverage of possible sequence combinations.

Objectives

To write an RCO program for Windows 95 for establishing an experimental global optimization methodology; to modify the RCO to apply to site-directed mutagenesis; and then to apply it for mutating one-site in the 16 amino acid peptide of active-site helix to maximize the thermostability of *B. stearothermophilus* protease.

METHODS

RCO Optimization

Figure 1 shows the menu for RCO optimization. The RCO computer program for Windows 95 was posted on the website of http://www.interchange.ubc.ca/agsci/foodsci/rco.htm for downloading to PC computers.

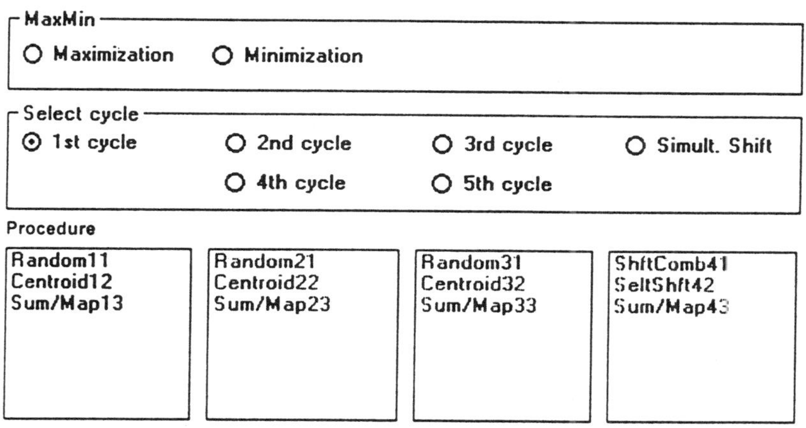

FIG. 1. OPERATION CHART

"MaxMin" are the option buttons for selecting maximization or minimization. "Select cycle" contains option buttons for selecting Cycle 1 to 5 and Simultaneous Shift. After clicking these option buttons, the processes in each procedure list should be followed step-by-step, for instance for Cycle 2, Random Search 21, Centroid Search 22, and Summary/Mapping 23. Two digits after each step are the identification number of the step in use.

Line-drawing on Maps

To draw lines on maps for approximating the response surfaces, the search space chosen for each factor is divided into three equal divisions in 3-factor optimization (Fig.

2C, D). Data points qualified to be linked, thereby forming trend lines for a factor (factor 2 in Fig. 2A, B), are those that belong to the same divisions for other factors (factors 1 and 3 in Fig. 2 C, D, respectively). In Fig. 2, data points to be linked are 1-2-3, 4-5 and 6-7 for factor 2. This is because they are in the same divisions for factor 1 (Fig. 2C) and factor 3 (Fig. 2D). When the number of trend curves is too small, some factors (factor 1 or 3 in the case of Fig. 2) are ignored in the line-drawing computation, on purpose, to increase the number of trend curves (intensified line-drawing).

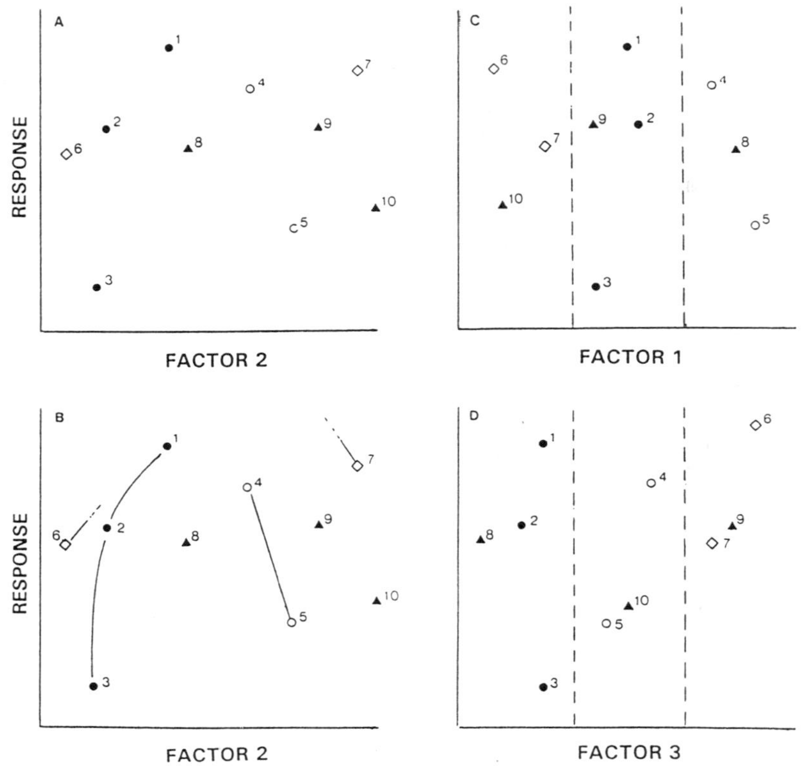

FIG. 2. HYPOTHETICAL GRAPHS FOR EXPLAINING THE MAPPING PRINCIPLE OF MAXIMIZATION OF A 3-FACTOR OPTIMIZATION

A: Before drawing trend curves on the scattergram of factor 2. The location of the maximum is unclear. B: After mapping. Lines are pointing toward the maximum. C and D: 3-Equal divisions of Factors 1 and 3 to find groups of data points common in these factors.

Randomization of Model Functions

To avoid an inadvertent influence of the knowledge on the optimum's location on setting search spaces for the succeeding cycle, the optimum level value of each factor was randomized. Wood's function (Reklaitis *et al.* 1983) for minimization used in this study is:

$$y = [100(x_2 - x_1^2)^2 + (1 - x_1)^2 + 90(x_4 - x_3^2)^2 + (1 - x_3)^2 + 10.1\{(x_2 - 1)^2 + (x_4 - 1)^2\} + 19.8(x_2 - 1)(x_4 - 1)] / 100 + 10 \quad (1)$$

Also an unconstrained 6-factor function unavailable in the literature was created by the method of Bowman and Gerard (1967) for maximization:

$$y = 33.6x_1 + 25x_2 + 41.4x_3 + 10.8x_4 + 8.4x_5 + 10.4x_6 - 4x_1x_2 - 12x_1x_3 - 10x_1x_4 - 4x_1x_5 - 16x_2x_3 - 12x_2x_4 - 6x_2x_5 - 10x_3x_6 + 16x_4x_6 - 2x_5x_6 - 15x_1^2 - 18x_2^2 - 20x_3^2 - 26x_4^2 - 10x_5^2 - 6x_6^2 \quad (2)$$

To make this function multimodal with 3 peaks, different locations of maxima were given (Fig. 3A).

Modification of RCO Program for Mutagenesis (RCG)

Factors 1, 3 and 5 were assigned for site numbers to be mutated in the peptide sequence. Then, factors 2, 4 and 6 were assigned for amino acid residues to substitute the residues at the sites selected. For selection of amino acid residues, the hydrophobicity scale of Wilce *et al.* (1995) is mostly employed. However, the helix and strand propensities of Muñoz and Serrano (1994) or the bulkiness of Gromiha and Ponnuswamy (1993) also can be used. Turn or loop is left blank.

Site-directed Mutagenesis of *B. stearothermophilus* Neutral Protease. The active site helix at sites 139-154 in total 319 amino acid residues of the enzyme was mutated one site at-a-time to maximize its thermostability. The mutation was conducted as reported by Nakamura *et al.* (1997). Throughout this mutagenesis, the hydrophobicity scale was employed for selecting amino acid residues to replace the residues at the site selected by RCG.

RESULTS AND DISCUSSION

RCO was applied to randomized multimodal functions to show that RCO could find the true optimum (global optimum) in biological projects without need for excessive experimentation. Then, RCO modified for site-directed mutagenesis (RCG) was applied to the active-site helix of *B. stearothermophilus* neutral protease to maximize the thermostability of the enzyme.

Application of RCO to Model Functions

Figure 3 shows the maps in Cycle 1 of maximization of the 6-factor function. Figure 3B is a result of the intensified line-drawing. A possibility of the presence of 3 peaks is shown. The true locations of maxima are at $x_3 = 0.7$, 0.5 and 0.1 (Fig. 3A). In contrast, when this function was unimodal at 0.8, 0.9, 0.7, 0.7, 0.8 and 0.9 for 6 factors, no trend of the presence of a peak other than that at $x_1 = 0.8$ is shown (Fig. 3C) even by using the intensified line-drawing.

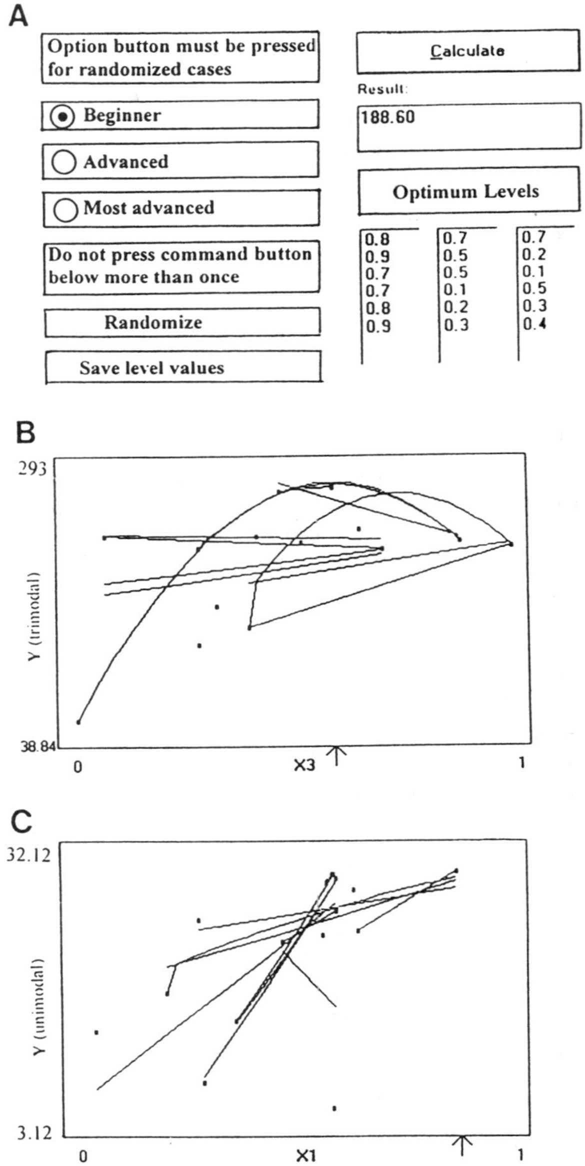

FIG. 3. MAPS IN CYCLE 1 OF THE RANDOMIZED 6-FACTOR MODEL FUNCTION
A: The program for response value computation. The optimum level values for 3 peaks in combination ratios of 5:3:3 for peak heights. B: x_3 is a mixture at level values of 0.7, 0.5 and 0.1. C: x_1 map of single 6-factor function.

In the case of minimization of a randomized Wood's function, the x_1 map in Cycle 1 (Fig. 4A) shows the presence of a minimum at around 0.4 although there is the possible existence of another minimum near 1.0. In Cycle 2 for continued search around 0.4, the x_1 map (Fig. 4B) showed more clearly the possible presence of another minimum at greater than 0.7. Therefore, the simultaneous shift process, manual shifts towards targets set (Fig. 1), was applied and obtained the x_1 map as shown in Fig. 4C. Certainly, there is another minimum at 0.7-0.9. A new search (Cycle 1) was initiated as a spot search which gave a minimum response of 12.77 at $x_1 = 0.85$ (Fig. 4D) after conducting a total of 38 runs. A minimum found in Cycle 2 of 18.99 at $x_1 = 0.29$ is a local minimum. The global minimum of this function was 10.0 at 0.8, 0.2, 0.9 and 0.8 for 4 factors. A computational optimization using Level-Set Program required over 5,000 iterations to reach the global minimum (Yassien 1993).

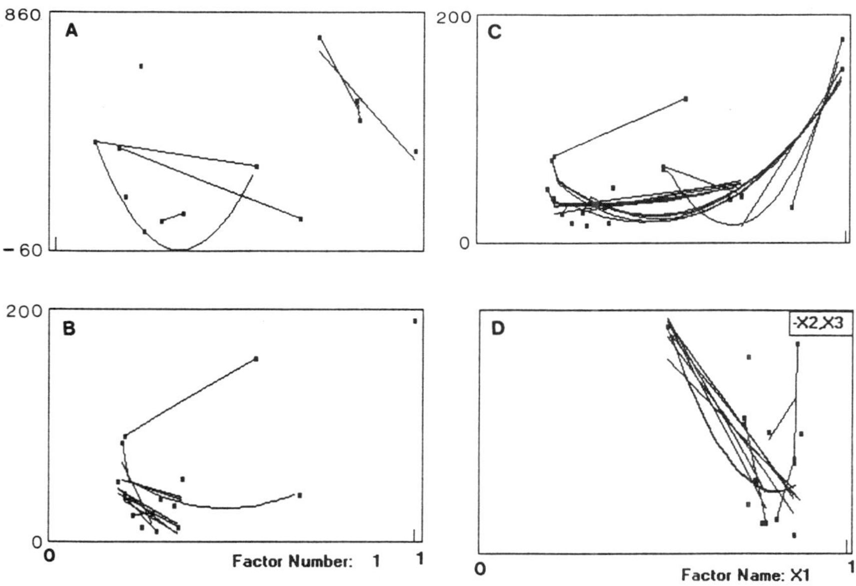

FIG. 4. X_1-MAPS FOR MINIMIZATION OF WOOD'S 4-FACTOR FUNCTION
A. Cycle 1. B. Cycle 2. C. Simultaneous shift. D. Spot search (repeated Cycle 1).

Application of RCO to other 3 multimodal functions was also successful. The functions used were the steep-sided helical valley of Fletcher and Powell (1963), Heese's function (Visweswaran and Floudas 1990) and a 2-factor function of Curtis (1994). Despite the fact that RCO is empirical, experimental global optimization such as RCO should be extremely valuable for biological experiments. Genetic work is usually very time-consuming and expensive; furthermore, it is difficult to derive working equations.

Application of the RCG to Mutate One Site of a 16-Amino Acid Peptide

The results are shown in Table 1 and Fig. 5. The mutant V143E (site 5) gave the greatest increase of 6.5°C in T_{50} from that of 68.3°C for the wild type enzyme with a 30% increase in proteolytic activity. In contrast, ΔT_{50} of 7.5°C was obtained in I140P (site 2) by proline introduction to the N-terminal side of active site helix (Nakamura *et al.* 1997).

TABLE 1.
RANDOM-CENTROID OPTIMIZATION OF MUTATION OF NEUTRAL PROTEASE

		Site	Mutation	ΔT_{50} (°C)	Proteolytic Activity (%)
Cycle 1	Random	13	V151D	5.7	45.2
		12	A150W	4.4	27.2
		7	H145G	1.7	−87.7
		3	D141P	5.0	76.3
		6	G144F	−0.7	82.9
		10	T148I	2.1	3.6
	Centroid	8	E146N	3.8	−96.3
		13	V151P	4.2	−12.8
Cycle 2	Random	11	H149W	3.5	−91.5
		7	H145K	6.0	−80.7
		5	V143E	6.5	32.1
		9	L147K	1.9	−1.2
		12	A150E	4.4	21.6

ΔT_{50}: difference in T_{50} (half-survival temperature in Nakamura *et al.* 1997) from that of wild type protease.

The map for mutation site (Fig. 5A) shows that the mutation of the N-terminal end is slightly more useful than that at the C-terminal end of active site sequence. Figure 5B is the map plotted by using the bulkiness as amino acid scale and shows the effect of bulkiness. The left-hand most data point is for glycine isolating far apart from the other amino acid data points. Within the bulkiness scale, except for glycine, the trend is the smaller in bulkiness the better. This result agrees with the conclusion of our proline introduction study (Nakamura *et al.* 1997) that greater rigidity in the N-terminal end is favorable for higher thermostability. Their conclusion was derived from α-chymotrypsin susceptibility and also the dihedral angle study of the computer-aided molecular models. Figure 5C shows a favorable trend towards low hydrophobicity. Figures 5D and 5E show almost no relevance of β-strand and α-helix with thermostability. This result is reasonable because sites 1-16 is originally a helix, thus no drastic changes in the structure and function by changing helix and strand can be expected. Figure 5 includes the data of Nakamura *et al.* (1997) to enhance the available information.

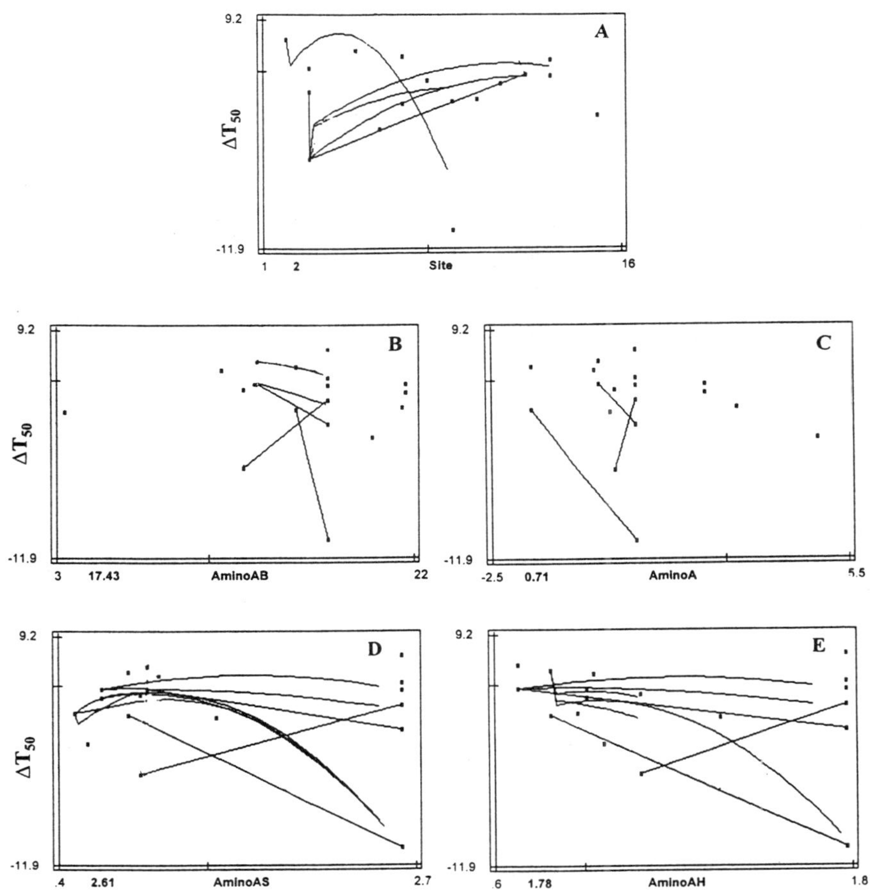

FIG. 5. MAPS FROM MAXIMIZATION OF THE THERMOSTABILITY OF NEUTRAL PROTEASE

AminoAG: amino acid scale for bulkiness, AminoA: amino acid scale for hydrophobicity, AminoAH: amino acid scale for α-helix propensity, AminoAS: amino acid scale for β-strand propensity, ΔT_{50}: see the footnote of Table 1.

In conclusion, the RCO approach may be useful in efficient mutation of protein molecules to find the best functions or even new functions. An advantage of this approach is that there is no need for information on molecular structure during the optimization experiments. Simultaneous mutation of two sites of cystatin C is under investigation in our laboratory.

ACKNOWLEDGMENT

The authors are grateful to the Natural Sciences and Engineering Research Council of Canada for Grants to support this study.

REFERENCES

AISHIMA, T. and NAKAI, S. 1986. Centroid mapping optimization: A new efficient optimization for food research and processing. J. Food Sci. *51,* 1297–1300.

BLUNDELL, T.L. 1994. Problems and solutions in protein engineering - towards rational design. Trends Biotechnol. *12,* 145–148.

BREAKER, R.R. and JOYCE, G.F. 1994. Inventing and improving ribozyme function: rational design versus iterative selection methods. Trends Biotechnol. *12,* 268–274.

BOWMAN, F. and GERARD, F.A. 1967. Higher Calculus. Cambridge University Press, London, pp. 227–246.

CURTIS, M.A. 1994. Optimization by simulated annealing theory and chemometric application. J. Chem. Educ. *71,* 775–778.

DELAGRAVE, S., GOLDMAN, E.R. and YOUVAN, D.C. 1993. Recursive ensemble mutagenesis. Protein Eng. *6,* 327–331.

DOU, J., TOMA, S. and NAKAI, S. 1993. Random-centroid optimization for food formulation. Food Res. Int. *26,* 27–37.

FLETCHER, R. and POWELL, M.L.D. 1963. A rapidly convergent descent method for minimization. Computer J. *6,* 163–168.

FUELLEN, G. and YOUVAN, D.C. 1994. Genetic algorithms and recursive ensemble mutagenesis in protein engineering. Complexity Int. *1,* (http://www.csu.edu.au/ci/voll/fuellen/REM.html).

GROMIHA, M.M. and PONNUSWAMY, P.K. 1993. Relationship between amino acid properties and protein compressibility. J. Theor. Biol. *165,* 87–100.

HOLLAND, J.H. 1975. Adaptation in Natural and Artificial Systems. Univ. Michigan Press, Ann Arbor.

HORST, R., PARDALOS, P.M. and THOAI, N.V. 1995. Introduction to Global Optimization. Kluwer Academic, Dordrecht, The Netherlands.

MUÑOZ, V. and SERRANO, L. 1994. Intrinsic secondary structure propensities of the amino acids, using statistical ϕ-ψ matrices: Comparison with experimental scales. Proteins *20,* 301–311.

NAKAI, S. 1982. Comparison of optimization techniques for application to food product and process development. J. Food Sci. *47,* 144–152.

NAKAI, S. 1990. Computer-aided optimization with potential application in biorheology. J. Jap. Biorheology Soc. *4,* 143–152.

NAKAI, S., KOIDE, K. and EUGUSTER, L. 1984. A new mapping super-simplex optimization for food product and processing development. J. Food Sci. *49,* 1143–1148, 1170.

NAKAMURA, S., TANAKA, T., YADA, R.Y. and NAKAI, S. 1997. Improving the thermostability of *B. stearothermophilus* neutral protease by introducing proline into the active site helix. Protein Eng. (In press).

REKLAITIS, B.V., RAVINDRAN, A. and RAGSDELL, K.M. 1983. Engineering Optimization: Methods and Application. Wiley-Interscience, New York.

SANDER, C. 1994. Design of protein structure: helix bundles and beyond. Trends Biotechnol. *12,* 163–167.

SCHWEFEL, H.-P. 1981. Numerical Optimization of Computer Models. John Wiley & Sons, New York. pp. 87–103.

VISWESWARAN, V. and FLOUDAS, C.A. 1990. A global optimization algorithm for certain classes of non convex NLPS. II. Application of theory and test problems. Computers Chem. Eng. *14*, 1419–1434.

WILCE, M.C.J., AGUILAR, M.-I. and HEAM, M.T. 1995. Physicochemical basis of amino acid hydrophobicity scales: Evaluation of four new scales of amino acid hydrophobicity coefficients derived from RP-HPLC of peptides. Anal. Chem. *67,* 1210–1219.

YASSIEN, H.A. 1993. A level set global optimization method for nonlinear engineering problems. Ph.D. Thesis, Univ. British Columbia, Vancouver, B.C. Canada. pp. 256–257.

CARCASS AND MEAT QUALITY CHARACTERISTICS OF FORAGE-BASED BEEF

G.K. FUKUMOTO[1], Y.S. KIM[2], K.H. KIM[2] and H. AKO[3]

[1]Cooperative Extension Service
Kealakekua, HI 96750
[2]Department of Animal Sciences
and [3]Department of Environmental Biochemistry
University of Hawaii at Manoa
Honolulu, HI 96822

ABSTRACT

There is a growing demand in the United States for meat products with a lower fat content because more and more consumers are informed about the adverse health implications of consuming excessive fat. In parallel to this trend, more consumers are demanding naturally produced, chemical-free products. Forage-based beef, which generally has a lower content of fat than grain-finished beef, may fill these consumer demands. In the Pacific Rim countries where grain production is limited, improving carcass and meat quality characteristics of forage-based beef will benefit the industry and the consumer. Six 9-month-old forage-based steers and six 36-month-old forage-finished heifers were slaughtered to investigate carcass and meat quality characteristics. Significant differences in carcass chilling rate, pH decline, and postmortem changes in muscle metabolites were observed between the two groups. Differences in fatty acid composition of the loin eye muscle were observed between the young steers and forage-finished heifers. Compared to grain-finished supermarket USDA Choice beef, the forage-based beef (9 and 36 months) had lower fat content. The shear value of loin eye muscle of 9-month old steer was lower than that of 36-month-old forage-finished heifers. The shear value of the 36-month-old forage-finished beef was higher than that of grain-finished beef, but the shear value of the 9-month-old beef was comparable to that of grain-finished beef.

INTRODUCTION

The recent trend of exporting feeder calves from Hawaii and importing grain-finished beef for consumption has generated a considerable concern about the long-term sustainability of the Hawaiian beef cattle industry. As a result, much attention has been focused on the marketing of forage-finished beef as an alternative marketing strategy. Furthermore, using lands available from the recent reduction of sugarcane and pineapple production for the production of high quality forage-based beef can improve the sustainability and productivity of these lands and the beef industry. In addition, forage-based beef production is an important component of the beef production in many of the Pacific Rim countries where grain production is limited.

While forage-finished beef has often been described as having less desirable flavor, less tenderness, and shorter retail shelf-life than grain-finished beef (Melton 1983; Kim 1995), forage-finished beef contains much lower levels of fat as compared to grain-finished beef (Bowling *et al.* 1977; Kim 1995). The lower fat content of forage-finished beef is likely to attract today's consumers seeking products with lower total and saturated fats. Also, forage-finished beef may appeal to consumers who are demanding naturally produced and chemical-free products. The objective of this study was to compare the carcass and meat quality characteristics of forage-based beef slaughtered at a young age (9 months) and at a normal market weight (36 months).

MATERIALS AND METHODS

Experimental Design and Sample Preparation

Six weaned, 9-month-old steers (Hereford × Santa Gertrudis cross) and six 36-month-old market heifers (Hereford × Brangus cross) raised without supplementary feed on two commercial ranches on the island of Hawaii were used. Animals were slaughtered at two commercial slaughterhouses on that island. The slaughtering and cooling processes were similar. The postmortem chilling rate of loin eye (LD) muscle was monitored with a metal meat thermometer inserted into the muscle at the 10th rib. Loin eye muscle samples (about 20 g) were taken from the 11 rib at 0, 1, 2, 4, 6 and 24 h after slaughter for the measurement of pH and ATP, glucose-6-phosphate, creatine phosphate, and glycogen concentrations, then immediately frozen in liquid nitrogen and stored in dry ice until subject to biochemical analysis. At 24-h postmortem, following the procedure of Boggs and Merkel (1990), we measured the rib eye area and backfat thickness at the 12th rib. On the same day, the short loins were removed and transported to the University of Hawaii, Manoa. Upon arrival, 1.5 cm thick slices of the frontal portion of LD muscle weighing about 150 g were excised, completely trimmed of subcutaneous fat, and ground for proximate analysis, determination of fatty acid composition, and cholesterol content. Steaks with 2.54 cm thickness were cut and trimmed to less than 2 mm of subcutaneous fat, then individually packaged in plastic trays with tight clear plastic wrapping. The steaks were assigned into two postmortem aging periods (10 and 14 d), then stored at −4°C until shear force measurement. About one cubic cm portions of loin eye muscle were frozen in dry-ice acetone (−78°C), and stored at −70°C for later histology.

Proximate Analysis, Fatty Acid and Cholesterol Assay

Moisture and lipid contents were determined according to AOAC methods (1980). Ash content was determined as the residue after combustion at 600°C for six h. Protein was estimated by the difference between the weight of moisture, ash, and lipid and the total sample weight. Cholesterol was extracted and determined colorimetrically by a commercially available enzymatic assay (Boeringer Mannheim, Indianapolis, IN). Fatty acid profiles were obtained using the procedure of Tamaru *et al.* (1992), involving Soxhlet extraction and measurement of fatty acid methyl esters by capillary, megabore gas chromatography on a Restek Stabilwax column.

Tenderness Measurement

Upon reaching each aging period, the steaks were gently dried with absorbent tissue paper, weighed, packed, and sealed with a semi-vacuum in Kapak pouches (Kapak Corporation, Minneapolis, MN). These packages were heated in water at 75°C for one h and cooled at room temperature for one h. The pouches were unwrapped, gently dried, and weighed again. Cooking loss was the difference in weight after heating. For measurement of tenderness, 3 to 4 core samples (1.8 cm diameter) were taken from the slice after cooking. Each core sample was cut with a Warner-Bratzler blade attached to a TA.XT2 Texture Analyzer (Texture Technologies Group, Scarsdale, NY) at a speed of 180 mm/min. The shear force requirement was the mean of the maximum forces required to shear each set of core samples.

Histology

Cross-sections (16 μm) of muscle were cut on a cryostat (−20°C) and mounted onto microscope slides, then stained for myofibrillar adenosine triphosphatase (ATPase) after acid incubation at pH 4.3 (Guth *et al.* 1970) and succinic dehydrogenase activity (SDH) as described by Pearse (1960). Images of stained sections were captured by a computer-based image analysis system, and analyzed for Type I (TI), Type IIa (TIIa) and IIb (TIIb) percentage. The ATPase positive fibers were identified as TI fibers representing slow-twitch oxidative fibers, and the ATPase negative fibers were identified as TII. TIIa and TIIb were separated by inspecting serial sections of ATPase and SDH. TII fibers that are positive to SDH were identified as TIIa fibers representing fast-twitching oxidative fibers, and TII fibers that are negative to SDH were identified as TIIb fibers representing fast-twitching glycolytic fibers. About 500 fibers were counted to estimate the distribution of fiber type.

Muscle Metabolites and pH Measurements

Frozen samples were pulverized cryogenically and stored at −70°C until all analyses were completed, a time of less than 2 weeks. Metabolites including glycogen, ATP, and creatine phosphate were determined by the method described by Passonneau and Lowry (1993). The pH was measured from the homogenates of 2.5 g muscle in 10 ml of 5 mM iodoacetate/150 mM KCL (adjusted to pH 7.0) according to Bendall (1973).

Statistical Analyses

Data were analyzed by the ANOVA procedure using the MINITAB (1989) program.

RESULTS AND DISCUSSION

Table 1 summarizes the carcass characteristics and proximate analysis of LD muscles from the young steers (YS) and forage-finished heifers (FFH). The carcasses from the YS group had less than 1 mm backfat thickness, while the carcasses from the FFH group had 11.6 mm backfat thickness. The LD muscle of the YS group had significantly higher moisture and lower lipid content than those from the FFH group. No difference in protein and ash content of the LD muscle was observed between the two groups. The carcass backfat thickness (11.6 mm) and lipid content of loin eye muscle (4.3%) of the FFH group in this study were significantly greater than those previously reported in forage-finished carcasses (3.8–9.4 mm backfat thickness and 1.3–3.6% lipid; a review by Kim 1995). The cholesterol content in the LD muscle of the YS group was significantly lower than that of the FFH group.

TABLE 1.
CARCASS CHARACTERISTICS AND PROXIMATE ANALYSIS OF LOIN EYE MUSCLE OF YOUNG AND FORAGE-FINISHED BEEF[a]

	Young Beef			Forage-finished Beef		
Hot carcass wt, kg	131.2	±	5.31	299.8	±	7.99
Backfat thickness, mm	<1.0			11.6	±	2.14
Rib eye area at 12th rib, cm²	50.7*	±	2.22	74.3	±	5.22
Proximate analysis						
Moisture, %	75.7*	±	0.20	72.3	±	0.89
Lipid, %	0.9*	±	0.12	4.3	±	0.97
Protein, %	22.5	±	0.16	22.5	±	0.38
Ash, %	1.0	±	0.03	0.9	±	0.04
Cholesterol, mg/100g muscle	47.8*	±	0.74	59.9	±	3.40

[a] The young and forage-finished beef were from 9 months and 36 months old cattle, respectively. Data are mean ± SEM (n= 6). * Means from young beef and forage-finished beef differ significantly ($P< 0.05$).

The results on shear force and cooking loss of LD muscle from the YS and FFH are summarized in Table 2. The shear force required to cut the cooked LD muscle from the YS was significantly lower than that from the FFH after aging for 10 and 14 d. Regardless of age, increasing aging period from 10 to 14 d enhanced tenderness. Even though statistically not significant, the enhancement was greater in FFH than in YS (27% and 13%, respectively). While increasing aging time decreased shear force requirement, the shear value of cooked LD aged 10 and 14 d (11.63 and 8.5) from the FFH was higher than the value (7.2) we observed from Choice grade grain-finished beef in a previous study (Fukumoto *et al.* 1995). In the YS group, the shear value of 10 d–aged cooked LD was higher than the shear value for Choice grade grain-finished beef, but for 14 d-aged cooked LD the shear value was lower than the Choice grade-grain-finished beef. The results suggest that improving tenderness needs to be considered in marketing forage-finished beef, and slaughtering at a younger age is an option to address the tenderness problem if other marketing conditions allow.

Since postmortem physical and biochemical processes influence meat quality, we measured changes in carcass temperature, muscle pH, and concentrations of muscle metabolites. Figure 1 shows the postmortem chilling rate of LD muscle from the YS and FFH groups. As expected from the smaller carcass and thin backfat, carcasses of the YS chilled significantly faster than carcasses of the FFH. At 6 h after slaughter, the carcass temperature of the YS passed 15°C, a critical temperature below which cold shortening is induced in pre-rigor muscle (Locker and Hagyard 1963). According to Newbold (1966), the cold shortening occurs when muscles containing more than 40% of the resting level of ATP are exposed to cold temperature. The ATP concentration of the loin eye muscle from the young steers at 6 h postmortem was more than 40% of the resting level of ATP (Fig. 3). Therefore, it is likely that the carcasses of the YS had undergone cold shortening. Since red fibers are more susceptible to cold shortening (Pearson 1987), the higher proportion of Type I fiber in young steers (Table 3) appears to make an additional contribution to cold shortening of the carcasses from the young steers. Given that muscle shortening progressively diminishes the improvement in tenderness incurred by aging (Davey *et al.* 1967), it is possible that the smaller improvement in tenderness during aging from 10 d to 14 d in the YS (13%) than in the FFH (27%) resulted from cold-shortening.

TABLE 2.
SHEAR FORCE AND COOKING LOSS OF LOIN EYE MUSCLE FROM YOUNG AND FORAGE-FINISHED BEEF[a]

	Young Beef		Forage-finished Beef		Statistical Significance		
	D10	D14	D10	D14	A	B	A×B
Shear Force[b]	7.68 (0.61)	6.69 (0.39)	11.63 (1.48)	8.50 (0.42)	*	*	NS
Drip Loss[c], %	25.2 (0.61)	25.9 (0.84)	25.5 (1.01)	25.7 (0.45)	NS	NS	NS

[a]The young and forage-finished beef were from 9 months and 36 months old cattle, respectively. Data are mean (SEM, n=6). [b]Expressed as kg/1.8 cm diameter core sample. [c]Weight difference before and after cooking. A, effect of age; B, effect of aging; A × B, effect of age and aging interaction;*, $P<0.05$

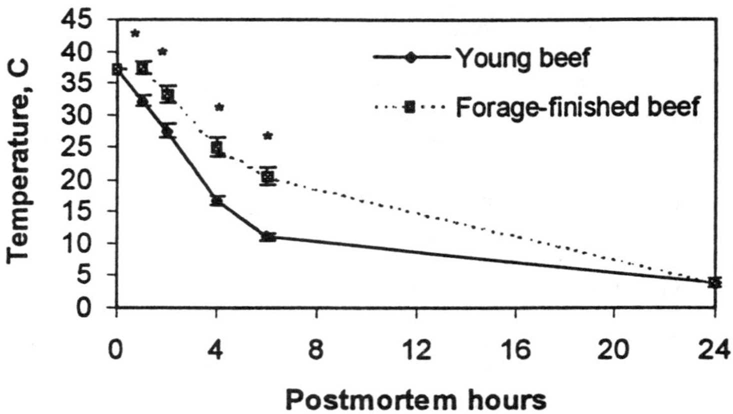

FIG. 1. POSTMORTEM CARCASS CHILLING RATE

Muscle fiber type is an important factor affecting qualitative characteristics of meat products (Ashmore 1974). The LD muscle of the YS had a significantly higher percentage of type I and significantly lower percentage of type IIb muscle fibers than that of the FFH (Table 3). Therefore, it is expected that in addition to the presumed impact of cold shortening mentioned above, the difference in muscle fiber type distribution between the two groups would result in differences in meat quality characteristics.

TABLE 3.
MUSCLE FIBER TYPE DISTRIBUTION OF LOIN EYE MUSCLES FROM YOUNG BEEF AND FORAGE-FINISHED BEEF[a]

	Young Beef			Forage-finished Beef		
Type I %	33.6*	±	2.95	21.3	±	1.60
Type IIa %	16.5	±	2.22	12.4	±	2.55
Type IIb %	49.9*	±	3.17	66.3	±	2.98

[a] The young and forage-finished beef were from 9 months and 36 months old cattle, respectively. Data are mean ± SEM (n= 6). *Means from young beef and forage-finished beef differ significantly ($P < 0.05$).

Figure 2 demonstrates the postmortem pH changes in LD muscle of the YS and FFH. Significant differences in the rate of pH drop and final pH were observed between the two groups of animals. In the LD muscle of the FFH, pH decline occurred rapidly before 1 h postmortem, followed by a gradual decline with the ultimate pH around 5.9. In the LD muscle of the YS, pH decline was gradual through the 24 h postmortem period with an ultimate pH around 5.7. Since postmortem pH changes are directly related to carcass temperature (Cassens and Newbold 1967), the rapid decline of carcass temperature would have played a significant role in the slower declining of pH in the YS. Other factors such as fiber type distribution are also expected to contribute to the difference in rate of pH decline between the two groups.

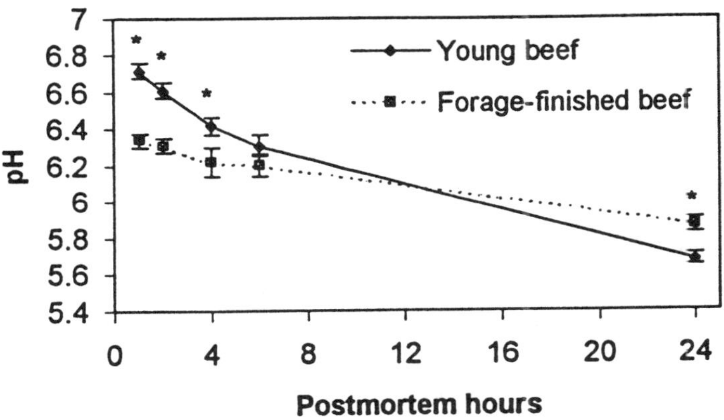

FIG. 2. CHANGES IN POSTMORTEM MUSCLE pH

The ultimate pH of LD muscle from the FFH (5.9) is higher than the normal ultimate pH of 5.4. Others also reported a higher ultimate muscle pH in forage-finished beef than in grain-finished beef (Schroeder *et al.* 1982). Postmortem muscle pH is related to meat tenderness, and the relationship is quadratic; at ultimate pH 6.0 meat is least tender, and above and below 6.0 tenderness improves (Lee 1986). The intermediate pH range (5.81–6.19) generally produces tough meat. Therefore, it is likely that the intermediate ultimate pH of the LD muscle from the FFH was an important factor leading to higher shear force requirement in cooked meat.

Figure 3 summarizes the postmortem changes in the concentrations of ATP, glucose-6-phosphate, creatine phosphate, and glycogen in LD muscles of the YS and FFH groups. The depletion of ATP was faster in FFH than in YS. The rise of glucose-6-phosphate in the LD during the first 4 h postmortem was faster in the YS than in the FFH, but the ultimate glucose-6-phosphate concentration was higher in the FFH than in the YS. Creatine phosphate in the LD was almost depleted at 6 h postmortem in both groups, but the concentration remained higher throughout the 24 h postmortem period in the FFH than in the YS. No difference in the change of glycogen concentration was observed. The results suggest that the pattern of postmortem muscle metabolism was different between the YS and FFH. The difference could be caused by extrinsic factors

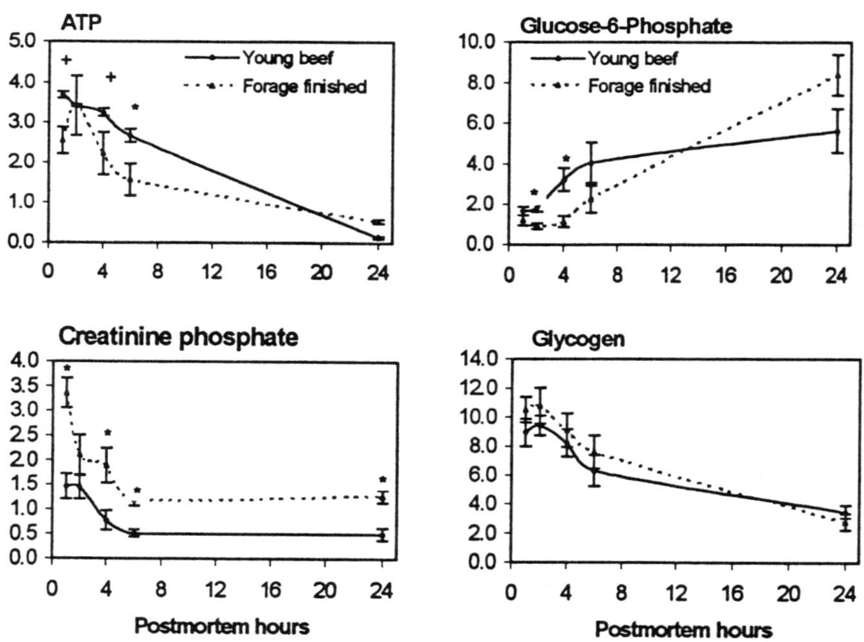

FIG. 3. CHANGE IN METABOLITE CONCENTRATIONS DURING THE 24 H POSTMORTEM PERIOD

The unit of metabolite concentration is μmoles/g muscle for ATP, glucose-6-phosphate, and creatine-phosphate, and mg/g muscle for glycogen.

such as carcass temperature or intrinsic factors such as muscle fiber type composition or a combination of both intrinsic and extrinsic factors.

Table 4 summarizes the data on fatty acid composition of the LD of the YS and FFH. Data from grain-finished beef obtained from our previous study is also included. The percentage of palmitate, palmitoleate, stearate, and oleate in the YS was significantly lower, but the percentage of linoleate, linolenate, octadecatetraenoate, and arachidonate was significantly higher than in the FFH. While it is well-known that there is a difference in fatty acid composition between forage-finished and grain-finished beef due to the difference in diet (Melton *et al.* 1982), the fatty acid composition in beef slaughtered at a young age is not well-documented. The current results demonstrate that the LD muscle of the YS group contains a higher percentage of omega-3 fatty acids than that of the FFH group or grain-finished beef. While the higher proportion of omega-3 and polyunsaturated fatty acids in young beef may appeal to health-conscious consumers, it may have an adverse effect on shelf-life characteristics due to a higher rate of lipid oxidation. Therefore, more studies are required to understand how the difference in fatty acid composition affects the sensory characteristics and shelf-life characteristics of beef produced from young animals.

TABLE 4.
FATTY ACID COMPOSITION (%) IN FAT FROM THE LOIN EYE MUSCLE OF YOUNG AND FORAGE-FINISHED BEEF[a]

Fatty Acids	Young	Forage-finished	Grain-finished[b]
14:0 myristate	4.50 ± 0.300	3.78 ± 0.165	3.56
16:0 palmitate	24.3* ± 0.46	31.1 ± 0.59	30.8
16:1n-7 palmitoleate	2.92* ± 0.087	3.47 ± 0.114	3.07
18:0 stearate	16.6* ± 0.41	19.0 ± 0.79	13.7
18:1n-9 oleate	31.7* ± 0.46	40.8 ± 0.84	42.3
18:2n-6 linoleate	6.70* ± 0.451	0.36 ± 0.023	4.6
18:3n-3 linolenate	3.27* ± 0.265	0.88 ± 0.162	0.40
18:4n-3 octadecatetraenoate	2.51* ± 0.162	0.12 ± 0.012	0.20
20:4n-6 arachidonate	4.56* ± 0.268	0.16 ± 0.037	0.92

[a]The young and forage-finished beef were from 9 months and 36 months old cattle, respectively. Data are mean ± SEM (n= 6). *Means from young beef and forage-finished beef differ significantly ($P<0.05$). [b]Data are from our previous study (Fukumoto *et al.* 1995).

ACKNOWLEDGMENTS

The authors acknowledge the County of Hawaii, Department of Research and Development for funding this study, and Hualalai Ranch, Kahuku Ranch, J.J. Andrade Slaughter House and Kulana Foods, Inc. for providing beef samples and assisting with sample collection. The authors also express their appreciation to Dr. Alvin Huang for use of his Texture Analyzer, and Dr. Halina Zaleski for her critical review of the manuscript.

REFERENCES

AOAC. 1980. Official Methods of Analysis (13th Ed.). Association of Official Analytical Chemists, Washington, D.C.

ASHMORE, C.R. 1974. Phenotypic expression of muscle fiber types and some implications to meat quality. J. Anim. Sci. *38*, 1158–1164.

BENDALL, J.R. 1973. Postmortem changes in muscle. *In* The Structure and Function of Muscle, 2nd Ed., Vol 2, G.H. Bourne (ed.) Academic Press, New York.

BOGGS, D.L. and MERKEL, R.A. 1990. Live Animal Carcass Evaluation and Selection Manual. Kendall/Hunt Publ. Co., Dubuque, IA.

BOWLING, R.A., SMITH, G.C., CARPENTER, Z.L., DUTSON, T.R. and OLIVER, W.M. 1977. Comparison of forage-finished and grain-finished beef carcasses. J. Anim. Sci. *45*, 209–215.

CASSENS, R.G. and NEWBOLD, R.P. 1967. Temperature dependence of pH changes in ox muscles postmortem. J. Food. Sci. *32*, 13–14.

DAVEY, C.L., KUTTEL, H. and GILBERT, K.V. 1967. Shortening as a factor in meat aging. J. Food Technol. *2*, 53–67.

FUKUMOTO, G.K., KIM, Y.S., OKUDA, D. and AKO, H. 1995. Chemical composition and shear force requirement of loin eye muscle of young, forage-fed steers. Hawaii Institute of Tropical Agriculture and Human Resources, Research Extension Series 161.

GUTH, Z., SAMAHA, F.J. and ALBERS, R.W. 1970. The neural regulation of some phenotypic difference between the fiber types of mammalian skeletal muscle. Exp. Neurol. *26*, 126–135.

KIM, Y.S. 1995. Carcass characteristics and meat quality in forage-finished and grain-finished beef — a mini review. RDA J. Agric. Sci. *37*, 573–582.

LEE, Y.B. 1986. Early postmortem measurements and conditioning in assessing and enhancing meat quality. J. Anim. Sci. *63*, 622–632.

LOCKER, R.H. and HAGYARD, C.J. 1963. A cold shortening effect in beef muscles. J. Sci. Food Agric. *14*, 787–793.

MELTON, S.L. 1983. Effect of forage feeding on beef flavor. Food Technol. *37*(5), 239–248.

MELTON, S.L., BLACK, J.M., DAVIS, G.W. and BACKUS, W.R. 1982. Flavor and selected chemical composition of ground beef from steers backgrounded on pasture and fed corn for up to 140 days. J. Food. Sci. *47*, 699–703.

MINITAB. 1989. Statistical Software. Minitab Inc., State College, PA 16801 USA.

NEWBOLD, R.P. 1966. Changes associated with rigor mortis. *In* The Physiology and Biochemistry of Muscle as a Food, p. 213. E.J. Briskey, R.G. Cassens and J.C. Trautman (eds.). Univ. of Wisconsin Press, Madison.

PASSONNEAU, J.V. and LOWRY, O.H. 1993. Enzymatic Analysis: A Practical Guide. Humana Press, Totowa, NJ.

PEARSE, A.G.E. 1960. Histochemistry, Theoretical and Applied, 3rd Ed. Churchill, London.

PEARSON, A.M. 1987. Muscle function and postmortem changes. *In* The Science of Meat and Meat Products. p. 155, J.F. Price and B.S. Schweigert (eds.). Food & Nutrition Press, Inc. Trumbull, CT.

SCHROEDER, J.W., CRAMER, D.A., BOWLING, R.A. and COOK, C.W. 1982. Postmortem muscle alterations in beef carcass temperature, pH and palatability from electrical stimulation. J. Anim. Sci. *54*, 549–552.

TAMARU, C.S., AKO, H. and LEE, C-S. 1992. Fatty acid and amino acid profiles of spawned eggs of striped mullet, *Mugil cephalus* L. Aquaculture *105*, 83–94.

QUANTITATIVE ASPECT FOR EFFECT OF LIPID HYDROPEROXIDES ON FISH MYOFIBRILLAR PROTEIN

TOORU OOIZUMI

Department of Marine Bioscience
Fukui Prefectural University
Obama, Fukui, 917 Japan

ABSTRACT

Treatment of myofibrils with autoxidized triglyceride caused ATPase activity changes, loss of protein extractability, and cross-linking of myosin heavy chains. The changes were all determined by the ratio of peroxide to myofibrils. The autoxidized triglyceride used in this study contained no secondary oxidation products such as malonaldehyde. Furthermore, hydroperoxides isolated from photoirradiated triglyceride caused essentially the same changes in ATPase activity and cross-linking of myosin heavy chains as the autoxidation products. Therefore, it was concluded that hydroperoxides in the autoxidized triglyceride were responsible for the protein denaturation.

INTRODUCTION

Fish lipid is characterized by its high content of highly unsaturated fatty acids (HUFA) which have favorable functions to human health. However, these HUFA are readily oxidized and result in deterioration in color and flavor of fish meat products during storage and processing. The interaction of lipid oxidation products with myofibrillar protein and its influences on the quality of muscle based products have been studied (Decker *et al.* 1993; Li and King 1996; Liu and Xiong 1996). We have also demonstrated that autoxidized fish lipid modifies the myofibrillar protein quantitatively by monitoring ATPase activity changes and cross-linking of myosin heavy chains (Kawasaki *et al.* 1991, 1992a,b). However, the components attributed to the protein denaturation were not fully understood. Buttkus (1967) stated that malonaldehyde, a secondary oxidation product of lipid, decreased protein solubility while Srinivasan and Hultin (1995) suggested the involvement of hydroxyl radicals in the modification of fish muscle protein.

The objective of this paper is to clarify whether hydroperoxides in autoxidized lipid induce protein denaturation. We employed photosensitized oxidation products of triglyceride as well as the autoxidized triglyceride. The former is known to generate hydroperoxides and no secondary products.

MATERIALS AND METHODS

Oxidation of Triglyceride

Triglyceride (TG) purified from sardine oil was allowed to oxidize in two oxidation systems. The first one was autoxidation, in which TG was incubated at 37°C in the dark. The other one was photosensitized oxidation, in which TG was irradiated with white light in the presence of methylene blue as a photosensitizer at 10°C. The oxidation process of TG was monitored by measuring peroxide value (PV) by the method of Bilinski *et al.* (1978).

Isolation of Oxidation Products

Oxidized TG in the two systems was submitted to thin layer chromatography (TLC) with developing solvent consisting of *n*-hexane:diethyl ether:acetic acid (85:15:1 or 80:70:1, v/v). Separated components were visualized by spraying the TLC plate with a solution consisting of 3% copper acetate/8% phosphate (w/v). Hydroperoxides separated on the TLC plate were detected by the potassium iodide-starch reaction. Thiobarbituric acid (TBA) reactive substances, such as malonaldehyde, were detected by spraying TBA reagent on the TLC plate. The oxidation products, as well as the unoxidized TG, separated on the TLC plate were extracted with chloroform:methanol(1:9,v/v) (for oxidation products) or with diethyl ether (for unoxidized TG), respectively. The oxidized TG and the isolated components were dissolved in dimethyl sulfoxide and used in this study.

Treatment of Myofibrils with Oxidation Products

Myofibrils were prepared from carp (*Cyprinus carpio*) by the method of Katoh *et al.* (1977). Myofibrils in a medium of 0.1 M KCl-20 mM Tris-HCl (pH 7.5) were mixed with either the whole oxidized TG or the isolated components, and the mixtures were incubated overnight at 0°C.

Evaluation of Protein Denaturation

The denaturation of myofibrils induced by treatment with the oxidation products was evaluated by measuring the ATPase activity, the cross-linking of myosin heavy chains and the protein extractability. The ATPase activity was assayed at 25°C in a medium of 0.5 M KCl-25 mM Tris-maleate (pH 7.0), 1 mM ATP and 5 mM either EDTA (for K-ATPase) or $CaCl_2$ (for Ca-ATPase). SDS gel electrophoresis was carried out by using 5% polyacrylamide gel. Protein bands were stained with Coomassie Brilliant Blue R250. Decrease in the staining intensity of myosin heavy chain was measured densitometrically as an indicator of the cross-linking reaction. Protein extractability was determined by measuring the amount of extracted protein from the myofibrils with 0.7 M KCl-20 mM Tris-HCl (pH 7.5). The Biuret method was used for the determination of protein concentration (Gornall *et al.* 1949).

RESULTS AND DISCUSSIONS

Peroxide-Induced Protein Denaturation

First, we analyzed the autoxidized TG used in this study by TLC. Unoxidized TG gave a spot with an R_f value of 0.34 while the oxidation products gave two additional spots, one at the original point (PF1) and the other with a very small R_f value (PF2) by using a developing solvent consisting of *n*-hexane:diethyl ether:acetic acid (85:15:1,v/v). No secondary oxidation products such as malonaldehyde, presumably generated from hydroperoxides, were detected in the autoxidized TG.

Quantitative effect of autoxidized TG on the protein denaturation was investigated by changing the ratio of peroxide to myofibrils. Various amounts of the autoxidized TG were mixed with myofibrils with three different concentrations and the mixtures were stored overnight at 0°C. Consequent ATPase activity changes, progress of myosin heavy chain cross-linking and loss of protein extractability were measured. The Ca- and K-ATPase activities were plotted as a function of the ratio of peroxide to myofibrils in the mixtures (Fig. 1 A,B). With all myofibrils concentrations, both the Ca- and K-ATPase activities changed along a respective single curve. Upon treatment with the autoxidized TG, myofibrillar Ca-ATPase activity increased, while K-ATPase activity decreased in response to the increase of the ratio of peroxide to myofibrils. Therefore, the modification of a thiol group in the ATPase active site of myosin was suggested.

The myofibrils treated with the autoxidized TG were submitted to SDS-PAGE to analyze the cross-linking of myosin heavy chains. Although the SDS-PAGE patterns are not presented, disappearance of myosin heavy chain was accompanied by the generation of a series of cross-linked heavy chains. With the increase of peroxide content in the mixtures, myosin heavy chain content decreased. The change was again well explained by the ratio of peroxide to myofibrils irrespective of myofibril concentrations (Fig. 2).

Upon treatment with autoxidized TG, protein extractability of myofibrils dropped drastically. The decrease in the extractability was also determined by the ratio of peroxide to myofibrils (Fig. 3). However, a full decrease occurred with a very small amount of peroxide (less than 1×10^{-6} meq/mg). This was much less than those for the half maximal decrease in the ATPase and the myosin heavy chain. The former and the latter occurred at 6×10^{-5} meq/mg and 1×10^{-3} meq/mg, respectively. These results suggest that hydroperoxides in the autoxidized TG interacted with myofibrillar protein leading to the modification of protein functions.

Effect of Hydroperoxides Isolated on Protein Denaturation

To prove that hydroperoxides were the components responsible for the modifying effect of autoxidized TG on myofibrillar protein, hydroperoxides were prepared by the photosensitized oxidation of TG. This oxidation system is known to generate no secondary products because no free radicals are involved in the reaction. When the photoirradiated TG was chromatographed on a TLC plate with the solvent consisting of *n*-hexane:diethyl ether:acetic acid (80:70:1, v/v), the main oxidation products were detected as spots with R_f values of 0.39 (HP1) and 0.61 (HP2), respectively. Unoxidized TG migrated near the top of the TLC plate (R_f 0.96). Since the chromatographic spot for HP1 heavily tailed from the original point, HP1 seemed to have a complicated composition. Since TG used in this study contained various molecular species and since all the oxidation products were positive for iodide-starch reaction, hydroperoxides with different polarity might be produced by the photosensitized oxidation of TG.

The hydroperoxides (HP1 and HP2) and the intact TG were isolated from photoirradiated TG by TLC. Their modifying effects on myofibrillar protein were compared with those of the isolated autoxidation products of TG (PF1 and PF2). Myofibrils were incubated with the isolated components overnight at 0°C. With the increase of the amount of hydroperoxides or autoxidation products, both the K-ATPase activity and the intact myosin heavy chain decreased while the intact TG caused no changes (Fig. 4 A,B). HP1 gave the same changes in both ATPase and cross-linking of

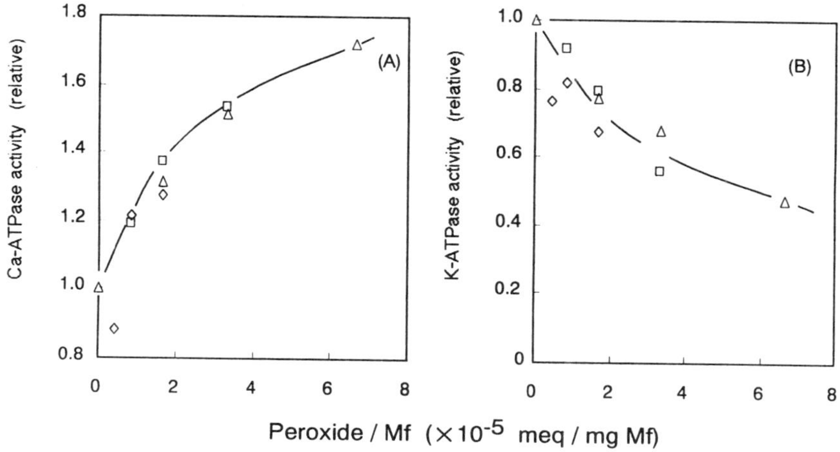

FIG. 1. PEROXIDE-INDUCED ATPase ACTIVITY CHANGES
Myofibrils at concentrations of 2.5 (△), 5.0 (□) and 10.0 (◇) mg/ml were incubated with autoxidized TG overnight at 0°C. Myofibrillar Ca- (A) and K-ATPase (B) were assayed.

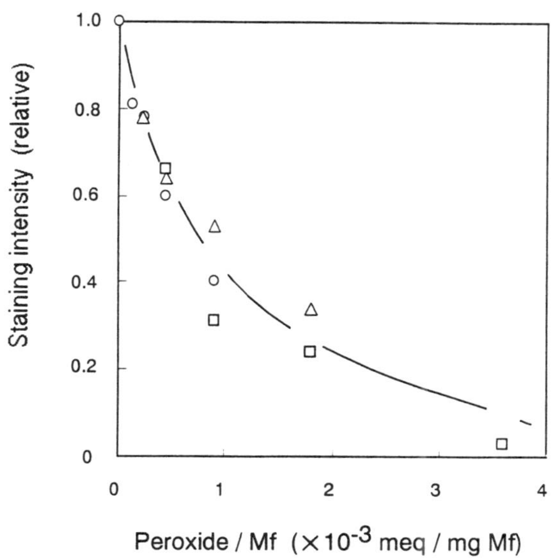

FIG. 2. PEROXIDE-INDUCED CROSS-LINKING OF MYOSIN HEAVY CHAINS
Myofibrils at concentrations of 22.4 (o), 11.2 (△) and 5.6 (□) mg/ml were incubated with autoxidized TG overnight at 0°C as in Fig. 1. Decrease in relative staining intensity of intact myosin heavy chain as a result of cross-linking reaction was measured by SDS-PAGE analysis.

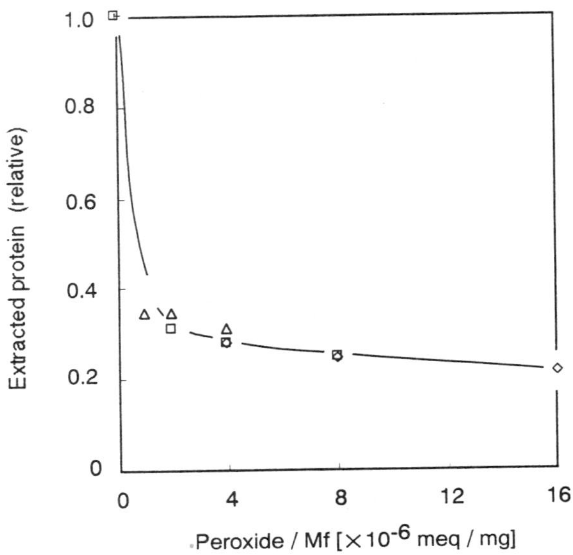

FIG. 3. PEROXIDE-INDUCED PROTEIN EXTRACTABILITY LOSS OF MYOFIBRILS
Myofibrils treated with the autoxidized TG as in Fig. 1 were used. Extracted protein with 0.7 M KCl-20 mM Tris-HCl (pH 7.5) was determined. The identical symbols as in Fig. 1 were used.

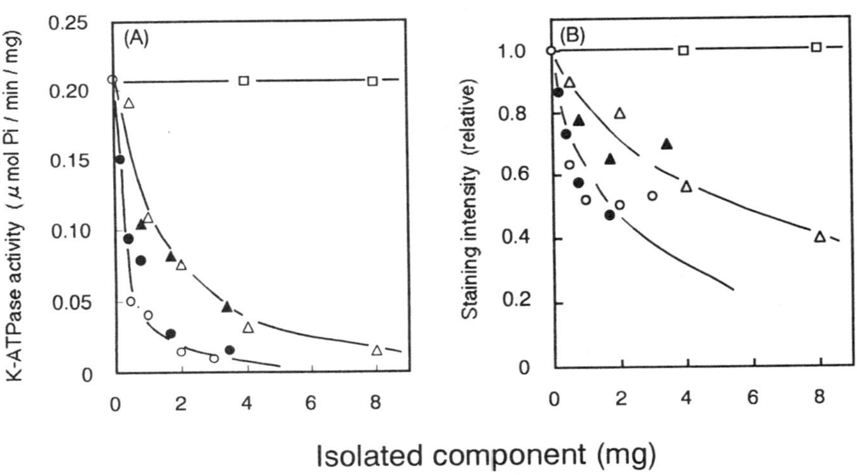

FIG. 4. COMPARISON OF MODIFYING EFFECTS OF HYDROPEROXIDES WITH AUTOXIDATION PRODUCTS
Myofibrils were incubated with hydroperoxides (HP1, ○; HP2, △) produced by photosensitized oxidation or autoxidation products (PF1, ●; PF2, ▲) and with the intact TG (□) under the same conditions as in Fig. 1. K-ATPase (A) and cross-linking of myosin heavy chains (B) were measured by the same methods as in Figs. 1 and 2.

myosin heavy chain as PF1, and HP2 did as PF2. However, the first more efficiently induced the changes than the latter components (HP2 and PF2). It was therefore proved that the autoxidation products were practically the same as the hydroperoxides produced by photosensitized oxidation in the modifying effects on myofibrillar protein.

Thus, the hydroperoxides present in autoxidized TG were concluded to be responsible for the protein denaturation. The conclusion was consistent with that in our previous paper, in which hydroperoxides produced by photosensitized oxidation of methyl oleate were used as model components (Kawasaki and Ooizumi 1996). It was reported that malonaldehyde as a secondary oxidation product of lipid decreased the solubility of trout myosin (Buttkus 1967) and that aldehydes such as glutaraldehyde formed cross-links with myosin (Hu *et al.* 1988). Nevertheless, we demonstrated that hydroperoxides rather than secondary oxidation products modified myofibrillar protein. It is well-known that the color and flavor of marine products deteriorate by secondary oxidation products such as carbonyl compounds rather than by hydroperoxides. Accordingly, hydroperoxides-induced protein denaturation as measured by the above indices seemed to occur even in a very early phase of lipid oxidation during the storage of fish meat. Research to correlate the hydroperoxides-induced protein denaturation with the quality of fish meat is in progress.

REFERENCES

BILINSKI, E., JONES, R.E.E. and LAU, Y. C. 1978. Chill storage and development of rancidity in frozen Pacific herring *clupea herengus pallasi*. J. Fish Res. Board Canada *35*, 473–477 .

BUTTKUS, H. 1967. The reaction of myosin with malonaldehyde. J. Food Sci. *32*, 432–434.

DECKER, E.A., XIONG, Y.L. and BLANCHARD, S.P. 1993. Chemical, physical, and functional properties of oxidized turkey white muscle myofibrillar protein. J. Agric. Food Chem. *41*, 186–189.

GORNALL, A.G., BARDAWILL, C.J. and DAVID, M.M. 1949. Determination of serum proteins by means of the biuret reaction. J. Biol. Chem. *177*, 751–766.

HU, D.H., KIMURA, S. and MARUYAMA, K. 1988. Cross-linking of native myosin forms, oligomers of myosin heavy chain dimers. J. Biochem. *104*, 509–511.

KATOH, N., UCHIYAMA, H., TSUKAMOTO, S. and ARAI, K. 1977. A biochemical study on fish myofibrillar ATPase. Nippon Suisan Gakkaishi *43*, 857–867. (in Japanese with English abstract)

KAWASAKI, K., OOIZUMI, T. and KONNO, K. 1991. Effect of peroxidized fish lipid on the ATPase activity of carp myofibrils. Nippon Suisan Gakkaishi *57*, 1185–1191. (in Japanese with English abstract)

KAWASAKI, K., OOIZUMI, T. and KONNO, K. 1992a. Cross-linking reaction of myosin heavy chain in carp myofibrils induced by peroxidized sardine oil. Nippon Suisan Gakkaishi *58*, 127–133. (in Japanese with English abstract)

KAWASAKI, K., OOIZUMI, T., KONNO, K. and HAYASHI, K. 1992b. Involvement of the polar fraction produced by autoxidation of triglyceride of sardine oil in the ATPase activity change and the cross-linking of myosin heavy chain of myofibrils. Nippon Suisan Gakkaishi *58*, 135–140. (in Japanese with English abstract)

KAWASAKI, K. and OOIZUMI, T. 1996. Effect of hydroperoxides produced by photosensitized oxidation of methyl oleate on carp myofibrillar protein. Fish. Sci. *62*, 69–72.

LI, S.J. and KING, A.J. 1996. Lipid oxidation and myosin denaturation in dark chicken meat. J. Agric. Food Chem. *44*, 3080–3084.

LIU, G. and XIONG, Y.L. 1996. Contribution of lipid and protein oxidation to rheological difference between chicken white and red muscle myofibrillar protein. J. Agric. Food Chem. *44*, 779–784.

SRINIVASAN, S. and HULTIN, H.O. 1995. Hydroxyl radical modification of fish muscle proteins. J. Food Biochem. *18*, 405–425.

HIGH FISCHER RATIO PEPTIDE MIXTURE

WENYING GU and MEI WANG

Food College, Wuxi University of Light Industry
Wuxi, Jiangsu, 214036, P.R. China

ABSTRACT

The ratio of BCAA (branched chain amino acids, Val, Ile, Leu) vs. AAA (aromatic amino acids, Phe, Tyr) was named as high Fischer (F) Ratio. High F Ratio protein hydrolysate, especially its peptide mixture, is available for patients with hepatic encephalopathy.

A process was proposed to produce a high F Ratio (>20) peptide mixture from corn gluten meal (CGM). It was mainly hydrolyzed at the peptide bond of AAA by protease A. Then the AAA on end of the peptide was liberated by protease B. Liberated AAA was adsorbed by activated charcoal and removed. The type of proteases and activated charcoal were optimized. No bitterness of the high F Ratio (F=38.92) peptide mixture was produced. The yield was more than 15% (based on N content in CGM).

Biological functions were tested in animals. The results proved that high F Ratio peptide mixture, produced by the proposed process, was available for protecting and curing of young male rats with hepatic disease.

INTRODUCTION

For patients with severe hepatic encephalopathy, it is generally observed that an amino acid imbalance state characterized by low levels of branched chain amino acids (BCAA) and high levels of aromatic amino acids (AAA) takes place in their systemic blood. The ratio of BACC molecules to AAA is named as the Fischer Ratio. In connection with this disease, Fischer *et al.* (1971) have reported that an increasing phenylalanine concentration in the brain inhibits the hydroxylation of tyrosine and the resulting increase in AAA level leads to a decrease in the normal neurotransmitters, dopamine and noradrenaline, as well as to an increase in the neurologically inactive phenylethanolamine and octopamine.

At present, the theory that such a monoamine imbalance in the brain is caused by hepatic encephalopathy is widely accepted. Fischer *et al.* (1971) have also reported that BCAA intake improves the plasma amino acid balance to mitigate the symptoms of hepatic encephalopathy. So a product of peptide formula with a high BCAA and low AAA character is needed for patients with hepatic encephalopathy. For hepatic patients, Fischer Ratio over 20 is expected (Okita *et al.* 1984).

Because CGM is not soluble in water (pH ~7), its utilization is limited in foods. So expanding its utilization is needed. Corn gluten meal (CGM) is a byproduct of wet milling corn starch. High level BCAA is contained in corn gluten. So CGM is a good source for producing high Fischer Ratio protein hydrolysate as shown in Table 1.

TABLE 1.
AMINO ACIDS OF SOME CEREALS

	Val (%)	Leu(%)	Ile(%)	BCAA(%)	Phe(%)
Rice	5.50	9.04	3.35	17.89	4.69
Wheat	4.22	7.11	3.58	14.91	4.53
Soybean	4.75	9.58	4.24	18.57	4.75
Broad bean	4.44	7.74	3.42	15.60	3.93
Pea	4.93	8.38	3.65	16.96	5.11
Corn	5.31	15.20	3.28	23.79	4.96
Sorghum	4.95	16.00	3.72	24.67	5.36

Preparation of High F Peptide Mixture

Most proteins found in CGM are zein. The amino acid sequence of zein is well known. For production of high Fischer Ratio product, some steps are needed:

1. Hydrolyze corn protein at the peptide bond of AAA, with other amino acids forming small peptides and a few free amino acids.
2. Reduce AAA from small peptide.
3. Remove AAA while keeping other amino acids, especially BACC, both in peptide and free form.

Procedure chosen was as follows:

CGM, enzymolysis by protease A; enzymolysis by protease B

(pH 10, 3 hr, 45 min) (pH 2.8, 2 hr, 25 min)

Centrifugation of peptide mixture with free AA filter to decolor and adsorb phenylalanine etc.; then the residue filtered on activated charcoal. Product was desalted and concentrated to give High F peptide mixture.

In the procedure, two proteases were chosen. One alkaline protease was chosen as protease A. Most of proteins in CGM are zein which could be dissolved in alcohol or alkaline solution. Alkaline protease was chosen to avoid use of and save cost. The purpose of protease B is to hydrolyze the peptide bonds adjacent to the aromatic amino acids. Conditions for one kind of proteases were optimized.

Free AAA was adsorbed by activated charcoal. Effect of activated charcoal type on efficiency of AAA adsorption was very significant. One type was optimum. CGM was treated by protease and activated charcoal. The results shown are as following.

Table 2 shows:

1. After treatment by protease A, the peptide mixture contained only a few free amino acids. In hydrolysate, free phenylalanine = 0.000, tyrosine = 0.075 mg/ml.
2. After treatment by protease B, some free AAA were increased (free phenylalanine = 0.1034, tyrosine = 0.1032).
3. After adsorption, AAA was decreased significantly.

4. Not only free AAA, but also some of AAA in peptide form was adsorbed significantly by activated charcoal. This result was confirmed by UV absorption spectrum.
5. A very high Fischer Ratio peptide mixture was obtained (F = 38.92). The high F peptide mixture was desalted and concentrated. About 8% nitrogen and some salt was contained in the finished mixture which was prepared for animal feeding tests.

TABLE 2.
AMINO ACID COMPOSITION AFTER PROTEASES AND ACTIVATED CHARCOAL TREATMENT

	Peptide mixture A (After protease A)		Peptide mixture B (After protease B)		After adsorption on activated charcoal	
	Free AA (mg/ml)	AA in peptide (mg/ml)	Free AA (mg/ml)	AA in peptide (mg/ml)	Free AA (mg/ml)	AA in peptide (mg/ml)
Val	0.0292	1.452	0.0640	1.7111	0.0632	0.4580
Ile	0.6292	0.592	0.6240	1.3460	0.0000	0.2420
Leu	0.0000	6.415	0.0182	7.7170	0.0326	1.1820
Tyr	0.0750	2.073	0.1032	2.3854	0.0220	0.0590
Phe	0.0000	2.244	0.1032	2.4610	0.0000	0.0000
Sum	0.7334	12.776	0.9126	15.6205	0.1178	1.9410
Total	13.5094		16.5331		2.0588	

Biological Function Test

Animal trial: 3 to 10 young male rats were divided into 3 groups randomly.

Group 1: Fed basic feeds with injections of 0.35 ml/100 g (body weight) CCl_4 with oil 2 times/week to cause hepatic disease.

Group 2: Fed basic feeds, with 10% (feed =100%) test peptide solution which was added and mixed; injection of CCl_4 was same as group 1.

Group 3: Control group. Fed basic feeds only.

The results of animal tests were the following:

The animals of control group (Group 3) grew well, from beginning to end. (32 days)

For Group 1, symptoms of hepatic disease were severe. Eleven days after beginning of trial, appetite of all ten rats was decreased and their fur had lost luster; after 15 days, 3 of ten rats had symptoms as above. After 19 days, all rats in this group lost half of appetite, and their fur became dark in no order. All ten rats showed effect of the cool temperature. After 32 days, 1 rat died, 2 rats did not take any feed.

Group 2, testing group, grew as well as group 3 (control group), although CCl_4 was injected same as in Group 1. Other data are shown in Table 3.

From Table 3, the results were as follows:

1. Group 1 was infected by hepatic disease due to injection of CCl_4. The symptoms of hepatic disease were severe, and data showed all rats were severely diseased.

2. Group 2 grew similar to Group 3. It means 10% test peptide solution added to basic feed can almost counteract the effect of CCl_4 injection.

TABLE 3.
RESULTS OF ANIMAL TESTS

	Group No.		
	1	2	3
Average W_1 (g/each)	182	180	178
Average W_2 (g/each)	210	265	282
Blood (at 32 days)			
Red blood cell ($\times 10^6$/ml)	0.46 ± 0.19	9.9 ± 1.3	8.4 ± 0.6
White blood cell ($\times 10^6$ml)	2.7 ± 0.9	1.5 ± 0.1	1.3 ± 0.2
Congealment time (sec)	88 ± 0.1	26 ± 0.7	27 ± 1.5
F Ratio of rat serum	2.23	2.81	2.62
Glu-Ala transaminase	79.0 ± 3	65 ± 3	64 ± 8
Time of swim to death (min)	—	101 ±14.4	75 ± 3.7

W_1, at beginning of test
W_2, 32 days later

Conclusion. The high Fischer Ratio peptide (F = 38.92, yield = 15.8% based on N of CGM) prepared in this trial is available for hepatic disease patients, even those with hepatic encephalopathy.

ACKNOWLEDGMENTS

The author thanks Ms. Wangmei, my Ph.D student, for help with this research work.

REFERENCES

FISCHER, J.E. and BALDESSARINI, R.J. 1975. Catechol amines and neurologic diseases. Neurotransmitter metabolism in hepatic encephalopathy. Comments. N. Engl. J. Med. *293*, 1152–1153.

OKITA, M., WATANABE, A., TAKEI, N., NAGASHIMA, H. and UBUKA, T. 1984. Effects of branched-chain α-beta acids on plasma amino acid concentrations in carbon tetrachloride-intoxicated rats. J. Nutr. *114*, 1235–1241.

ZHOU, S. and ZHONG, L. 1986. Chinese Commercial Publishing House, p. 149.

SDS-PAGE IN TRIS-GLYCINE BUFFER FOR SEPARATION OF PROTEINS OF LOW MOLECULAR WEIGHT

PING-FAN RAO, RU-MING CHEN, LI NI, JIAN-CAI LI, SHU-TAO LIU, RONG-ZHEN ZHANG, BI-HONG SHI, GONG-RUI CHEN, YU-QIANG ZHENG and WEN-HONG GAO

Institute of Biotechnology
Fuzhou University
523, Gong-ye Road, Fuzhou, Fujian
P.R. China 350002

ABSTRACT

Polyacrylamide gel electrophoresis in the presence of sodium dodecyl sulfate (SDS) is an extremely important means in the analysis and molecular weight determination of proteins and polypeptides. Most systems, however, fail to obtain reasonable separation of small proteins and polypeptides of molecular weight lower than 10,000 daltons, which is especially important in the protein studies of fermented food products. The only system which can be used to separate polypeptides as small as 3,000 daltons employs tris-tricine buffer. The system is an improved version of the Laemmli method that involves a discontinuous buffer system. The other concern with this system is that tricine is fairly expensive.

An improved SDS-PAGE system was developed by this group, in which a simple continuous buffer of 0.05 M tris-glycine is used as buffer for both separation gel and stacking gel as well as electrode buffer. Polypeptides with molecular weights as low as 3,000 daltons can be satisfactorily separated. Protein bands are as sharp and clear as those of the most widely used Laemmli system, in which a front band is formed in the process of electrophoresis to ensure uniformity of electric field and prevent band broadening, and the linearity between the protein mobility and its molecular weight is as good as the Weber-Osborn system, which is known for its reliability in molecular weight estimation because of its simple ion system. It is an SDS-PAGE system with advantages both of the most widely used system with greater ease at lower expense, and it is very useful in protein study of fermented foods.

INTRODUCTION

Polyacrylamide gel electrophoresis (PAGE) in the presence of sodium dodecyl sulfate (SDS) is a very important method in the analysis subunit and molecular weight determinations of proteins and polypeptides. Most (SDS-PAGE) systems, however, fail to obtain reasonable separation of small proteins and polypeptides of molecular weight lower than 10,000 daltons, which is especially important in protein studies of fermented food products and other studies involving enzymatic hydrolysis of proteins.

The most widely used Laemmli method, employing a discontinuous buffer system, is well known for the sharp protein bands but fails to separate proteins with molecular weight lower than 10,000 from its electrophoretic front even with 15% separation gel (Laemmli 1970). Another well-known method is that of Weber-Osborn which employs a simple continuous buffer throughout the electrode cell, stacking gel and separation gel and works very well to separate proteins according to their molecular weights. Serious diffusion of the protein bands with the Weber-Osborn method, however, has hindered its application to the separation of small proteins and polypeptides. The more the protein band migrates in the gel and the longer the time, the more the band expands, and the bands of smaller molecular weight proteins can hardly be recognized (Weber and Osborn 1969).

A modified Laemmli method suitable for separation of polypeptides as small as 3,000 daltons has been proposed (Schagger and Von Jagow 1987). Separation is satisfactory and the protein bands are sharp and clear. It employs, however, a discontinuous tris-tricine buffer system. The apparent disadvantage for a discontinuous buffer system is inconvenience in preparing the electrophoresis. Another disadvantage can be inconvenience in preservation of the precast gel of this Tris-tricine system. An additional concern with this system is that tricine is fairly expensive, and tricine concentration in the electrode buffer is as high as 0.1 M.

A novel SDS-PAGE method for small polypeptides is proposed here on the basis of investigation of the differences between the Laemmli method and the Weber-Osborn method. It is an SDS-PAGE system including advantages of the both systems, enabling excellent performance on SDS-PAGE of small proteins at reasonable cost.

EXPERIMENTAL

Sodium dodecyl sulfate polyacryamide gel electrophoresis (SDS-PAGE) throughout this work was performed on a protein mini slab apparatus (Atto Co., Japan) connected to an Atto 1000 electrophoretic power supply. Gel size was $8 \times 7 \times 0.7$ (cm), with 1 cm stacking gel and 6 cm separation gel. The separation gel and the stacking gel were prepared basically according to the procedure of Laemmli, except that the final buffer in both gels was 0.46 M Tris-0.047 M glycine, pH 9.57, which was also the electrode buffer.

SDS of electrophoretic grade was purchased from BDH (Shanghai, China). Ultra-pure acrylamide was a product of BRL (Gaithersburg, Md.). TEMED was a product of SERVA (Heidelberg, Germany), and low molecular weight protein standard kit (2.5-31 KDa) was a product of Pharmacia Biotechonology. All the other reagents used in this work were of analytical grade.

RESULTS AND DISCUSSION

An electrophoretogram of the standard proteins with low molecular weights is shown in Fig. 1. All seven proteins with molecular weights ranging from 2.5 to 31 KDa were satisfactorily separated, and even the smallest protein of myoglobin fragment with molecular weight of 2.5 KDa shows a very sharp band on the electrophoretogram with characteristic patterns of protein bands of the Laemmli system.

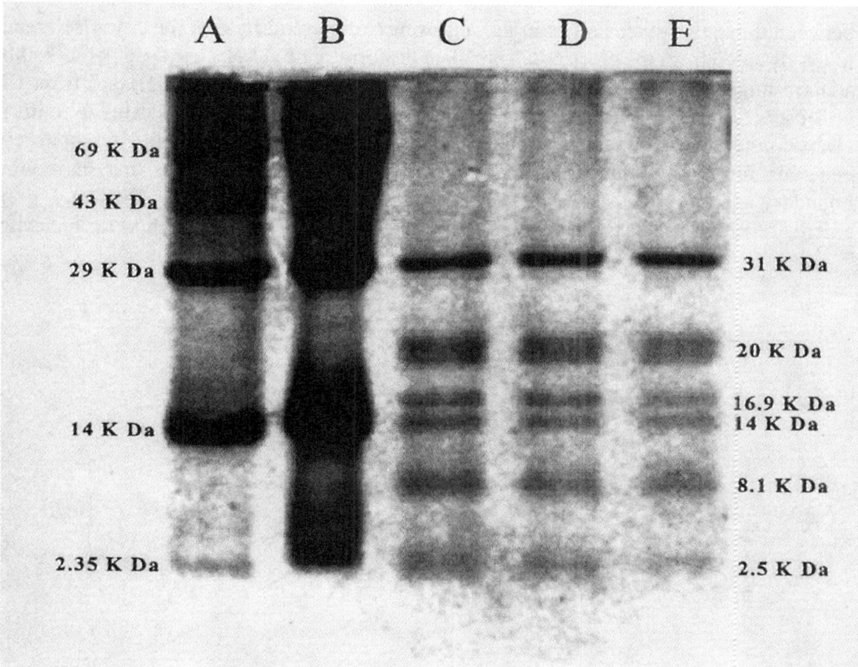

FIG. 1. PHOTOGRAPH OF A 15% ACRYLAMIDE, 3% BIS-ACRYLAMIDE GEL
The channels contain: (A,B) Molecular-weight standards (5 μl, 3 μl); (C,D,E) Promega low-molecular-weight standards (3 μl, 2 μl, 1 μl).

Among all the SDS-PAGE systems, the Laemmli system is most widely used because of protein band sharpness and the consistency of the sharpness of protein molecules irregardless of migration distance. It is apparent that protein bands obtained by this new method are equally good as those obtained by the Laemmli system in terms of consistent sharpness of the bands of various molecular weights.

A major shortcoming of the Laemmli method is that small proteins cannot be separated from the electrophoretic front which consists of SDS micelles of relatively large molecular weights. Another less important problem with the system is that it is difficult to determine molecular weight with both large proteins and small ones because only the center part of the plot is linear. Our new method apparently has overcome those two shortcomings.

Figure 2 shows a plot of logarithm of protein molecular weights vs. their relative migration rates. The proteins used and their molecular weights are shown in Table 1. The Weber-Osborn system is known for its good linear correlation between the migration rate and the logarithm of molecular weight. Satisfactory linearity was given with our new continuous buffer system, permitting an accurate estimation of molecular weights.

A convenient and easy method with great performance for its simple buffer and easy availability of common reagents used, our new SDS-PAGE procedure assumes advantages of both the two most important SDS-PAGE systems. The greatest difference between those two systems lies in the uniformity of electric field in the gel in reference to the distance from the electrode. Excellent uniformity of gel electric field is marked by a sharp migration front (Takagi *et al.* 1987); on the other hand no migration front can be observed in the Weber-Osborn system. The migration front indicates a uniform electric potential perpendicular to the migration direction, suggesting an electrophoretic behavior for electrolytes present in the Laemmli system more like that in moving boundary electrophoresis. A moving boundary can narrow protein bands to a great extent, resulting in sharp protein bands just as in the case of electrophoretic focusing.

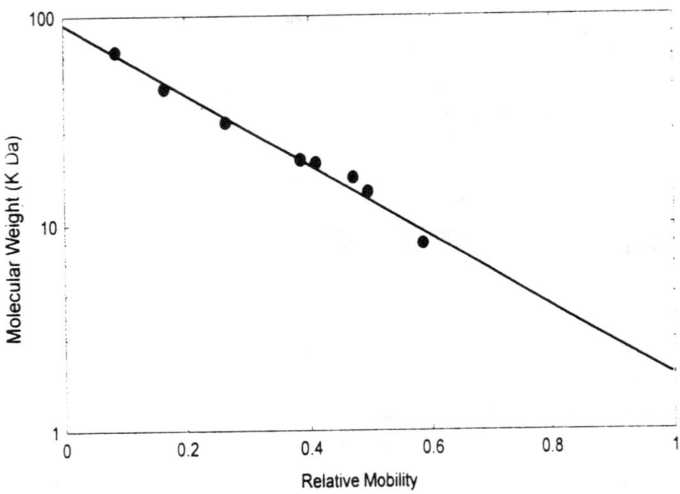

FIG. 2. CALIBRATION CURVES FOR 15% ACRYLAMIDE, 3%C BIS-ACRYLAMIDE

Small protein separation on the Weber-Osborn system in a slab gel is satisfactory with a good correlation between molecular weights and mobility. The greatest problem is the serious diffusion of the bands, especially with small proteins which have migrated a longer distance; this fatal shortcoming has literally eliminated the Weber-Osborn system from daily application. On comparing the Weber-Osborn system in slab gel and in tube gel, we found that it is very clear that this problem of the blurred protein bands with the system does not exist with the latter. This is apparently attributed to the difference in uniformity of the electric field in the gel. The sample well of the tube gel is surrounded by electrically charged glass while that of the slab gel is by electrically active gel. Actually it was observed that the shape of sample wells greatly affect electrophoretic patterns (Mae 1989) in the Weber-Osborn system. As stated above, a migration front indicates a uniform electric field perpendicular to the migration direction. Introduction of such a front into the Weber-Osborn system could possibly turn the whole slab gel into a thin but long tube with a uniform electric field, thus solving the blurred band problem and creating a system assuming advantages of the both systems.

TABLE. 1.
MOLECULAR WEIGHTS OF PROTEINS AND PEPTIDES

Protein or peptide	Molecular weight
Bovine serum albumin	69,000
Egg albumin	45,000
Carbonic anhydase[a]	31,000
Soybean Trypsin Inhibitor (doublet)[a]	20,400/19,700
Horse Heart Myoglobin[a]	16,900
Lysozyme[a]	14,000
Myoglobin Fragment F_1[a]	8,100
Myoglobin Fragment F_2[a]	6,200
Insulin, B chain	3,400
Myoglobin Fragment F_3[a]	2,500
Insulin A chain	2,350

[a]These proteins are the Promega low-molecular-weight standards

Factors determining the formation of the front were investigated such as species of cation and anion of the buffer, different combinations of buffers in the stacking gel and separation gel. We found that a low mobility of anion of the buffer is required for formation of a migration front. High mobility of sodium ion in the phosphate buffer of the Weber-Osborn system creates a charge flux against the SDS-protein complex migration, which causes SDS-protein complexes to be less important charge carriers and can possibly disturb the complexes' migration. Tris is one of the very few anions with low mobility.

The effect of cation, or the tailing ion species, on the migration was studied with acetate, borate, chloride and glycine. Mobilities of all the tailing ions except glycine were found to be too large in comparison with the SDS-protein complex; cation concentration in the cathode buffer reservoir could be consumed before the SDS-protein complex migrates sufficiently. Separation of small proteins from the SDS micelle, which forms a front, is as good as the system of Tris-tricine, if not any better. The proposed explanation of successful separation of small proteins from the SDS micelle when glycine is replaced with tricine is that tricine migrates much faster than glycine ion at the same pH, slowing the SDS-protein complex migration (Schagger and Von Jagow 1987). Our successful separation with glycine as the tailing ion sounds odd in light of the above explanation but there are some other factors which was neglected in the above model. The molecular size of SDS-protein complexes and SDS micelle can be close (Rao and Takagi 1989), but their electrophoretic mobilities can be totally different due to the totally different mass/charge ratio, and thus should be able to be separated with any kind of tailing ions, even the glycine ion, which is surely not the case with the Laemmli system. What is missing here is the stacking gel at pH 6.8, which limits the migration velocity of glycine. It is the slow glycine which pushes the SDS-protein complexes to approach or even merge into the SDS micelle front.

What is different with our new system is the consistent alkaline pH 9.57 throughout the stacking and separation gel, ensuring fast enough migration of glycine ions. It will be very helpful that expensive tricine can be replaced with glycine without any compromise in separation performance.

This proposed new system includes merits of both the Laemmli and Weber-Osborn systems, and can be applied to separate proteins of a range of molecular weights, especially with smaller proteins and peptides. Application of the method in our protein studies of several traditional Chinese foods has proved it to be a convenient and useful tool.

SUMMARY

When phosphate buffer in the Weber-Osborn method of SDS-PAGE was replaced with 0.46 M Tris-0.047 M glycine buffer, pH 9.57, while other constituents remained the same, usually blurred protein bands obtained became as sharp as those obtained by the Laemmli method. This improved SDS-PAGE method can be used to achieve satisfactory separation of small proteins with good linearity between the migration rate and the logarithm of molecular weight while retaining sharp protein band patterns. It is an SDS-PAGE system with advantages of both of the most widely used systems (Laemmli and Weber-Osborn) with greater ease and lower cost, very useful in protein study in fermented foods.

REFERENCES

LAEMMLI, U.K. 1970. Cleavage of structural proteins during the assembly of the head of bacteriophage T4. Nature (London) *227,* 680–685.

MAE, H. 1989. Differences in Electrophoretic Patterns between Weber-Osborn Method and Laemmli Method. Graduate Thesis of Polymer Science, Faculty of Science, Osaka University, Japan, pp. 9–16.

RAO, P.F. and TAKAGI, T. 1989. Reassessment of the viscosity behavior of sodium dodecyl sulfate-protein polypeptide complexes. J. Biochem. (Tokyo) *106*(3), 365–371.

SCHAGGER, H. and VON JAGOW, G. 1987. Tricine-sodium dodecyl sulfate-polyacrylamide gel electrophoresis for the separation of proteins in the range from 1 to 100 KDa. Anal. Biochem. *166,* 368–379.

TAKAGI, T., RAO, P.F. and KUBOTA, H. 1987. Real-time monitoring of polyacrylamide gel electrophoresis by Schlieren optics. J. Biochem. (Tokyo) *102*(4), 681–684.

WEBER, K. and OSBORN, M. 1969. The reliability of molecular weight determinations by dodecyl sulfate-polyacrylamide gel electrophoresis. J. Biol. Chem. *244*(16), 4406–4412.

ISOLATION AND CHARACTERIZATION OF PEPTIDES WITH ANGIOTENSIN CONVERTING ENZYME INHIBITORY ACTIVITY FROM VINEGAR EGG TONIC

SHU-TAO LIU, FANG FAN, LONG LI, RONG-ZHEN ZHANG, RU-MING CHEN, BI-HONG SHI, GONG-RUI CHEN, YU-QIANG ZHENG, WEN-HONG GAO and PING-FAN RAO

Institute of Biotechnology
Fuzhou University
Fuzhou, Fujian, 350002, P.R. China

ABSTRACT

Vinegar egg tonic is a traditional folk remedy in China with a history of hundreds of years. It is readily prepared by soaking a raw whole hen egg in three egg volumes of rice vinegar for 48 h, then mixing the egg contents with the vinegar. The tonic is widely used in China today by more than three million people as remedies for many kinds of chronic diseases such as cardiovascular diseases, diabetes, arteriosclerosis and asthma. It is especially well-known for its hypotensive effect.

Great efforts have been made to elucidate the biochemical mechanism of this folk remedy by our group. Acetic acid hydrolysis of proteins in the presence of high concentration of calcium ion, which is what vinegar egg tonic is in terms of its biochemical nature, was found to be specific rather than non-specific as is widely believed of acidic hydrolysis of proteins. Peptides with powerful superoxide activity were identified in the vinegar egg tonic. It is very possible that bioactive peptides generated as products of protein hydrolysis are one of the determining factors of the clinical effectiveness of the vinegar egg tonic.

The objective of this work was to isolate and identify peptides exhibiting angiotension converting enzyme inhibitory activity, which is linked to the hypotensive effect of the vinegar egg tonic. The soluble fraction of the tonic was fractionated by anion-exchange chromatography on a Porous 50 HQ column and by reverse phase chromatography on a Porous 50 R2 column. Improved Cushman's method was employed to screen the fractions with angiotension-converting enzyme activity. The isolated peptides with activity were further purified by capillary liquid chromatography on ABI 173A before being subjected to sequence determination on ABI 476A. Amino acid sequence and IC50 of each peptide obtained were determined.

INTRODUCTION

Vinegar egg tonic (VET) is a traditional folk remedy in China with a history of hundreds of years. It is readily prepared by soaking a fresh whole hen egg in 180 mL of rice vinegar for 48 h, then thoroughly mixing the egg contents with the vinegar. The tonic is widely used in China today by more than 3 million people as a remedy for many kinds of chronic diseases such as cardiovascular diseases, diabetes, arteriosclerosis and asthma. It is especially well-known for its hypotensive effect.

Many efforts have been made to elucidate the biochemical mechanism of this folk remedy by this group. Acetic acid hydrolysis of proteins in the presence of a high concentration of calcium ion, which is what vinegar egg tonic is in terms of its biochemical nature, was found to be specific rather than non-specific as is widely believed of acidic hydrolysis of proteins (Rao *et al.* 1997). Peptides with powerful superoxide activity were identified in the vinegar egg tonic (Wei *et al.* 1994). The most likely explanation for the reported clinical effectiveness of the vinegar egg tonic is that bioactive peptides may exist in the tonic as products of protein hydrolysis. Isolation and characterization of these peptides are the key to elucidation of the biochemical mechanism of the remedy.

Among all the reported effectiveness of the vinegar egg tonic, the hypotensive effect is most well-known, and one of the reasons why more than a million Chinese are taking the tonic every day. Angiotensin converting enzyme (ACE) is an enzyme linked to hypertension. Captopril, the most effective medicine for the condition, ACE's best inhibitor, successfully designed on the basis of full knowledge of the enzyme's structure (Brunner *et al.* 1978). Peptides which act as ACE inhibitors have been successfully prepared and identified in proteolytic products of numerous kinds of foods (Matsuda *et al.* 1983; Lantz *et al.* 1991; Matsumura and Shimazu 1992; Yoshikawa *et al.* 1992; Fujida *et al.* 1993; Kinoshita *et al.* 1993; Yamamoto *et al.* 1994). ACE inhibitory properties of the tonic were investigated in this work as the first effort for elucidation of the tonic's hypotensive effect.

EXPERIMENTAL

Preparation of Vinegar Egg Tonic

Vinegar egg tonic was prepared according to the traditional procedures. A fresh shell chicken egg was suspended in 180 ml of 9% rice vinegar purchased from Guangzhou Jinyuan Food Factory (Guangdong, China) for two days when the shell was dissolved. The egg membrane was subsequently broken and the egg was mixed with the vinegar; the mixture obtained was the vinegar egg tonic sample used in this study.

Isolation of Peptides with ACE Inhibitory Activity Using Anion-Exchange Chromatography

Anion-exchange chromatography of the vinegar egg tonic was carried out with a Tosoh 8000 CCPD liquid delivery pump (Tokyo, Japan) at 25°C. The flow rate was 0.5 ml/min, and the eluate was monitored with a Tosoh UV 8000 monitor (Tokyo, Japan) at 220 nm. The vinegar egg tonic sample was first centrifuged at 10,000 rpm for 10 min to remove precipitated proteins; the supernatant obtained was diluted 10 fold with pH 8.3 boric acid/borax buffer and filtered through a 0.45 μm cellulose acetate membrane. The filtrate was subsequently heated at 100°C for 5 min and filtered through a 0.22 μm cellulose acetate membrane after it was cooled to remove proteins and other precipitated substances. The filtrate (7.5 mL) was applied to a 0.75 $\times$ 3 cm stainless steel column of anion-exchanger Source 30Q purchased from Pharmacia Biotech (Uppsala, Sweden), which was equilibrated with the same boric acid/borax buffer. The column was then washed with the same buffer until the A_{220} of the effluent returned to the baseline value.

Then a linear NaCl gradient was applied to the column to elute the adsorbed components. The linear NaCl gradient was made from 15 ml of borate buffer and 15 ml of borate buffer containing 0.5 M NaCl. Peaks of the eluted fraction were collected, and ACE inhibitory activity was determined with both eluted samples and the un-adsorbed fraction to the column.

Determination of ACE Inhibitory Activity

Determination of ACE inhibitory activity was carried out according to a modified Cushman method. Briefly, it was conducted based on satisfactory separation of hippuric acid from ACE activity assay reaction system and its precise quantification by HPLC on a Toyopearl HW-40S column (Liu *et al.* 1997).

Capillary Liquid Chromatography

The fractions obtained from the anion-exchange chromatography of the chromatographic fractions from the vinegar egg tonic was carried out on a Perkin-Elmer capillary liquid chromatograph (CLC) with a 0.5 × 150 mm C18 column. This chromatograph consisted of a 140 D solvent delivery system, a 112A Oven/Injector and a 785A programmable absorbance detector (CA, USA). The eluate was an acetonitrile gradient from 5% to 45% in 0.1% trifluoroacetic acid. The flow rate was 5 μl/min, and the applied sample volume was 25 μl.

Peptide Sequence Determination

Amino acid sequence of the ACE inhibitory peptides obtained was determined automatically on an ABI 476A Protein Sequencer (CA, USA).

RESULTS AND DISCUSSION

Anion-Exchange Chromatography of Vinegar Egg Tonic

Shown in Fig. 1 is an anion-exchange chromatogram of the vinegar egg tonic on a Source S30 column. A large portion of the tonic components were not adsorbed to the column, and the adsorbed components were fractionated into 6 peaks. While it was not difficult to conclude that the adsorbed components were peptides or polypeptides, it was not easy to decide what the greatest amount of the vinegar egg tonic components not adsorbed to the column were. Capillary liquid chromatography was carried out to analyze the non adsorbed fraction, and the results are shown in Fig. 2. It is clear from the chromatogram that the component(s) of largest amount in the fraction was eluted at the void volume of the column, indicating the strong polarity of the component(s). According to its quantity and chemical nature, the component was identified as the calcium ion from the vinegar egg tonic. Some peaks were eluted at rather high concentrations of acetonitrile. They were minor proteins or peptides with relatively long chains, because hardly any egg protein remained in the vinegar egg tonic sample after acid denaturation in the course of vinegar egg tonic preparation and removal of proteins by heating and filtering.

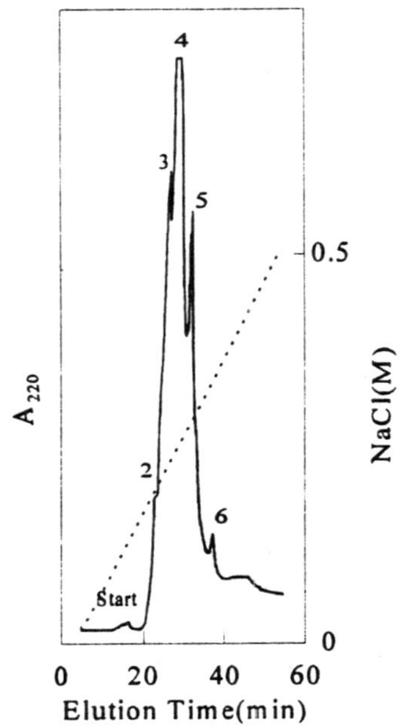

FIG. 1. ANION-EXCHANGE CHROMATOGRAM OF VINEGAR EGG TONIC SAMPLE
Conditions are described in the Experimental Section. AUFS = 0.64.

Determination of ACE Inhibitory Activity

Of all the fractions collected from anion-exchange chromatography of the vinegar egg tonic sample, only two fractions were determined to display ACE inhibitory activity. The un-adsorbed fraction exhibited an inhibitory activity of 50% while the inhibitory activity for the 6th peak of Fig. 1 was determined to be 13%. The ACE inhibitory activity of the un-adsorbed fraction can be attributed to the high concentration of calcium ion in the un-adsorbed fraction because ACE is an enzyme containing zinc ion (Meng and Suzanne 1996).

Peptide Sequencing

Twenty μL of the 6th fraction exhibiting 13% ACE inhibitory activity was directly applied to an ABI 476A protein sequencer through a blotter membrane. It was determined to contain only one tripeptide of 0.194 μmole/L, as determined by comparison of amino acid peak with the standard. Its amino acid sequence was Pro-Ser-Lys. IC_{50} peptide concentration at which ACE activity is inhibited by 50%, was determined to be 1.51 μM.

Major properties of the ACE inhibitory peptide obtained from the vinegar egg tonic are listed in Table 1.

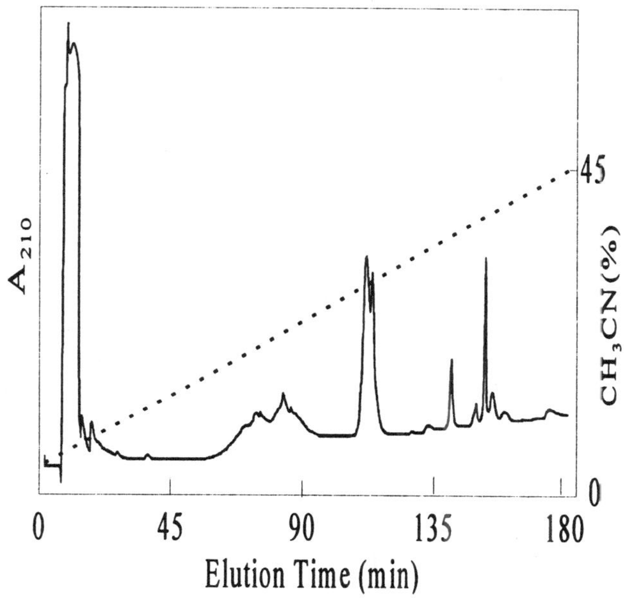

FIG. 2. CAPILLARY LIQUID CHROMATOGRAM OF UN-ADSORBED FRACTION ON ANION-EXCHANGE CHROMATOGRAPHY
Conditions are described in the Experimental Section. AUFS = 0.300.

TABLE 1.
MAJOR PROPERTIES OF THE ACE INHIBITORY PEPTIDE FROM THE VINEGAR EGG TONIC

Amino Acid Sequence	Concentration in the Tonic (μmole/ L)	IC_{50} (μM)
Pro-Ser-Lys	0.06	1.51

Only one peptide with ACE inhibitory activity was isolated from the vinegar egg tonic (VET), unusually few in comparison with ACE inhibitory peptides prepared by protein hydrolysis where much more peptides are present. There are reports about identification of peptides with ACE inhibitory activity from both rice vinegar (Tsuzuki *et al.* 1992) and egg white protein (Fujida *et al.* 1993), but none of them shares the same amino acid sequence with the peptide identified in this work. Furthermore, the inhibitory activity of this obtained peptide is much higher than those reported to be isolated from vinegar and egg white hydrolysate. As a matter of fact, the inhibitory activity of this peptide is comparable to the reported peptides with the highest activity derived from food proteins.

Identification of the peptide with ACE inhibitory activity in the vinegar egg tonic has in part helped elucidate the hypotensive effect of the tonic. Its effectiveness, however, should be very limited because its concentration in the vinegar egg tonic is extremely low. What needs to be done is monitoring of content variation of the hypotensive peptides in the course of the vinegar egg tonic preparation. It would also be interesting to further determine other factors in the VET which are really responsible for the hypotensive effect.

REFERENCES

BRUNNER, H.R., WAEBER, B., WAUTERS, J.P., TURIN, G., McKINSTRY, D. and GAVRAS, H. 1978. Inappropriate renin secretion unmasked by Captopril (SQ 14 225) in hypertension of chronic renal failure. Lancet *2*, (8092), Pt 1, 704-707.

FUJIDA, Y., USUI, H., KURAHASHI, W. and YOSHIKAWA, M. 1993. Ovokinin: An artery relaxing peptide derived from ovalbumin. Nippon Nogeikagaku Kaishi. *67*, 290.

KINOSHITA, E., YAMAKOSHI, J. and KIKUCHI, M. 1993. Purification and identification of an angiotensin I-converting enzyme inhibitor from soy sauce. Biosci. Biotechnol. Biochem. *57*, 1107–1110.

LANTZ, I., GLAMSTA, E.L., TALBACK, L. and NYBERG, F. 1991. Hemorphins derived from hemoglobin have an inhibitory action on angiotensin converting enzyme activity. FEBS Lett *287*, 39–41.

LIU, S.-.T, CHEN, G.-R., SHI, B.-H., ZHANG, R.-Z., LI, J.-C., CHEN, R.-M., LI, L., GAO, W.-H., CHEN, T.-B., ZHENG, Y.-Q. and RAO, P.-F. 1997. HPLC determination of angiotensin-converting enzyme activity on Toyopearl HW-40S column. 3rd International Conference of Food Science and Technology, October 19-23, Davis, U.S.A. (In press).

MATSUDA, H., NAGAOKA, T., MORITA, H., OSAJIMA, K. and OSUJIAM, Y. 1983. Angiotensin I converting enzyme inhibitory peptides generated from sardine muscle by protease for food industry. Nippon Shokuhin Kogyo Gakkaishi *39*(8), 678–683.

MATSUMURA, N. and SHIMAZU, T. 1992. Angiotensin I Converting Enzyme Inhibitory Peptides and Their Manufacture. Jpn. Kokai Tokkyo Koho JP 04, 149, 196.

MENG, Q.C. and SUZANNE, O. 1996. Purification and assay methods for angiotensin-converting enzyme. J. Chromatog. A. *743*, 105–122.

RAO, P.-F., CHEN, R.-M. and LIU S.-T. 1997. Acetic acid hydrolysis of proteins in the presence of metallic ion. (In preparation).

TSUZUKI, W., KIKUCHI, Y., KAZUKI, S. and SUZUKI, T. 1992. Fluorometric assay of angiotensin I-converting enzyme inhibitory activity of vinegars. Nippon Shokuhin Kogyo Gakkaishi *39*(2), 188–192.

WEI, Z., LI, J.-C., LIU, S.-T., CHEN, R.-M., ZHENG, Y.-Q., CHEN, G.-R. and RAO, P.-F. 1994. Identification of bioactives from vinegar egg tonic. Presented at 2nd International Conference on Food Science and Technology, September 27–30, Wuxi, Jiangsu, P.R. China.

YAMAMOTO, N., AKINO, A. and TAKANO, T. 1994. Anti-hypertensive effect of the peptides derived from casein by an extracellular proteinase from *Lactobacillus helveticus*. J. Dairy Sci. *77*(4), 917–922.

YOSHIKAWA, M., SASAKI, M. and CHIBA, H. 1992. Bioactive Peptides and Their Salt, Jpn. Kokai Tokkyo Koho JP 04, 154, 798.

DISCUSSION ON THE MULTIFUNCTIONAL CONVERSION OF DIETARY FIBER[1]

JIANXIAN ZHENG[2] and XIAOLIN DING[3]

[2]South China University of Technology and
[3]Wuxi University of Light Industry
Wuxi, Jiangsu
214036 P.R. China

ABSTRACT

With the help of physical or chemical methods, the chemical structures of some composed polymeric fractions and their relative contents in natural dietary fiber are adjusted and optimized, so that some new properties are brought about or some original but very weak properties are strengthened, including both technological and nutritional properties. As a result, a number of physiological functions in promoting body health are strengthened; positive technological characteristics in food applications are presented also. Multifunctional conversion of dietary fiber is achieved and additional values are increased.

INTRODUCTION

Multifunctional conversion of dietary fiber is used to bring about some new properties or to strengthen some original but weak properties for dietary fiber, including both technological and nutritional behaviors. The multifunctionally converted dietary fiber is not only a kind of effective physiological active substance, but also a kind of practical dough improver. This is a completely new concept and completely new theory, which may increase the application values of dietary fiber and engender inevitably economic effects.

NATURAL BEHAVIORS OF DIETARY FIBER

Definition and Constituent of Dietary Fiber

Dietary fiber (DF) is defined as "all the polysaccharides and lignin that are undigested by endogenous secretions of human digestive tract". In terms of structure, the constituents of dietary fiber fall into three groups: a) the fibrillar polysaccharide cellulose; b) the matrix polysaccharides pectin, pectin substances, hemicellulose, etc.; and c) the encrusting lignin substances.

Based on the detailed polymeric constituents, dietary fiber contains arabinogalactan, arabinan, galactan, glucomannan, β-glucan, xylan, arabinoxylan, polygalacturonic acid, xyloglucan, glycoprotein, cellulose, lignin, etc. Some of these polymers are soluble in water, so called water soluble dietary fiber (SDF); the others are water insoluble dietary fiber (IDF). Various kinds of dietary fibers from different materials differ in detailed polymeric constituents and their relative contents in the total fiber.

[1] The Project was supported by the Chinese Postdoctoral Science Foundation and Gangdong Provincial Natural Science Foundation of China.

While the constituents of dietary fiber are not affected by our endogenous enzymes, they can be metabolized by the intestinal microflora in the gut and absorbed or utilized to some extent; thus dietary fiber is not completely noncaloric.

Physiological Effects of Dietary Fiber

A number of physiological effects have been attributed decisively to dietary fiber which are: a) to protect against constipation and colorectal cancer; b) to lower serum cholesterol, and prevent diverticular disease; c) to improve glucose tolerance, and stabilize the blood glucose level in diabetes; d) to be noncaloric, and prevent obesity; and e) the deficiency or lack of dietary fiber is considered to cause hiatus, hernia, appendicitis, gall-stones, varicose veins, hemorrhoids, Crohn's disease, pelvic phleboliths, gastroesophageal reflux, deep-vein thrombosis, ischaemic heart disease and breast cancer.

Adequate dietary fiber can prevent the above diseases. But the different kinds of dietary fiber produce different physiological effects. Not all kinds of dietary fibers have all of above effects (Zheng 1995). Therefore, we propose for the first time that dietary fiber can be divided into two varieties: a) common dietary fiber as only the noncaloric bulk additive, and high quality dietary fiber as the physiologically active substance.

With exploitation of dietary fiber, the fiber material which has good physiological effects itself must be chosen as far as possible at first. But for the second variety, some advanced techniques (physical or chemical) can be used to strengthen the nutritional effects in promoting body health.

Technological Behaviors of Dietary Fiber

Here, the technological behaviors refer to the application behaviors when dietary fiber is incorporated into dough foods. As a foreign matter, dietary fiber is quite different from the natural constituents of wheat flour; when incorporated it dilutes the protein content of wheat flour and reduces the content of gluten network. As a result, the dough framework structure is less concentrated, and the dough rheological characteristics, loaf baking properties and noodle cooking properties are weakened. The more the incorporation level of fiber, the more significant the weakening.

The constituents of soluble polysaccharide dietary fiber can form a continuous, viscoelastic, three-dimensional network through noncovalent linkages such as hydrogen bonds between chains, which can have similar functions of gluten network and therefore improve the dough properties (Zheng *et al.* 1994). The natural content of these fractions in dietary fiber is usually too low to cause improvement. In accordance with a specially designated kind of dietary fiber, the relative content of these soluble fractions can be adjusted and increased after special treatment with advanced techniques, and the improvement can be large.

MULTIFUNCTIONAL CONVERSION OF DIETARY FIBER

Based on the natural characteristics of dietary fiber, advanced techniques may be used to achieve multifunctional conversion, by transforming the chemical structure and relative content of partial constituents in natural dietary fiber. As a result, some new functions are shown or some original but very weak functions are strengthened, including both physiological functions on body health and application functions when incorporated into dough foods.

The practical conversion methods include extrusion cooking, pneumatic puffing, partial explosion, wet thermal treatment, acid thermal treatment, enzyme treatment and microbiological conversion technology. The modern extruder performs several operational units of conveying, mixing, heating and pressurizing, which can cause the direct or indirect chemical conversion of high molecular polymers within a very short time. For this reason extrusion cooking technology is an effective method when used in the multifunctional conversion of dietary fiber.

Extrusion cooking treatment cannot cause extensive degradation of dietary fiber polymeric structure, but some partial solubilization or fragmentation occurs in the water-insoluble arabinoxylan or pectin substances, which increase the corresponding water-soluble polymers. For example, the content of water soluble fractions in natural soybean fiber is 3 to 6%; it increases up to 10 to 16% after extrusion cooking. Besides, extrusion cooking treatment affects the polymerization degree, molecular weight, monosugar constituents and relative content of the various polymeric constituents in total soybean fiber, such as arabinogalactan, galactan, arabinan, arabinoxylan, xyloglucan, etc., and increases the physiochemical properties such as water-holding, water-binding, expanding and cation-exchange capacity (Zheng 1996a,b).

Up to now, the relationships among the chemical structure, physicochemical properties and physiological functions of dietary fiber remain vague. The effects of the above various treatments on physiological functions of dietary fiber cannot be deduced from the analysis of chemical structure variations. But the insoluble fiber fraction is known to have a mechanical effect on the intestinal tract, whereas the soluble fraction seems to be more responsible for metabolic effects which affect primarily carbohydrate and lipid metabolism. The results in Table 1 show that soybean fiber, after multifunctional conversion (MSF), can lower serum lipids, total serum cholesterol and serum low density lipoprotein cholesterol level more than that of natural soybean fiber (NSF). It is clear that the dietary fiber after conversion has more manifest physiological effects on health.

After treatment with the above modern techniques, the soluble fraction in soybean fiber increased greatly. All these soluble fractions are aqueous polysaccharide gels, which form a viscoelastic three-dimensional network, and have similar functions of the gluten network, improving the dough rheological characteristics. Due to the increasing content of such fractions in multifunctionally converted dietary fiber, their improved effects on dough rheological properties can exceed the weakening effects by the gluten dilution. At this time, the comprehensive effects on dough functions caused by the dietary fiber's incorporation into flour would be positive (improving) but not negative (weakening). In other words, at this time the dietary fiber is also a kind of dough improver. As a result, it would greatly increase the practical values of fiber-enriched dough foods.

Tables 2 and 3 show that the natural soybean fiber (NSF) improves the farinograph properties when supplemented into dough. While it reduced the extensograph curve, the ratio of resistance to extension increased sharply and exceeded the optimum scope. As a result, the dough became too stiff and fragile, and its original viscoelastic properties were decreased. Generally speaking, the dough rheological characteristics are weakened or softened by the incorporation of NSF. But the results were quite different with soybean fiber after multifunctional conversion (MSF). At the same incorporation level,

TABLE 1.
THE EFFECTS OF SOYBEAN DIETARY FIBER ON SERUM LIPIDS

Groups	Total Cholesterol (mg/dl)	HDL Cholesterol (mg/dl)
Basal + 1% Cholesterol (BC Control)	278.4 ± 20.3	47.3 ± 3.5
BC + 10% NSF (Experiment I)	228.2 ± 28.7*	40.5 ± 7.0
BC + 10% MSF (Experiment II)	188.6 + 30.2**	46.8 ± 5.8

Groups	LDL Cholesterol (mg/dl)	Total Triglyceride (mg/dl)
Basal + 1% Cholesterol (BC Control)	128.7 ± 6.3	100.3 ± 7.6
BC + 10% NSF (Experiment I)	86.2 ± 5.4*	83.7 ± 6.2*
BC + 10% (Experiment II)	68.2 ± 3.8**	68.3 ± 5.4**

* $p<0.01$, compared with Control group;
** $p<0.01$, compared with Control group; $p<0.05$, compared with Experiment I group.

TABLE 2.
THE EFFECTS OF SOYBEAN DIETARY FIBER ON FARINOGRAPH PROPERTIES

Additive	Water Absorption (%)	Dough Development (min)
Control (0%)	60.1	2.2
NSF (3%)*	63.6	2.5
NSF (6%)	67.2	4.0
MSF (3%)	65.5	3.0
MSF (6%)	71.7	5.8

Additive	Dough Stability (min)	Dough Softening (Bu)	Valorimeter Value
Control (0%)	4.6	90	43
NSF (3%)*	6.2	90	45
NSF (6%)	5.6	120	50
MSF (3%)	7.6	80	50
MSF (6%)	8.4	40	58

* NSF, natural soybean fiber; MSF, soybean fiber after multifunctional conversion.

TABLE 3.
THE EFFECTS OF SOYBEAN DIETARY FIBER ON EXTENSOGRAPH PROPERTIES

Rest Period 45 min				
Additive	Energy (cal)	Res.[a] (Bu)	Ext.[b] (Bu)	Ratio[c]
Control (0%)	85	335	14.0	23.9
NSF (3%)	73	370	11.7	31.6
NSF (6%)	54	420	8.7	48.3
MSF (3%)	82	350	13.6	25.7
MSF (6%)	80	360	12.8	28.1
Rest Period 45 min				
Additive	Energy (cal)	Res.[a] (Bu)	Ext.[b] (Bu)	Ratio[c]
Control (0%)	99	480	12.6	38.1
NSF (3%)	77	610	9.5	64.2
NSF (6%)	71	630	8.1	77.8
MSF (3%)	100	500	12.2	41.0
MSF (6%)	105	520	10.8	48.1
Rest Period 135 min				
Additive	Energy (cal)	Res.[a] (Bu)	Ext.[b] (Bu)	Ratio[c]
Control (0%)	100	580	12.0	48.3
NSF (3%)	72	670	8.3	80.7
NSF (6%)	65	710	7.3	97.2
MSF (3%)	105	600	10.9	55.1
MSF (6%)	98	630	10.1	62.4

[a]Res, Resistance; [b]Ext., Extension; [c]Ratio, Ratio of Resistance to Extension

MSF clearly improved the farinograph properties. At the same time, it did not reduce the extensograph curve, and therefore it did not increase the ratio of resistance to extension above the optimum range. A suitable increase of ratio of resistance and extension contributed to a strengthening of the dough extensograph curve. The dough energy after incorporation of MSF is evidently greater than after incorporation of NSF. All these results indicated that the MSF supplemented dough had improved viscoelastic properties. In conclusion, soybean dietary fiber after multifunctional conversion improves dough rheological properties, which appear to be a practical improver.

CONCLUSION

Advanced techniques were adopted to adjust and optimize the constituents and extensive polymeric structures of natural dietary fiber, through multifunctional conversion of dietary fiber. As a result, it not only strengthened the physiological effects on body health, but also improved the application function of fiber-enriched food production. The dietary fiber, after multifunctional conversion, is not only an effective physiologically active substance, but also a practical dough improver. Multifunctional conversion of dietary fiber is a completely new concept and a new theory proposed for the first time.

In conclusion, we would say that not all natural dietary fiber can be multifunctionally converted.

REFERENCES

ZHENG, J.X. 1995. Functional Foods. Chinese Light Industry Publishing House, Beijing, China.

ZHENG, J.X. and DING, X.L. 1994. Studies on a multifunctional additive of dietary fiber. Proceedings Second Intern. Conf. Food Sci. Technol. Wuxi, China.

ZHENG, J.X. 1996a. Studies on the extrusion modification of dietary fiber-I. J. South China Univ. Technol. *12*, 59–63.

ZHENG, J.X. 1996b. Studies on the extrusion modification of dietary fiber-II. J. South China Univ. Technol. *12*, 64–68.

THE CARBOHYDRATE COMPOSITION OF COTYLEDONS AND HULLS OF THREE CHINESE INDIGENOUS LEGUME SEEDS

PETER C.K. CHEUNG and CHI-FAI CHAU

Department of Biology
The Chinese University of Hong Kong, Shatin
New Territories, Hong Kong

ABSTRACT

As one of the major constituents of legume seeds, legume carbohydrate has significant nutritional values. Different carbohydrates including sugars, oligosaccharides, starch and non-starch polysaccharides (NSP) can be found in the hulls and cotyledons of the legume seeds. The carbohydrate composition of the hulls and cotyledons from Phaseolus angularis, Phaseolus calcaratus *and* Dolichos lablab *seeds indigenous to China were studied. Appreciable amounts of oligosaccharides of the raffinose family were found mainly in the cotyledons. The cotyledons contained 45.9 to 51.4% of starch by weight with relatively low content of cellulose. The NSP of the cotyledons (7.84 to 9.93% by weight) were dominated by the water-insoluble fraction (WIF). Hulls were predominantly NSP (74.6 to 78.8% by weight) for which the WIF was also the major fraction. The bulk of water-soluble fraction of the NSP for the cotyledons and the hulls mainly consisted of pectins. While xylans and cellulose were the major NSP present in the WIF of the hulls, xyloglucans and arabinose-rich pectic substances were the principal NSP in the WIF of the cotyledons. The three legume seeds studied here may have considerable value as sources of digestible complex carbohydrate and dietary fiber in human diet.*

INTRODUCTION

Legume seeds are good sources of dietary carbohydrates (Reddy *et al.* 1984). Carbohydrates in legumes contain a digestible fraction (which includes simple sugars and starch) and a nondigestible fraction (oligosaccharides and non-starch polysaccharides) (Schneeman 1994). More than half of the energy requirements beyond infancy was provided by digestible carbohydrates which could help limit the intake of fat (Schneeman 1994). Legume seeds contain appreciable amounts of nondigestible oligosaccharides of the raffinose family such as raffinose and stachyose which are responsible for the problem of flatulence (Vidal-Valverde *et al.* 1993). Dietary fiber or non-starch polysaccharides (NSP) can be divided into a water-soluble fraction (WSF) and a water-insoluble fraction (WIF), both of which are known to affect gastrointestinal functions and provide health benefits to humans (Hughes 1991).

The seeds of *Phaseolus angularis*, *Phaseolus calcaratus* and *Dolichos lablab* indigenous to China have not been used as sources of dietary carbohydrate in China in the past. These three legume seeds are only traditionally used as soup ingredients for therapeutic purposes such as driving away dropsy, relieving diarrhea and tonic to the viscera (Li 1973). The present study was aimed at evaluating the potential of these three legume seeds as new sources of digestible carbohydrate and dietary fiber.

MATERIALS AND METHODS

P. angularis, P. calcaratus and *D. lablab* seeds were imported from mainland China. Cleaned seeds of these three legume seeds were manually dehulled after soaking. The hulls and cotyledons of the legume samples were separately freeze-dried and finely ground (0.5 mm in size) using a Cyclotec mill. Disaccharides and oligosaccharides in the hulls and cotyledons of the legume seeds were extracted with 80% ethanol and analyzed by HPLC (Vidal-Valverde *et al.* 1993).

The NSP of the legume samples were determined by the enzymatic-gravimetric method for dietary fiber of the Official Methods of Analysis (32.1.17; AOAC 1995). The water-soluble fraction (WSF) and water insoluble fraction (WIF) of the legume NSP were equivalent to the soluble and insoluble dietary fiber measured by the above AOAC method, respectively. Procedures for the determination of starch were those described by Theander and Westerlund (1986).

Using the method of Englyst and Cummings (1988), the alditol acetate derivatives of the sugar residues released by 12 M sulfuric acid hydrolysis in the WSF and WIF of the legume NSP samples were quantified by capillary gas chromatography. For non-cellulosic glucose determination, NSP of the hulls and cotyledons of the legume samples were hydrolyzed with 2 M sulfuric acid before GC analysis. Uronic acids in the acid hydrolysates of the above samples were measured colorimetrically by the Official Methods of Analysis method (45.4.11; AOAC 1995). All measurements were done in duplicate.

RESULTS AND DISCUSSION

Table 1 shows the carbohydrate composition of the cotyledons and hulls from the seeds of *P. angularis, P. calcaratus* and *D. lablab*. As the major fraction, the cotyledons of the three legume seeds contained 45.9 to 51.4% dry weight of starch which accounted for 98.2 to 99.7% of total starch in the whole seeds. The starch contents (40.1 to 46.8% dry weight of the whole seed) were comparable to those of other common legume seeds such as black gram, lentil and cowpea (Reddy *et al.* 1984). The amounts of sucrose and oligosaccharides (raffinose and stachyose) (4.31 to 5.91% dry weight of the whole seed), which were mainly found in the cotyledons, were comparable to those of soybean, broad bean and navy bean, but lower than those of wrinkled peas, cowpea and lupin seeds (Evans *et al.* 1993; Reddy *et al.* 1984).

The amount of total NSP in the cotyledons of *P. angularis, P. calcaratus* and *D. lablab* (which were 7.84, 9.93 and 9.84% dry weight of the seeds, respectively) was much less than that of the hulls (74.6, 78.7 and 77.4%, respectively) (Table 1). In spite of being a minor seed fraction, the hulls from *P. angularis, P. calcaratus* and *D. lablab* seeds contributed 49.5, 55.6 and 67.3% of the total NSP in the whole seed, respectively. The WIF was the dominant component in the NSP of both the cotyledons (92.2 to 94.8%) and the hulls (85.9 to 90.8%).

The monosaccharide compositions of the WIF and WSF of the NSP in the cotyledons from *P. angularis, P. calcaratus* and *D. lablab* seeds are shown in Table 2.

TABLE 1.
CARBOHYDRATE COMPOSITION OF COTYLEDONS AND HULLS FROM *P. ANGULARIS*, *P. CALCARATUS* AND *D. LABLAB* SEEDS[a]

	Cotyledons			Hulls		
	P. angularis	*P. calcaratus*	*D. lablab*	*P. angularis*	*P. calcaratus*	*D. lablab*
Proportion of seed[b]	90.8	86.6	82.9	9.20	13.4	17.1
Starch	51.4±0.84	45.9±1.06	49.1±1.08	1.31±0.09	2.50±0.07	4.30±0.14
Sucrose	1.57±0.10	1.44±0.04	1.49±0.06	0.78±0.05	0.83±0.03	0.35±0.02
Raffinose	1.19±0.10	1.03±0.01	0.84±0.03	0.60±0.05	0.60±0.02	0.28±0.01
Stachyose	3.53±0.07	3.34±0.06	2.68±0.13	0.74±0.02	0.99±0.02	0.28±0.02
Water-insoluble NSP[c]	7.00±0.26	9.02±0.13	8.45±0.47	70.7±0.03	74.0±0.35	71.4±0.00
Water-soluble NSP	0.84±0.06	0.91±0.12	1.39±0.13	3.88±0.19	4.75±0.06	6.04±0.15

[a] All values are on % dry weight of the samples and are means ± SD of duplicate determinations.
[b] Percentage of the whole legume seed
[c] Non-starch polysaccharides

TABLE 2.
MONOSACCHARIDE COMPOSITION OF THE WATER-INSOLUBLE AND -SOLUBLE NON-STARCH POLYSACCHARIDES (NSP) FROM COTYLEDONS OF *P. ANGULARIS*, *P. CALCARATUS* AND *D. LABLAB* SEEDS[a]

	Fucose	Rhamnose	Ribose	Arabinose	Xylose	Mannose	Galactose	Glucose	Uronic acids	Glucos-amine
Water-insoluble NSP										
P. angularis	1.45	0.59	0.45	44.0	5.58	0.91	6.00	29.8	9.06	2.16
P. calcaratus	1.56	0.40	0.39	40.5	5.00	1.22	4.19	33.8	10.3	2.64
D. lablab	1.43	0.45	0.22	27.2	4.71	0.49	9.17	44.3	9.68	2.35
Water-soluble NSP										
P. angularis	1.00	0.37	1.57	24.9	4.63	13.5	10.5	12.7	21.2	9.63
P. calcaratus	0.99	0.27	1.69	24.4	4.28	16.4	10.3	12.5	23.1	6.07
D. lablab	1.13	0.35	0.66	24.9	5.30	11.5	15.9	14.7	21.8	3.76

a Expressed as a percentage of the total polysaccharide sugars.

TABLE 3.
MONOSACCHARIDE COMPOSITION OF THE WATER-INSOLUBLE AND -SOLUBLE NON-STARCH POLYSACCHARIDES (NSP) FROM HULLS OF *P. ANGULARIS*, *P. CALCARATUS* AND *D. LABLAB* SEEDS[a]

	Fucose	Rhamnose	Ribose	Arabinose	Xylose	Mannose	Galactose	Glucose	Uronic acids	Glucos-amine
Water-insoluble NSP										
P. angularis	0.83	tr[b]	--	5.98	22.2	0.24	1.61	62.6	4.88	1.58
P. calcaratus	0.95	tr	--	5.42	18.3	0.41	1.24	63.2	8.02	2.37
D. lablab	0.97	tr	--	3.69	16.0	0.48	1.74	67.7	7.45	1.88
Water-soluble NSP										
P. angularis	3.68	0.23	0.16	21.1	5.55	6.99	14.5	3.63	39.8	4.36
P. calcaratus	3.37	0.34	tr	16.9	9.90	8.40	10.0	7.51	40.3	3.19
D. lablab	3.08	0.16	tr	11.3	20.2	4.58	10.8	3.95	42.8	3.05

a Expressed as a percentage of the total polysaccharide sugars.
[b] tr, trace amount (< 0.1).

Pectic polysaccharides, on the basis of the relative abundance of arabinose, galactose and uronic acids, were the major noncellulosic polysaccharides (56.6 to 62.6%) in the WSF of the NSP in all cotyledons. The WIF of the NSP in the cotyledons from *P. angularis* and *P. calcaratus* possessed a higher level of arabinose-rich pectic polysaccharides than that of *D. lablab*. The noncellulosic glucose released from the WIF of the NSP of the *P. angularis, P. calcaratus* and *D. lablab* seed cotyledons by 2 M sulfuric acid hydrolysis were 33.3, 38.7 and 61.5% of the total glucose, respectively (data not shown).

The monosaccharide compositions of the WIF and WSF of the NSP in the hulls from *P. angularis, P. calcaratus* and *D. lablab* seeds are given in Table 3. The monosaccharide composition of the NSP from the hulls was different from that of the cotyledons. Among the NSP of the hulls, the bulk of WSF mainly consisted of pectic polysaccharides rich in arabinose and galactose while the WIF had lower levels of pectic polysaccharides. Glucose (62.6 to 67.7%) and xylose (16.0 to 22.2%) were the major components of the WIF in the NSP of the hulls (Table 3). Compared to the NSP of the cotyledons, the proportion of glucose in the WIF of hulls susceptible to 2 M sulfuric acid hydrolysis was low (2.81 to 4.03%) (data not shown). Since the noncellulosic glucose of all three seed hulls was low, the bulk of the xylose would mainly come from xylan rather than xyloglucan. Similar results on the NSP composition of the hulls has been reported for mung bean (Gooneratne *et al.* 1994) and pea (Ralet *et al.* 1993). The presence of different levels of mannose and glucosamine in both the WIF and WSF of the NSP from the hulls and cotyledons suggests that some intracellular glycoproteins are strongly associated with the NSP (Racusen and Foote 1971).

Other than the protein fraction, the digestible carbohydrate and NSP are the major food ingredients targeted in legume processing. The presence of a large amount of starch and NSP in the three legume seeds under study indicated the potential uses of these seeds in the food industry.

REFERENCES

AOAC 1995. Official Methods of Analysis, 16th Ed., Association of Official Analytical Chemists, Washington, DC.

ENGLYST, H.N. and CUMMINGS, J.H. 1988. Improved method for measurement of dietary fiber as non-starch polysaccharides in plant foods. J. Assoc. Off. Anal. Chem. *71*, 808–814.

EVANS, A.J., CHEUNG, P.C-K. and CHEETHAM, N.W.H. 1993. The carbohydrate composition of cotyledons and hulls of cultivars of *Lupinus angustifolius* from Western Australia. J. Sci. Food Agric. *61*, 189–194.

GOONERATNE, J., MAJSAK-NEWMAN, G., ROBERTSON, J.A. and SELVENDRAN, R.R. 1994. Investigation of factors that affect the solubility of dietary fiber, as non-starch polysaccharides, in seed tissues of Mung bean (*Vigna radiata*) and Black gram (*Vigna mungo*). J. Agric. Food Chem. *42*, 601–611.

HUGHES, J.S. 1991. Potential contribution of dry bean dietary fiber to health. Food Technol. *9*, 122–126.

LI, S.-C. 1973. Chinese Medical Herbs. (Translated by F.P. Smith and G.A. Stuart), Georgetown Press, San Francisco, USA.

RACUSEN, D. and FOOTE, M. 1971. The major glycoprotein in germinating bean seeds. Can. J. Bot. *49*, 2107–2111.

RALET, M.C., SAULNIER, L. and THIABAULT, J.F. 1993. Raw and extruded fiber from pea hulls. Part II. Structural study of the water soluble polysaccharides. Carbohydr. Polym. *20*, 25–34.

REDDY, N.R., PIERSON, M.D., SATHE, S.K. and SALUNKHE, D.K. 1984. Chemical, nutritional and physiological aspects of dry bean carbohydrates - A review. Food Chem. *13*, 25–68.

SCHNEEMAN, B.O. 1994. Carbohydrates: Significance for energy balance and gastrointestinal function. J. Nutr. *124*, 1747S–1753S.

THEANDER, O. and WESTERLUND, E. 1986. Studies on dietary fiber 3. Improved procedures for analysis of dietary fiber. J. Agric. Food Chem. *34*, 330–336.

VIDAL-VALVERDE, C., FRIAS, J. and VALVERDE, S. 1993. Changes in the carbohydrate composition of legumes after soaking and cooking. J. Amer. Diet. Assoc. *93*, 547–550.

CULTURE OF *DIOSCOREA ALATA* L. VAR. *PURPUREA* M. POUCH

MING C. WEN, LIR-WAN FAN and TIEN-KEN HSU

Graduate Institute of Food Science
Tunghai University
Taichung, Taiwan, R.O.C

ABSTRACT

Response surface methodology with a central composite design was used to search for the optimum composition of media for the production of anthocyanins by the tissue culture of Dioscorea alata L. var. purpurea M. Pouch. *Over the ranges used in this experiment, 2,4-D very significantly affected the percentage of purple calli initiation and degree of purple callusing. The optimum medium for the purple calli initiation included a modified MS media containing 1.1% sucrose, 2,475 mg/l ammonium nitrate, 2,850 mg/l potassium nitrate, 130 mg/l potassium dihydrogen phosphate, 30.97 μM 2,4-D and 0.64 μM kinetin. This medium proved to be valid in the later experiment.*

INTRODUCTION

Plant tissue culture offers great potential in the production of useful natural products (Ilker 1987). Following routine subculturing, plant tissues and cells can be maintained for years. These tissues and cells can provide year-round supply of products without the limitation of climate, politics or geographic location. The production can be free of contamination from pests or microorganisms, and the genetic expression and metabolism of cultured tissues and cells can be strictly controlled to obtain maximum yield.

Tubers of *Dioscorea alata* L. var. *purpurea* M. Pouch are rich in anthocyanins which are pH-stable and heat-stable and thus good sources of natural food pigments (Yeh and Tsai 1994). A seven factor, two-level fractional factorial experimental design was used to analyze the effect of charcoal, type of vessel, concentration of sucrose, ammonium nitrate, potassium nitrate, potassium dihydrogen phosphate, 2,4-dichloroacetic acid (2,4-D) and kinetin on the initiation of purple calli. After analyzing the results of the above design, the last five factors which showed significant effects on the percentage of purple calli initiation and degree of purple callusing were chosen in the five-level central composite design (Cochran and Cox 1957).

The use of response surface technology (Cochran and Cox 1957; Giovanni 1983) provides researchers with an efficient means of obtaining optimum conditions. This investigation was undertaken to optimize the cultural conditions for the initiation of purple calli by the explants of *Dioscorea alata* L. var. *purpurea* M. Pouch.

MATERIALS AND METHODS

Tubers of *Dioscorea alata* L. var. *purpurea* M. Pouch were purchased from a local farmer. They were washed, surface sterilized and rinsed in sterile water. Segments (0.5

cm × 4 cm) of the tubers were aseptically removed with a scalpel and placed on semisolid modified MS medium (Murashige and Skoog 1962) solidified with 0.8% agar and sterilized by autoclaving at 121°C for 15 min. The explants were maintained at 25°C under fluorescent lights with an intensity of 3,000 lux.

Response surface methodology with a central composite design (Cochran and Cox 1957) was used to optimize the composition of media for maximization of initiation of purple calli. The variables tested were: concentration of sucrose, nitrate, phosphate, 2,4-dichloroacetic acid and kinetin (Table 1). The design is shown in Table 2, in which the first sixteen points were the points in an ordinary 2^5 factorial design used to fit a first-order surface. The seven center points gave us an augmented 2^5 factorial, while the ten axial points enabled us to fit the second-order surface. The responses included: 1) percentage of explants initiating purple calli; and 2) degree of purple callusing. The latter was determined by the area of purple calli initiated, i.e. from 0 point for none initiated to 5 points for 6.25 cm^2 of calli initiated. The relationship between the factors and the response parameters could be described mathematically by a second-order equation by the SAS statistic software (SAS Institute, Raleigh, North Carolina). The optimal combinations were derived from calculations and from two-dimensional contour plots of the three-dimensional response curves, by slicing the surface at different levels for the response parameters.

TABLE 1.
LEVELS OF FACTORS OF THE CENTRAL COMPOSITE DESIGN FOR STUDYING THE EFFECTS OF COMPOSITION OF MEDIA ON THE INITIATION OF PURPLE CALLI FROM *DIOSCOREA ALATA* L. VAR. *PURPUREA* M. POUCH.

Variables	Level				
	-2	-1	0	+1	+2
Sucrose (%)	0.1	1.2	2.3	3.4	4.5
Nitrogen					
NH_4NO_3 (mg/l)	825	1650	2475	3300	4125
KNO_3 (mg/l)	950	1900	2850	3800	4750
Phosphate					
KH_2PO_4 (mg/l)	10	70	130	190	250
2,4-D (μM)	2	10	18	26	34
Kinetin (μM)	0.04	0.34	0.64	0.94	1.24

RESULTS AND DISCUSSION

The resulting design points and responses (percentage of explants initiating purple calli and degree of purple callusing) are shown in Table 3. The analyses of variance of the responses are presented in Tables 4 and Table 5. For both responses, the lack of fit was insignificant; however, the linear terms were significant and quadratic terms were

TABLE 2.
THE CENTRAL COMPOSITE DESIGN FOR STUDYING THE EFFECTS OF THE COMPOSITION OF MEDIA ON THE INITIATION OF PURPLE CALLI FROM *DIOSCOREA ALATA* L. VAR. *PURPUREA* M. POUCH[a]

	Design point					Experiment condition					
							nitrogen		phosphate		
Treatment	X1	X2	X3	X4	X5	sucrose (%)	NH_4NO_3 (mg/l)	KNO_3 (mg/l)	KH_2PO_4 (mg/l)	2,4-D (M)	kinetin (M)
1	-1	-1	-1	-1	1	1.2	1650	1900	70	10	0.94
2	1	-1	-1	-1	-1	3.4	1650	1900	70	10	0.34
3	-1	1	-1	-1	-1	1.2	3300	3800	70	10	0.34
4	1	1	-1	-1	1	3.4	3300	3800	70	10	0.94
5	-1	-1	1	-1	-1	1.2	1650	1900	190	10	0.34
6	1	-1	1	-1	1	3.4	1650	1900	190	10	0.94
7	-1	1	1	-1	1	1.2	3300	3800	190	10	0.94
8	1	1	1	-1	-1	3.4	3300	3800	190	10	0.34
9	-1	-1	-1	1	-1	1.2	1650	1900	70	26	0.94
10	1	-1	-1	1	1	3.4	1650	1900	70	26	0.94
11	-1	1	1	1	1	1.2	3300	3800	70	26	0.94
12	1	1	1	1	-1	3.4	3300	3800	70	26	0.94
13	-1	-1	1	1	1	1.2	1650	1900	190	26	0.34
14	1	-1	1	1	-1	3.4	1650	1900	190	26	0.34
15	-1	1	1	1	-1	1.2	3300	3800	190	26	0.34
16	1	1	1	1	1	3.4	3300	3800	190	26	0.94
17	0	0	0	0	0	2.3	2475	2850	130	18	0.64
18	0	0	0	0	0	2.3	2475	2850	130	18	0.64
19	0	0	0	0	0	2.3	2475	2850	130	18	0.64
20	0	0	0	0	0	2.3	2475	2850	130	18	0.64
21	0	0	0	0	0	2.3	2475	2850	130	18	0.64
22	0	0	0	0	0	2.3	2475	2850	130	18	0.64
23	0	0	0	0	0	2.3	2475	2850	130	18	0.64
24	-2	0	0	0	0	0.1	2475	2850	130	18	0.64
25	2	0	0	0	0	4.5	2475	2850	130	18	0.64
26	0	-2	0	0	0	2.3	825	950	130	18	0.64
27	0	2	0	0	0	2.3	4125	4750	130	18	0.64
28	0	0	-2	0	0	2.3	2475	2850	10	18	0.64
29	0	0	2	0	0	2.3	2475	2850	250	18	0.64
30	0	0	0	-2	0	2.3	2475	2850	130	2	0.64
31	0	0	0	2	0	2.3	2475	2850	130	34	0.64
32	0	0	0	0	-2	2.3	2475	2850	130	18	0.04
33	0	0	0	0	2	2.3	2475	2850	130	18	1.24

[a]Experimental runs were performed in random order.

TABLE 3.
THE CENTRAL COMPOSITE DESIGN FOR STUDYING THE EFFECTS OF THE COMPOSITION OF MEDIA ON THE INITIATION OF PURPLE CALLI FROM *DIOSCOREA ALATA* L. VAR. *PURPUREA* M. POUCH

	Design point					Experiment condition							Response	
							nitrogen		phos-phate					
Treat-ment	X_1	X_2	X_3	X_4	X_5	su-crose (%)	NH_4-NO_3 (mg/l)	KNO_3 (mg/l)	KH_2PO_4 (mg/l)	2,4-D (M)	kine-tin (M)	% of explants initiation purple calli	degree of purple callusing
1	-1	-1	-1	-1	1	1.2	1650	1900	70	10	0.94	60.0	1.07
2	1	-1	-1	-1	-1	3.4	1650	1900	70	10	0.34	60.0	1.67
3	-1	1	-1	-1	-1	1.2	3300	3800	70	10	0.34	80.0	2.20
4	1	1	-1	-1	1	3.4	3300	3800	70	10	0.94	80.0	2.00
5	-1	-1	1	-1	-1	1.2	1650	1900	190	10	0.34	86.7	2.67
6	1	-1	1	-1	1	3.4	1650	1900	190	10	0.94	86.7	1.87
7	-1	1	1	-1	1	1.2	3300	3800	190	10	0.94	73.3	2.13
8	1	1	1	-1	-1	3.4	3300	3800	190	10	0.34	80.0	2.00
9	-1	-1	-1	1	-1	1.2	1650	1900	70	26	0.34	86.7	2.93
10	1	-1	-1	1	1	3.4	1650	1900	70	26	0.94	66.7	2.67
11	-1	1	-1	1	1	1.2	3300	3800	70	26	0.94	93.3	3.27
12	1	1	-1	1	-1	3.4	3300	3800	70	26	0.34	86.7	2.20
13	-1	-1	1	1	1	1.2	1650	1900	190	26	0.94	73.3	2.80
14	1	-1	1	1	-1	3.4	1650	1900	190	26	0.34	73.3	2.40
15	-1	1	1	1	-1	1.2	3300	3800	190	26	0.34	100.0	3.93
16	1	1	1	1	1	3.4	3300	3800	190	26	0.94	86.7	2.33
17	0	0	0	0	0	2.3	2475	2850	130	18	0.64	100.0	3.31
18	0	0	0	0	0	2.3	2475	2850	130	18	0.64	81.3	2.81
19	0	0	0	0	0	2.3	2475	2850	130	18	0.64	75.0	2.69
20	0	0	0	0	0	2.3	2475	2850	130	18	0.64	93.8	3.06
21	0	0	0	0	0	2.3	2475	2850	130	18	0.64	100.0	2.40
22	0	0	0	0	0	2.3	2475	2850	130	18	0.64	93.3	2.93
23	0	0	0	0	0	2.3	2475	2850	130	18	0.64	91.1	2.83
24	-2	0	0	0	0	0.1	2475	2850	130	18	0.64	100.0	1.87
25	2	0	0	0	0	4.5	2475	2850	130	18	0.64	73.3	1.53
26	0	-2	0	0	0	2.3	825	950	130	18	0.64	80.0	2.00
27	0	2	0	0	0	2.3	4125	4750	130	18	0.64	93.3	2.47
28	0	0	-2	0	0	2.3	2475	2850	10	18	0.64	93.3	2.33
29	0	0	2	0	0	2.3	2475	2850	250	18	0.64	86.7	2.93
30	0	0	0	-2	0	2.3	2475	2850	130	2	0.64	53.3	0.67
31	0	0	0	2	0	2.3	2475	2850	130	34	0.64	93.3	3.13
32	0	0	0	0	-2	2.3	2475	2850	130	18	0.04	93.3	2.40
33	0	0	0	0	2	2.3	2475	2850	130	18	1.24	93.3	2.93

TABLE 4.
ANALYSIS OF VARIANCE OF THE CENTRAL COMPOSITE DESIGN FOR STUDYING THE EFFECTS OF COMPOSITION OF MEDIA ON THE PERCENTAGE OF PURPLE CALLI FROM *DIOSCOREA ALATA* L. VAR. *PURPUREA* M. POUCH FOUR WEEKS AFTER CULTURING

Source	Degree of freedom	Sum of squares	Mean square	F-ratio
Regression				
Linear	5	0.2246	0.0449	6.156**
Quadratic	5	0.1099	0.0220	3.013*
Crossproduct	10	0.0673	0.0067	0.922 N.S.
Residual				
Lack of fit	6	0.0378	0.0063	0.782 N.S.
Pure error	8	0.0644	0.0081	
Total error	14	0.1022	0.0073	

* : significant at the 5% level.
** : significant at the 1% level.
N.S. : non-significant

TABLE 5.
ANALYSIS OF VARIANCE OF THE CENTRAL COMPOSITE DESIGN FOR STUDYING THE EFFECTS OF COMPOSITION OF MEDIA ON THE DEGREE OF PURPLE CALLUSING FROM *DIOSCOREA ALATA* L. VAR. *PURPUREA* M. POUCH FOUR WEEKS AFTER CULTURING

Source	Degree of freedom	Sum of squares	Mean square	F-ratio
Regression				
Linear	5	111.4111	22.2822	10.379**
Quadratic	5	42.4322	8.4864	3.960*
Crossproduct	10	31.0333	3.1033	1.448 N.S.
Residual				
Lack of fit	6	16.6084	2.7681	1.296 N.S.
Pure error	502	1072.1180	2.1357	
Total error	508	1088.7264	2.1432	

* : significant at the 5% level.
** : significant at the 1% level.
N.S. : non-significant

significant. Thus, quadratic equations were then fitted to the resulting data listed in Table 3 in an attempt to describe the response surface as a function of five coded variables. The regression coefficients are presented in Table 6. The fitted equations are:

$$Y_1 = 0.9138 - 0.0361X_1 + 0.0472X_2 - 0.0028X_3 + 0.0750X_4 - 0.0139X_5 + 0.0042X_1X_2 - 0.0125X_1X_3 - 0.0042X_1X_4 + 0.0459X_1X_5 - 0.0042X_2X_3 + 0.0042X_2X_4 + 0.0042X_2X_5 - 0.0292X_3X_4 - 0.0292X_3X_5 + 0.0125X_4X_5 - 0.0190X1^2 - 0.0190X_2^2 - 0.0107X_3^2 - 0.524X_4^2\ 0.0024X_5^2$$

$$Y_2 = 2.8076 - 0.1700X_1 + 0.1222X_2 + 0.1389X_3 + 0.4944X_4 - 0.0333X_5 - 0.1333X_1X_2 - 0.1250X_1X_3 - 0.1750X_1X_4 + 0.1917X_1X_5 - 0.0417X_2X_3 - 0.0083X_2X_4 + 0.0417X_2X_5 - 0.0833X_3X_4 - 0.1167X_3X_5 + 0.0667X_4X_5 - 0.2123X_1^2 - 0.1040X_2^2 - 0.0040X_3^2 - 0.1837X_4^2 + 0.0043X_5^2$$

where

Y_1 = expected percentage of explants initiating purple calli
Y_2 = expected degree of purple callusing
X_1, X_2, X_3, X_4, X_5 = coded levels of sucrose, nitrate, phosphate, 2,4-D and kinetin, respectively

These equations provide an adequate description of the response surface over the range of variables used in this study. There is no indication that a more complex equation is required over the range of variables studied here.

TABLE 6.
REGRESSION COEFFICIENTS OF THE RESULTS OF THE CENTRAL COMPOSITE DESIGN FOR STUDYING THE EFFECTS OF THE INITIATION OF PURPLE CALLI FROM *DIOSCOREA ALATA* L. VAR. *PURPUREA* M. POUCH

Term	Coefficient	
	% of explants initiating purple calli	Degree of purple callusing
Intercept	0.9138	2.8076
X_1	-0.0361	-0.1700
X_2	0.0472	0.1222
X_3	-0.0028	0.1389
X_4	0.0750	0.4944
X_5	-0.0139	-0.0333
X_1X_1	-0.0190	-0.2123
X_2X_1	0.0042	-0.1333
X_2X_2	-0.0190	-0.1040
X_3X_1	-0.0125	-0.1250
X_3X_2	-0.0042	-0.0417
X_3X_3	-0.0107	-0.0040
X_4X_1	-0.0042	-0.1750
X_4X_2	0.0042	-0.0083
X_4X_3	-0.0292	-0.0833
X_4X_4	-0.0524	-0.1873
X_5X_1	0.0459	0.1917
X_5X_2	0.0042	0.0417
X_5X_3	-0.0292	-0.1167
X_5X_4	0.0125	0.0667
X_5X_5	-0.0024	0.0043

From the statistical analysis (Tables 7 and 8), 2,4-D was shown to be the most important factor among the five factors affecting the response variables. Sucrose had a significant effect on degree of purple callusing but did not affect the percentage of explants initiating purple calli. The same conclusion could also be drawn on considering the magnitudes of the coefficients of the regression equations. By holding the level of nitrogen, phosphate and kinetin at 0, the above polynomial approximations can be simplified to develop contour plots (Fig. 1) to illustrate the relationships among the response variables, Y_1 and Y_2 and concentrations of sucrose and 2,4-D. Figure 1 shows that percentage of explants initiating purple calli and degree of purple callusing increased as concentration of 2,4-D increased. These results agree with studies on *Dimorphotheca auriculata* (Harbone *et al.* 1970) and *Rosa* sp. (Davies 1972). In our study, the optimum 2,4-D concentration for the percentage of purple calli was 26.63 μM and the optimum 2,4-D concentration for the degree of purple callusing was 35.31 μM. By averaging the above two concentrations, the final 2,4-D concentration was determined to be 30.97 μM.

Lowering the sucrose concentration from 4.5% to 1.1% increased the degree of purple callusing (Fig. 1a), although the effect was not found on the percentage of purple calli (Fig. 1b). High concentration of sucrose was found to inhibit the production of anthocyanins in the culture of *Dimorphotheca sinuata* (Ball and Arditti 1974) and *Petunia hybrida* (Colijn *et al.* 1981). In our study the optimum sucrose concentration for the percentage of purple calli was 1.39% and the optimum sucrose concentration for the degree of purple callusing was 0.81%. By averaging the above two concentrations, the final sucrose concentration was determined to be 1.10%. Since the other three independent variables, i.e., nitrogen, phosphate and kinetin did not affect the initiation of purple calli within the experimental ranges, their concentrations were kept at level 0 in the optimum medium. Thus the major medium composition was optimized to be 1.1%

TABLE 7.
ANALYSIS OF VARIANCE OF THE CENTRAL COMPOSITE DESIGN FOR STUDYING THE EFFECTS OF COMPOSITION FACTORS OF MEDIA ON THE PERCENTAGE OF PURPLE CALLI FROM *DIOSCOREA ALATA* L. VAR. *PURPUREA* M. POUCH FOUR WEEKS AFTER CULTURING

Source	Degree of freedom	Sum of squares	Mean square	F-ratio
Sucrose	6	0.0794	0.0132	1.814 N.S.
Nitrogen				
NH_4NO_3	6	0.0660	0.0110	1.508 N.S.
KNO_3				
Phosphate				
KH_2PO_4	6	0.0338	0.0056	0.770 N.S.
2,4-D	6	0.2381	0.0397	5.439**
Kinetin	6	0.0548	0.0091	1.252 N.S.

** : significant at the 1% level.
N.S. : non-significant

TABLE 8.
ANALYSIS OF VARIANCE OF THE CENTRAL COMPOSITE DESIGN FOR STUDYING THE EFFECTS OF COMPOSITION FACTORS OF MEDIA ON THE DEGREE OF PURPLE CALLUSING FROM *DIOSCOREA ALATA* L. VAR. *PURPUREA* M. POUCH FOUR WEEKS AFTER CULTURING

Source	Degree of freedom	Sum of squares	Mean square	F-ratio
Sucrose	6	56.2683	9.3781	4.376**
Nitrogen				
NH_4NO_3	6	15.6303	2.6050	1.216 N.S.
KNO_3				
Phosphate				
KH_2PO_4	6	16.0521	2.6753	1.248 N.S.
2,4-D	6	114.7742	19.1290	8.926**
Kinetin	6	13.9756	2.3293	1.087 N.S.

** : significant at the 1% level.
N.S. : non-significant

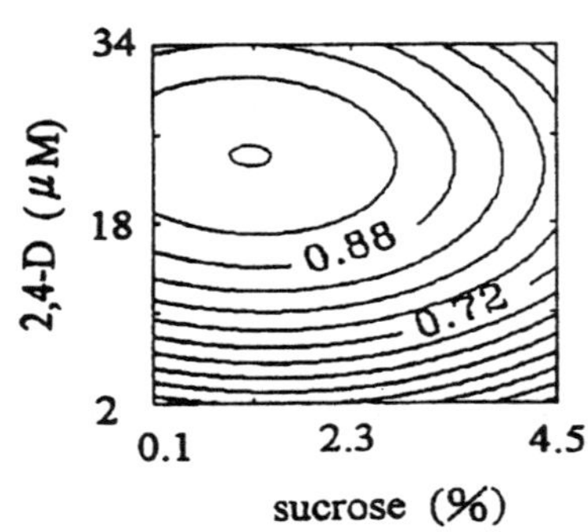

(a)

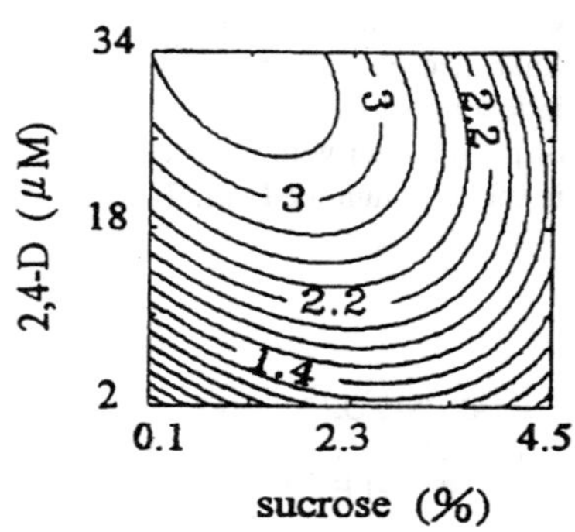

(b)

FIG. 1. CONTOUR PLOTS OF THE INITIATION OF PURPLE CALLI OF *DIOSCOREA ALATA* L. *VAR. PURPUREA* M. POUCH AT VARIOUS CONCENTRATIONS OF SUCROSE AND 2,4-D.
(a) For the percentage of purple calli and (b) for the degree of purple callusing. (X2, X3, X5 = 0).

sucrose, 2,475 mg/l ammonium nitrate, 2,850 mg/l potassium nitrate, 130 mg/l potassium dihydrogen phosphate, 30.97 μM 2,4-D and 0.64 μM kinetin. Adequacy of the model equations for predicting optimum response values was tested in this laboratory. The predicted percentage of explants initiating purple calli by the optimum medium was 100% and the predicted degree of purple callusing for the same medium was 3.50.

The experimental values for the predicted percentage of explants initiating purple calli by the optimum medium was 100% and the predicted degree of purple callusing for the same medium was 3.61 suggesting the validity of the equations and the effectiveness of the optimum medium on the initiation of purple calli.

ACKNOWLEDGMENTS

The authors gratefully acknowledge the financial support of the National Science Council, Taiwan (NSC84-2321-B-029).

REFERENCES

BALL, E.A. and ARDITTI, J. 1974. The relationship of sugar concentration in the culture medium to anthocyanin accumulation in a plant callus culture. Am. J. Bot. *61*, 5–33.

COCHRAN, W.G. and COX, G.M. 1957. Experimental Design. John Wiley & Sons, Inc., New York. pp. 335–369.

COLIJN, C.M., JONSSON, L.M.V., SCHRAM, A.W. and KOOL A.J. 1981. Synthesis of malvidin and petunidin in pigmented tissue cultures of *Petunia hybrida*. Protoplasma *107*, 63–68.

DAVIES, M.E. 1972. Polyphenol synthesis in cell suspension cultures of Paul's scarlet rose. Planta *104*, 50–65.

GIOVANNI, M. 1983. Response surface methodology and product optimization. Food Technol. *37*, 41–45.

HARBORNE, J.B., ARDITTI, J. and BALL, E. 1970. The anthocyanins of a callus culture from the stem of *Dimorphotheca auriculata*. Am. J. Bot. *57*, 763.

ILKER, R. 1987. In-vitro pigment production: an alternative to color synthesis. Food Technol. *41*, 70–72.

MURASHIGE, T. and SKOOG, F. 1962. A revised media for rapid growth and bioassays with tobacco tissue cultures. Physiol. Plant *15*, 473–497.

YEH, P. and TSAI, T. 1994. Stability of three natural anthocyanin extracts: *Dioscorea alata, Dioscorea batatas* and *Ipomoea batatas*. Tunghai J. *35*, 161–175.

"EFFICIENT, ECONOMIC AND CLEAN" ETHANOL PRODUCTION

GUIYANG SHI, LIXIN ZHANG and KECHANG ZHANG

School of Biotechnology
Wuxi University of Light Industry
Wuxi, Jiangsu 214036, P.R. of China

ABSTRACT

In this study, milled starch material such as corn and sweet potato was liquefied at low temperature (80-85 °C) followed by simultaneous saccharification and fermentation at 30-37 °C with Saccharomyces cerevisiae. *In a commercial scale ethanol concentration as high as 15% with a conversion rate from starch to ethanol of 90% was obtained. This clearly indicated that high alcohol concentrations could still be produced industrially through very high gravity (V.H.G) technology at a certain condition. The effluent pollution was completely eliminated by "totally recycling technology" (TRT). The objective — "efficient, economic and clean" was fully reflected in the system.*

INTRODUCTION

In recent years research on ethanol production has focused on all phases of the process from raw materials to by-product recovery and is ultimately directed toward improving the efficiency of fermentation and reducing the cost of ethanol production (Ryu *et al.* 1984, Alison and Ingledew 1994, Hahn-Hagerdal *et al.* 1994). The cost of raw materials, capital equipment, and processing all influence greatly the profitability of fuel alcohol manufacture. Further improvement can be achieved only with a technology which will help in reducing the fermentation time (increasing the rate of production) and increasing the concentration of alcohol by fermenting greater amounts of sugar (Kazuyoshi *et al.* 1993). These include energy consumption and conversion, effluent pollution control and protection of the environment (Ingledew 1993, Hahn-Hagerdal *et al.* 1994).

The amount of carbohydrate that can be fermented at elevated temperatures is limited because of deleterious osmotic effect coupled with an increased toxicity of higher level of ethanol to yeast growth and metabolism. Industrial or fuel alcohol is produced at temperatures in the range of 30-35 °C. Temperatures of this range are preferred because the metabolic activities of the yeast are maximal, and this normally results in the completion of fermentation in a shorter time and less cooling requirement.

To enhance the ethanol concentration in fermented mash, most scientific researchers have focused in strain selection, uncooking technology and low fermentation temperature use (Matin and Ingledew 1985). But no satisfactory results were reported in industrial application. In our laboratory, the emphasis on process technological researches shows very good results. To lower some substances inhibiting yeast activity and to promote the tolerant ability on ethanol with certain additives are much more efficient than the other methods attempting VHG (very high gradient) ethanol fermentation.

On the other hand, VHG consists greatly of organic substances in distillate. Its BOD usually is as high as 30,000 mg/l. By VHG the amount of distillate is reduced from 12-15 to less than 8 tons per ton ethanol production. The distillate was treated by "totally recycling technology" (TRT).

MATERIALS AND METHODS

Microorganism And Cultivation Conditions

Saccharomyces cerevisiae was maintained on agar slant medium containing 15 g/l agar, 20 g/l glucose, 5 g/l yeast extract, and 5 g/l peptone. Inoculum cultures were grown at 35 °C for 36 h with periodic shaking. The cells were collected by centrifugation (Himac Centrifuge Hitachi SCR 20 BC) at 2,000 × g for 20 min. The number of cells in 1 gram precipitate was determined by direct microscopic counting on a Thomas haemacytometer. The precipitate was not washed and was used straight away for fermentation.

Starch Materials

Ground corn or sweet potato used throughout the study was received from Wuxi Bioproducts Company (Wuxi, P.R. of China). The size of particles was almost 20 mesh which did not require any further treatment before using.

Chemicals

α-Amylase of 6,000 units per gram (optimum pH 6.5, temperature 80 °C), and glucoamylase of 100,000 units per gram (optimum pH 4.5, temperature 60 °C) were received from Wuxi Bioproducts Company. All routinely used chemicals and microbial medium ingredients were purchased from local suppliers. Ash was obtained by incinerating yeast extract (Difco Laboratories, Detroit, Michigan) at 550 °C for 4 h.

Mash Preparation

Ground corn or sweet potato was dispensed in the water with constant agitation, the pH was therefore adjusted to 6.5-6.7 using 5 N NaOH. Five units α-amylase per gram corn or sweet potato was added. The temperature was raised to 85 °C and held at this temperature for 60 min with continuous stirring. The temperature was lowered to 60 °C. The mash thus prepared, the pH was adjusted to 4.3 with 6 N HCl and then saccharified using glucoamylase (150 units per gram corn or sweet potato) and fermented directly.

Fermentation Tests

An additive for fermentation was sterilized by autoclaving at 120 °C for 20 min. The pH of the fermentation medium was adjusted to 4.3 with HCl, and it was inoculated with a proper amount of cell density at 35 °C until fermentation ceased.

TRT Process

Distillate from first turn fermentation was separated by a rotating filter. The filtrate then was used for mash preparation in a second turn fermentation which would be called one recycling. The same process was repeated to two recycling, three recycling and so on.

Analytical Methods

The reducing sugar was analyzed by DNS (dinitrosalicylic acid agent) method. A standard curve for this volumetric assay was calculated by linear regression. Total sugars at the beginning and at the end of fermentation were determined as reducing sugars after acid hydrolysis (0.54 N HCl, 60 min, 100°C) and neutralization with 20% NaOH. The ethanol content was determined by distillation and gas chromatography with a flame ionization detector. The carrier gas was N_2. Butanol was used as the internal standard.

Calculation of Some Parameters

$$\text{Ethanol yield} = \frac{\text{ethanol content}}{\text{total sugar content}}$$

$$\text{Starch utilization rate} = \frac{\text{Ethanol yield}}{0.511} \times 100\%$$

RESULTS AND DISCUSSION

Effect of Minerals

Mash containing 22.15% (w/w) sugar was prepared and fermented at 35°C with and without 0.1% (w/w) ash as a nutrient supplement. The results showed that minerals had no stimulatory effect on fermentation. It suggested that enough minerals were already present in the mash. In fact, proximate analysis of corn or sweet potato showed that they contain 1 to 3.9% ash on dry basis. The minerals are essential for the yeast, especially in VHG fermentation (24). It is therefore rare for corn or sweet potato mash as well as other grain mashes to be deficient in minerals.

Effect of Amino Nitrogen

Evidence for the stimulatory role of amino nitrogen is presented in Table 1. It shows that X, yeast extract and peptone enhanced considerably the rate of fermentation. X is the cheapest one among them. The results for further investigation of X is presented in Fig. 1. It points out that the best yield appeared at 0.2%X, and concentration in excess of 0.2%X did not further benefit the rate of fermentation.

25 Liter and 1500 m^3 Fermentation

Figure 2 presents the results for scale-up test and industrial application. Comparison with the normal batch fermentation, the productivity using VHG nearly reached 3 to 5 times higher. The starch utilization rate was about 90%.

TABLE 1.
EFFECT OF AMINO NITROGEN ON FERMENTATION

Additive	control	0.5%X	0.5% yeast extract	0.5% peptone
Sugar consumed %	77.8	99.2	97.6	98.3
Ethanol concentration %(v/v)	11.5	14.4	14.1	14.0

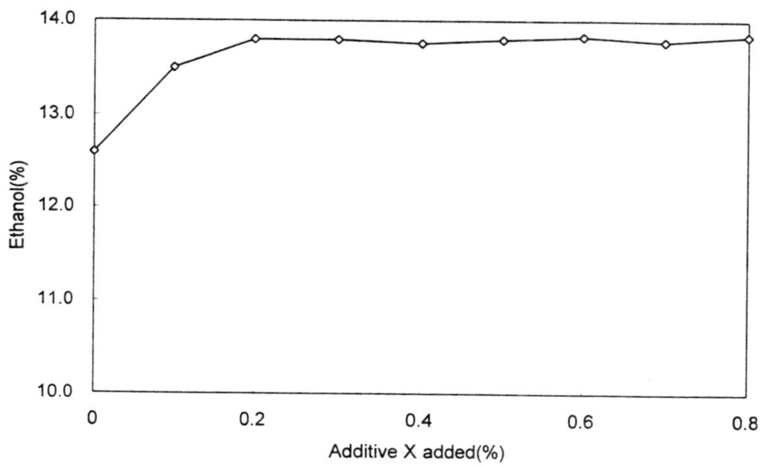

FIG. 1. EFFECT OF ADDITIVE X ON FERMENTATION

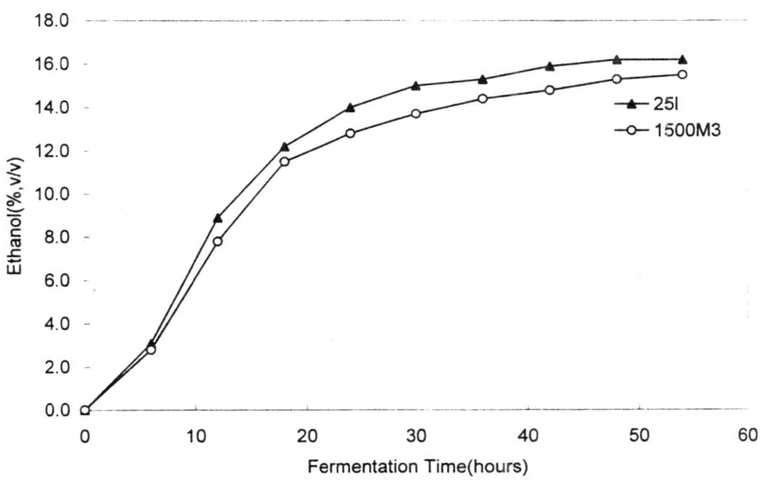

FIG. 2. 25 LITER AND 1500 m³ FERMENTATION

Theoretical Analysis for TRT

If: The amount of distillate N(kg)
Solid content (soluble and insoluble) in distillate S (%,w/w)
Solid content (soluble and insoluble) in filtrate F (%,w/w)
Solid content (soluble and insoluble) in dregs Q (%,w/w)

Then the filter rate $R = \frac{S\ (kg)}{F\ (kg)}$

Calculation data for each recycling are given as follows:

Recycling Times	Solid in Distillate (kg)	Solid in Filtrate (kg)	Solid in Dregs (kg)
0 recycling	NS	NSR	NS(1-R)
1 recycling	NS+NSR =NS(1+R)	NS(1+R)R $=NS(R+R^2)$	$NS(1+R)-NS(R+R^2)$ $=NS(1-R^2)$
2 recycling	$NS+NS(R+R^2)$ $=NS(1+R+R^2)$	$NS(1+R+R^2)R$ $=NS(R+R^2+R^3)$	$=NS(1-R^3)$
3 recycling	$NS+NS(R+R^2+R^3)$ $=NS(1+R+R^2+R^3)$	$NS(1+R+R^2+R^3)R$ $=NS(R+R^2+R^3+R^4)$	$NS(1-R^4)$
...	...	...	...
n recycling	$NS(1+R+R^2+...+R^n)$ $NS(1-R^{n+1})/(1-R)$	$NS(R+R^2+R^3+...+R^{n+1})$ $=NSR(1-R^{n+1})/(1-R)$	$NS(1-R^{n+1})$
$n\rightarrow\infty$	NS/(1-R)	NSR/(1-R)	NS

After n recycling the solid content S (soluble and insoluble) in distillate could be expressed: $S = S_0(1-R^{n+1})/(1-R)$. For certain filter and distillate, R is almost a constant. So the solid content will not expand without limit with the recycling increase.

Effect of Recycling Times on Some Important Parameters

With continuously recycling operation, some important parameters were determined during the fermentation. See Figs. 3-6. Starch utilization rate, total sugar of fermentation mash, acidity and total solid content were oscillated within a range during 15 recycling. The experimental data coincided with the theoretical calculation. It proved that TRT is practical and efficient to eliminate the pollution caused by distillate from ethanol production.

CONCLUSIONS

Milled starch material, such as corn and sweet potato, was liquefied at low temperature (80-85°C) which reduces the toxic substances to yeast. A commercial scale ethanol concentration as high as 15% with a conversion rate from starch to ethanol of 90% was obtained. This clearly indicates that high alcohol concentrations could still be produced industrially through very high gravity (VHG) technology at a certain condition without strain mutation and selection. The "totally recycling technology" (TRT) is one of the best choices for complete elimination of an effluent pollution of ethanol factory.

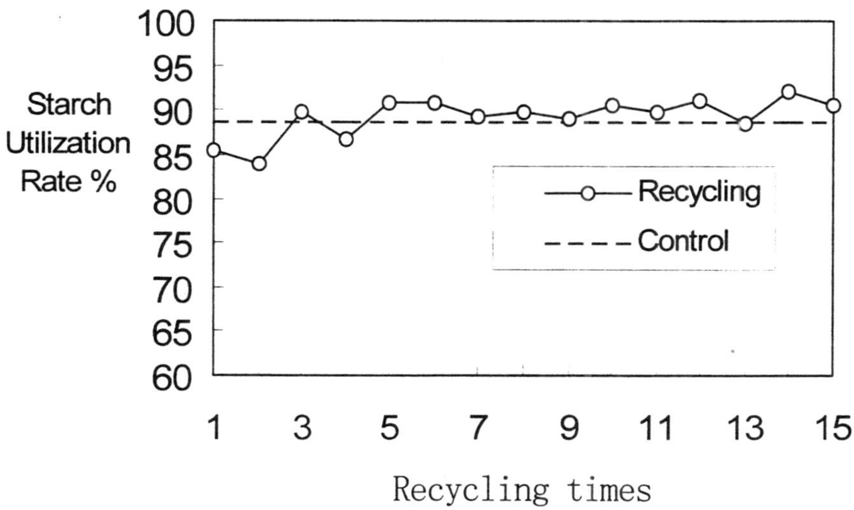

FIG. 3. EFFECT OF RECYCLING TIMES ON STARCH UTILIZATION RATE

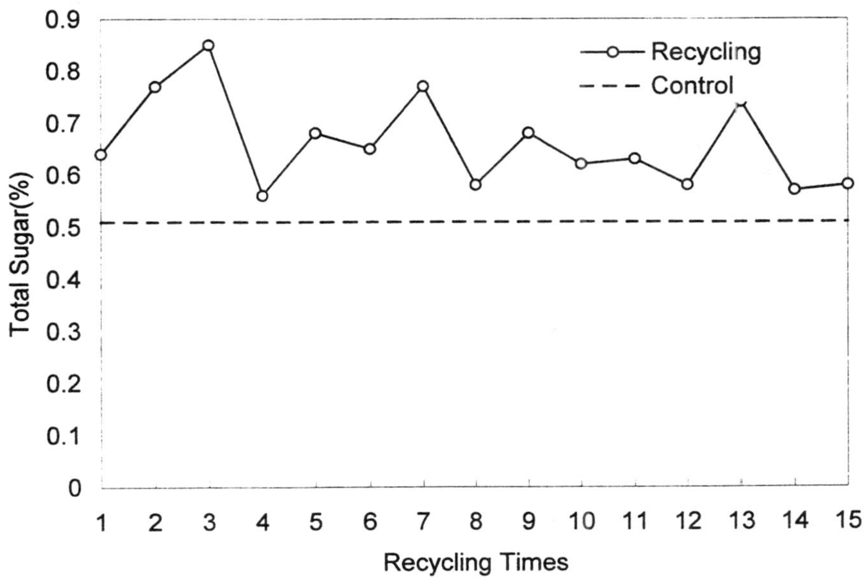

FIG. 4. EFFECT OF RECYCLING TIMES ON TOTAL SUGAR OF FERMENTATION MASH

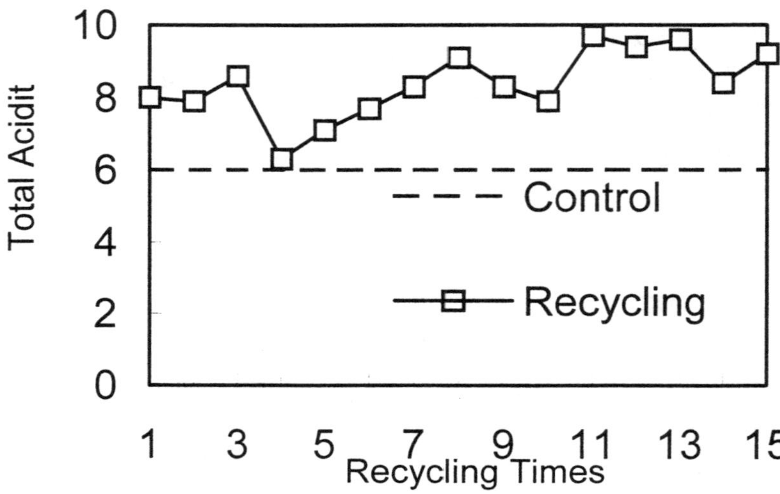

FIG. 5. EFFECT OF RECYCLING TIMES ON ACIDITY OF FERMENTATION

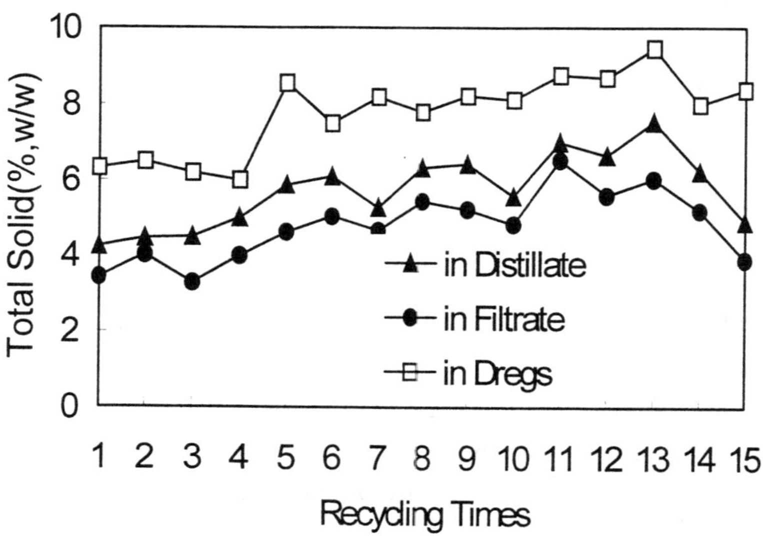

FIG. 6. EFFECT OF RECYCLING TIMES ON TOTAL SOLID CONTENT

REFERENCES

ALISON, M.J. and INGLEDEW, W.M. 1994. Fuel alcohol production: appraisal of nitrogenous yeast food for very high gravity wheat mash fermentation. Process Biochem. *29*, 483–488.

HAHN-HAGERDAL, B., JEPPSSON, H., OLSSON, L. and MOHAGHEGHI, A. 1994. An interlaboratory comparison of the performance of ethanol producing microorganisms in a xylose-rich acid hydrolysate. Appl. Microbiol. Biotechnol. *41*, 62–72.

INGLEDEW, W.M. 1993. Yeasts for production of fuel ethanol. pp. 245–287. In Rose, A.H. and Harrison, J.S. (eds). The Yeasts. Vol. 5, 2nd edition: Yeast Technology. London, Academic Press.

KAZUYOSHI, O., HAMADA, S. and NAKAMURA, T. 1993. Production of high concentration of ethanol from inulin by simultaneous saccharification and fermentation using *Aspergillus niger* and *Saccharomyces cerevisiae*. Applied Environ. Microbiol. *59*(1), 729–733.

MATIN, L.K. and INGLEDEW, W.M. 1985. Evaluation of ethanol tolerance in selected *Saccharomyces cerevisiae* strains. J. Am. Soc. Biochem. *43*(4), 189–196.

RYU, -D.D.Y., KIM, -Y.J. and KIM, -J.H. 1984. Effect of air supplement on the performance of continuous ethanol fermentation system. *Saccharomyces cerevisiae* Biotechnol. Bioeng. *26*, 12–16.

EFFECT OF α-TOCOPHEROL ON LIPOXYGENASE-CATALYZED OXIDATION OF HIGHLY UNSATURATED FATTY ACIDS

BONNIE SUN PAN, HSIU-HUA HSU, SUSAN CHEN and HUA-MING CHEN

Marine Food Science Department
National Taiwan Ocean University
2 Pei-Ning Rd.
Keelung, Taiwan, R.O.C.

ABSTRACT

Lipoxygenase (LOX) activities were found in blood of cultured grey mullet (Mugil cephalus). *Platelets had the highest activity, followed by plasma and erythrocytes. 12-LOX was identified with the highest activity followed by 5-, and 15-LOX using arachidonic acid as substrate. When the grey mullet was cultured with diet containing increased content of α-tocopherol acetate, 12-LOX activity in platelets was reduced, while total polyenoic acids increased in erythrocytes. When isolated blood platelets were preincubated with α-tocopherol acetate in the range of 0 to 1500 μM, LOX activity was significantly reduced. Both* in-vivo *and* in-vitro *results indicated the inhibitory effect of α-tocopherol on LOX-catalyzed oxidation of highly unsaturated fatty acids. Apparent viscosity of blood was reduced, indicative of higher deformability of the erythrocytes in mullet fed with vitamin E fortified diets.*

INTRODUCTION

Deficiency in dietary vitamin E resulted in reduction of mean corpuscular volume (MCV), mean corpuscular hemoglobin concentration (MCH), and increased hemolysis, poikilocytosis and anisocytosis in salmonids (Cowey *et al.* 1983; Halver 1982; Watanabe *et al.* 1981). Hemoglobin and membrane of red blood cells became oxidized by molecular oxygen while vitamin E stabilized membrane by interacting with the unsaturated fatty acids of the phospholipid bilayer (Mino *et al.* 1982; Urano *et al.* 1987). α-Tocopherol inhibits the membrane impairment of erythrocytes, thus it prevents hemolysis in the presence of oxidizing agents (Niki *et al.* 1988). Grey mullet fed with basal diets containing vitamin E at 90 mg/kg showed slightly more spontaneous hemolysis than those fed with diets fortified with 100 or 200 mg/kg vitamin E (Shyu and Pan 1993).

The objectives of this study were to examine the *in vivo* effect of dietary vitamin E on the polyenoic acids of erythrocytes and the blood viscosity which is an indication of the erythrocyte deformability and the fluidity of blood.

Since LOX activities were identified in mullet gill (Hsu and Pan 1996) which consists of sanguineous tissues, LOX is likely to occur in blood and to catalyze the peroxidation of blood tissues. To identify the types of LOX and the interrelationship between vitamin E, the LOX-catalyzed oxidation in mullet blood, and the blood viscosity so affected was also a goal of interest in this investigation.

MATERIALS AND METHODS

Cultured Grey Mullet

An experimental pond of 9400 m^2 was divided with nylon net into divisions of 25 m × 8 m × 2.1 m at the Experimental Station of Hanaqua International Corp., Tainan, Taiwan. The culture density was 0.5 mullet/m^2. Salinity was controlled at 11 ± 2 ppt. At the start of the feeding experiment, about 100 one-year-old grey mullets *Mugil cephalus* (450 g per fish) were put into each pond division.

Experimental Diet

A commercial feed (Hanaqua International Corp.), composed of fish meal, full-fat soybean meal, peanut meal and linseed meal as protein sources; wheat bran, wheat flour middling and cassava flour as carbohydrate sources and binder; and rice bran as filler, was used as basal diet with an energy level of 3200 kcal/kg. Different levels of vitamin E (α-tocopherol acetate) were supplemented to the basal diet. Ethoxyquin (0.02%) was added to the diets to inhibit the oxidation of lipid and α-tocopherol. Diets were mechanically mixed to ensure homogeneity and pelleted, then fed to fish throughout the 12 month period. Proximate composition and vitamin E of the diets (Table 1) were analyzed by AOAC methods (1984).

TABLE 1.
PROXIMATE COMPOSITION AND VITAMIN E CONTENT OF EXPERIMENTAL DIETS FOR CULTURED 1 YEAR GREY MULLET

Vitamin E added (mg/kg)	Moisture (%)	Crude Protein (%)	Crude fat (%)	Ash (%)	Vitamin E (mg/kg)
basal	11.45	30.30	9.84	9.73	90±3
100	11.46	32.95	10.11	10.71	190±7
200	12.68	33.80	10.50	10.64	290±11
400	11.49	31.08	9.32	11.68	471±13

Separation of Platelets Plasma and Erythrocytes

Ten ml of blood samples were taken from the caudal vein of each fish and immediately mixed with 143 U.S.P units of sodium heparin powder (Sigma Chemical Co., St. Louis, Mo), and kept in ice to be analyzed within a half h. For serum preparation, blood samples in 5 ml were put into separate tubes and frozen at -20°C until used.

Mullet blood was centrifuged at 1000 rpm for 10 min to separate the erythrocytes from the platelet rich plasma. The supernatant was again centrifuged at 3000 rpm for 10 min. The supernatant was the plasma and the precipitant consisted of platelets (Ho *et al.* 1977; Wallach and Brown 1981).

Determination of α-Tocopherol Content in Diets and Plasma

The α-tocopherol content in plasma was measured with Emmerie and Engel's method modified by Augustin *et al.* (1985) using 0.3-0.6 ml plasma. The method is based on the oxidation of xylene-extracted plasma tocopherols by ferric chloride. The pink complex of ferrous ions with bathophenathroline was measured at 536 nm using dl-α-tocopherol (Wako Pure Chemical Industries, Japan) as a standard.

Lipid was extracted from 10 g diets by the method of Folch *et al.* (1957). Accurately weighed lipid was diluted with *n*-hexane to 10 ml and filtered with a 0.45 μm millipore, then analyzed for α-tocopherol content (Ueda and Igarashi 1990) by HPLC (Hitachi F-1050) equipped with a fluorescence spectrophotometer (Model: 050-0702) and Shimadzu integrator C-R5A. The HPLC chromatographic column was Spheris S5ODS2 stainless steel, 150 × 4.6 mm id. Methanol:water (99:1, v/v) was used as mobile phase at a flow rate of 2.0 ml/min. Excitation and emission wavelengths were 290 nm and 330 nm, respectively. dl-α-Tocopherol was used as a standard.

Preparation of Lipoxygenase (LOX) Crude Extract

Platelets were dissolved in 0.05 M Tris buffer, pH 7.4, as the crude LOX extract according to the method of Wallach and Brown (1981). The extract was immersed in liquid nitrogen to freeze and was stored at -40°C until used.

Determination of Apparent Viscosity of Whole Blood

A volume of 1.4 ml whole blood was applied to a Haake Cone and Plate Microviscometer (Model PK 45) and measured at a cone angle of 4°C and a shear rate ranging from 1 to 300 sec^{-1} at a constant temperature of 15 and 25°C, respectively.

Determination of Hydroxyeicosatetraenoic Acid (HETE)

The LOX extract was incubated with arachidonic acid (100 μM) at 25°C for 5 min. The reaction was terminated by adjusting the pH to 3.0 with 6 N HCl. The reaction products were extracted with 2 volumes of ethyl acetate and methylated with diazomethane (Ayorinde *et al.* 1989). The methylated compounds were adsorbed on a solid phase extraction column (J&W Scientific, Folsom, CA) (German and Berger 1990). The HETE products were eluted with a hexane/ether mixture (75:25, v/v) and were subjected to HPLC analysis according to the method of Hsu and Pan (1996).

High-pressure liquid chromatographic analyses were performed on a Lichrospher 100 RP-18 column (25 cm × 4 mm, 5 μM) equipped with a pump (Waters, Model 510, Milford, MA) and a UV detector (Waters, Model 490E), monitored at 235 nm. The compounds were eluted using a solvent system of methanol/water (75:25, v/v) buffered with 5 mM ammonium acetate containing 0.5 mM EDTA to an apparent pH of 5.7. Retention times were compared with standards of 5(S)-, 12(S)-, and 15(S)-HETE (Cayman Chemical Co., Ann Arbor, MI).

Statistical Analysis

A test of variation among treatments was done using the Kruskal-Wallis one way analysis (Daniel 1974). If the variations were significant, Kruskal-Wallis multiple comparison was further tested.

RESULTS AND DISCUSSION

α-Tocopherol in Blood Plasma

The level of α-tocopherol in blood plasma of one year old cultured grey mullet showed seasonal changes reaching maximal in November and minimal in December regardless of being feminized with estradiol (H1+) or without (1+) (Fig. 1). The timing was coincidental with the maximal gonad development and atresia (Pan *et al.* 1992). Increases in dietary vitamin E fortification (400 and 200 mg/kg) resulted in significantly higher concentration of α-tocopherol ($p<0.05$) in blood plasma than those fed with the control and the 100 mg/kg throughout the year (Fig. 1). The peak time for the 2 year old (2+) fed with fortified vitamin E diet appeared in October, a month sooner than that sampled from mullet fed with basal diet. Therefore, α-tocopherol in blood plasma reflected the dietary intake of vitamin E.

Changes of Polyenoic Acids in Erythrocyte

The lipid contents of erythrocytes did not show significant changes with dietary vitamin E intakes ranging from 0 to 400 mg/kg fortification after 10 months of feeding tests. The one year old (1+, and H1+) had 0.72 to 1.20% lipid in erythrocytes, while the 2+ had 1.01 to 1.87% (data not shown). However, the total content of polyenoic fatty acids in erythrocyte correlated with the dietary intake of vitamin E (Fig. 2). $C_{18:2}$ and $C_{22:6}$ were the major polyenoic fatty acids. Each of these two was at a concentration higher than 10 g/100 g lipid (data not shown). The presence of α-tocopherol in blood is likely to enhance the stability of polyenoic acid of erythrocytes, since α-tocopherol has been considered an efficient antioxidant against radical-mediated oxidation of low-density lipoprotein especially in the presence of suitable reducing agent (Thomas *et al.* 1995; Olsson and Yuan 1996). The *in vivo* cause of the loss of polyenoic acids in erythrocytes was then examined.

Lipoxygenase Activities in Blood

Erythrocytes, platelets, and plasma were incubated with arachidonic acid, respectively. Their HPLC chromatograms showed peaks with retention times equivalent to those of the 5-, 12-, and 15- HETE standards (Hsu and Pan 1996). Based on the peak areas, platelets showed LOX activities including 5-, 12-, and 15-LOX significantly higher than the respective LOX in plasma followed by erythrocytes (Table 2). Among the 3 LOX, 12-LOX was the highest assayed at pH 6.5 and 25°C. Therefore in the following experiments, platelet 12-LOX was used as an indicator to study the vitamin E effects.

Effect of Dietary Vitamin E on Platelet 12-LOX

One year old grey mullet were fed with 828 and 1851 mg/kg vitamin E for 6 months under the same experimental conditions otherwise as the previous experiments. Blood samples were drawn in September. Activity of platelet 12-LOX was reduced by 25% as dietary vitamin E was fortified and increased from 828 to 1851 mg/kg (Table 3). Similar inhibitions of 5-HETE and 12-HETE formation were observed in human platelet and leukocytes when vitamin E was added (Goetzl 1980). Since the effect was concluded

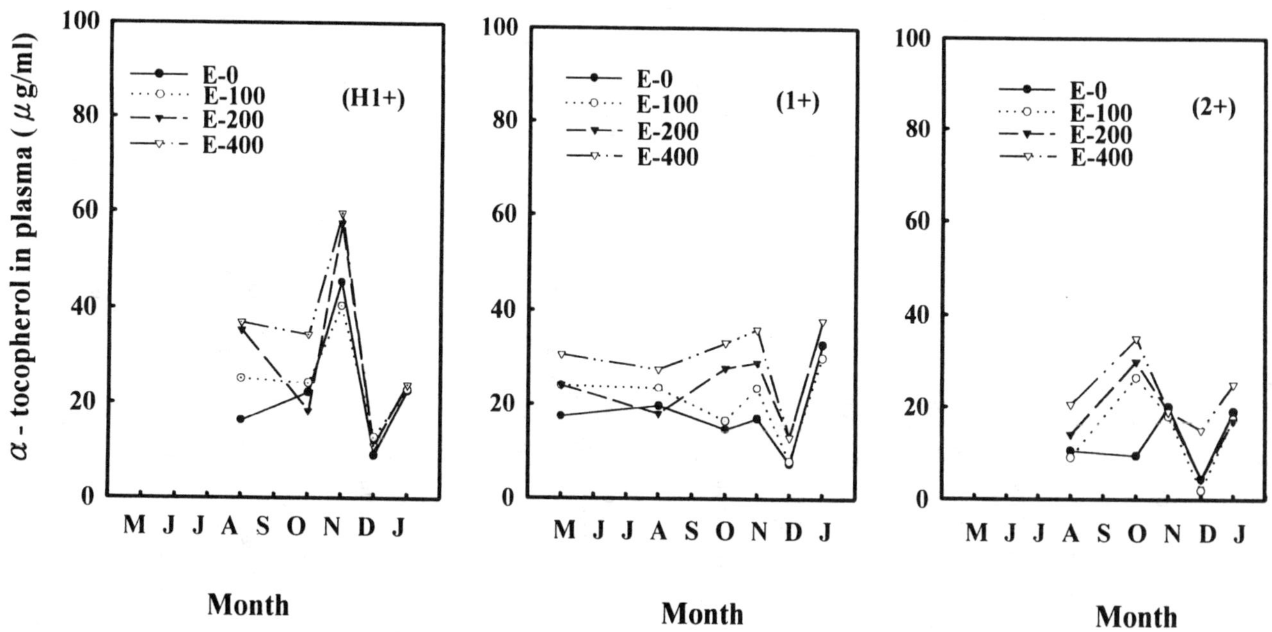

FIG. 1. α-TOCOPHEROL CONTENT IN PLASMA OF CULTURED MULLET OF ONE YEAR FEMINIZED WITH ESTRADIOL (H1+), ONE YEAR (1+), TWO YEAR (2+), ALL FED WITH DIETS FORTIFIED WITH VITAMIN E AND REARED FROM MARCH TO JANUARY

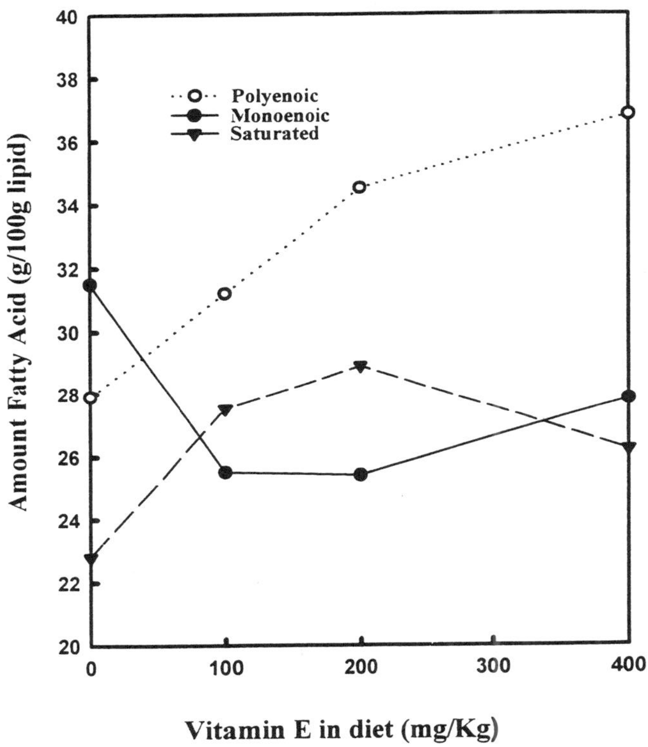

FIG. 2. CHANGES IN POLYENOIC, MONOENOIC AND SATURATED FATTY ACIDS (G/100 G) IN ERYTHROCYTE OF CULTURED MULLET OF ONE YEAR (H1+) FED WITH DIETS FORTIFIED WITH VITAMIN E AND ESTRADIOL 17 β FOR 10 MONTHS (SAMPLED IN JANUARY)

TABLE 2.
LIPOXYGENASE ACTIVITY[1] OF ERYTHROCYTES, PLATELETS AND BLOOD PLASMA OF CULTURED GREY MULLET (*MUGIL CEPHALUS*)

Mullet blood	lipoxygenase activity 5-HETE	12-HETE (pmole/min/mg protein)	15-HETE
erythrocyte	1.1	4.2	0.3
platelet	139.0	2817.0	94.8
plasma	2.0	27.8	1.4

[1] Lipoxygenase activity was assayed on 100 μM arachidonic acid as substrate in 0.2 M phosphate buffer (pH 6.5) at 25°C for 30 min. Products were analyzed with HPLC.

TABLE 3.
EFFECT OF DIETARY VITAMIN E ON PLATELET 12-LIPOXYGENASE ACTIVITY[1] OF CULTURED GREY MULLET (SAMPLED IN SEPTEMBER)

diet		platelet 12-LOX activity
Fish oil (%)	Vitamin E (ppm)	12-HETE (nmole/min/mg protein)
1	828	1.261
	1851	0.838
5	828	1.252
	1851	0.946

[1]Lipoxygenase activity was assayed as shown in Table 2

based on measurements of the hydroxy products reduced from hydroperoxy radicals, the modulation of lipoxygenase-catalyzed peroxidation could be a result of the free radical scavenger function of vitamin E. Therefore a test was designed to preincubate the platelet 12-LOX with vitamin E ranging up to 1500 μM at 25°C in 0.2 M phosphate buffer, pH 6.5 for 30 min, then assayed for 12-HETE.

The platelet 12-LOX preincubated with vitamin E (1500 μM) showed a 12-HETE content down to 26.9% of the control, while that preincubated without the vitamin E but which was added during assay showed a reduction of 12-HETE to 55.1% (Fig. 3). Both treatments formed 12-HETE inversely proportional to vitamin E addition. The proportionate ratio was more pronounced in the treatment preincubated with vitamin E. These observations suggest that the effects of the α-tocopherol on LOX-catalyzed peroxidation were two fold. It not only served as a peroxide scavenger but also partially inhibited the LOX enzyme.

Since the dietary vitamin E requirement of blue tilapia increased by 3 to 4 ppm for every percent of increase in corn oil in the diet (Roem *et al.* 1990), the experiment was done at two levels of fish oil, 1 and 5% (Table 3). No significant difference was found between these two levels on the modulation of 12-LOX catalysis.

Effect of Dietary Vitamin E on Blood Viscosity

Since vitamin E was found to inhibit the LOX-catalyzed oxidation of polyunsaturated fatty acids in blood cells of cultured mullet (Table 3, Fig. 2 and 3), and it reduced hemolysis in vitro (Shyu and Pan 1993), the flow behavior of blood was also expected to change with tocopherol concentration. The apparent viscosity of mullet blood was measured at 15 and 25°C over a range of shear rate (0.3 to 300 S^{-1}). The apparent viscosity was shear dependent at both temperatures (Fig. 4). The blood viscosity of mullet fed with diet fortified with 400 mg/kg vitamin E was significantly lower than that fed with the basal diet indicating α-tocopherol present in blood has a blood thinning effect possibly by reducing the oxidation of the polyunsaturated fatty acids in blood cell membrane and maintaining a better deformability of erythrocytes.

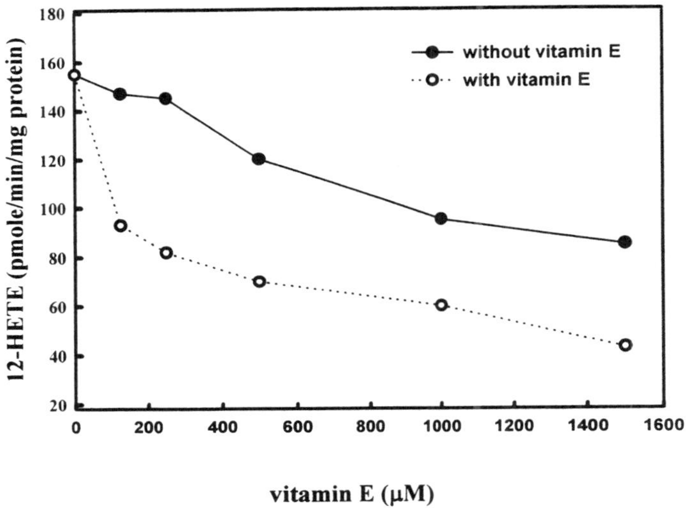

FIG. 3. EFFECT OF VITAMIN E CONCENTRATION ON THE ACTIVITY OF MULLET PLATELET 12-LIPOXYGENASE USING ARACHIDONIC ACID AS SUBSTRATE

(1) Platelets (10 mg protein/ml) were preincubated in 0.2 M phosphate buffer (pH 6.5) with vitamin E at 25°C for 30 min, then assayed for 12-lipoxygenase activity. (2) Platelet was preincubated in 0.2 M phosphate buffer (pH 6.5) at 25°C for 30 min, then added with vitamin E and assayed immediately for 12-lipoxygenase activity.

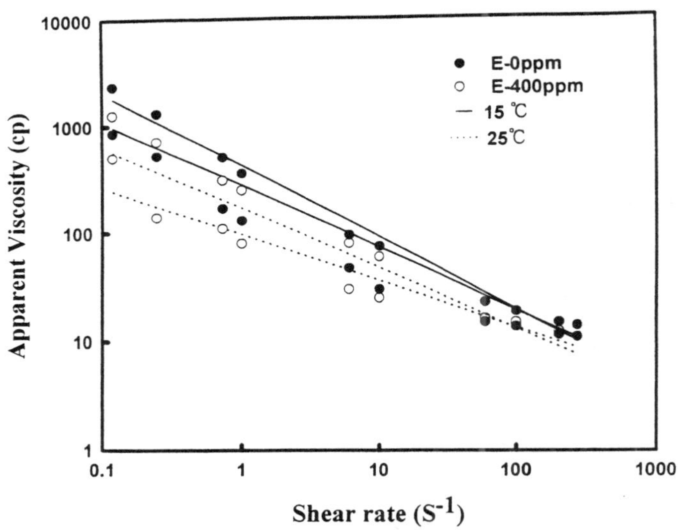

FIG 4. EFFECTS OF TEMPERATURE AND SHEAR RATE ON THE VISCOSITY OF CULTURED MULLET OF ONE YEAR (1+) FED WITH DIETS FORTIFIED WITH VITAMIN E FOR 10 MONTHS

(hematocrit: 50 ± 1%; sampled in January)

ACKNOWLEDGMENT

This project was supported by the National Science Council of the Republic of China with a grant NSC 82-0409-B-019-018.

REFERENCES

AOAC (Association of Official Analytical Chemists). 1984. W. Horwitz (ed.), Official Methods of Analysis, 13th Ed. Washington, D.C., U.S.A.

AUGUSTIN, J., KLEIN, B.P., BECKER, D. and VENUGOPAL, P.B. 1985. Methods of Vitamin Assay. 4th Ed. John Wiley and Sons Press, New York.

AYORINDE, F.O., OLOGUNDE, M.O., NANA, E.Y., BERNARD, B.N., AFOLABL, O.A. and SHEPARD, F.O. 1989. Determination of fatty acid composition of Amaranthus species. J. Am. Oil Chem. Soc. *66*, 1812–1814.

COWEY, C.B., ADRON, J.W. and YOUNGSON, A. 1983. The vitamin E requirement of rainbow trout (*Salmo gairdmer*) given diets containing polyunsaturated fatty acids derived from fish oil. Aquaculture *30*, 85–93.

DANIEL, W.W. 1974. Kruskal-Wallis One-way Analysis of Variance by Ranks. Applied Nonparametric Statistics. Houghton Mifflin Co. New York. pp. 201–206.

FOLCH, J., LEES, M. and SLOANE, S.G.H. 1957. A simple method for the isolation and purification of total lipids from animal tissues. J. Biol. Chem. *226*, 497–509.

GERMAN, J.B. and BERGER, R. 1990. Formation of 8, 15-dihydroxyeicosatetraenoic acid via 15- and 12-lipoxygenase in fish gill. Lipids *25*, 849–853.

GOETZL, E.J. 1980. Vitamin E modulates the lipoxygenase of arachidonic acid in leukocytes. Nature *288*, 183–185.

HALVER, J.E. 1982. The vitamins required for cultivated salmonids. Comp. Biochem. Physiol. *73B*, 43–50.

HO, P.P.K., WALTERS, C.P. and SULLIVAN, H.R. 1977. A particulate arachidonate lipoxygenase in human blood platelets. Biochem. Biophys. Res. Commun. *76*, 398–405.

HSU, H.H. and PAN, B.S. 1996. Effects of protector and hydroxyapatite partial purification on stability of lipoxygenase from grey mullet gill. J. Agric. Food Chem. *44*(3), 741–745.

MINO, M., NAKAGAWA, S., TAMSI, H. and MIKI, M. 1982. Clinical evaluation of red blood cell tocopherol. Ann. N.Y. Acad. Sci. *393*, 175–178.

NIKI, E., KOMURO, E., TAKAHASHI, M., URANO, S., ITO, E. and TERAO, K. 1988. Oxidative hemolysis of erythrocytes and its inhibition by free radical scavenger. J. Biochem. *263*(36), 19809–19814.

OLSSON, A.G. and YUAN, X.M. 1996. Antioxidants in the prevention of atherosclerosis. Curr. Opin. Lipidol. *7*(6), 374–380.

PAN, B.S., SHEEN, S.-S., SHEW, S.-H., CHEN, C.-M. and HUNG, J. 1992. Difference in sex ratio and physiological indices of cultured and wild grey mullet *Mugil cephalus* in Taiwan. Nippon Suisan Gakkaishi *58*(7), 1229–1235.

ROEM, A.J., KOHLER, C.C. and STICKNEY, R.R. 1990. Vitamin E requirements of the blue tilapia *Oreochromis aureus*, in relation to dietary lipid level. Aquaculture *87*, 155–164.

SHYU, J.F. and PAN, B.S. 1993. Influence of dietary vitamin E on the content of vitamin E in blood plasma, ovary tissue and on hemolysis of cultured female grey mullet (*Mugil cephalus*). J. Food Drug Analysis *1*(2), 155–163.

THOMAS, S.R., NEUZIL, J., MOHR, D. and STOCKER, R. 1995. Co-antioxidants make alpha-tocopherol an efficient antioxidant for low-density lipoprotein. Am. J. Clin. Nutr. *62*(6), 1357s–1364s.

UEDA, T. and IGARASHI, O. 1990. Determination of vitamin E in biological specimens and foods by HPLC. Pretreatment of samples and extraction of tocopherols. J. Micronut. Anal. *7*, 79–96.

URANO, S., IIDA, M., OTANI, I. and MATSUO, M. 1987. Membrane stabilization of vitamin E interactions of alpha-tocopherol with phospholipid in bilayer liposomes. Biochem. Biophys. Res. Commun. *146*, 1413–1418.

WALLACH, D.P. and BROWN, V.R. 1981. A novel preparation of human platelet lipoxygenase. Biochim. Biophy. Acta. *663*, 361–372.

WATANABE, T., TAKEUCHI, T., WADA, M. and UEHARA, R. 1981. The relationship between dietary lipid levels and alpha-tocopherol requirement of rainbow trout. Bull. Jpn. Soc. Sci. Fish *47*, 1463–1471.

APPLICATION OF DIPHASIC DIALYSIS EXTRACTION IN ETHYL CARBAMATE ANALYSIS

FUU SHEU and YUAN-TAY SHYU

Department of Horticulture
National Taiwan University
Taipei, Taiwan R.O.C.

ABSTRACT

Application of diphasic dialysis in the extraction of ethyl carbamate (as model mid-polar compound) was developed. The dialysis times as well as sample-to-solvent volume ratio were also determined. n-Propyl carbamate was used as internal standard and the calibration curve was referred for quantitation. Use of dichloromethane as dialysis solvent resulted in the highest recovery. The lowest detectable level was 5 μg/L and the linearity was acceptable. Eleven domestic wines were analyzed and the ethyl carbamate contents and relative recoveries ranged between 0-249.6 μg/L and 75.4-96.4%, respectively. The quantitation results between traditional methods and diphasic dialysis were similar, but diphasic dialysis extraction method had the advantage of solvent saving.

INTRODUCTION

Diphasic dialysis is a new and developing technique for sample preparation in the 1990s. It is usually applied in the extraction of low molecular weight substances which are soluble in organic solvents from aqueous sample. Two immiscible phases, such as water and organic solvent, are separated by a semipermeable membrane in a classic diphasic dialysis apparatus. During the diphasic dialysis, the desired compounds will pass through the membrane and move toward the organic solvent phase, while larger molecular weight or more polar substances are retained in water phase by the membrane. Thus, the extraction based on the molecular weight and the solubility in organic solvent is classified as a selective technique (Dominguez *et al.* 1992).

Miere *et al.* (1977) used polyethylene film for dialysis of nonpolar compounds from water into organic solvents. Later, Byrne and Aylott (1980) patented a device which separated a nonpolar organic solvent from water by semipermeable membranes that concentrated organic molecules from water. Heindorf and Zabik extended this concept to solvent filled bags of polymeric films, designed for field monitoring of organic aqueous contaminants (Huckins *et al.* 1990). Tuinstra *et al.* (1990) developed an on-line monitoring approach for aflatoxin M1 determination in milk; however the recoveries were about 50%. Huckins *et al.* (1990) reported the application of membrane dialysis for the determination of nonpolar organochlorine analytes from fish oil, and 93% of tested analytes were removed from water. Dominguez *et al.* (1992), Diaz *et al.* (1993), and Bayo *et al.* (1994) reported more applications of this technique in the analysis of aflatoxin M1 from milk, patulin from apple juice, clenbuterol from urine, and heptachlor from water. They extended the applications, achieved better recoveries, and named this technique as "diphasic dialysis".

The theories and kinetic mechanisms of this complex two-phase dialysis system are not clear, neither are some of the factors used in classic dialysis. In literature, the efficiency of diphasic dialysis and the recovery of target compound are influenced by the properties of interest compound, the selected organic solvent, the type of semipermeable membrane, the volume ratio of sample to organic solvent, the adjusted pH of sample, and the dialysis time (Dominguez *et al.* 1992; Diaz *et al.* 1993). Compared with the traditional liquid-liquid extraction, diphasic dialysis not only avoids the problems such as protein precipitation and lipid emulsions, but also comprises the advantages of labor and solvent saving (Diaz *et al.* 1993; Bayo *et al.* 1994).

Ethyl carbamate was recognized as a carcinogen, and commonly found in various fermented beverages. The official procedure of ethyl carbamate analysis is composed of dichloromethane extraction, concentration, and gas chromatography determination. Our previous work (Sheu *et al.* 1994) showed that ethyl carbamate was a hydrophilic compound with low extraction efficiency (the partition ratio in water/dichloromethane = 1 is 1.69), and the solutes within the tested samples such as ethanol and sugar would significantly influence the recovery. Thus, calibration with spiked internal standard is necessary for ethyl carbamate analysis.

We then intended to adapt diphasic dialysis technique for the extraction of ethyl carbamate as a model for mid-polar compound extraction. Parameters affecting the efficiency and calibration methods of diphasic dialysis were examined and the ethyl carbamate contents of some alcoholic beverages sold in Taiwan were determined.

MATERIALS AND METHODS

Effect of dialysis time on the recoveries of ethyl carbamate and n-propyl carbamate in simulation sample is shown in Fig. 1(a) and (b). The recoveries of both ethyl carbamate and n-propyl carbamate increased with time. After 12 h of dialysis, the recovery of ethyl carbamate achieved 95% of the equilibrium state (48 h). Figure 1(a) and (b) showed that the recoveries for both ethyl carbamate and n-propyl carbamate are higher in dichloromethane system than in ethyl acetate system. Higher level of solvent recovery was obtained when dichloromethane was used as extraction solvent rather than ethyl acetate (69.98% to 61.51%, figure not shown). The result indicated that dichloromethane was more suitable than ethyl acetate for ethyl carbamate extraction when using diphasic dialysis method.

Figure 2 shows the recovery of ethyl carbamate decreased when the volume ratio of sample to dichloromethane increased, but the decrease of the ethyl carbamate recovery seemed to slow down when the sample volume is more than 4 times of the solvent volume. Six repeats were performed to test the dialysis conditions while the sample to solvent volume ratio was fixed at 4, and the results of ethyl carbamate recovery (22.9 ± 0.4%) and detection limit (5 ppb) in simulation sample were reproducible.

Due to the hydrophilic characteristic of ethyl carbamate, the absolute recovery of ethyl carbamate (ca. 23%) was too low to be quantitated by diphasic dialysis method. The methods developed for accuracy improvement included (a) using calibration curve as reference curve instead of standard curve during quantitation, (b) using spiked internal standard, (c) using standard addition method for relative recovery calibration.

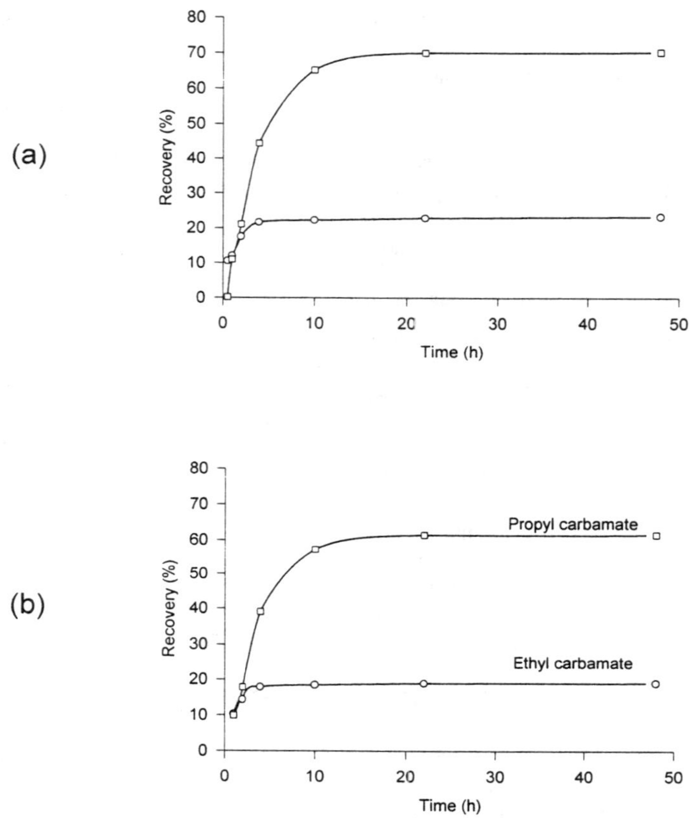

FIG. 1. EFFECT OF DIALYSIS TIME ON THE RECOVERIES OF ETHYL CARBAMATE (EC) AND PROPYL CARBAMATE (PC) IN SIMULATION SAMPLE
(a) dichloromethane used as extraction solvent; (b) ethyl acetate used as extraction solvent. All experiments were performed in triplicate.

Figure 3 is the calibration curve of simulation samples after dialysis extraction, concentration and analysis. The high linear regression correlation (0.9979) indicated that the method we developed had good linearity and high reproducibility with a 0.235 RRF value. The lowest detectable concentration was 5 ppb with 91.7% relative recovery (Table 1).

The method used for ethyl carbamate analysis in alcoholic beverage was based on the results of simulation experiments. Figure 4 was the chromatogram of Shao-Hsing wine after diphasic dialysis and GC/MS determination. The retention time of ethyl carbamate was 15.94 min. Table 2 shows the results of spike and recovery test using diphasic dialysis for 11 alcoholic beverages with 500 ppb ethyl carbamate spiked. The relative recoveries (75.44-96.36%) and the coefficient of variation (2.8-6.8%) among samples were acceptable.

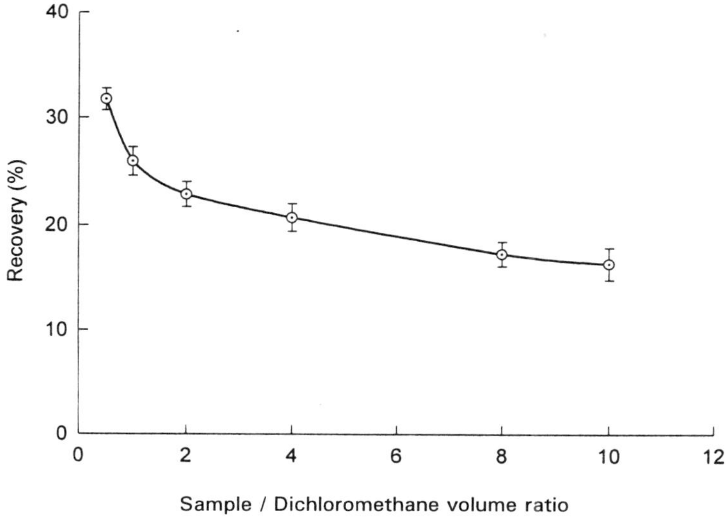

FIG. 2. EFFECT OF THE VOLUME RATIO OF SAMPLE TO DICHLOROMETHANE ON THE RECOVERY OF ETHYL CARBAMATE IN STIMULATION SAMPLE
All experiments were performed in triplicate.

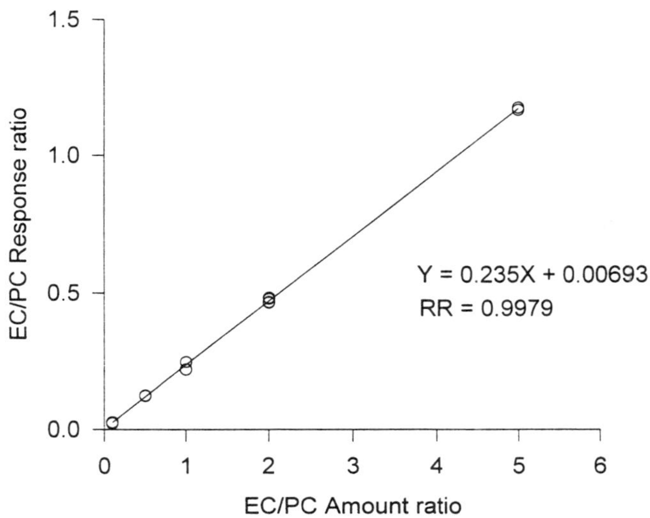

FIG. 3. CALIBRATION CURVE OF ETHYL CARBAMATE TO PROPYL CARBAMATE

TABLE 1.
LOWEST QUANTITATIVELY DETERMINABLE CONCENTRATION OF ETHYL CARBAMATE IN SIMULATION SAMPLE AFTER DIPHASIC DIALYSIS BY GAS CHROMATOGRAPHY WITH MS DETECTOR

Ethyl carbamate content (ppb)	Detectability	Relative recovery[a] (%)	S.D.[b] (%)
100	Yes	100.4	1.1
50	Yes	98.8	4.8
10	Yes	96.3	7.4
5	Yes	91.7	21.6
2	No	-	-
1	No	-	-

[a] Blank and spiked samples were quantitated by calibration curve. Recovery calculated by traced amount divided by spiked × 100.
[b] Coefficient of variation (cv%).
All experiments were performed in triplicate.

According to our previous studies, the interference of solutes distributed in alcoholic beverage, such as ethanol and sugars would decrease the recovery of ethyl carbamate. This unavoidable problem explained why the relative recoveries were not 100%. Table 3 shows the comparisons of ethyl carbamate levels determined by diphasic dialysis to other classical methods in some alcohol beverages. Results indicated that diphasic dialysis technique could be applied on the analysis of mid-polar compound in aqueous samples.

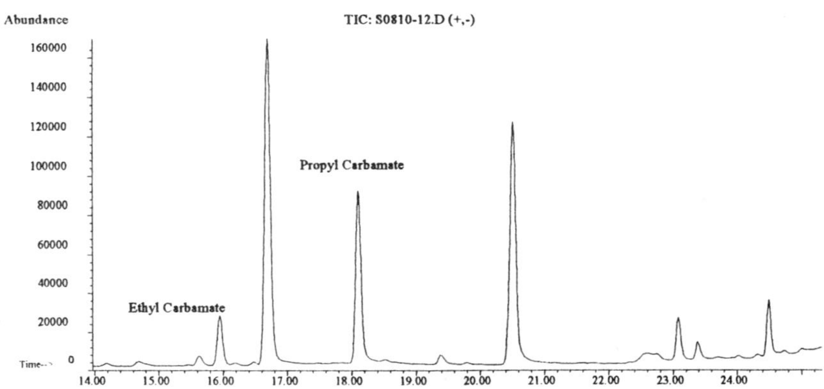

FIG. 4. CHROMATOGRAM OF SHAO HSING WINE AFTER DIPHASIC DIALYSIS BY MASS SPECTRUM DETECTOR
(SIM mode, target ions:44, 62,74).

TABLE 2.
CONTENTS AND RELATIVE RECOVERIES OF ETHYL CARBAMATE FROM ALCOHOLIC BEVERAGES BY DIPHASIC DIALYSIS

Sample	Ethyl carbamate found[a] (ppb)	Found after spiked ethyl carbamate[b] (ppb)	Relative recovery[c] (%)	S.D.[d] (%)
Shao Hsing wine	249.6	658.8	81.84	5.1
Rose wine	11.5	394.2	76.54	6.8
Red wine	9.1	368.3	75.44	6.4
Plum liqueur	28.2	432.1	80.78	3.6
Rice wine	240.1	696.3	91.24	4.1
White wine	0	460.3	92.06	5.8
Light grape liqueur	7.8	420.3	82.50	4.4
Honey grape wine	6.4	446.0	86.92	5.2
Rum	34.5	516.3	96.36	6.1
Premium plum liqueur	0	384.2	76.86	6.7
Apple vinegar	66.9	492.3	85.08	2.8

[a] Original ethyl carbamate content in each sample.
[b] 500 ppb of ethyl carbamate was added to each sample.
[c] (b - a) / 500
[d] Coefficient of variation (cv%).
All experiments were performed in triplicate.

TABLE 3.
COMPARISON OF ETHYL CARBAMATE IN SOME ALCOHOLIC BEVERAGES BY DIFFERENT METHODS

	Ethanol (%)	Ethyl carbamate content (ppb)		
		Method A[a]	Method B[b]	Method C[c]
Rose wine	10	11.5	9	14
Plum wine	15	28.2	24	26
Rice wine	22	240.1	296	274
Light grape liqueur	2	7.8	n.d.	11
Premium plum liqueur	19	66.9	68	65

[a] Diphasic dialysis.
[b] Solvent extraction and calibration quantitation (Sheu 1994; Canas 1988; Conacher 1987).
[c] Solvent extraction and standard addition quantitation (Sheu 1994).
All experiments were performed in triplicate.

ACKNOWLEDGMENT

We express our appreciation to Dr. On Lee for his helpful suggestions.

REFERENCES

BAYO, J., MORENO, M.A., PRIETA, J., DIAZ, S., SUAREZ, G. and DOMINGUEZ, L. 1994. Chloramphenicol extraction from milk by using the diphasic dialysis method followed by liquid chromatographic determination. J. Assoc. Offic. Anal. Chem. *77*, 854–856.

BLANCO, J.L., DOMINGUEZ, L., RODRIGUEZ, E.F. and SUAREZ, G. 1987. Determination of aflatoxin M1 in milk and milk products contaminated at low level. J. Assoc. Offic. Anal. Chem. *70*, 470–472.

BYRNE, G.A. and AYLOTT, R.I. 1980. British patent 1566253, Concentrator for Removing Organic Materials from Aqueous Systems.

CANAS, B.J., HAVERY, D.C. and JOE, F.L. 1988. Rapid gas chromatographic method for determining ethyl carbamate in alcoholic beverages with thermal energy analyzer detection. J. Assoc. Offic. Anal. Chem. *71*, 509–511.

CONACHER, H.S.B. 1987. Capillary column gas chromatographic determination of ethyl carbamate in alcoholic beverages with confirmation by gas chromatography/mass spectrometry. J. Assoc. Offic. Anal. Chem. *70*, 749–751.

DIAZ, S., MORENO, M.A., DOMINGUEZ, L., SUAREZ, G. and BLANCO, J.L. 1993. Application of a diphasic dialysis technique to the extraction of aflatoxins in dairy products. J. Dairy Sci. *76*, 1845–1849.

DOMINGUEZ, L., BLANCO, J.L., MORENO, M.A., DIAZ, S.D., PRIETA, J., CAMARA, J.M., BAYO, J. and SUAREZ, G. 1982. Diphasic dialysis: a new membrane method for a selective and efficient extraction of low molecular weight organic compounds from aqueous solutions. J. Assoc. Off. Anal. Chem. *75*, 854– 857.

HUCKINS, J.N., TUBERGEN, M.W., LEBO, J.A., GALE, R.W. and SCHWARTZ, T.R. 1990. Polymeric film dialysis in organic solvent media for cleanup of organic contaminants. J. Assoc. Off. Anal. Chem. *73*, 290–293.

MIERE, J.P., MAPPES, G.W., TUCKER, E.S. and DIETRICH, M.W. 1977. Identification and Analysis of Organic Pollutants in Water, L.H. Keith (ed.), Ann Arbor Science Publisher, Inc., Ann Arbor, MI, pp. 113–133.

PIERCE, W.M., CLARK, A.O. and HURST, H.E. 1980. Determination of ethyl carbamate in distilled alcoholic beverages by gas chromatography with flame ionization or mass spectrometric detection. J. Assoc. Offic. Anal. Chem. *71*, 781–784.

SHEU, F., CHEN, M.Y. and SHYU, Y.T. 1994. Studies on the methodology of ethyl carbamate analysis in foods(1) - Selection of internal standards and reference curves as well as the effects of ethanol and glucose on the extraction. J. Chinese Soci. Hort. Sci. *40*, 287–296.

TUINSTRA, L.M., KIENHUIS, P.G. and DOLS, P. 1990. Automated liquid chromatography determination of aflatoxin M1 in milk using on-line dialysis for sample preparation. J. Assoc. Off. Anal. Chem. *73*, 969–973.

ZIMMERLI, B. and SCHLATTER, J. 1991. Ethyl carbamate: analytical methodology, occurrence, formation, biological activity and risk assessment. Mutation Res. *259*, 325–350.

MOLECULAR BASIS OF ALCOHOLIC AROMA FORMATION DURING TEA PROCESSING

KANZO SAKATA, NAOHARU WATANABE and TAIICHI USUI

Faculty of Agriculture
Shizuoka University
836 Ohya, Shizuoka 422, Japan

ABSTRACT

Alcoholic tea aroma compounds, such as geraniol and linalool, are known to mainly contribute to the floral aroma of oolong and black tea, and to be produced during the fermentation process in their manufacturing. We were very interested in oolong tea which is processed via the most complicated processing to be rich in floral aroma. Recently we have isolated and identified the alcoholic tea aroma precursors as well as the specific enzyme (β-primeverosidase) concerned with the aroma formation.

*From the tea leaves (*Camellia sinensis *var.* sinensis cvs. *Shuixian and Maoxie) to be processed to oolong tea, we have isolated and identified alcoholic aroma precursors of geraniol, linalool, 2-phenylethanol, benzyl alcohol, linalool oxides I and II* (trans- *and* cis-*linalool 3,6-oxide), and methyl salicylate as β-primeverosides (6-O-β-D-xylopyranosyl-β-D-glucopyranosides), guided by an enzymatic hydrolysis (with the acetone powder prepared from cv. Yabukita) and followed by GC and GC-MS analyses. Aroma precursors of linalool oxides III and IV* (cis- *and* trans-*linalool 3,7-oxides) and (Z)-3-hexenol were found to be present particularly as 6-O-β-D-apiofuranosyl-β-glucopyranoside and β-D-glucopyranoside, respectively.*

We have also purified β-primeverosidases from fresh leaves of cv. Yabukita for Japanese green tea, cv. Shuixian for oolong tea and a cultivar of C. s. var. assamica *for black tea. The molecular weight of each enzyme was shown to be 60.5, 60.2 and 60.3 kDa by TOFMS, respectively. The enzymatic characteristics (optimum temperature, 45 °C; stable temp., 40-45 °C; optimum pH, 4; pH stability, pH 3-5; specific activity, 0.90-0.99 unit/mg) were very similar to each other. The enzyme was confirmed to hydrolyze the aroma precursors, β-primeverosides as well as 6-O-β-D-apiofuranosyl-β-D-glucopyranoside, into disaccharides and each aglycon (alcoholic tea aroma) without further hydrolysis.*

As a consequence, the alcoholic aroma formation during processing of fermented tea (oolong and black tea) has been substantiated on a molecular basis that most of the alcoholic tea aroma compounds are stored mainly as disaccharide glycosides (β-primeverosides and 6-O-β-D-apiofuranosyl-β-D-glucopyranosides) and generated by the action of a specific enzyme, β-primeverosidase, during fermentation process in tea manufacturing.

INTRODUCTION

Any tea leaves can basically be processed to green, oolong or black tea, although suitable cultivars for each tea have been developed. Floral tea aroma compounds are known to be generated during the fermentation process in the tea manufacturing (Withering and Turn over processes in oolong tea production and Withering and Fermentation processes in black tea production; Fig. 1) and is one of the most important factors to determine the quality of each tea type, especially oolong and black tea (Yamanishi 1995).

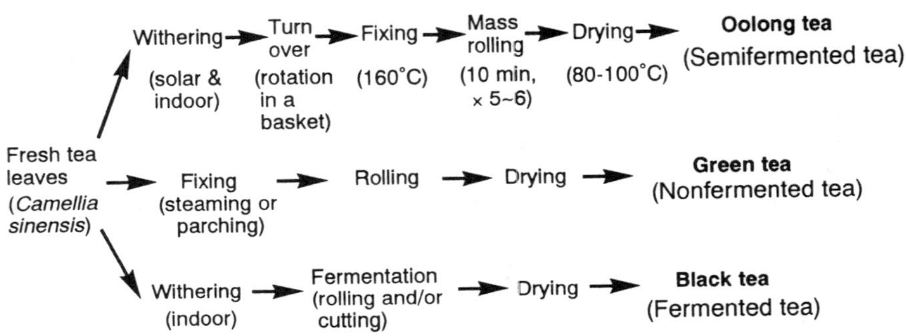

FIG. 1. TEA MANUFACTURING PROCESS

In the course of our study on the molecular basis of the alcoholic aroma formation in oolong tea, we isolated aroma precursors of most of the alcoholic aroma compounds as glycosides. Most of them were β-primeverosides (6-0-β-D-xylopyranosyl-β-D-glucopyranosides) (Guo *et al.* 1993; Guo *et al.* 1994; Moon *et al.* 1994; Sakata *et al.* 1995a; Moon *et al.* 1996). But the aroma precursors of linalool oxides III and IV (*cis*- and *trans*-linalool 3,7-oxides) and (Z)-3-hexenol were especially isolated as 6-O-β-D-apiofuranosyl-β-D-glucopyranosides and β-D-glucopyranoside, respectively (Moon *et al.* 1996).

Kobayashi *et al.* (1994) had, for the first time, isolated and identified (Z)-3-hexenyl and benzyl β-D-glucopyranosides as aroma precursors from cv. Yabukita (see also Yano *et al.* 1991). Recently, they also found geranyl β-primeveroside as well as geranyl β-vicianoside (6-O-α-L-arabinopyranosyl-β-D-glucopyranoside) in cv. Yabukita (Nishikitani *et al.* 1996). Figure 2 summarizes all the alcoholic aroma precursors isolated from tea leaves by us and Kobayshi's group.

Quite recently we have purified a β-primeverosidase from fresh tea leaves (cvs. Yabukita and Shuixian) (Guo *et al.* 1996; Sakata *et al.* 1995b; Ogawa *et al.* 1997). Here we describe the purification of β-primeverosidase from fresh leaves of a cultivar for black tea (C. *sinensis* var. *assamica*) to compare its enzymatic and chemical properties with those of the β-primeverosidases from green and oolong tea leaves (cvs. Yabukita and Shuixian), together with its substrate specificity toward several kinds of disaccharide glycosides which were mainly isolated as aroma precursors.

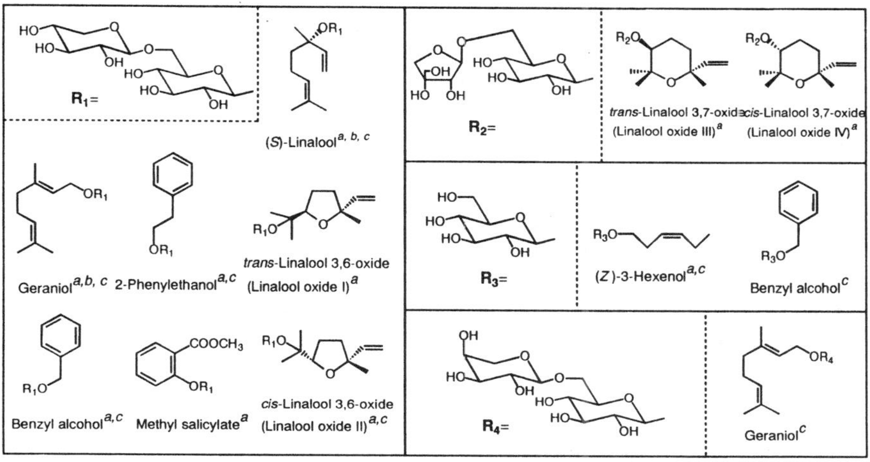

FIG. 2. ALCOHOLIC AROMA PRECURSORS ISOLATED FROM TEA LEAVES
a: from oolong tea leaves (cv. Maoxie); *b*: from oolong tea leaves (cv. Shuixian);
c: from green tea leaves (cv.Yabukita)

MATERIALS AND METHODS

Purification of β-Primeverosidase

From var. assamica. All operations were carried out at 4°C unless otherwise stated. Fresh tea leaves of *C. sinensis* var. *assamica*, which were plucked at the Makurazaki Station of the National Institute of Vegetables, Ornamental Plants and Tea (NIVOT), Kagoshima, Japan, in November, 1996, were subjected to the conventional preparation process for acetone powder. The acetone powder (20 g, equivalent to 100 g of fresh tea leaves) was suspended in 0.1 M citrate buffer (pH 6.0, 800 mL) containing 2 mM DTT (dithiothreitol), 5 mM EDTA, Polyclar SB-100 (30 g) and ascorbic acid (1 g), stirred for 1.5 h, and centrifuged at 35,000 g for 20 min. To the combined supernatant (ca. 570 mL), chilled acetone (-4°C) was added up to 50% with stirring and left overnight at 4°C. The precipitate obtained by centrifugation at 35,000 g for 20 min was dissolved in 0.1 M citrate buffer (pH 6.0, 200 mL) containing 2 mM DTT and subjected to conventional ammonium sulfate precipitation. The crude enzyme separated between 40 to 80% ammonium sulfate saturation was dissolved in 32 mL of 20 mM citrate buffer (pH 6.0) and then dialyzed overnight against the same buffer. The dialyzed enzyme was placed on a CM-Toyopearl 650M column (ϕ32 × 140 mm, ca. 110 mL) equilibrated with 20 mM citrate buffer (pH 6.0). The adsorbed protein was eluted by a linear gradient elution of NaCl from 0 to 0.5 M in 500 mL each of 20 mM citrate buffer (pH 6.0) at a flow rate of 2 mL/min. Fractions of 10 mL were collected. Glycosidase activities were measured using several kinds of *p*-nitrophenyl (*p*NP) glycosides as previously reported (Ogawa *et al.* 1997).

The primeverosidase fractions were combined and concentrated using an ultrafiltration module (Amicon PM-10). A primeverosidase fraction obtained by the CM-Toyopearl column chromatography was further purified by FPLC on a column of Mono S HR (ϕ0.5 × 50 mm) equilibrated with 20 mM citrate buffer (pH 6.0). The enzyme was eluted by a linear gradient elution of NaCl from 0 to 0.2 M in the same buffer at a flow rate of 1 mL/min. Fractions of 1 mL were collected.

From cvs. Yabukita and Shuixian. Fresh leaves of cvs. Yabukita and Shuixian were plucked at NIVOT, Shizuoka, Japan, in May, 1995 and at the Species Garden of the Department of Tea Science, Zhejiang Agricultural University, Hangzhou, Zhejiang, P.R. China, in May, 1995. After plucking, the leaves were conventionally treated to prepare acetone powder and stored in a freezer (-20°C) before use. Purification of β-primeverosidases was carried out in the same manner as previously reported (Guo *et al.* 1996; Ogawa *et al.* 1997).

SDS-PAGE analysis, molecular weight measurement, isoelectric point measurement and effects of temperature and pH on the enzymic activity and stability were performed as described by Ogawa et al. 1997.

Peptide Mapping of β-Primeverosidases from Tea Leaves

Digestion of β-Primeverosidases by Trypsin. Each β-primeverosidase purified by FPLC was further purified by HPLC (Column: YMC-Pack C8; ϕ4.6 × 150 mm; equilibrated with H_2O containing 0.1% TFA). The adsorbed protein was eluted by a gradient elution of MeCN from 0 to 80% at a flow rate of 0.8 mL/min at 40°C. Each primeverosidase was eluted at 64 min, while a β-glucosidase from almond was eluted at 38 min under these conditions. Each primeverosidase fraction was evaporated to dryness by a centrifugal concentrator. The β-primeverosidase dissolved in a mixture of H_2O (120 μL) and PBS (40 μL) was denatured for 10 min at 100°C and reacted with 2-5 μg of trypsin for 24 h at 37°C.

HPLC Analysis of the Trypsin Hydrolysate of β-Primeverosidases. The hydrolysate of each β-primeverosidase obtained by hydrolysis by trypsin was concentrated with a centrifugal concentrator and analyzed by HPLC (BMLC-10, Shimadzu Co. Ltd.) equipped with a capillary column (FUS-15-03-C18; ϕ0.3 × 150 mm, equilibrated with 5% MeCN containing 0.1% TFA). Eluates were obtained by a gradient elution of MeCN from 5 to 90% at a flow rate of 2.5 μL/min at 40°C and monitored at 220 nm.

Substrate Specificity of the β-Primeverosidase from cv. Yabukita. GC Analysis of the Liberated Alcoholic Aroma (Ogawa *et al.* 1997)

Determination of the Liberated Sugars. The resulting aqueous phase after the extraction of the liberated aroma compounds was subjected to centrifugation with a Centricon-10 (Grace Japan, Co. Ltd., Tokyo) to remove proteins. The supernatant was analyzed by HPLC equipped with a Shodex SUGAR KS-801 (Φ8 × 300 mm) column (H_2O at flow rate of 0.5 mL/min; 70°C). Detection of sugars was performed at 415 nm by a post labelling method using 0.1 M H_3BO_3, 50 mM guanidine hydrochloride, 0.5 mM $NaIO_4$ and 20% MeCN (pH 12) at flow rate 0.5 mL/min at 170°C.

RESULTS AND DISCUSSION

Purification of β-Primeverosidase from *C. sinensis* var. *assamica* and Comparison with Those from var. *sinensis* cvs. Yabukita and Shuixian

First, we purified β-primeverosidase from cv. Yabukita (Guo *et al.* 1996), and then confirmed its presence in cv. Shuixian for oolong tea (Ogawa *et al.* 1997). Here, we attempted to purify the β-primeverosidase from a cultivar for black tea (var. *assamica*) and compare its enzymic and chemical characteristics with those of the primeverosidases from tea leaves for green and oolong tea. As oxidative enzyme activity is known to be more potent in black tea leaves than in oolong and green tea leaves, crude enzymes from black tea leaves were extracted from the acetone powder with 0.1 M citrate buffer (pH 6.0) containing 2 mM DTT, 5 mM EDTA, Polyclar SB100 and ascorbic acid, and subjected to acetone precipitation followed by 40-80% ammonium sulfate precipitation. The crude enzyme was applied onto a column of CM-Toyopearl in the same way, and glycosidase activities of each fraction were measured with *p*NP β-D-glucoside and *p*NP β-primeveroside (synthesized by enzymatic transglycosylation; unpublished). The β-primeverosidase from var. *assamica* was eluted just before the main glucosidase (Fig. 3). The elution pattern was similar to those of cvs. Yabukita and Shuixian (Ogawa *et al.* 1997). The β-primeverosidase fractions which were almost devoid of other glycosidases were purified by FPLC with a column of Mono S-HR (Fig. 4). The peak showing high

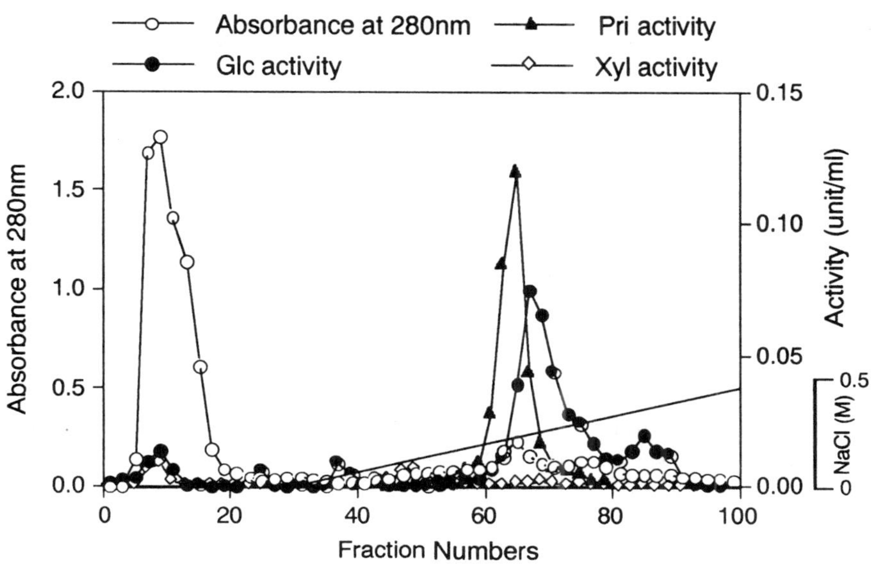

FIG. 3. CM-TOYOPEARL 650M COLUMN CHROMATOGRAPHY OF ENZYMES FROM BLACK TEA LEAVES (*CAMELLIA SINENSIS* VAR. *ASSAMICA*)
Elution: 20 mM citrate buffer (pH 6.0); NaCl gradient elution; flow rate, 2 ml/min.

primeverosidase activity and very low apparent β-glucosidase activity overlapped with the peak of absorption at 280 nm. The β-primeverosidase from var. *assamica* was shown to be a single protein of 61 kDa by SDS-PAGE analysis and identical to those of cvs. Yabukita (Guo *et al.* 1996; Sakata *et al.* 1995b) and Shuixian (Ogawa *et al.* 1997).

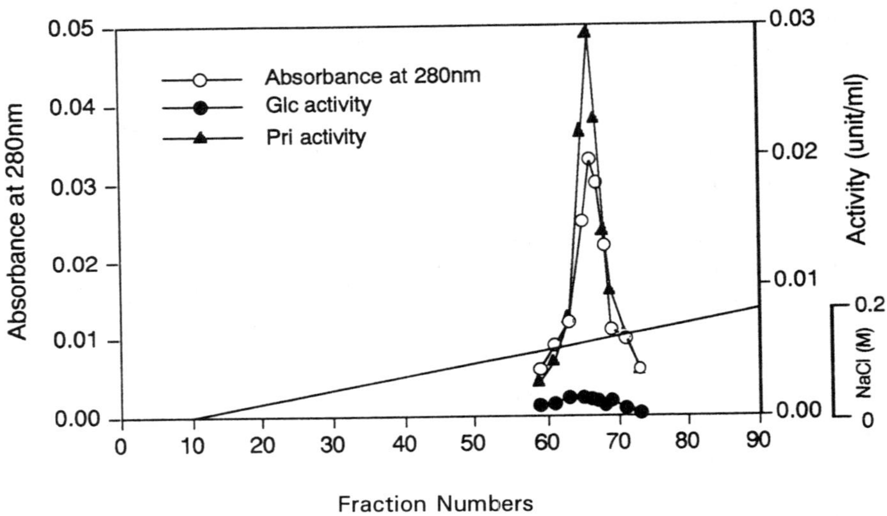

FIG. 4. FPLC OF A PRIMEVEROSIDASE FRACTION ON MONO S COLUMN FROM BLACK TEA LEAVES (*CAMELLIA SINENSIS* VAR. *ASSAMICA*)
Column: Mono S HR 5/5. Elution: 20 mM citrate buffer (pH 6.0); NaCl gradient elution; flow rate, 1 ml/min.

The β-primeverosidase showed maximal activity at 45°C and pH 4.0. It was stable at temperatures up to 40°C and between pH 4 and 5 (Fig. 5). The specific activity of the β-primeverosidase is 0.99 unit/mg which is very close to those of β-primeverosidases from cvs. Yabukita and Shuixian (Ogawa *et al.* 1997). The isoelectric point of the β-primeverosidase from var. *assamica* was found to be 9.5, which is very similar to those of the primeverosidases from cvs Yabukita (pI, 9.4) and Shuixian (pI, 9.5) (Guo *et al.* 1996; Ogawa *et al.* 1997). These analytical results suggest that β-primeverosidase from var. *assamica* is identical or quite similar to the enzymes from cvs. Yabukita and Shuixian.

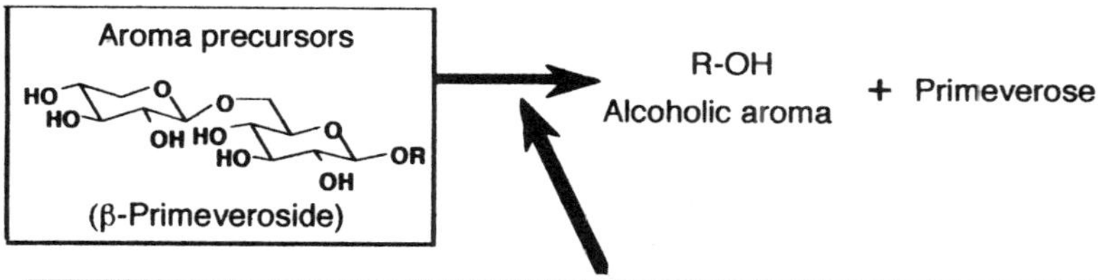

	β-Primeverosidase		
	From black tea	oolong tea	green tea
M.W.(kDa)	60.3	60.2	60.5
pI	9.5	9.5	9.4
Optimum temp.(℃)	45	45	45
Stable temp.(℃)	40	40	45
Optimum pH	4	4	4
pH stability	4~5	3~5	4~5
Specific activity (unit/mg)	0.99	0.98	0.90

FIG. 5. ENZYMATIC CHARACTERISTICS OF β-PRIMEVEROSIDASES FROM TEA LEAVES OF CULTIVARS FOR GREEN, OOLONG AND BLACK TEA AND A PROPOSED MECHANISM FOR THE MAIN ALCOHOLIC TEA AROMA FORMATION

The slight molecular weight differences among these three β-primeverosidases (60.3 kDa, 60.5 kDa and 60.2 kDa, respectively) shown by TOFMS analysis were suggested to be due to one or two amino acid residues based on an error range of 15-80 mμ in this mass region around 0-70 kDa. Each β-primeverosidase finally purified by HPLC with a YMC-Pack C8 column showed the same retention time. Each of them was digested by trypsin at 37°C for 24 h and analyzed by HPLC equipped with a capillary column of FUS-15-03-C18 (5 to 90% MeCN in 0.1% TFA). Each chromatogram showed a very similar elution profile (Fig. 6), however, that of var. *assamica* was a little different from those of cvs. Yabukita and Shuixian. This indicates that each enzyme from the green, oolong or black tea cultivar has a very similar molecular composition.

Substrate Specificity of β-Primeverosidase

β-Primeverosidases from tea leaves for green, oolong and black tea were shown to be enzymatically identical. The acetone powder from cv. Yabukita was treated in the same manner as shown above for var. *assamica* to give an elution profile of glycosidases (Fig. 7). Each fraction was measured for glucosidase and primeverosidase activities and then combined into Fractions A to H according to β-glucosidase activities. Several kinds of disaccharide glycosides (Fig. 8), which were mostly isolated as aroma precursors from tea leaves and some flower buds, were reacted with Fr. (fraction) C [primeverosidase (Pri)], Fr. E [glucosidase (Glc) II)], Frs. A + G (Glcs I and III) and Frs. A + E + G (Glcs I, II and III), respectively, and the generated aroma constituents were analyzed by GC.

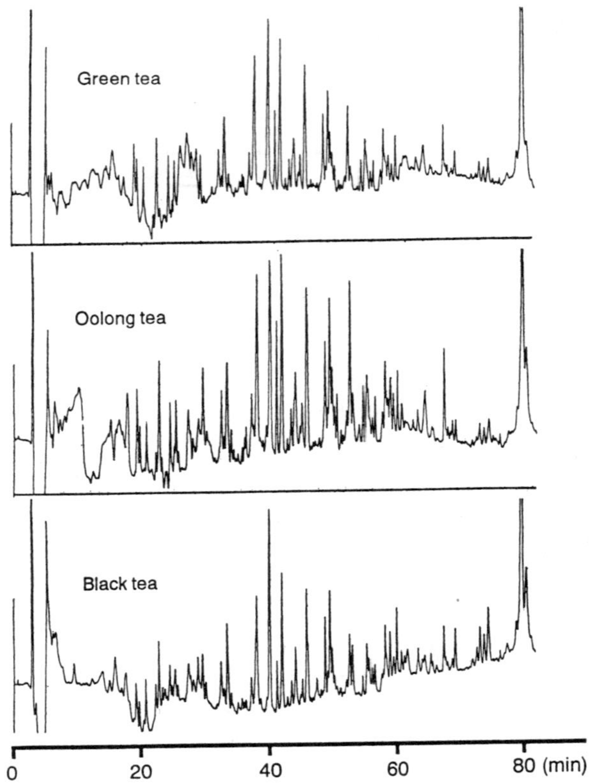

FIG. 6. PEPTIDE MAPPING OF EACH PRIMEVEROSIDASE FROM CULTIVARS FOR GREEN, OOLONG AND BLACK TEA

The Pri-fraction showed high substrate specificity toward linalyl and benzyl β-primeverosides as well as benzyl 6-O-β-D-apiofuranosyl-β-D-glucopyranoside (Table 1). The Glc-fractions (Frs. A, E and G) hydrolyzed the substrates much less effectively than the Pri-fraction. The Pri-fraction also hydrolyzed both geranyl 6-O-α-L-arabinofuranosyl-β-D-glucopyranoside and linalyl β-vicianoside. But the amounts of the liberated alcoholic aroma were much less than those produced by Glcs I + II + III which liberated arabinose, glucose and the corresponding aglycons (Fig. 9).

As a vicianoside was hydrolyzed much less effectively than primeverosides (Table 1), the axial hydroxyl group at C-4″ of the arabinose moiety (Fig. 8) may be responsible for the low reactivity; in other words, the lack of a substituent at C-4″ may be important for the recognition of a disaccharide moiety by the primeverosidase. We can guess that

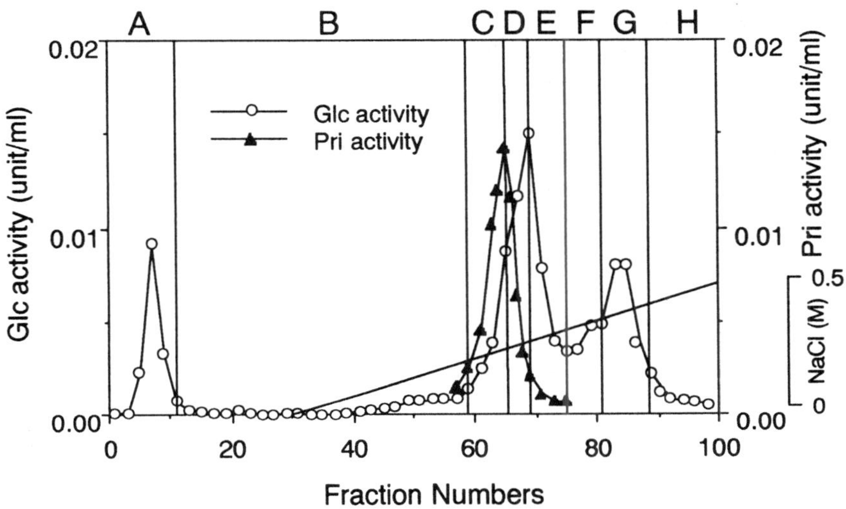

FIG. 7. CM-TOYOPEARL 650M COLUMN CHROMATOGRAPHY OF ENZYMES FROM TEA LEAVES (CV. SHUIXIAN)

Elution: 20 mM citrate buffer (pH 6.0); NaCl gradient elution; flow rate 2 mL/min. Glucosidase (Glc) and primeverosidase (Pri) activities were measured using *p*NP β-D-glucopyranoside and *p*NP β-primeveroside, respectively.

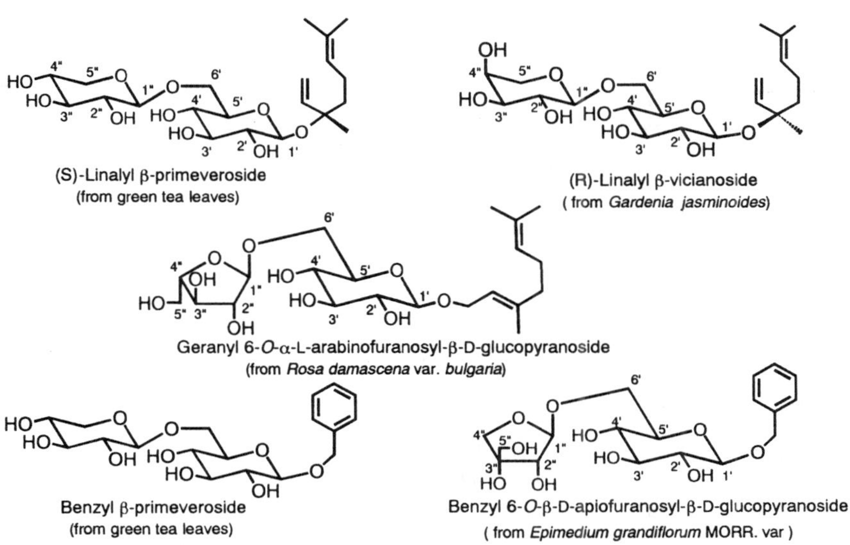

FIG. 8. STRUCTURES OF DISACCHARIDE GLYCOSIDES TESTED FOR THE ENZYMATIC HYDROLYSIS

TABLE 1.
HYDROLYSIS ACTIVITIES OF THE GLYCOSIDASES FROM TEA LEAVES (CV. YABUKITA) TOWARDS SEVERAL KINDS OF DISACCHARIDE GLYCOSIDES

Aroma precursor	Alcoholic aroma	Enzymes			
		Pri (Fr. C)	Glc II (Fr. E)	Glc I+III (Fr. A+G)	Glc I+II+III (Fr. A+E+G)
Benzyl β-primeveroside	Benzyl alcohol	100[a]			45
Linalyl β-primeveroside	Linalool	100	69	18	87
Benzyl 6-*O*-β-D-apiofuranosyl-β-D-glucopyranoside	Benzyl alcohol	100	4	5	9
Geranyl 6-*O*-α-L-arabinofuranosyl-β-D-glucopyranoside	Geraniol	50			100
Linalyl β-vicianoside (6-*O*-α-L-arabinopyranosyl-β-D-glucopyranoside)	Linalool	39			100

Pri, β-Primeverosidase fraction; Glc, β-Glcosidase fraction

[a] Activities are expressed as relative activities.

the β-primeverosidase recognizes a disaccharide unit, in which a monosaccharide is attached to the C-6′ hydroxyl group of the glucose moiety, to show a rather broad substrate specificity to these disaccharide glycosides.

Next, the remaining saccharide constituents in the residual aqueous layer in the enzymatic hydrolysates were analyzed by HPLC (Fig. 9). The peak observed at t_R 22 min in all the chromatograms was found to be a contaminate glycerol from the centrifugation equipment. The β-primeverosidase was clearly shown to recognize disaccharide units of benzyl β-primeveroside and benzyl 6-O-β-D-apiofuranosyl β-D-glucopyranoside to hydrolyze these disaccharide glycosides into aglycone and disaccharide. Both disaccharides were only slightly further hydrolyzed into monosaccharides by the β-primeverosidase. When benzyl β-primeveroside was reacted with a mixture of Glcs I, II and III, considerable amounts of monosaccharide (glucose and xylose) were liberated. But a lot of primeverose still remained, suggesting that the xylose moiety in either β-primeveroside or primeverose is difficult to be cleaved by other glycosidases. Based on these experimental results, the β-primeverosidase can be concluded to be the same from all three types of tea leaves.

As shown above, β-primeverosidase was shown to be the most important glycosidase in the floral alcoholic aroma formation in tea leaves and to be a glycosidase having a fairly broad substrate specificity toward disaccharide glycosides with a 1→6 glycosyl linkage.

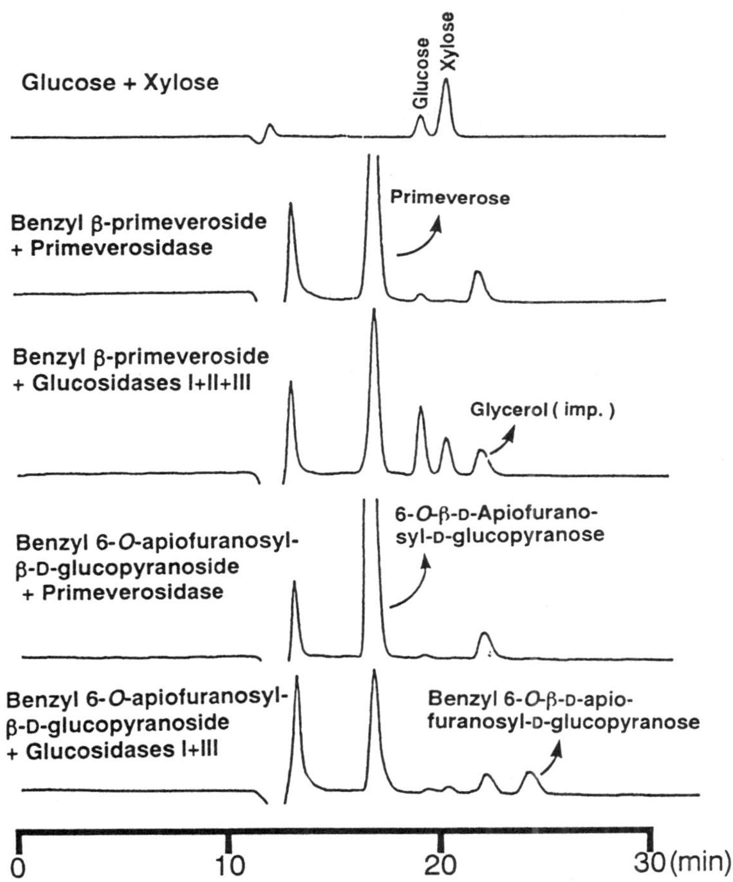

FIG. 9. HPLC SUGAR ANALYSIS OF THE ENZYMATIC HYDROLYSATES OF EACH DISACCHARIDE GLYCOSIDE

ACKNOWLEDGMENTS

The authors thank Dr. Hakamada and Mr. Y. Sawai of the National Research Institute of Vegetables, Ornamental Plants and Tea (Shizuoka, Japan), and Dr. Y. Takeda of its Makurazaki Station (Kagoshima, Japan) and Prof. Q. Tong of Department of Tea Science, Zhejiang Agricultural University, Hangzhou, P.R. China, for provision of the fresh tea leaves of cv. Yabukita, var. *assamica* sp. and cv. Shuixian, respectively. They thank Drs. M. Ohnishi-Kameyama and T. Nagata of National Food Research Institute, Ministry of Agriculture, Forestry and Fisheries (Tsukuba, Japan) and Ms. C. Sakai of Mitsuinorin Co. Ltd. (Fujieda, Japan) for MALDI-TOFMS measurements and isoelectric focusing analysis, respectively. They are indebted to Prof. T. Miyase of the School of Pharmaceutical Sciences, University of Shizuoka, for his generous gift of benzyl 6-O-β-D-apiofuranosyl-β-D-glucopyranoside.

This work was supported in part by a Grant-in-Aid for Scientific Research (B) (No. 07456060) to K.S. from the Ministry of Education, Science, Sports and Culture of Japan and by a Grant-in-Aid for the Joint Industry-University Project sponsored by Shizuoka Prefectural Government.

REFERENCES

GUO, W., SAKATA, K., WATANABE, N., NAKAJIMA, R., YAGI, A., INA, K. and LUO, S. 1993. Geranyl 6-O-β-D-xylopyranosyl-β-D-glucopyranoside isolated as an aroma precursor from tea leaves for oolong tea. Phytochemistry *33*, 1373–1375.

GUO, W., HOSOI, R., SAKATA, K., WATANABE, N., YAGI, A., INA, K. and LUO, S. 1994. (S)-Linalyl, 2-phenylethyl, and benzyl disaccharide glycosides isolated as aroma precursors from oolong tea leaves. Biosci. Biotech. Biochem. *58*, 1532–1534.

GUO, W., OGAWA, K., YAMAUCHI, K., WATANABE, N., USUI, T., LUO, S. and SAKATA, K. 1996. Isolation and characterization of a β-primeverosidase concerned with alcoholic aroma formation in tea leaves. Biosci Biotech. Biochem. *60*, 1810–1814.

KOBAYASHI, A., KUBOTA, K., JOKI, Y., WADA, E. and WAKABAYASHI, M. 1994. (Z)-3-Hexenyl-β-D-glucopyranoside in fresh tea leaves as a precursor of green odor. Biosci. Biotech. Biochem. *58*, 592–593.

MIYASE, T., UENO, A., TAKIZAWA, N., KOBAYASHI, H. and OGUCHI, H. 1988. Studies on the glycosides of *Epidemium grandiflorum* MORR. var. *thunbergianum* (MIQ.) NAKAI III. Chem. Pharm. Bull. *36*, 2475–2484.

MOON, J.-H., SAKATA, K., WATANABE, N., YAGI, A., INA, K. and LUO, S. 1994. *trans*- and *cis*-Linalool 3,6-oxides and methyl salicylate 6-O-β-D-xylopyranosyl-β-D-glucopyranosides isolated as aroma precursors from leaves for oolong tea. *In* Abstracts of the 38th Symposium on the Chemistry of Terpenes, Essential Oils and Aromatics in Niigata, Japan pp. 63–65.

MOON, J.-H., WATANABE, N., IJIMA, Y., YAGI, A., INA, K. and SAKATA, K. 1996. *cis*- and *trans*-Linalool 3,7-oxides, methyl salicylate glycosides and (Z)-3-hexenyl β-D-glucopyranoside as aroma precursors from tea leaves for oolong. Biosci. Biotech. Biochem. *60*, 1815–1819.

NISHIKITANI, M., KUBOTA, K., KOBAYASHI, A. and SUGAWARA, F. 1996. Geranyl 6-O-α-L-arabinopyranosyl-β-D-glucopyranoside isolated as an aroma precursor from leaves of a green tea cultivar. Biosci. Biotech. Biochem. *60*, 929–931.

OGAWA, K., MOON, J.-H., GUO, W., YAGI, A., WATANABE, N. and SAKATA, K. 1995. A study on tea aroma formation mechanism. Alcoholic aroma precursor amounts and glycosidase activity in part of the tea plant. Z. Naturforsch. *50C*, 493–498.

OGAWA, K., IJIMA, Y., GUO, W., WATANABE, N., USUI, T., DONG, S., TONG, S. and SAKATA, K. 1997. Purification of a β-primeverosidase concerned with alcoholic aroma formation in tea leaves (cv. Shuixian) to be processed to oolong tea, J. Agric. Food Chem. *45*, 877–882.

OKA, N., OHKI, M., IKEGAMI, A., SAKATA, K. and WATANABE, N. 1997. First isolation of geranyl disaccharide glycosides as aroma precursors from rose flowers. Natl. Prod. Lett. in press.

SAKATA, K., GUO, W., MOON, J.-H., WATANABE, N., USUI, T. and LUO, S. 1995a. Alcoholic aroma formation mechanism of oolong tea. *In* Proceedings of the 13th International Congress of Flavours, Fragrances and Essential Oils in Istanbul, Anadolu University Press, pp. 283–302.

SAKATA, K., GUO, W., MOON, J.-H., WATANABE, N., USUI, T. and LUO, S. 1995b. Molecular basis of alcoholic aroma formation in oolong tea. *In* Proceedings of '95 International Tea - Quality - Human Health Symposium in Shanghai. pp. 175–187.

WATANABE, N., NAKAJIMA, R., WATANABE, S., MOON, J-H., INAGAKI, J., SAKATA, K., YAGI, A. and INA, K. 1994. Linalyl and bornyl disaccharide glycosides from *Gardenia jasminoides* flowers. Phytochemistry *36*, 457–459.

YAMANISHI, T. 1995. Flavor of tea. *Food Rev. Int. 11*, 477–525.

YANO, M., JOKI, Y., MUTOH, H., KUBOTA, K. and KOBAYASHI, A. 1991. Benzyl glucoside from tea leaves. Agric. Biol. Chem. *55*, 1205–1206.

INHIBITORY MECHANISMS OF HUMAN PLATELET AGGREGATION BY ONION AND GARLIC

YASUJIRO MORIMITSU, S. KAWAKISHI and T. OSAWA

Laboratory of Food and Biodynamics
Nagoya University School of Agricultural Sciences
Nagoya 464-01, Japan

ABSTRACT

*Ten kinds of α-sulfinyldisulfides (**AC** series) have been isolated from onion as inhibitors of human platelet aggregation. We found that the **AC** series inhibited platelet aggregation induced by collagen, arachidonic acid (AA), ADP and PAF (platelet activating factor), but had minimal effect on platelet aggregation induced by U46619 (an analog of PGH_2), STA_2 (an analog of TXA_2), A23187 (a calcium ionophore), thrombin, PMA (phorbol 12-myristate 13-acetate) and OAG (an analog of diacylglycerol). Especially, the **AC** series showed the potent inhibitory activity of platelet aggregation induced by collagen and AA. The **AC** series strongly inhibited prostaglandin endoperoxide synthase (PGH synthase) of rabbit renal microsomes, indicating that the antiaggregation is caused by an impairment of AA metabolism. From the results of inhibitory activity of platelet aggregation by structurally related compounds of the **AC** series, both sulfinyl and disulfide groups of the **AC** series seem to play an important role in the inhibition of PGH synthase.*

INTRODUCTION

Garlic (*Allium sativum* L.) and onion (*A. cepa* L.) have been extensively studied for their physiological, pharmaceutical or therapeutical effects, and especially for their antithrombotic activities (Phillips and Poyser 1978; Apitz-Castro *et al.* 1983; Block 1992). As for one of the possible mechanisms of their antithrombotic effect, their extracts have been examined for the ability of inhibiting AA metabolism. They were ascertained to possess a strong inhibitory activity for PGH synthase in human platelet (Makheja *et al.* 1979; Srivastava 1984, 1986). Ajoene (4,5,9-trithiadodeca-1,6,11-triene 9-oxide) and MATS (methyl allyl trisulfide), the major antiplatelet compounds isolated from garlic, were also observed to have direct inhibition of the arachidonic acid metabolism (Ariga *et al.* 1981; Sendl *et al.* 1992). On the contrary, Apitz-Castro *et al.* (1986a,b; Rendu *et al.* 1989) have investigated the other mode of action of ajoene.

We have isolated and identified potent inhibitors of platelet aggregation termed **AC** series, analogs of α-sulfinyldisulfides, from the methanol extract of onion (Kawakishi and Morimitsu 1988; Morimitsu and Kawakishi 1990). Bayer *et al.* (1988, 1989) have also isolated anti-asthmatic and antiplatelet compounds named cepaenes, which can be regarded as homologs of the **AC** series, from the chloroform extract of onion. The cepaenes were reported to depress the activities of both PGH synthase of sheep seminal microsomes and 5-lipoxygenase of porcine leukocytes (Bayer *et al.* 1988).

The present study examined the inhibitory effect of the **AC** series on platelet aggregation induced by various agonists and quantitative analyses of AA metabolites using PGH synthase of rabbit renal microsomes. In addition, structurally related compounds of the **AC** series were prepared and evaluated for their inhibitory activity of platelet aggregation.

MATERIALS AND METHODS

Measurement of Antiaggregation Activity

Antiaggregation activity was measured by the reported method (Morimitsu and Kawakishi 1990) using a dual-channel aggregometer (NKK, Hematracer I). Platelet aggregation was induced by various agonists at minimum concentrations as follows (final conc.): collagen (1 μg/mL), AA (0.5 mM), ADP (10 μM), PAF (5 μM), A23187 (13.2 μM), U46619 (5 μM), STA_2 (5 μM), PMA (25 μM), OAG (200 μM) and thrombin (0.5 units/mL). (*E*)- and (*Z*)-Ajoenes were isolated from garlic by the method of Block *et al.* (1984). TTHO (2,3,5-trithiahexane 5-S-oxide) was prepared by the MCPBA oxidation of TTH (2,3,5-trithiahexane).

Inhibitory Assay for PG Biosynthesis

The preparation of rabbit renal microsomes and the inhibitory assay were carried out using the procedure of Sankawa *et al.* (1982) with a slight modification. The reaction mixture (0.2 mL) contained 0.1 M sodium phosphate buffer (pH 7.5), 10 mM tryptophan, 0.25 μM hemoglobin, 4.0 mM reduced glutathione, 20 μM [1-^{14}C] arachidonic acid (1.35 μCi), rabbit renal microsomes (100 μg protein) and a test sample (DMSO solution). The reaction (37°C, 20 min) was started by the addition of microsomes and terminated by the addition of 1 N HCl (50 μL). The reaction mixture was then extracted with ether. After the ether was removed, the residue was dissolved in acetone and applied to a TLC plate. The TLC plate was developed with a solvent mixture [$CHCl_3$/MeOH/AcOH = 90/5/5 (V/V)], and radioactivities of PGE_2, $PGF_{2\alpha}$ and arachidonic acid were measured by an imaging plate reader (Bio-Image Analyser, FUJIX BA-100).

RESULTS AND DISCUSSION

The AC Series and Their Inhibitory Activities for Platelet Aggregation Induced by Various Agonists

The **AC** series isolated from onion (Fig. 1), showed a potent inhibitory activity of platelet aggregation induced by collagen, particularly **AC-11a**, **AC-11b**, **AC-12a** and **AC-12b** (Table 1). Indeed, the inhibitory activity of **AC-12b** was stronger than that of indomethacin. Platelet aggregation induced by U46619, STA_2, A23187, thrombin, PMA and OAG was not appreciably affected by **AC-11a** even in high concentration (200 μM). In contrast, **AC-11a** inhibited platelet aggregation induced by collagen, AA, ADP and PAF (Table 2). Thus, intact platelets treated with **AC-11a** significantly affected the rate and amplitude of platelet aggregation by collagen and AA. Platelet aggregation induced by A23187, PMA and OAG involves mobilization of Ca^{2+} from intracellular stores leading to stimulation of contractile reactions in platelets, and activation of protein kinase C (PKC) by increasing its affinity for Ca^{2+}, respectively. Thrombin is also known to elevate intracellular Ca^{2+} concentration and thereby activates intracellular Ca^{2+} dependent thiol proteases (calpains). Our results suggest that the **AC** series do not inhibit the Ca^{2+} mobilization, PKC activation, and subsequent platelet activations which were caused by elevating the intracellular Ca^{2+} concentration. Platelet aggregation induced by U46619 and STA_2 stimulates the release reaction from platelets (ADP, serotonin and so on), and the **AC** series had no effect. Our results are consistent with the fact that the **AC** series significantly inhibited platelet aggregation induced by collagen and AA, which directly or indirectly involve activating of AA metabolic pathway. So inhibition of platelet aggregation by the **AC** series is most likely due to the suppression of the enzymes related to the AA cascade in platelets. In addition, the **AC** series were found to potently inhibit PAF-induced platelet aggregation (**AC-11a**: 80% inhibition at 50 μM). These properties can account in part for the pharmaceutical activities of onion. But the inhibition mechanism of PAF-induced platelet aggregation is uncertain.

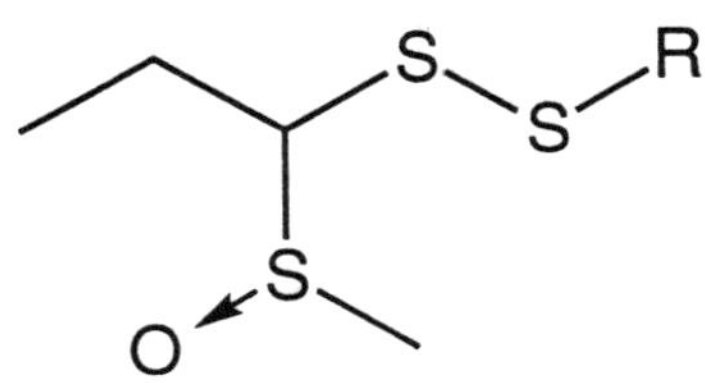

R= methyl (**AC-1a, b**)
trans-1-propenyl (**AC-11a, b**)
cis-1-propenyl (**AC-12a,b**)

FIG. 1. CHEMICAL STRUCTURES OF THE AC SERIES

TABLE 1.
INHIBITORY ACTIVITY OF THE AC SERIES FOR HUMAN PLATELET AGGREGATION AND PG BIOSYNTHESIS

	IC_{50} (μM)	
	platelet aggregation	PG biosynthesis
AC-1a	6.1	ND[a]
AC-1b	1.4	ND
AC-11a	48.9	1.2
AC-11b	11.7	1.6
AC-12a	6.1	ND
AC-12b	1.4	ND
indomethacin	2.1	0.75

[a]ND, not determined.

TABLE 2.
INHIBITORY EFFECT OF AC-11A ON HUMAN PLATELET AGGREGATION BY VARIOUS AGONISTS

AC-11a	Inhibition (%)									
	collagen	AA	ADP	U46619	STA_2	PAF	A23187	thrombin	PMA	OAG
200μM	100	100	100	51	35	100	93	50	24	0
100μM	100	100	80							
50μM	73	45	29	17	0	80	5	0		
25μM	46	15				19				

Inhibitory Effect of the AC Series on PG Biosynthesis

AC-1a was tested for inhibitory activity of the enzymatic formation of malondialdehyde (MDA) in washed human platelets measured by the TBA (2-thiobarbituric acid) method as described by Okuma *et al.* (1970). A part of the exogenously added arachidonic acid was metabolized to MDA, 12(S)-hydroxy-5,8,10-heptadecatrienoic acid (HHT) and TXA_2 in equal amounts by TX synthase of human platelets (Haurand and Ullrich 1985). **AC-1a** mildly inhibited the formation of MDA (Morimitsu and Kawakishi, unpublished data). This result suggested that the **AC** series would possibly inhibit the platelet cyclooxygenase pathway, including PGH synthase. Therefore, **AC-11a** and **AC-11b** were directly examined for inhibition of PG biosynthesis using rabbit renal microsomes (Table 1). They inhibited PG biosynthesis potently and their IC_{50} values were nearly twice that of indomethacin. The **AC** series could be considered strong inhibitors of PG biosynthesis, probably inhibitors of PGH synthase just like cepaenes (Bayer *et al.* 1989).

Relationships between Structure and Antiaggregation Activity of α-Sulfinyldisulfides

Some analogs of α-sulfinylsulfides and α-sulfinyldisulfides were prepared to study their structure-activity relationship (Fig. 2). The analogs of α-sulfinylsulfides had no inhibitory activity on platelet aggregation (Kawakishi and Morimitsu 1994). However, there is a noticeable tendency for the structure-activity relationship among the analogs of α-sulfinyldisulfides (Table 3). α-Alkylthio-disulfides (n=0) did not have inhibitory

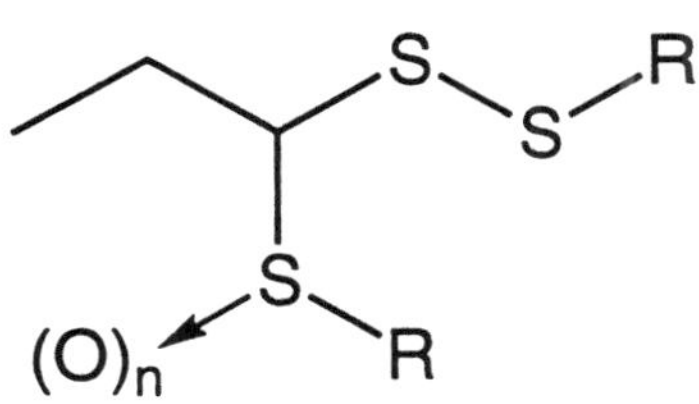

FIG. 2. CHEMICAL STRUCTURES OF A-SULFINYLDISULFIDE DERIVATIVES

TABLE 3.
STRUCTURE-ACTIVITY RELATIONSHIP OF A-SULFINYLDISULFIDE INHIBITION OF HUMAN PLATELET AGGREGATION

R	IC_{50} (μM)		
	n=0	n=1	n=2
methyl	465	67.6 18.4	126.2
ethyl	>1000	26.8 12.0	40.6
propyl	>1000	5.1 3.0	13.0

activity against platelet aggregation, but both α-sulfinyldisulfides (n=1) and α-sulfonyldisulfides (n=2) exhibited strong inhibitory activities. The oxidation of sulfide (n=0) to a sulfinyl side chain (n=1) converted the inactive compounds to significantly strong active compounds. Furthermore, the activity is reduced by one more oxidation of sulfinyl (n=1) to a sulfonyl side chain (n=2) by about 1/6 - 1/2. These data suggest that both sulfinyl and disulfide groups in the **AC** series are essential for the development of antiaggregation activity.

The α-sulfinyldisulfides structure in the **AC** series is related to ajoene from garlic in possessing the sulfinyl and disulfide groups. Therefore, ajoene and a more simple compound of α-sulfinyldisulfide, TTHO (2,3,5-trithiahexane 5-S-oxide) were prepared to assess the antiaggregation activity (Fig. 3). (*E*)- and (*Z*)-ajoenes showed inhibitory activity of platelet aggregation similar to that of **AC-1a** and **AC-11a** (Table 4). TTHO exhibited the lower inhibitory activity of platelet aggregation, but TTH (2,3,5-trithiahexane) was an inactive compound. In conclusion, the presented results suggest that the **AC** series in onion are structurally similar to ajoene in garlic, regarding its sulfinyl and disulfide groups. These sulfur-containing groups may play an important role in the inhibition of PGH synthase of cyclooxygenase pathway in platelets. The sulfinyl group can be deduced to be the reactive function for the active site (*cf.* tyrosine radical) of PGH synthase. Since onion is a widely consumed vegetable, physiological characteristics of onion components as inhibitors of this enzyme have an important meaning for human health from the viewpoint of the possible prevention of thrombosis and coronary diseases.

ACKNOWLEDGMENTS

The authors thank Drs. T. Matsuzaki and M. Ninomiya of Japan Tobacco Inc. for their supply of rabbit renal microsomes. The author Morimitsu gratefully acknowledges Research Foundation for the Electrotechnology of Chubu of Japan (REFEC) for financial support of his attending this conference at U.C. Davis, California.

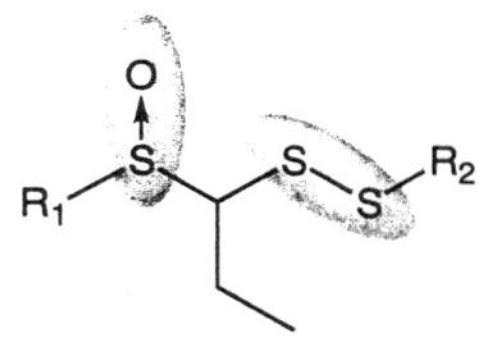

AC series/cepaenes

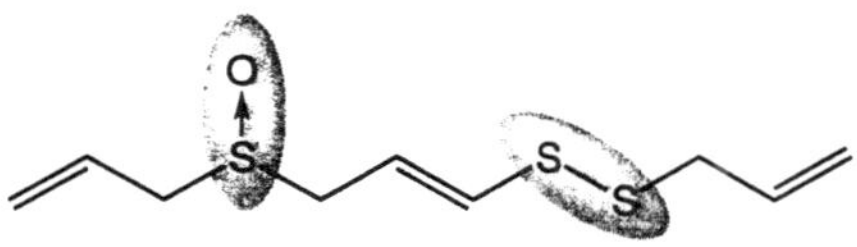

(*E*)-ajoene

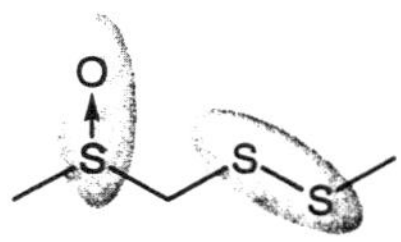

TTHO

FIG. 3. CHEMICAL STRUCTURES OF THE **AC** SERIES, CEPAENES, (*E*)-AJOENE AND TTHO

TABLE 4.
INHIBITORY ACTIVITY OF HUMAN PLATELET AGGREGATION BY THE AC SERIES AND AJOENES

	IC_{50} (μM)
(*E*)-ajoene	65.1
(Z)-ajoene	53.8
TTHO	194
TTH	>1000
AC-1a	67.6
AC-11a	48.9
AC-12b	1.2
indomethacin	2.1

REFERENCES

APITZ-CASTRO, R., CABRERA, S., CRUZ, M.R., LEDEZMA, E. and JAIN, M.K. 1983. Effects of garlic extract and of platelet aggregation, arachidonate metabolism, release reaction and platelet ultrastructure. Thrombosis Res. *32*, 155–169.

APITZ-CASTRO, R., LEDEZMA, E., ESCALANTE, J. and JAIN, M.K. 1986a. The molecular basis of the antiplatelet action of ajoene: Direct interaction with the fibrinogen receptor. Biochem. Biophys. Res. Commun. *141*, 145–150.

APITZ-CASTRO, R., ESCALANTE, J., VARGAS, R. and JAIN, M.K. 1986b. Ajoene, the antiplatelet principle of garlic, synergistically potentiates the antiaggregatory action of prostacyclin, forskolin, indomethacin and dipyridamole on human platelets. Thrombosis Res. *42*, 303–311.

ARIGA, T., OSHIBA, S. and TAMADA, T. 1981. Platelet aggregation inhibitor in garlic. Lancet, Vol. 1, No. 8212, 150–151.

BAYER, T., WAGNER, H., WRAY, V. and DORSCH, W. 1988. Inhibitors of cyclo-oxygenase and lipoxygenase in onions. Lancet, Vol. 2, No. 8616, 906.

BAYER, T., BREU, W., SELIGMANN, O., WRAY, V. and WAGNER, H. 1989. Biologically active thiosulfinates and α-sulfinyldisulfides from *Allium cepa*. Phytochemistry *28*, 2373–2377.

BLOCK, E., AHMAD, S., JAIN, M.K., CRECELY, R.W., APITZ-CASTRO, R. and CRUZ, M.R. 1984. (*E,Z*)-Ajoene: a potent antithrombotic agent from garlic. J. Am. Chem.Soc. *106*, 8295–8296.

BLOCK, E. 1992. The organosulfur chemistry of the genus *Allium* - Implications for the organic chemistry of sulfur. Angew. Chem. Int. Ed. Engl. *31*, 1135–1178.

HAURAND, M. and ULLRICH, V. 1985. Isolation and characterization of thromboxane synthase from human platelets as a cytochrome P-450 enzyme. J. Biol. Chem. *28*, 15059–15067.

KAWAKISHI, S. and MORIMITSU, Y. 1988. New inhibitor of platelet aggregation in onion oil. Lancet, Vol. 2, No. 8606, 330.

KAWAKISHI, S. and MORIMITSU, Y. 1994. Food phytochemicals for cancer prevention I. *In* Chapter 8: Sulfur Chemistry of Onions and Inhibitory Factors of the Arachidonic Acid Cascade. ACS Symposium Series No. 546, pp. 120–127, M.-T. Huang, T. Osawa, C.-T. Ho and R.T. Rosen (eds.). American Chemical Society, Washington, D.C.

MAKHEJA, A.N., VANDERHOEK, J.Y. and BAILEY, J.M. 1979. Inhibition of platelet aggregation and thromboxane synthesis by onion and garlic. Lancet, Vol. 1, No. 8119, 781.

MORIMITSU, Y. and KAWAKISHI, S. 1990. Inhibitors of platelet aggregation from onion. Phytochemistry *29*, 3435–3439.

OKUMA M., STEINER, M. and BALDINI, M. 1970. Studies on lipid peroxides in platelets. I. Method of assay and effect of storage. J. Lab. Clin. Med. *75*, 283–296.

PHILLIPS, C. and POYSER, N.L. 1978. Inhibition of platelet aggregation by onion extracts. Lancet, Vol. 1, No. 8072, 1051–1052.

RENDU, F., DAVELOOSE, D., DEBOUZY, J.C., BOURDEAU, N., LEVY-TOLEDANO, S., JAIN, M.K. and APITZ-CASTRO, R. 1989. Ajoene, the antiplatelet compound derived from garlic, specifically inhibits platelet release reaction by affecting the plasma membrane internal microviscosity. Biochem. Pharmacol. *38*, 1321–1328.

SANKAWA, U., SHIBUYA, M., EBIZUKA, Y., NOGUCHI, H., KINOSHITA, T. and IITAKA, Y. 1982. Depside as potent inhibitor of prostaglandin biosynthesis: A new active site model for fatty acid cyclooxygenase. Prostaglandins *24*, 21–34.

SENDL, A., ELBL, G., STEINKE, B., REDL, K., BREU, W. and WAGNER, H. 1992. Comparative pharmacological investigations of *Allium ursinum* and *Allium sativum*. Planta Med. *58*, 1–7.

SRIVASTAVA, K.C. 1984. Aqueous extracts of onion, garlic and ginger inhibit platelet aggregation and alter arachidonic acid metabolism. Biomed. Biochim. Acta *43*, 335–346.

SRIVASTAVA, K.C. 1986. Onion extracts antiaggregatory effects by altering arachidonic acid metabolism in platelets. Prostaglandins Leukotrienes Med. *24*, 43–50.

PLATELET AGGREGATION INHIBITORY ACTIVITY OF VINYLDITHIINS AND THEIR DERIVATIVES FROM JAPANESE DOMESTIC *ALLIUM (A. VICTORIALIS)*

HIROYUKI NISHIMURA[1], C. HANNY WIJAYA[2], ATSUSHI SATOH[1] and TOYOHIKO ARIGA[3]

[1]Department of Bioscience and Technology
School of Engineering, Hokkaido Tokai University
Sapporo 005, Japan

[2]Faculty of Agricultural Technology
Bogor Agricultural University
P.O. Box 122, Bogor, Indonesia

[3]Department of Nutrition and Physiology
School of Agriculture and Veterinary Medicine
Nihon University
Setagaya, Tokyo 154, Japan

ABSTRACT

The leaves and stems of Japanese domestic Allium *plant, caucas* (A. victorialis *L.), which are widely distributed in the northern part of Japan, especially Hokkaido, under the name "Gyaja ninniku" is a nutritious vegetable. The significant flavor compounds of caucas are methyl allyl disulfide (Chinese chive-like odor), diallyl disulfide (garlic-like odor) and methyl allyl trisulfide (pickles-like odor) among more than 85 peaks on the gas chromatogram. 1-Propenyl-containing disulfide which is responsible for the onion flavor was identified in caucas, one of garlic-like* Allium *species. Furthermore, 2-vinyl-4*H*-1,3-dithiin and 3,4-dihydro-3-vinyl-1,2-dithiin as platelet aggregation inhibitors were found in a dichloromethane extract of caucas. These vinyldithiins and derivatives (sulfoxides, sulfones, alkyl derivatives) were synthesized to compare the inhibitory activity. As a result, sulfur-oxidized compounds exhibited more potent inhibitory activity than original vinyldithiins.*

INTRODUCTION

Caucas (*Allium victorialis* L.) is one of the *Allium* species that grows well wild in Hokkaido, the northern part of Japan. The Ainu, the native people of Hokkaido, have eaten the leaves and stalks of caucas as a vegetable for a long time. Although it has not been as well-known as other *Allium* species such as onion and garlic, it seems to have potential in terms of the utilization of nutritious vegetables.

Yurugi *et al.* (1954) gave the first report about the ingredients of caucas in studies on the reaction between thiamine (vitamin B_1) and thiosulfinates of the *Allium* species. The present authors have investigated the identification of volatile components responsible for caucas flavor and the enzymatic development of the *Allium* volatiles (Nishimura *et al.* 1971; Akashi *et al.* 1975). The significant flavor components of caucas were presumed to be 1-propenyl-containing disulfides and 2-methyl-2-pentenal, one of the breakdown products of propanethial S-oxide in addition to methyl allyl disulfide, diallyl disulfide, and so on.

Garlic is reputed to offer protection against strokes, coronary thrombosis, atherosclerosis, and platelet aggregation (Adamu *et al.* 1982; Samson 1982; Qureshi *et al.* 1983). Ariga *et al.* (1981) have isolated a platelet aggregation inhibitor identified as methyl allyl trisulfide from garlic. Recently, it was reported that garlic had potent antithrombotic agents identified as 2-vinyl-4*H*-1,3-dithiin, 3,4-dihydro-3-vinyl-1,2-dithiin, diallyl trisulfide, and a compound named ajoene; these compounds were nonenzymatically derived from allicin ($CH_2=CHCH_2S(O)SCH_2CH=CH_2$, allyl 2-propenylthiosulfinate) (Apitz-Castro *et al.* 1983; Apitz-Castro *et al.* 1986; Block *et al.* 1984; 1986).

The discovery of vinyldithiins in caucas volatiles, which have antithrombotic activity, is also of great interest in terms of the search for more useful vegetables. This paper deals with the identification of vinyldithiins in caucas extracts as well as volatile flavor components, synthesis of vinyldithiin derivatives, and food processing of caucas.

MATERIALS AND METHODS

Sample Preparation

Young caucases were collected from several places in Hokkaido, Japan. Both leaves and stalks were cut into small pieces. One part was placed in a three-necked flask, and volatile flavor components were distilled off by passing through nitrogen gas as a carrier at approximately 40 °C and absorbing into an isopentane trap cooled with dry ice-ethanol. This process is called headspace gas distillation extraction. Extraction from the other part was made by placing it in methylene chloride for 2 weeks at room temperature and is called direct solvent extraction. The sample obtained by headspace gas distillation extraction was concentrated and directly used for analysis. However, the direct one had to be separated from chlorophyll and some other pigments by column chromatography (Florisil column; 0-5% ether/hexane, v/v) before further analysis.

Isolation of Vinyldithiins

The vinyldithiins were isolated from the direct-extraction sample. The total concentrate was chromatographed over a SiO_2 column using ether and hexane as gradient eluants to give several fractions (each 5 mL). The fractions suspected to contain vinyldithiins **1** and **2** (R_f 0.24 and 0.12 on TLC in n-pentane; also detected by GC and GC-MS) were pooled separately. Purification by HPLC (hexane) gave rise to two fractions each containing pure vinyldithiin. The structures were confirmed by spectral data as mentioned later.

Authentic Vinyldithiins

3,4-Dihydro-3-vinyl-1,2-dithiin (**1**) and 2-vinyl-4*H*-1,3-dithiin (**2**) were derived from allicin by modification of the method of Block *et al.* (1984). In this experiment, allicin was prepared by the oxidation of diallyl disulfide with *m*-chloroperbenzoic acid in chloroform.

The decomposition of allicin in methanol at room temperature for 7 days gave vinyldithiins as well as diallyl disulfide and diallyl trisulfide. The synthesized vinyldithiins were isolated by SiO_2 column chromatography and preparative HPLC (hexane). Physicochemical data are as follows.

3,4-Dihydro-3-vinyl-1,2-dithiin (1). IR (film) 1630 (C=C), 985 and 915 cm^{-1} (vinyl double bond); ^1H NMR (270 MHz, $CDCl_3$) δ 2.41-2.68 (m, 2H, allylic methylene), 3.68-3.76 (m, 1H, methine proton), 5.23-5.32 (m, 2H, CH_2=C), 5.94 (dd, 1H, exo olefinic =CH), 6.04 (m, 1H, endo olefinic SC=CH), 6.37 (dt, 1H, J=9 and 2 Hz, endo olefinic SCH=C); ^{13}C NMR (67.5 MHz, $CDCl_3$) δ 30.3 (C4), 44.1 (C3), 117.5 (C8), 120.6 (C7), 126.0 (C5), 136.4 (C6); MS m/z (relative intensity, %) 144 (M^+, 78), 111 (100), 103 (51), 97 (70), 85 (17), 79 (43), 77 (48), 72 (57), 71 (55), 45 (59), 39 (40).

2-Vinyl-4*H*-1,3-dithiin (2). IR (film) 1630 (C=C), 982 and 918 cm^{-1} (vinyl double bond); ^1H NMR (270 MHz, $CDCl_3$) δ 3.23 and 3.40 (two ddd, 2H, J=17, 5, and 2 Hz, allylic methylene), 4.73 (d, 1H, J=7 Hz, methine proton), 5.30 and 5.40 (two d, 2H, J=17 and 10 Hz, CH_2=C), 5.92-6.05 (m, 2H, exo olefinic =CH and endo olefinic SC=CH), 6.31 (dt, 1H, endo olefinic SCH=C); ^{13}C NMR (67.5 MHz, $CDCl_3$) δ 25.1 (C4), 45.1 (C2), 117.2 (C8), 118.3 (C7), 122.2 (C5), 134.3 (C6); MS m/z (relative intensity, %) 144 (M^+, 45), 111 (35), 103 (10), 97 (16), 85 (7), 79 (11), 72 (100), 71 (78), 45 (41), 39 (23).

Instrumental Analysis

Gas chromatography (GC) was carried out on a Hitachi 263-30 instrument equipped with a flame ionization detector and a 50 m $\times$ 0.35 mm (i.d.) PEG-20M-bonded capillary column at a helium flow rate of 1.2 mL/min; the column temperature was programmed linearly from 40 to 220°C at 2 °C/min; the injection port temperature was 250 °C. Mass spectrometry (MS) using electron impact (EI; JEOL JMS-DX 300) and field ionization (FI; JEOL JMS-01SG-2) was performed to identify the purified components. In the case of EI-MS, the operating parameters were as follows: inlet temperature, 30-70°C; ion source pressure 10^{-6} Torr; ion source temperature 250°C; acceleration voltage, 3kV; chamber voltage, 70 eV. In FI-MS, the operating parameters were as follows: inlet temperature, 25°C; ion source pressure 0.2 $\times$ 10^{-6} Torr; acceleration voltage, 9kV; cathode high voltage, 4 kV. The method of GC-MS combination (JMS-DX 300 GC-MS) was preferred for obtaining the mass spectral data of mixtures and/or trace amounts of components. The operating parameters were as follows. Gas chromatograph: column, a 30 m $\times$ 0.28 mm (i.d.) PEG-HT SCOT capillary column; flow rate, helium carrier gas at 1.2 mL/min; temperature, 40-220°C at 4°C/min; injection port temperature, 230°C. Mass spectrometer: inlet temperature, 30-70°C; ion source pressure 10^{-6} Torr; ionization current, 300 μA; total emission, 160μA; chamber voltage, 70 eV. Proton nuclear magnetic resonance (^1H NMR) spectra were recorded on a JEOL JNM-GX FT (270 MHz) spectrometer: solvent, $CDCl_3$; internal standard, Me_4Si. Infrared (IR) and ultraviolet (UV) absorption spectrometry was performed on a Hitachi 285 infrared spectrometer and Hitachi EPS-3T UV spectrometer, respectively. High-performance liquid chromatography (HPLC) was carried out on a

Jasco PG-350 D with a Shodex RI SE-31 refractometer and a Unisil Q 100-5 (30 cm × 16.7 mm (i.d.)) or Lichrospher SI 60/II super 250-4 column (24 cm × 4 mm (i.d.)).

Measurement of Antiaggregation Activity

Platelet-rich plasma (PRP) was prepared from citrated human or rabbit blood. Platelet aggregation was induced by various agonists at concentrations designated in the text, and measured by an aggregation meter (Aggregometer DP-247E, Sienco Inc., U.S.A.). To assay antiaggregation activity, the *Allium* oil or its component was diluted with ethanol or acetone and added as a 1 μl aliquot to 300 μl PRP to avoid solvent inhibition. Aggregation curves were analyzed for maximum aggregation and disaggregation. For the former, inhibition percent was obtained as described elsewhere, and for the latter, disaggregation percent was taken as the negative slope (-%/min) appearing just after the maximum aggregation was obtained.

RESULTS AND DISCUSSION

Flavor Components

The gas chromatographic separation of volatile flavor components of caucas (*A. victrialis* L.) is shown in Fig. 1. Identification was accomplished by comparing their gas chromatographic retention times and mass spectra with those of authentic compounds and published data. The compounds identified are summarized in Table 1.

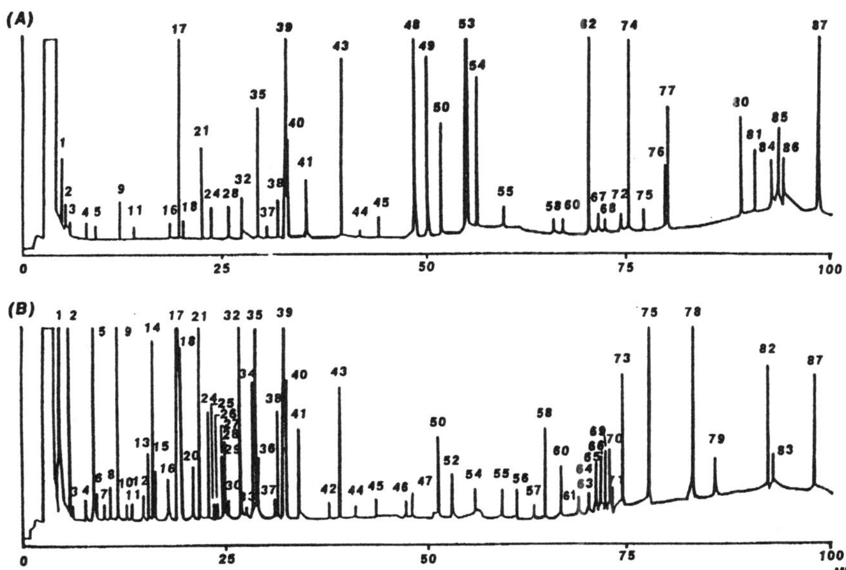

FIG. 1. GAS CHROMATOGRAMS OF THE VOLATILE COMPONENTS OF FRESH CAUCAS (*A. VICTRIALIS* L.)

The oils were prepared by either direct extraction with dichloromethane (A) or headspace gas distillation extraction (B).

TABLE 1.
IDENTIFICATION OF VOLATILE COMPONENTS FOUND IN CAUCAS

Peak	Compound	M^+, m/z	Identification[a]	Extraction[b]
1	$CH_2{=}CHCH_2SH$	74	MS, Rt, A	S, D
2	$CH_3SCH_2CH{=}CH_2$	88	MS, Rt, A	S, D
3	$CH_3COCH{=}CHCH_3$	84	MS, Rt, T	S, D
5	CH_3SSCH_3	94	MS, Rt, A	S, D
7	$CH_2{=}CHCH_2SCH_2CH_2CH_3$	116	MS, Rt, A	S
8	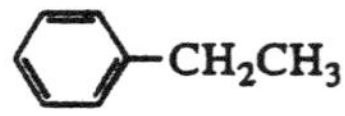	108	MS, T	S
9	$CH_2{=}CHCH_2SCH_2CH{=}CH_2$	114	MS, Rt, A	S, D
12	$CH_3CH{=}CHCH(OH)CH_3$	86	MS, R, T	S
13		106	MS, T	S
14	$CH_3CH_2CH{=}C(CH_3)CHO$	98	MS, Rt, A	S
15	$CH_3SSCH_2CH_2CH_3$	122	MS, Rt, A	S
16	*cis*-$CH_3SSCH{=}CHCH_3$	120	MS, Rt, A	S, D
17	$CH_3SSCH_2CH{=}CH_2$	120	MS, Rt, A	S, D
18	*trans*-$CH_3SSCH{=}CHCH_3$	120	MS, Rt, A	S, D
20		108	MS, T	S
21	CH_3SSSCH_3	126	MS, Rt, A	S, D
24		134	MS, Rt, A	S
28	$CH_3CH_2CH_2SSCH_2CH_2CH_3$	150	MS, Rt, A	S, D
32	$CH_3SSO_2CH_3$	126	MS, Rt, A	S, D
34	*cis*-$CH_3CH_2CH_2SSCH{=}CHCH_3$	148	MS, Rt, A	S, D
35	$CH_3CH_2CH_2SSCH_2CH{=}CH_2$	148	MS, Rt, A	S
38	$CH_3CH{=}CHSSCH{=}CHCH_3$[c]	146	MS, Rt, A	S, D
39	$CH_2{=}CHCH_2SSCH_2CH{=}CH_2$	146	MS, Rt, A	S, D
40	*trans,trans*-$CH_3CH{=}CHSSCH{=}CHCH_3$	146	MS, Rt, A	S, D
41	$CH_3SSSCH_2CH_2CH_3$	154	MS, Rt, A	S, D
42	*cis*-$CH_3SSSCH{=}CHCH_3$	152	MS, Rt, A	S, D
43	$CH_3SSSCH_2CH{=}CH_2$	152	MS, Rt, A	S, D
44	*trans*-$CH_3SSSCH{=}CHCH_3$	152	MS, Rt, A	S, D
45	$CH_2SCH_2SSCH_3$	140	MS, T	S, D
48	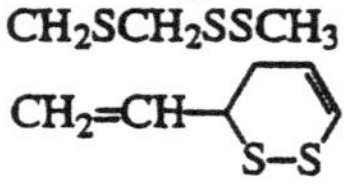	144	MS, Rt, A	D
49		146	MS, Rt, A	D
50	$CH_2{=}CHCH_2SSSCH_2CH{=}CH_2$	178	MS, T	S, D
52		167	MS, T	S
53	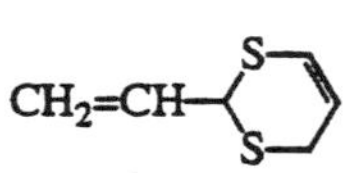	144	MS, Rt, A	D
54		166	MS, T	S, D
62–67	Polymeric hydrocarbons			

[a] MS = mass spectrometry; Rt = gas chromatographic retention time; T = tentative; A = authentic compound.
[b] S = steam distillation; D = direct.
[c] *cis,cis* or *cis,trans*

The major components responsible for the caucas flavor have been reported: methyl allyl disulfide (peak 17, Chinese chive-like odor), diallyl disulfide (peak 39, garlic-like odor), and dimethyl disulfide and methyl allyl trisulfide (peaks 5 and 43, pickles-like odor) (Nishimura *et al.* 1971). These disulfides have also been thought to be produced via thiyl radicals (anisotropic signals of ESR, g=2.00-2.05) formed in the first stage of the enzymatic reaction of S-alk(en)yl-L-cysteine sulfoxide with alliinase (Akashi *et al.* 1975).

Interestingly, a considerable number of 1-propenyl-containing disulfide and 2-methyl-2-pentenal, one of the breakdown products of propanethial S-oxide (a lachrymatory substance), were found in the caucas volatiles as shown in Table 1, although caucas belongs to the garlic-like *Allium* species and those volatiles have never been found so far in garlic type plants. The occurrence of these compounds in caucas is of interest in terms of chemotaxonomy.

Isolation and Identification of the Vinyldithiins (Nishimura *et al.* 1988).

When the two chromatograms shown in Fig. 1 are compared, the significant difference is the appearance of the relatively large peaks 48 and 53 around 50 min on the GC trace. These peaks were found in the direct extracted sample but not in the headspace gas extracted one. The two peaks were suspected to represent vinyldithiins **1** and **2** detected by GC-MS. To confirm the structure of the peaks, isolation and identification were carried out. Both were obtained as pale yellow oils with a characteristic sulfur odor.

A high-resolution MS (M^+ 144.0056) of the earlier eluted product (compound I) suggested $C_6H_8S_2$. The ^1H NMR spectral datum of compound I agreed well with the known 3,4-dihydro-3-vinyl-1,2-dithiin structure (Brodnitz *et al.* 1971; Baslin 1983). A 2D-COSY experiment was performed in an effort to establish proton connectivities through J coupling. The 2D ^1H-^1H NMR spectrum of compound I is shown in Fig. 2.

The spectrum revealed the existence of the following spin-spin interactions: A coupled to B, G, and H; B coupled to A, G, and H; C coupled to D-H; D coupled to C, E, and F; E coupled to C, D, and F; F coupled to C-E, G, and H; G coupled to A-C, F, and H; H coupled to A-C, F, and G. From these data, there is no doubt that the isolated compound I is 3,4-dihydro-3-vinyl-1,2-dithiin (**1**). Compound I was confirmed by comparing with mass and NMR spectra of the synthetic compound. The mass spectral fragmentation of 3,4-dihydro-3-vinyl-1,2-dithiin is proposed as shown in Fig. 3. The evidence of the fragmentation mechanism was obtained by the observation of metastable ion peaks (Nishimura *et al.* 1988).

On the other hand, a high-resolution MS (M^+ 144.0071) of the later eluted product (compound II) also suggested $C_6H_8S_2$. Compound II has a vinyl double bond, i.e. IR νmax 982 and 918 cm^{-1}. The decoupling data of ^1H NMR are as follows: Irradiation at δ 4.73 changes δ 5.92-6.05, a complex multiplet, to simply a multiplet. Irradiation at δ 5.96 changes δ 3.23-3.40, two double double doublets, to two double doublets, δ 4.73, a doublet, to a singlet; and δ 6.31, a double triplet, to a singlet. Furthermore, the 2D ^1H-^1H NMR spectrum of compound II is shown in Fig. 4. The spectrum revealed the existence of the following spin-spin interactions: A coupled to C, G, and H; B coupled to D-F; C coupled to A, G, and H; D coupled to B, E, and F; E coupled to B, D, and F; F coupled to B, D, and E; G coupled to A, C, and H; H coupled to A, C, and G. As a result, compound II was identified as 2-vinyl-4H-1,3-dithiin (**2**). The NMR and mass

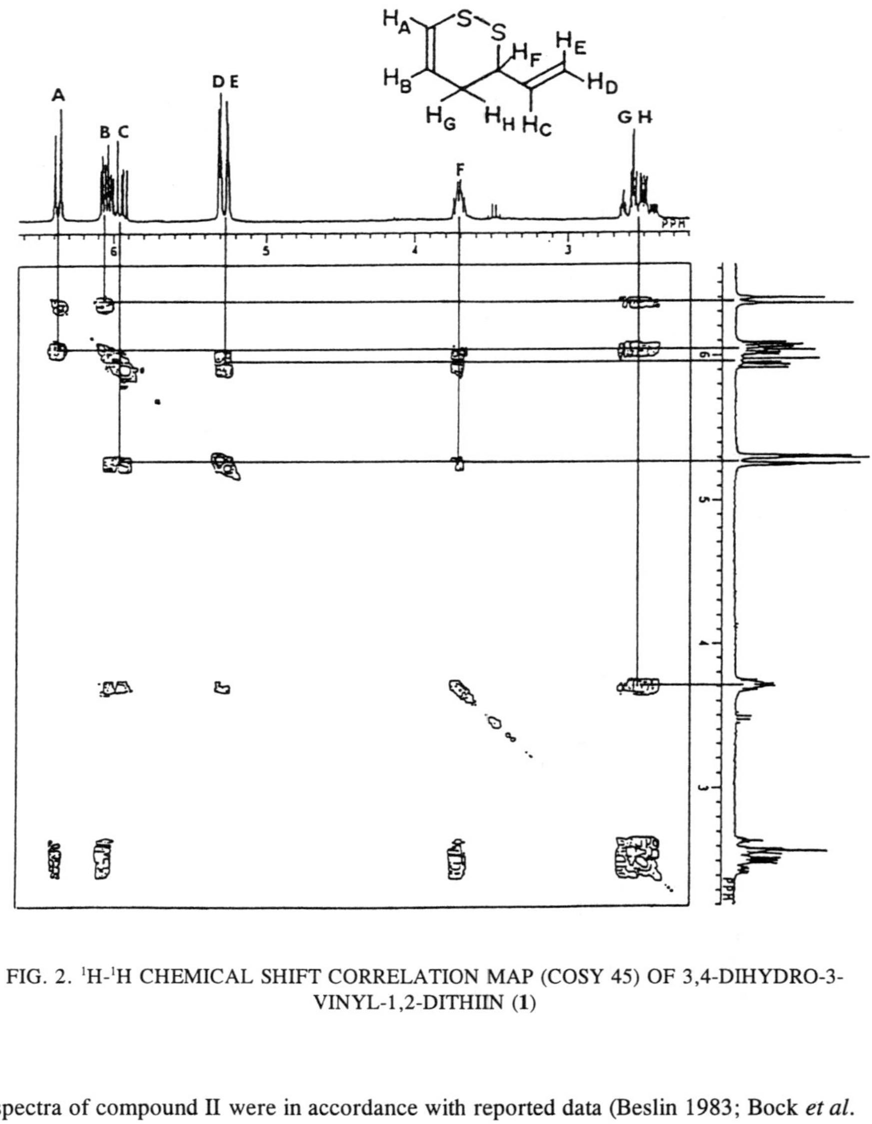

FIG. 2. ^{1}H-^{1}H CHEMICAL SHIFT CORRELATION MAP (COSY 45) OF 3,4-DIHYDRO-3-VINYL-1,2-DITHIIN (**1**)

spectra of compound II were in accordance with reported data (Beslin 1983; Bock *et al.* 1982). The mass spectral fragmentation of 2-vinyl-4*H*-1,3-dithiin was elucidated by the observation of metastable ion peaks as shown in Fig. 5.

Neither of the vinyldithiins was detected in the headspace gas of caucas (see Table 1). However, these compounds were found in the ether extract of residue after removal of the volatile components (Nishimura *et al.* 1988) and in the cooked caucases (Wijaya *et al.* 1991).

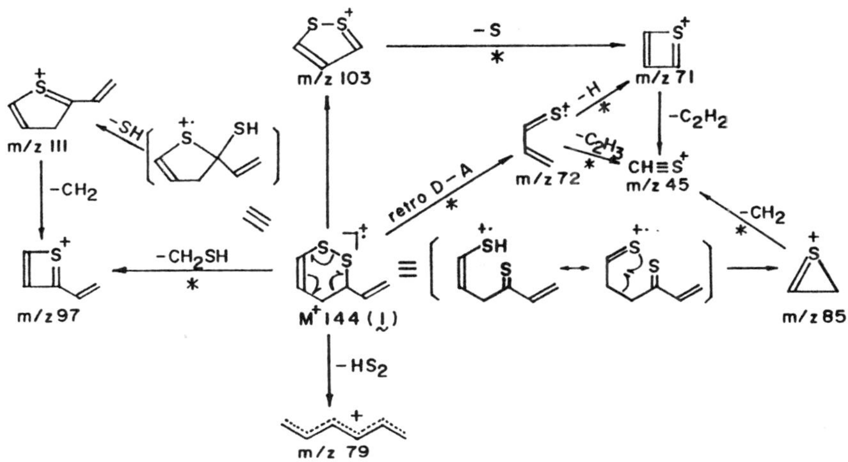

FIG. 3. MASS SPECTRAL FRAGMENTATION OF 3,4-DIHYDRO-3-VINYL-1,2-DITHIIN (**1**)

* indicates observed metastable ion.

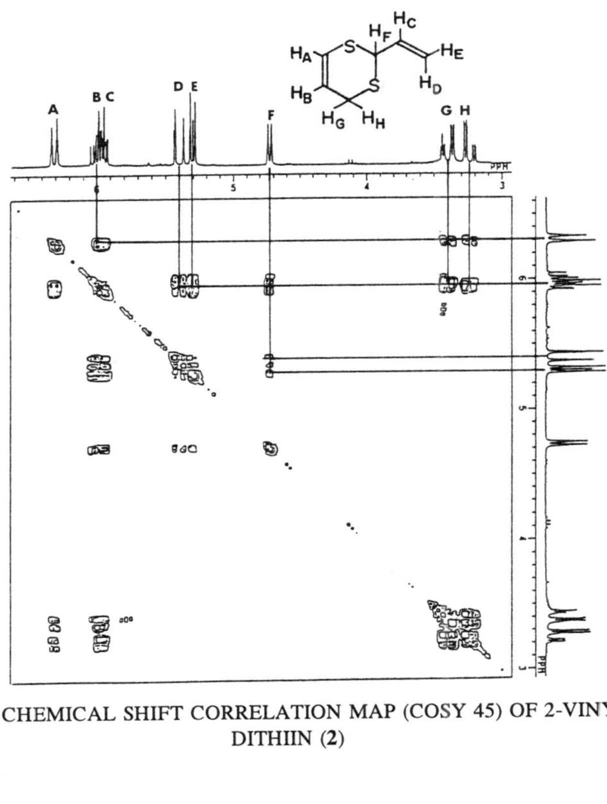

FIG. 4. [1]H-^{1}H CHEMICAL SHIFT CORRELATION MAP (COSY 45) OF 2-VINYL-4*H*-1,3-DITHIIN (**2**)

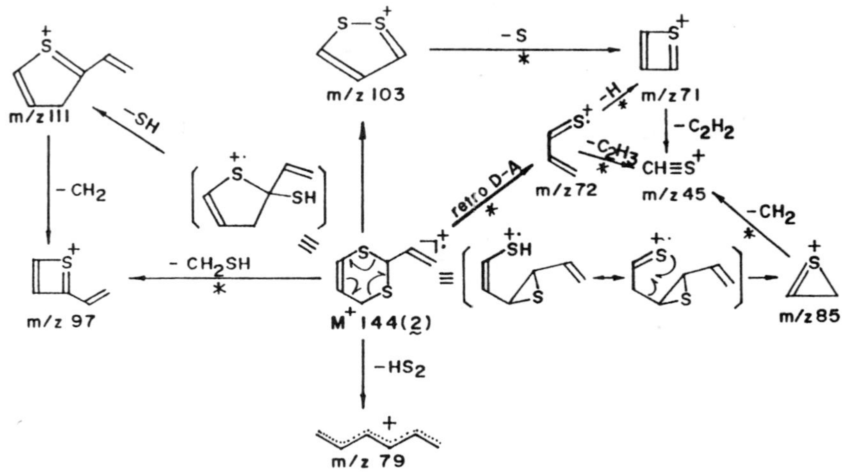

FIG. 5. MASS SPECTRAL FRAGMENTATION OF 2-VINYL-4*H*-1,3-DITHIIN (**2**)
* Indicates observed metastable ion.

Synthesis and Activity of Vinyldithiin Derivatives

To examine the structure-activity relationship for the platelet aggregating inhibition, vinyldithiin derivatives were synthesized as shown in Fig. 6.

As a result, sulfur-oxidized compounds shown in Fig. 7 exhibited more potent inhibitory activity than the non-oxidized dithiins.

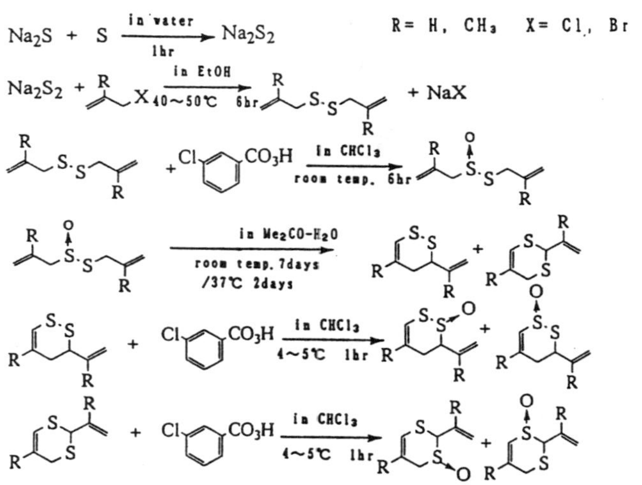

FIG. 6. SYNTHESIS OF VINYLDITHIIN DERIVATIVES

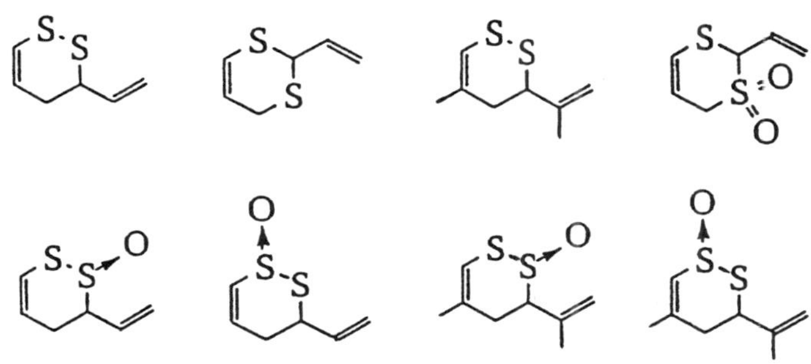

FIG. 7. VINYLDITHIINS AND SULFUR-OXIDIZED COMPOUNDS

REFERENCES

ADAMU, I., JOSEPH, P.K. and AUGUSTI, K.T. 1982. Hypolipidemic action of onion and garlic unsaturated oils in sucrose fed rats over a two-month period. Experientia *38*, 899–901.

AKASHI, K., NISHIMURA, H. and MIZUTANI, J. 1975. Precursors and enzymatic development of caucas flavor components. Agric. Biol. Chem. *39*, 1507–1508.

APITZ-CASTRO R., CABRERA S., CRUZ M.R., LEDEZMA, E. and JAIN, M.K. 1983. Effects of garlic extract and of three pure components isolated from it on human platelet aggregation arachidonate metabolism, release reaction and platelet ultrastructure. Thromb. Res. *32*, 155–169.

APITZ-CASTRO, R., ESCALANTE, J., VARGAS, R. and JAIN, M.K. 1986. Ajoene, the antiplatelet principle of garlic, synergistically potentiates the antiaggregatory action of prostacyclin, foskolin, indomethacin and dypiridamole on human platelets. Thromb. Res. *42*, 303–311.

ARIGA, T., OSHIBA, S. and TAMADA, T. 1981. Platelet aggregation inhibitor in garlic. Lancet *1*, 150–151.

BESLIN, P. 1983. A facile synthesis of two thioacrolein dimers. A new entry to a flavor component in asparagus. J. Heterocycl. Chem. *20*, 1753–1754.

BLOCK, E., AHMAD, S., JAIN, M.K., CRECELY, R.W., APITZ-CASTRO, R. and CRUZ, M.R. 1984. The chemistry of alkyl thiosulfinate esters. 8. (*E*, *Z*)-Ajoene; a potent antithrombotic agent from garlic. J. Am. Chem. Soc. *106*, 8295–8296.

BLOCK, E., AHMAD, S., CATALFAMO, J.L., JAIN, M.K. and APITZ-CASTRO, R.C. 1986. The chemistry of alkyl thiosufinate esters. 9. Antithrombotic organosulfur compounds from garlic; structural, mechanistic and synthetic studies. J. Am. Chem. Soc., *108*, 7045–7055.

BOCK, H., MOHMAND, S., HIRABAYASHI, T. and SEMKOV, A. 1982. Thioacrolein: Das stabilste C_3H_4S-Isomere und sein PE-spektroskopischer Nachweis in der Gasphase. Chem. Ber. *115*, 1339–1348.

NISHIMURA, H., FUJIWARA, K., MIZUTANI, J. and OBATA, Y. 1971. Volatile flavor components of caucas. J. Agric. Food Chem. *19*, 992–994.

NISHIMURA, H., WIJAYA, C.H. and MIZUTANI, J. 1988. Volatile flavor components and antithrombotic agent; vinyldithiins from *Allium victorialis L.* J. Agric. Food Chem. *36*, 563–566.

QURESHI, A.A., ABUIRMEILEH, N., DIN, Z.Z., ELSON, C.E. and BURGER, W.C. 1983. Inhibition of cholesterol and fatty acid biosynthesis in liver enzymes and chicken hepatocytes by polar fraction of garlic. Lipids *18*, 343–348.

SAMSON, R.R. 1982. Effect of dietary garlic and temporal drift on platelet aggregation. Atherosclerosis *44*, 119–120.

YURUGI, S., MATSUOKA, M. and TOGASHI, M. 1954. Vitamin B_1 and related compounds. LXI. Reactions between thiamine and constituents of Allium and related plants. J. Pharm. Soc. Jpn. *74*, 1017–1021.

WIJAYA, C.H., NISHIMURA, H., TANAKA, T. and MIZUTANI, J. 1991. Influence of drying methods on volatile sulfur constituents of caucas (*Allium victorialis* L.). J. Food Sci. *56*, 72–75.

CANCER PREVENTIVE PHYTOCHEMICALS FROM TROPICAL ZINGIBERACEAE

AKIRA MURAKAMI[1], YOSHIMASA NAKAMURA[2], YOSHIMI OHTO[2], TAKUJI TANAKA[3], HIROKI MAKITA[3], KOICHI KOSHIMIZU[1], and HAJIME OHIGASHI[2]

[1]Department of Biotechnological Science
Faculty of Biology-Oriented Science and Technology
Kinki University
Iwade-Uchita, Wakayama 649-64, Japan

[2]Division of Applied Life Sciences
Graduate School of Agriculture
Kyoto University
Kyoto 606-01, Japan

[3]First Department of Pathology
Gifu University School of Medicine
40 Tsukasa-machi, Gifu 500, Japan

ABSTRACT

*Screening tests for inhibitory activities of the methanol extracts from edible southeast Asian plants toward 12-O-hexadecanoylphorbol 13-acetate (HPA)-induced Epstein-Barr virus (EBV) activation suggested a high potentiality of such plants, especially the Zingiberaceae, for cancer chemoprevention. Activity-guiding separation of the extracts from Zingiberaceae samples resulted in the isolation and identification of cardamonin (*Boesenbergia pandurata*), curcumin (*Zingiber cassumunar*), and 1'-acetoxychavicol acetate (ACA) (*Languas galanga*). Notably, ACA showed powerful inhibitory effects on 4-nitroquinoline 1-oxide (4-NQO)-induced rat tongue carcinogenesis in the initiation or post-initiation phase as well as on 12-O-tetradecanoylphorbol 13-acetate (TPA)-induced skin tumor promotion in ICR mice initiated with 7,12-dimethylbenz[a]anthracene (DMBA). ACA, previously reported to be a xanthine oxidase (XOD) inhibitor, exhibited noticeable inhibition toward TPA-induced superoxide ($O_2^{\cdot-}$) generation in DMSO-differentiated HL-60 cells. Suppression of TPA-induced hydrogen peroxide (H_2O_2) production in mouse skin was then confirmed in the two-dose treatment model. Lacking radical scavenging potential, ACA may be recognized as an intrinsic antioxidant which specifically blocks both the XOD and NADPH oxidase systems generating $O_2^{\cdot-}$.*

INTRODUCTION

It is no longer a subject of controversy that food habits are closely related to the onset of "life style-related diseases", e.g., cardiovascular disease or cancer. We have been focusing on anti-tumor promotion with food phytochemicals as a strategy for cancer chemoprevention (Murakami *et al.* 1996a). The tumor promotion stage, caused by phorbol esters or other chemicals in experimental rodents and probably by high fat or salt intake in humans, is a reversible process at least in its earlier stages, and takes a long time to occur (Pitot and Dragan 1991). Inhibition of tumor promotion, thus, is predicted to be a more practical and effective means of cancer control in humans. In our continuing studies of anti-tumor promoting food items, ingredients, or agents, edible Thai plants, most of which have been traditionally used as condiments, flavors and concurrently as folk medicines, exhibited a high potentiality for cancer prevention (Murakami *et al.* 1993). In particular, the Zingiberaceae from Thailand were implied to contain potent chemopreventive agents when screened for inhibitory activities toward tumor promoter 12-O-hexadecanoylphorbol 13-acetate (HPA)-induced Epstein-Barr virus (EBV) activation in Raji cells (Murakami *et al.* 1994, 1995). In this article, we describe: 1) the high applicability of the Zingiberaceae from southeast Asian countries for chemoprevention; 2) some of their active constituents; 3) cancer preventive activities *in vivo*, and 4) possible action mechanisms.

RESULTS AND DISCUSSION

Zingiberaceae Plants as a Promising Source of Chemopreventive Agents

A total of 398 methanol extracts from edible plants collected at local markets in Thailand, Indonesia and Malaysia were tested for the inhibitory assay of HPA-induced EBV activation in Raji cells, which is a short-term assay measuring anti-tumor promoting activities *in vitro* (Koshimizu *et al.* 1988). Their inhibitory activities at a concentration of 200 μg/mL were divided into the following four ranks: +++, strongly active [inhibitory rate (IR) ≥ 70%]; ++, moderately active (70% > IR ≥ 50%); +, weakly active (50% > IR ≥ 30%); -, inactive (30% > IR). As summarized in Fig. 1, the Zingiberaceae plants tested in the present study were found to be promising sources of chemopreventive agents as compared with plants from other families.

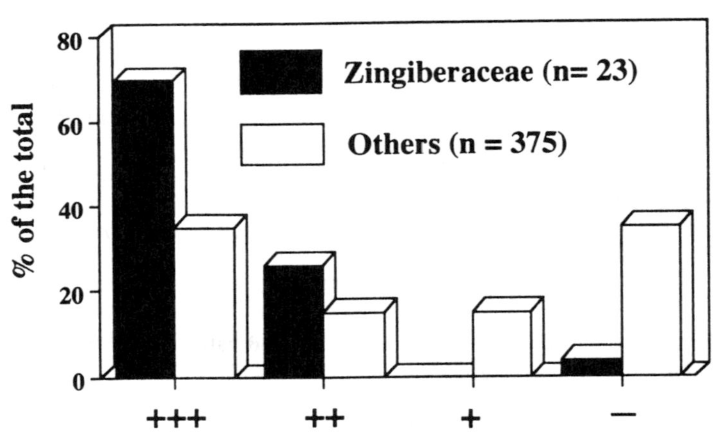

FIG. 1. INHIBITORY PROPORTIONS OF THE ZINGIBERACEAE AND OTHER SPECIES TOWARD EBV ACTIVATION

In vitro Active Constituents

So far, activity-guiding separation of the EBV activation inhibitors of the Zingiberaceae plants resulted in the isolation and identification of cardamonin (*Boesenbergia pandurata*, IC_{50} = 3.1 μM) (Murakami *et al.* 1993), curcumin (*Zingiber cassumunar*, IC_{50} = 5.4 μM) (Murakami *et al.* 1994), and 1′-acetoxychavicol acetate (ACA) (*Languas galanga*, IC_{50}= 1.3 μM) (Kondo *et al.* 1993) (Fig. 2).

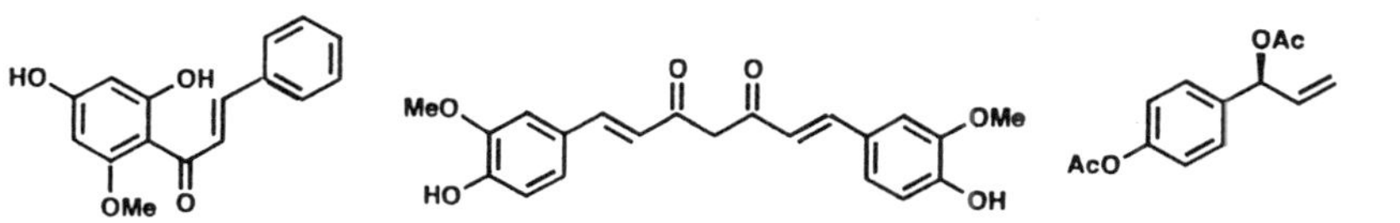

cardamonin (*Boesenbergia pandurata*) — curcumin (*Zingiber cassumunar*) — 1′-acetoxychavicol acetate (*Languas galanga*)

FIG. 2. STRUCTURES OF ACTIVE CONSTITUENTS FROM ZINGIBERACEAE

Curcumin is a yellow pigment used as a food additive and has been reported to inhibit carcinogenesis in several animal models (Huang *et al.* 1988, 1994; Tanaka *et al.* 1994). Curcumin has diverse biological activities, i.e., inhibition of enzymes involved in the tumor promotion stage (ornithine decarboxylase, lipoxygenase, cyclooxygenase, etc.), anti-oxidative, anti-inflammatory activities, and so forth (Sharma 1976; Rao *et al.* 1982; Lu *et al.* 1988; Kelley *et al.* 1996). ACA, occurring in the rhizomes of *Languas galanga* at a level of 0.09% in the rhizomes (Murakami *et al.* 1994), was first identified as an anti-ulcer agent by Mitsui *et al.* (1976). The IC_{50} value of ACA (1.3 μM) in the EBV assay was evaluated to be much lower (18-52 times) than those of representative chemopreventive agents from edible plants: α-linolenic acid (IC_{50} = 27 μM), β-carotene (IC_{50} = 30 μM), (-)-epigallocatechin gallate (IC_{50} = 68 μM), and quercetin (IC_{50} = 23 μM) (Murakami *et al.* 1994).

Chemopreventive Effect of ACA on 4-NQO-induced Rat Tongue Carcinogenesis

Chemopreventive effect of ACA on 4-nitroquinoline 1-oxide (4-NQO)-induced rat tongue carcinogenesis was examined in the initiation and post-initiation phases (Ohnishi *et al.* 1996). The experimental protocol and results after 32 weeks are shown in Fig. 3. While 58% of rats in Group 1 (4-NQO alone) bore tongue tumors (17% papilloma and 54% carcinoma), no tumors were observed in Groups 2, 4, and 5, and only 9% (2 rats) developed tumors in Group 3. Incidence of preneoplastic lesions (hyperplasia and dysplasia) were also reduced in Groups 2-5. These results definitely indicate that oral administration of ACA at 100 or 500 ppm in the initiation or post-initiation phase is highly effective for 4-NQO-induced oral carcinogenesis. In the tests, biomarkers for proliferation indices such as polyamine levels, silver-stained nucleolar organizer regions' protein (AgNORs) and 5-bromodeoxyuridine (BrdU)-labeling indices were also significantly reduced in Groups 2-5 compared with those in Group 1 (data not shown) (Ohnishi *et al.* 1996).

Anti-tumor-promoting Activity of ACA in Mouse Skin

The anti-tumor-promoting activity of ACA was examined by a standard initiation-promotion protocol with 7,12-dimethylbenz[a]anthracene (DMBA) and TPA as previously reported (Murakami *et al.* 1996b). The mice at 7 weeks old were initiated with topical application of DMBA (0.19 μmol). One week after initiation, the mice were promoted

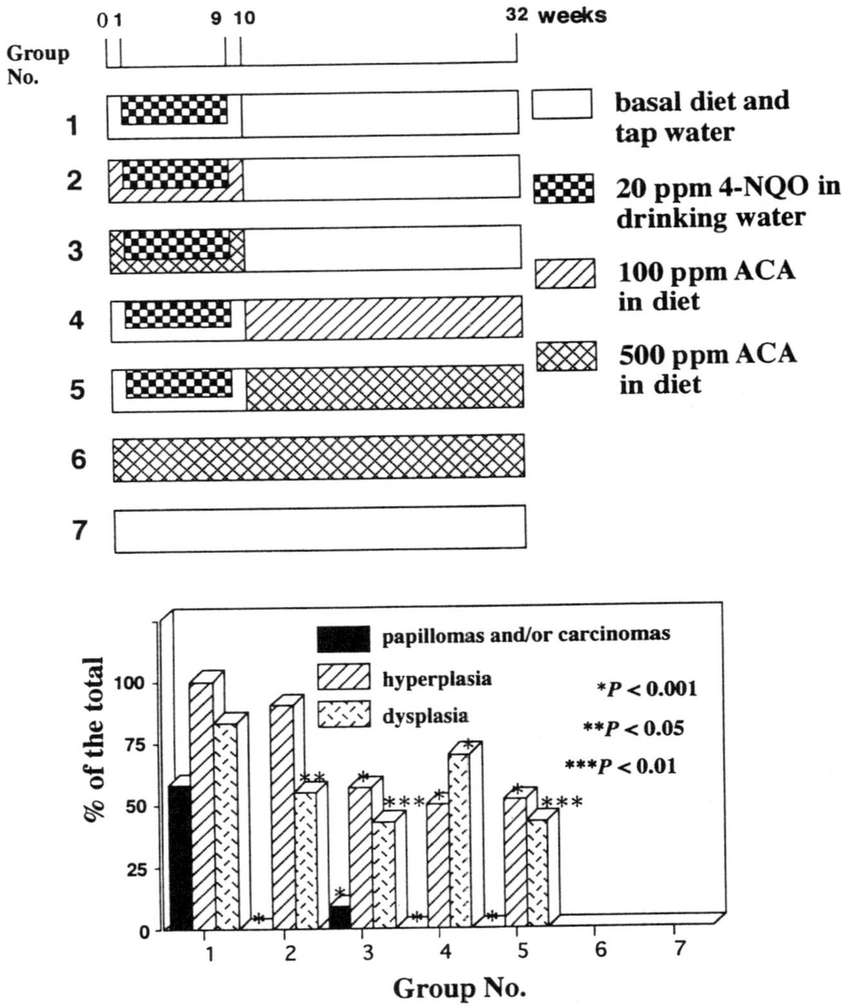

FIG. 3. EXPERIMENTAL PROTOCOL (ABOVE) AND RESULTS (BELOW) OF 4-NQO-INDUCED RAT TONGUE CARCINOGENESIS TEST

with TPA (1.6 nmol) twice a week for 20 weeks. In two other groups, the mice were treated with topical application of ACA (1.6 nmol or 160 nmol) 40 min before each TPA treatment. As shown in Fig. 4, the rate of tumor-bearing mice and the average number of tumors per mouse in the control group reached 88% and 16.0, respectively, at 20 weeks into the experiment. In the group pretreated with 160 nmol of ACA, the average number of tumors per mouse and the ratio of tumor-bearing mice were reduced by 90% and 42%, respectively. ACA, even at an equal dose (1.6 nmol) to TPA, significantly reduced the average number of tumors per mouse by 44%.

Suppressive Effect of ACA on Superoxide Generation *In Vitro*

ACA was previously reported to be a xanthine oxidase (XOD) inhibitor. This was reconfirmed in our recent study (Murakami *et al.* 1996b). XOD, a versatile enzyme occurring widely in epidermal cells, converts xanthine (XA) into uric acid, and this reaction is conjugated with superoxide ($O_2^{\cdot-}$) generation. On the other hand, the NADPH oxidase system is also known to be responsible for $O_2^{\cdot-}$ generation in leukocytes. Promyelocytic HL-60 cells are differentiated into granulocyte-like cells by treatment with DMSO, generating $O_2^{\cdot-}$ with TPA stimulation. Figure 5 shows the inhibitory effect of ACA and genistein, a tyrosine kinase inhibitor used as a positive control, on TPA-induced extracellular $O_2^{\cdot-}$ generation in differentiated HL-60 cells. Because extracellular test compounds were removed by washing with PBS, the inhibition observed here would not be due to $O_2^{\cdot-}$ scavenging effect but might be attributable to the blocking of $O_2^{\cdot-}$ generation pathway(s) in the NADPH oxidase system. In fact, ACA has no $O_2^{\cdot-}$ scavenging effect in the XA/XOD system (Murakami *et al.* 1996b).

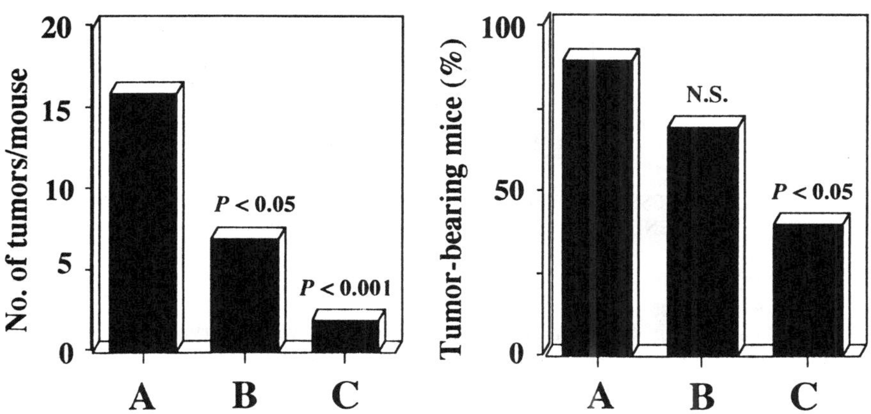

FIG. 4. ANTI-TUMOR-PROMOTING ACTIVITY OF ACA IN ICR MOUSE SKIN
A: TPA (1.6 nmol) alone
B: TPA (1.6 nmol) + ACA (1.6 nmol)
C: TPA (1.6 nmol) + ACA (160 nmol)

Suppressive Effect of ACA on Hydrogen Peroxide Production *In Vivo*

A strong inhibitory activity of ACA toward $O_2^{\cdot-}$ generation led us to examine *in vivo* anti-oxidative activity using the two-dose treatment model (Wei *et al.* 1992, 1993), in which first application of TPA to mouse skin recruits leukocytes such as neutrophils by chemical mediators to the TPA-applied inflammatory regions. Superoxide is then drastically generated with a second TPA application through the NADPH oxidase system of leukocytes to form reactive oxygen species (ROS) such as hydrogen peroxide (H_2O_2), hydroxyl radical, or hydroperoxides. Also, TPA application reduces the activity of reactive oxygen scavenging or decomposing enzymes such as superoxide dismutase (SOD), glutathione peroxidase, or catalase. These lines of evidence raise the possibility that oxidative stress, resulting from an altered balance between production and deactivation of ROS, would be a critical step for the tumor promotion stage.

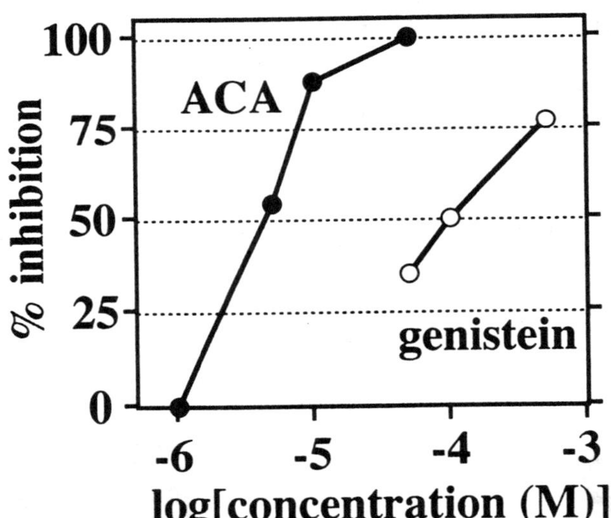

FIG. 5. SUPPRESSIVE EFFECT OF ACA AND GENISTEIN ON SUPEROXIDE GENERATION IN DIFFERENTIATED HL-60 CELLS

As shown in Fig. 6, remarkable production of H_2O_2 was observed ($0.36 \pm 0.25 \rightarrow 10.46 \pm 1.84$ nmol/6 mm punch in diameter) with the second TPA treatment (8.1 nmol) in mouse skin. Pretreatment with 810 nmol ACA, 30 min prior to TPA treatment restored this to basal levels of H_2O_2 (0.79 ± 0.38 nmol/punch). Thus, ACA was proven to mitigate TPA-induced oxidative stress possibly through suppression of leukocyte activation. In addition to relevance of the NADPH oxidase system to oxidative stress, topical application of TPA in mouse skin also elevates the level of XOD. Therefore, XOD inhibition by ACA could contribute to mitigation of oxidative stress in mouse skin.

Overall, suppressive effects of ACA on TPA-induced oxidative stress would, at least in part, be involved in the action mechanisms by which ACA inhibits tumor promotion in mouse skin.

CONCLUSIONS

The present study demonstrated the appropriateness of our criterion for plant selection, i.e., directed to edible southeast Asian plants, for the discovery of new highly effective types of chemopreventers. The screening data revealed that there are a considerable number of promising Zingiberaceae plants. In this regard, systematic phytochemical surveys are requisite to locate and prove the beneficial aspects of such plants for chemoprevention.

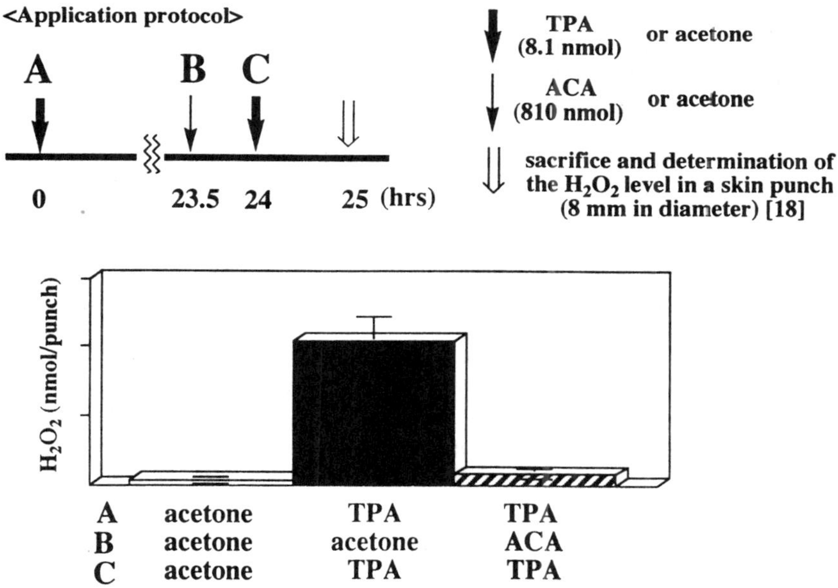

FIG. 6. EXPERIMENTAL PROTOCOL (ABOVE) AND SUPPRESSIVE EFFECT OF ACA ON TPA-INDUCED H_2O_2 PRODUCTION IN MOUSE SKIN (BELOW)

ACKNOWLEDGMENTS

This study was partly supported by a Grant-in-Aid from the Ministry of Health and Welfare for the Second Term Comprehensive 10-Year Strategy for Cancer Control, Japan, and Takeda Food Products, Ltd. We thank M.A. Huffman for his continued enthusiasm of our work and helpful comments on earlier versions of this manuscript.

REFERENCES

HUANG, M.-T., SMART, R.C., WONG, C.Q. and CONNEY, A.H. 1988. Inhibitory effect of curcumin, chlorogenic acid, caffeic acid, and ferulic acid on tumor promotion in mouse skin by 12-*O*-tetradecanoylphorbol-13-acetate. Cancer Res. *48*, 5941–5946.

HUANG, M.-T., LOU, Y.-R., MA, W., NEWMARK, H.L., REUHL, K.R. and CONNEY, A.H. 1994. Inhibitory effects of dietary curcumin on forestomach, duodenal and colon carcinogenesis in mice. Cancer Res. *54*, 5841–5847.

KELLEY, D.J., SACK, P.G., RAMONETTI, J.T., SCHANTZ, S.P. and DANNENBERG, A.J. 1996. Curcumin inhibits prostaglandin synthesis and cyclooxygenase-2 expression in oral epithelial cells. Proc. Amer. Assoc. Cancer Res. *37*, 598.

KONDO, A, OHIGASHI, H., MURAKAMI, A., SURATWADEE, J. and KOSHIMIZU, K. 1993. A potent inhibitor of tumor promoter-induced Epstein-Barr virus activation, 1′-acetoxychavicol acetate from *Languas galanga*, a traditional Thai condiment. Biosci. Biotech. Biochem. *57*, 1344–1345.

KOSHIMIZU, K., OHIGASHI, H., TOKUDA, H., KONDO, A. and YAMAGUCHI, K. 1988. Screening of edible plants against anti-tumor promoting activity. Cancer Lett. *39*, 247–257.

LU, Y.-P., CHANG, R.L., HUANG, M.-T. and CONNEY, A.H. 1988. Inhibitory effect of curcumin on 12-*O*-tetradecanoylphorbol-13-acetate-induced increase in ornithine decarboxylase mRNA in mouse epidermis. Carcinogenesis *14*, 293–297.

MITSUI, S., KOBAYASHI, S., NAGAHORI, H. and OGISO, A. 1976. Constituents from seeds of *Alpinia galanga* Wild. and their anti-ulcer activities. Chem. Pharm. Bull. *24*, 2377–2382.

MURAKAMI, A., KONDO, A., NAKAMURA, Y., OHIGASHI, H. and KOSHIMIZU, K. 1993. Possible anti-tumor promoting properties from edible plants of Thailand, and identification of an active constituent, cardamonin, of *Boesenbergia pandurata*. Biosci. Biotech. Biochem. *57*, 1971–1973.

MURAKAMI, A., OHIGASHI, H. and KOSHIMIZU, K. 1994. Possible anti-tumour promoting properties of traditional Thai food items and some of their active constituents. Asia Pacific J. Clin. Nutr. *3*, 185–191.

MURAKAMI, A., JIWAJINDA, S., KOSHIMIZU, K. and OHIGASHI, H. 1995. Screening for *in vitro* anti-tumor promoting activities of edible plants from Thailand. Cancer Lett. *95*, 139–146.

MURAKAMI, A., OHIGASHI, H. and KOSHIMIZU, K. 1996a. Anti-tumor promotion with food phytochemicals: a strategy for cancer chemoprevention. Biosci. Biotech. Biochem. *60*, 1–8.

MURAKAMI, A., OHURA, S., NAKAMURA, Y., KOSHIMIZU, K. and OHIGASHI, H. 1996b. 1′-Acetoxychavicol acetate, a superoxide anion generation inhibitor, potently inhibits tumor promotion by 12-*O*-tetradecanoylphorbol-13-acetate in ICR mouse skin. Oncology *53*, 386–391.

OHNISHI, M., YANAKA, T., MAKITA, H., KAWAMORI, T., MORI, H., SATOH, K., HARA, A., MURAKAMI, A., OHIGASHI, H. and KOSHIMIZU, K. 1996. Chemopreventive effect of a xanthine oxidase inhibitor, 1′-acetoxychavicol acetate, on rat oral carcinogenesis. Jpn. J. Cancer Res. *87*, 349–356.

PITOT, H.C. and DRAGAN, Y.P. 1991. Facts and theories concerning the mechanisms of carcinogenesis. FASEB J. *5*, 2280–2286.

SHARMA, O.P. 1976. Antioxidant activity of curcumin and related compounds. Biochem. Pharmacol. 25, 1811–1812.

RAO, T.S., BASU, N. and SIDDIQUI, H.H. 1982. Anti-inflammatory activity of curcumin analogs. Indian J. Med. Res. *75*, 574–578.

TANAKA, T., MAKITA, H., OHNISHI, M., HIROSE, Y., WANG, A., MORI, H., SATOH, K., HARA, A. and OGAWA, H. 1994. Chemoprevention of 4-nitroquinoline 1-oxide-induced oral carcinogenesis by dietary curcumin and hesperidine: comparison with the protective effect of β-carotene. Cancer Res. *54*, 4654–4659.

WEI, H. and FRENKEL, K. 1992. Sarcophytol a suppresses the oxidative events and DNA damage in vivo: A possible mechanism of anti-tumor promotion. Cancer Res. *52*, 2298–2303.

WEI, H., WEI, L., BOWEN, R., FRENKEL, K. and BARNES, S. 1993. Inhibition of tumor promoter-induced hydrogen peroxide production *in vitro* and *in vivo* by genistein. Nutr. Cancer. *20*, 1–12.

HIGH PRESSURE PRESERVED FOODS: COMMERCIAL DEVELOPMENT CHALLENGES

DANIEL F. FARKAS

Department of Food Science and Technology
Oregon State University
Corvallis, OR 97331-6602

ABSTRACT

Foods preserved by high pressure processes (HPP) are available in Japan and are entering the market in the United States and Europe. HPP technology can be used as a pasteurization process to extend the shelf life of refrigerated foods and with acid foods can yield commercially sterile, shelf stable, products. Because HPP will inactivate vegetative microbes with minimal effects on enzyme activity, pressure preserved foods may require additional treatments to reduce or block degrading enzyme activity. Products which use heat in their preparation cannot be distinguished from non-treated controls when preserved by HPP. High pressure preserved foods can lose their fresh character after several weeks of storage at room temperature. Packaging to reduce quality loss includes careful removal of oxygen followed by packaging in a superior oxygen barrier flexible container. HPP preservation treatments must be determined for each product based on expected microbiological contamination. Commercial equipment for the cost effective HPP preservation of foods is undergoing rigorous development.

INTRODUCTION

Preserving foods by high hydrostatic pressures above 100 MPa (1000 atmospheres) is designated as high pressure processing (HPP). Currently commercial HPP processes operate in the range of 400 to above 680 MPa (4000 to 6800 atmospheres). Since HPP does not cause changes in covalent bonds in foods, operating pressures near 680 MPa are used to reduce the treatment time needed to inactivate microbes. This is an economic advantage rather than a quality advantage and is in contrast to heat preservation in which high-temperature-short-time (HTST) heat treatments are used to take advantage of the differences in activation energies between microbial inactivation and the reaction rates leading to the loss of food flavors, colors and nutrients.

Research on the HPP of foods during the last 15 years has differentiated the mechanism of microbial inactivation by HPP from that of heat. Vegetative microbes lose their ability to reproduce due to HPP damage to their cell membranes. This damage appears to reduce the cell's ability to control the transport of ions and water, causing the cell to collapse. HPP damaged cells may be able to repair themselves when held under favorable conditions of nutrient media composition and temperature. Holding times for repair may be as long as 60 days at refrigerated temperatures (Nadathur *et al.* 1997). Further information on HPP technology can be found in books edited by Ledward *et al.* (1995) and Ohlsson (1996).

HPP APPLICATIONS TO FOOD PROCESSING

HPP, like heat, can be used in the preservation of foods and to create improved food structures by gelling proteins and starches. Because HPP does not break covalent bonds HPP treated foods can be rendered free of vegetative microbes without changing the flavor of the food. HPP is not effective in inactivating spores of *Clostridium botulinum* and other heat resistant spores including non-proteolytic types of C. *botulinum* such as Type E. HPP treatments may be only marginally effective in the inactivation of food spoilage enzymes. These constraints must be overcome if HPP is to be used to extend the shelf-life of low acid foods.

Peck (1997) reviewed the safety of low acid foods preserved by refrigeration and summarized published values for storage times to form toxins for Type B, E, and F *C. botulinum* (non-proteolytic) in foods held at several refrigerated temperatures. Salmon and cod were found to form toxins in 21 days at 4°C and in 6-8 days at 8°C when inoculated with 1-100 spores. Peck listed eight procedures which, if incorporated into the product formulation, the distribution procedure, or the preservation process, would ensure the safety of low acid HPP treated foods against the production of *C. botulinum* toxin. Procedures applicable to HPP technology include limiting the shelf life to less than 5 days if the product is held at 5-10°C, adjusting the pH of the product to less than 5.0, and reducing the water activity to below 0.97.

USING HPP IN COMBINATION WITH REFRIGERATION TO EXTEND THE SHELF LIFE OF LOW ACID FOODS

Low acid foods (with a pH greater than 4.5) in hermetically sealed containers must be held below 10°C (50°F) to prevent the production of proteolytic *C. botulinum* toxin and below 3°C (37°F) to prevent the growth of non-proteolytic *C. botulinum* toxin. Because there is no assurance that the temperature of a refrigerated low acid food will be below 3°C during distribution, the food processor should employ pH reduction to below 5.0 or water activity reduction to below 0.97 to ensure the safety of the food. If these procedures are followed, HPP treated low acid foods may achieve a refrigerated shelf-life of more than 30 days.

The actual pressure-time treatment needed to achieve a desired refrigerated shelf life must be determined experimentally because the product composition and types and numbers of microbes will determine these values. At this time the only product to have been HPP treated and distributed commercially under refrigeration is guacamole. Thus it is not possible to specify typical pressures and times to achieve a useful and safe shelf life extension for low acid foods in general. Background microbial counts (plate count agar) of several hundred per gram typically can be achieved with pressure time combinations of 550-650 MPa in the range of 5-10 min. These counts reflect germinated spores.

Research is needed to develop process conditions for the safe shelf life extension of low acid foods by HPP. Microbial challenges using 10^6 to 10^7 pathogens or spoilage species must be performed. Ideally an HPP treatment that can inactivate 10^6 cells of non-proteolytic *C. botulinum* is required. As in heat process development, the results of this research would be product specific.

COMMERCIAL STERILIZATION AND PASTEURIZATION OF ACID FOODS BY HPP

Naturally acid and directly acidified foods (with a pH of 4.5 or lower) are well suited to preservation by HPP. Values of pH of 4.5 or lower will block the germination of proteolytic and non-proteolytic *C. botulinum* spores. Pathogenic and spoilage vegetative microbes appear to be reasonably susceptible to inactivation by HPP treatments. However, those spores which may germinate below a pH of 4.5 such as *Bacillus coagulans* spores may not be inactivated by the pressures and times needed to inactivate vegetative microbes (Roberts and Hoover 1996).

HPP treated acid foods have been marketed in Japan for over five years and represent an ideal application of this technology to the preservation of foods. Commercial sterility of acid foods can be achieved with a wide range of pressure-time processes. Process optimization is needed to deliver a shelf stable product at the lowest process cost. The food processor can formulate a product to take advantage of hurdles such as pH and nisin together with pressure level and time to reduce the overall cost of the preservation process. Lower pressures allow lower equipment and operating costs, but may reduce product production rates due to longer treatment times. Process costs are related to the hourly cycle rate of a high pressure system.

HPP treatments can be used for the pasteurization of acid foods to render the food free of vegetative microbial pathogens without changing its fresh sensory profile. Fruit juices, fruits for yogurt or ice cream, and fresh or frozen fruits can be rendered pathogen free for safe addition to products in which no further heat or other microbial inactivation treatment is possible or desirable. For example HPP treatment could eliminate the need for preservatives in fresh fruit mixes sold refrigerated from vending machines.

OPTIMIZING HPP MANUFACTURING TECHNOLOGIES LIQUID FOODS

The technology for HPP preservation of liquid and solid acid foods is under intense development. Equipment for the semi-continuous HPP treatment of liquid foods is based on pumping products into one or more small volume pressure vessels, holding the liquid at the desired pressure for a specified time, and releasing the treated product under controlled de-pressurizing conditions to a sterile holding tank for subsequent aseptic or clean filling. The design of pumps, valves, seals, piping, and pressure vessels compatible with foods and capable of long term aseptic operation at pressures over 500 MPa is challenging. Flow International (Kent, Washington) has prototype equipment under development in conjunction with the U.S. Army Natick RD&E Center at Natick, Massachusetts. Initial tests indicate that pilot plant scale units can pasteurize fruit juices using operating pressures between 400 to 540 MPa. Microbiological challenges are in progress using *Listeria*, *Salmonella*, yeasts, molds, and lactic acid spoilage bacteria inoculated at 10^7 microbes per gram of test food.

Pressurization of liquid and solid foods results in a heating on compression of several degrees centigrade per 100 MPa pressure increase. There is a volume decrease of up to 15% at 680 MPa (100,000 psi). On decompression both the volume and temperature of the food return to their initial state. Compression is not a major concern in liquid foods treated in a pumped system and filled aseptically after HPP treatment.

Volume compression of pre-packaged foods treated in batch systems is a packaging issue because the package must withstand compression of up to 15%.

SOLID FOODS

HPP treatment of solid foods consists of placing the food in a suitable package without a headspace after thorough vacuum de-gassing. The package is hermetically sealed and pressure treated for the time needed to achieve the needed shelf life of the product. The fresh sensory attributes of HPP stabilized foods dictates that products should be held at refrigerated temperatures prior to use. Storage studies on the sensory qualities of HPP stabilized foods all have shown the quality advantages of refrigerated storage even though the products themselves are microbiologically stable. Sensory studies have shown that products stored at 27°C can be differentiated from those held at 5°C in as little as 30 days and show lower sensory ratings for freshness (Young *et al.* 1997). Aseptically processed products show a similar loss in sensory quality when held at temperatures above 5°C.

PACKAGING

HPP treated foods must be packaged to accommodate compression of the food which can be as high as 15% at 680 MPa. Polymer packaging structures for HPP treated foods must protect against oxygen and not scalp aromas or be stained by natural pigments. The structure must maintain an hermetic seal during possible distortion under compression. These requirements can be met using existing high oxygen barrier polymer structures. The microwaveable Omni™ bowl (Silgan Container Co., Chicago, Illinois) with a double seamed, easy-open, aluminum lid has proved to be a useful semirigid package for HPP treated foods. The Omni™ bowl must be filled completely to prevent compression damage.

All packaging used in HPP must be filled and sealed without a headspace. Any residual gas requires substantial additional compression work and the gas is driven into the food. On standing any residual gas accumulates in the headspace of the package. If oxygen is present it can discolor the product in the headspace area.

Packaging for HPP must make maximum use of the available treatment volume in the pressure vessel since volumetric efficiency (package volume/vessel volume) is a critical part of HPP treatment costs. This will be discussed in the section on process costs.

PROCESS COSTS

Research is underway on batch and semi-continuous pumped HPP systems to reduce capital, operating, and maintenance costs for equipment operating at pressures up to 680 MPa.

Semi-Continuous Pumped Systems

Equipment is being tested at operating pressures up to 545 MPa for the semi-continuous treatment of foods that can be pumped (Flow International, Kent, Washington). The advantages of a pumped system include minimum pressure vessel cost and potentially long vessel life since multiple small vessels can be filled, pressurized, and de-pressurized automatically using a single pump. A pumped system uses the entire volume of the pressure vessel and process temperatures can be measured and controlled in a conventional manner. The treated product can be accumulated in a sterile holding tank for aseptic filling in a variety of aseptic packages and filling systems. Labor costs are usually lower with an automated, pumped system.

Pumped systems represent a mechanical challenge because seals, valves, and pumping equipment must run safely and without cross contamination for extended periods of time at pressures over 500 MPa. The engineering demands of these operating pressures require state-of-the-art advances in metallurgy and high pressure engineering. It is too early in the development cycle to determine the cost per kilogram for pumped HPP treated foods treated in semi-continuous systems.

Batch Isostatic Press Systems

The isostatic press, used to form powders into high strength parts, has been adapted for food processing use. Isostatic pressing systems consist of a pressure vessel, a pump designed to deliver oil at pressures in the range of 100 MPa or less to an intensifier, an intensifier, and appropriate controls for process pressure, temperature, and time. The cost of the pressure vessel is a function of operating pressure, useful cycle life, vessel volume, and method of sealing. The cost of other components is related to the operating pressure and their ability to resist wear due to the flow of water and potential corrosiveness of water at pressures up to 680 MPa.

Systems operating below 400 MPa are less costly to construct because relatively long-vessel cycle life can be obtained without multiple wall or wire wound structures. Operating pressures above 400 MPa require wire wound or multiple wall vessels to achieve useful cycle lives of over 100,000 cycles. Current pressure vessel design efforts are aimed at useful cycle lives of 1,000,000 cycles. The operating cost of a pressure vessel with a useful cycle life of one million cycles will be much less than a unit with a cycle life of one hundred thousand cycles even if the capital cost for the million cycle unit is two or three times greater.

HPP costs per kilogram of food treated include equipment capital, operating, and maintenance costs. HPP systems using pressures above 400 MPa may incur high maintenance costs as regular inspection is required of pumps, valves, seals, vessel closures, intensifier and process piping. The pressure vessel liner must be inspected for potential cracks after a predetermined number of cycles. Even a minute leak of high pressure water must be repaired immediately. Operating costs include labor, utilities and related plant and business costs.

HPP treatment cost per kilogram of food is the yearly operating of the HPP system divided by the kilograms of food treated per year. If all food treated is sold, then the cost per kilogram of food will be directly related to the number of cycles the high pressure system can deliver per year. Multiple daily shifts are favored to increase product throughput.

The remaining variable affecting the processing cost per kilogram of food is the volumetric efficiency (volume of packages/volume of pressure chamber) of the process chamber for the mix of packaged products treated. Volumetric efficiencies can range from over 0.8 for food packaged in five kilogram plastic bags to 0.25 for food packaged in Omni™ bowls holding 0.24 kg. All things being equal the treatment cost per kg of the product in bowls could be three times the bulk pack.

Because per kg treatment costs are so sensitive to cycle rate per h and volumetric efficiency, there is a large incentive to design isostatic presses with rapid cycling capability for packages that occupy 0.8 or more of the available process volume. A desirable target would be a batch isostatic press that can be loaded, sealed, pressurized, depressurized, opened and unloaded in less than a min.

REFERENCES

LEDWARD, D.A., JOHNSTON, D.E., EARNSHAW, R.G. and HASTING, A.P.M. (eds.) 1995. High Pressure Processing of Foods. Nottingham University Press, Nottingham.

NADATHUR, S.R., ALEMAN, G.D., FARKAS, D.F. and RAGHUBEER, E.V. 1997. Inactivation and long term regeneration of vegetative microbes in high pressure treated ranch style salad dressing. Paper 59E-22, Institute of Food Technologists Annual Meeting, June 14-18, Orlando, FL.

OHLSSON, T. (ed.) 1996. High Pressure Processing of Foods and Food Components — A Literature Survey and Bibliography. SIK, Swedish Institute for Food and Biotechnology, Goteborg, Sweden.

PECK, M.W. 1997. *Clostridium botulinum* and the safety of refrigerated processed foods of extended durability. Trends Food Sci. Technol. *8* (6), 186–192.

ROBERTS, C.M. and HOOVER, D.G. 1996. Sensitivity of *Bacillus coagulans* spores to combinations of high hydrostatic pressure, heat, acidity and nisin. J. Appl. Bact. *81*, 363–368.

YOUNG, S.L., WALKER, M.K., LEDERER, C.L. and McDANIEL, M.R. 1997. Effect of high pressure treatment on sensory properties of a vegetable mix (tomato, green pepper, and onion). Paper 67-9, Institute of Food Technologists Annual Meeting, June 14-18, Orlando FL.

HIGH PRESSURE-TEXTURIZED PRODUCTS FROM FROZEN SURIMI AND SARDINE LIPID

YASUHIRO FUNATSU[1], YUKAKO NABESHIMA-ITO[1], KEN-ICHI KAWASAKI[1] and KUNIHIKO SAMEJIMA[2]

[1]Toyama Prefectural Food Research Institute
360 Yoshioka
Toyama 939, Japan

[2]Rakuno Gakuen University
582 Midori-cho, Bunkyodai
Ebetsu, Hokkaido 069, Japan

ABSTRACT

We investigated the breaking strength (BS) and breaking strain (Bs) of pressure-induced gels and pressure-induced, heated gels with different lipid contents and different size and distribution of lipid droplets in salt-ground meats. When the protein concentration in salt-ground meat was high, a tough gel having high BS and Bs and containing a small quantity of lipid was formed. The lipid droplets in the gel had a length of about 2.8 ± 1.01 μm and were distributed uniformly. In contrast, at low protein concentration, a soft gel was formed which showed low values of BS and Bs and contained a large quantity of lipid. The lipid droplets were closely distributed with a length of about 4.7 ± 2.08 μm. Under the conditions of grinding, high pressure, heating and storage, fish lipid was little separated from the gels and the deterioration of their gel forming ability was not observed when the lipid droplets were at the above length ranges. These results suggest that the quality of food materials containing EPA and DHA may be assessed by measuring the size and distribution of their lipid droplets.

INTRODUCTION

Previous investigators have reported that eicosapentaenoic acid (EPA) may play an important role in reducing blood platelet aggregation and thereby lower the risk of a heart attack (Dyerberg *et al.* 1978; Kobatake *et al.* 1984). Dokosahexaenoic acid (DHA) has also been found to have an effect on learning ability and on the visual process (Yamamoto *et al.* 1987; Hashimoto and Okuyama 1987). With present day advances in medical science, there has also been corresponding advances in food science, such as the use of high pressure techniques in food processing (Hayashi 1989; Ikeuchi *et al.* 1992). Such a high pressure technique has been reported for surimi-based products by Shoji *et al.* (1990). A strong gel was formed when the meat of walleye pollack was ground with 2.5% NaCl and subjected to high hydrostatic pressure. When stored at low temperature, this gel was converted to a tough gel. High pressure techniques, therefore, many contribute significantly in the future in improving food quality and human health.

The present study was undertaken to assess the quality of various food materials texturized under high pressure with surimi and sardine lipid rich in EPA and DHA (Kawasaki *et al.* 1996).

MATERIALS AND METHODS

Frozen Surimi from Walleye Pollack

The SA grade frozen surimi from walleye pollack was produced by Nippon Suisan Co. (Tokyo). It contained 4% sucrose, 4% sorbitol and 0.2% polyphosphate. It was stored for about 6 months at -20°C before use. The pH, water content and lipid content were 7.3, 74.3% and 0.2%, respectively.

Fatty Acid Composition and Quality of Sardine Lipid

The refined sardine lipid was obtained from Nippon Oil Co. (Tokyo). The fatty acids consisted mainly of C16:0 (palmitic acid, 17.2%), C16:1 (palmitoleic acid, 7.1%), C18:0 (stearic acid, 3.2%), C18:1 (oleic acid, 14.0%), C18:2 (linoleic acid, 1.%), C20:5n3 (EPA, 13.4%) and C22:6n3 (DHA, 9.0%). The lipid was stored at -60°C and used within a period of 1 year after being produced.

Preparation of Pressure-induced, Heated Gels

Frozen surimi of walleye pollack was ground with 2.5% NaCl and 0-20% sardine lipid at a protein concentration of 70 and 130 mg/g wet wt. of surimi, respectively, in a speed cutter (National MK-K7) for 5 min at a temperature of 10°C or less. The salt-ground meat was stuffed into a stainless ring (diam, 30 mm × length, 30 mm) coated with a film of polyvinylidene chloride, and texturized under a pressure of 300 MPa at about 13°C for 10 min. After the pressure treatment, the gel was stored at 5°C for use in preparing "pressure-induced gels." The gel was subsequently heated at 90°C for 20 min to prepare the "pressure-induced, heated gels."

Penetration Test with Rheometer

After cooling the gels in ice water and removing the rings, the load values at breaking points were measured with a rheometer (Rheoner RE-3305, Yamaden Co., Tokyo) equipped with a cylindrical plunger (diam, 5 mm; depression speed, 30 mm/min). The load values were expressed in g and penetrating distance in mm at the breaking point below 5°C.

Extraction of Lipid

Lipids in the samples were extracted with a mixture of chloroform/methanol (2:1, v/v) according to the method of Folch *et al.* (1957).

Microscopic Observation

Tissue staining with OsO4 was performed according to Mallory (1938). The gels were cut into 3-5 mm cubes and placed in 20% formalin in neutral buffer solution (pH 7.4) for about 12 hours and fixed with 1.0% OsO4 in 0.1 M phosphate buffer (pH 7.0) for about 24 hours and dehydrated in a graded series of ethanol (50%, 60%, 70%, 90% and 100%). After dehydration, they were transferred to xylene and embedded in paraffin, after which they were cut in a microtome to give thin sections (thickness, 3 μm). They were then placed in xylene to dissolve the paraffin and mounted on slides using permount. The slides were observed under an optical microscope (OPTIPHOT, Nikon) with a 40 × objective and a 10 × ocular. Photographic images were reproduced with a color video printer (Mavigraph, SONY).

Measurement of Size and Distribution of Lipid Droplets in the Gels

The outlines of lipid droplets in the color prints from the optical microscopic observations were traced on tracing paper using a lead pencil (lead size, diam, 0.5 mm). Afterwards, the tracings were copied onto white bond paper. The size and distribution of lipid droplets per 56 × 56 mm^2 area were determined by computer image analysis (Gohtani *et al.* 1992).

RESULTS AND DISCUSSION

Effect of Sardine Lipid Content and Protein Concentration on Gel Forming Ability of Salt-Ground Meats

In a previous paper, we reported that breaking strength and breaking strain had the largest values when carried out at 300 MPa (Kawasaki *et al.* 1996). Fig. 1 shows the changes in breaking strength and breaking strain in the salt-ground meats texturized at 300 MPa with 0, 5, 10, 15 and 20% sardine lipid at protein concentrations of 70 and 130 mg/g wet wt. of surimi, respectively. At high protein concentration (Fig. 1A), it was found that as the lipid content of the pressure-induced gels was increased above 5%, the lower was the breaking strength even though the breaking strength was increased during storage (Fig. 1a). Similarly, the breaking strength decreased in the case of the pressure-induced, heated gels when the lipid content was increased above 5% (Fig. 1b). However, the breaking strength of the pressure-induced, heated gels increased more rapidly and to a higher level than in the case of the pressure-induced gels, even though the lipid content was the same in both gels (Figs 1a, b). At low protein concentration (Fig. 1B), the rate of increase in breaking strength of the gels in storage was considerably less than that of the gels at high protein concentration (Fig. 1B e,f). The lipid content did not affect the rate of increase in breaking strength of the pressure-induced gels (Fig. 1B e). However, there was a decrease in the rate of increase in the breaking strength of the pressure-induced, heated gel when the lipid content was 20% (Fig. 1B f). At either high (Fig. 1A c, d), or low protein concentration (Fig. 1B g, h), the effect of lipid content on breaking strain and breaking strength resembled each other.

Changes in Lipid Content of Gels During Storage

Figure 2 shows the changes in lipid content during storage at 5°C in salt-ground meat texturized at protein concentrations of 70 and 130 mg/g wet wt. of surimi with 0, 5, 10, 15 and 20% sardine lipid at 300 MPa. At high protein concentration (Fig. 2A), the addition of 0% and 5% lipid during grinding resulted in the lipid contents of the gels, regardless of storage time, to be about 0.2% and 5%, respectively (Fig. 2A a, b). On

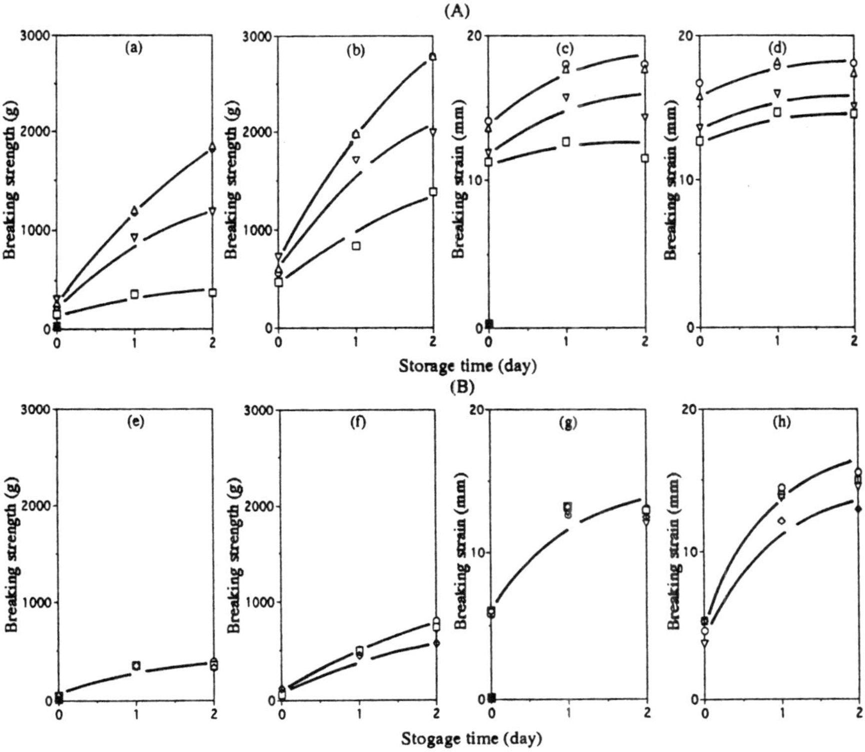

FIG. 1. EFFECT OF SARDINE LIPID ON BREAKING STRENGTH AND BREAKING STRAIN IN PRESSURE-INDUCED GELS AND PRESSURE-INDUCED, HEATED GELS ON STORAGE AT 5°C

Sardine lipid content, 0% (○), 5% (Δ), 10% (▿), 15% (□) and 20% (◇).
Protein conc., 130 mg/100 g (A), 70 mg/100 g (B).
Before pressure, 0% (●), 5% (▴), 10% (▾), 15% (■) and 20% (◆).
Breaking strength, a, b, e, f. Breaking strain, c, d, g, h.

increasing the lipid content to 10%, the lipid contents in the pressure-induced gel and the pressure-induced, heated gel were both about 8% resulting in a net loss in lipid content from the grinding (Fig. 2A c). Increasing the lipid content in the gels to 15% caused an increase in the loss from the grinding and heating, regardless of storage time, so that the lipid contents in the pressure-induced gel and the pressure-induced, heated gel were about 11% and 8%, respectively (Fig. 2A d). At low protein concentration (Fig. 2B), the addition of 0%, 10% and 15% lipid during grinding caused the lipid contents of the gels, regardless of storage time, to be about 0.1%, 8.5% and 13.2%, respectively (Fig. 2B e, f, g). On increasing the lipid content in the gels to 20%, the lipid content of the gel was 19.5%, regardless of storage time (Fig. 2B h). Thus, except for 0% lipid content, the

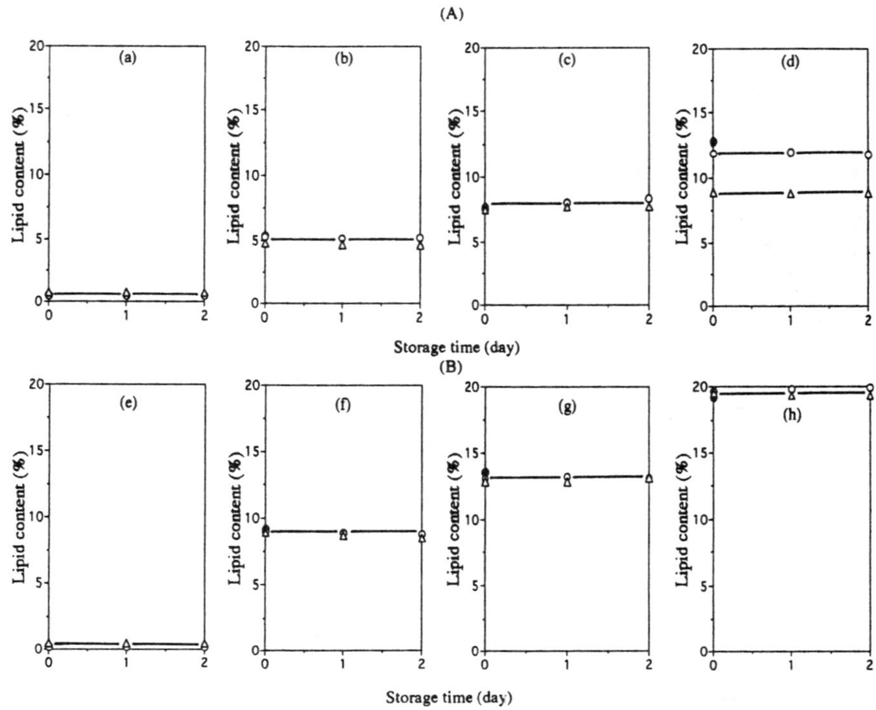

FIG. 2. CHANGES IN LIPID CONTENT OF PRESSURE-INDUCED GELS AND PRESSURE-INDUCED, HEATED GELS DURING STORAGE AT 5°C

Sardine lipid content, 0% (a, e), 5% (b), 10% (c, f), 15% (d, g) and 20% (h). Protein conc., 130 mg/100 g (A), 70 mg/100 g (B). Before pressure, 0% (●), 5% (▲), 10% (▼), 15% (■) and 20% (♦). Pressure-induced gel, (○). Pressure-induced, heated gel, (Δ).

results indicate that lower the protein concentration in the salt-ground meat, the larger will be the lipid content in the gel. Under these experimental conditions, the lipids were not separated from the gels by texturizing with surimi and lipid, but the lipid content was nevertheless decreased from not using an emulsifying agent.

Microscopic Observation of Size and Distribution of Lipid Droplets in the Gels

Figure 3 shows the size and distribution of lipid droplets in the salt-ground meats observed by optical microscopy. At high protein concentration, small lipid droplets were found dispersed in the salt-ground meats containing 5% and 10% sardine lipid, but the lipid droplets were absent in salt-ground meats containing 0% lipid (Fig. 3a, b, c). But, as seen for the sample containing 15% sardine lipid, large masses of lipids and small-size lipid droplets are dispersed throughout (Fig. 3d). Except for density, the distribution of lipid droplets in pressure-induced, heated gels containing 5%, 10% and 15% lipid appeared to resemble each other (Fig. 3 b vs f, c vs g, d vs h). In contrast, at low protein concentration, as the lipid content in salt-ground meats became higher, the more closely the lipid droplets were distributed and larger was their size, whereas no lipid was found in meat containing 0% sardine lipid (Fig. 3i, j, k, l). The tendency for lipid droplets to be distributed in pressure-induced, heated gels containing 10% and 15% lipid was the same in meats (Fig. 3 m, n, o). As seen in Fig. 3p, pressure-induced, heated gels containing 20% sardine lipid contained a relatively large mass of lipids.

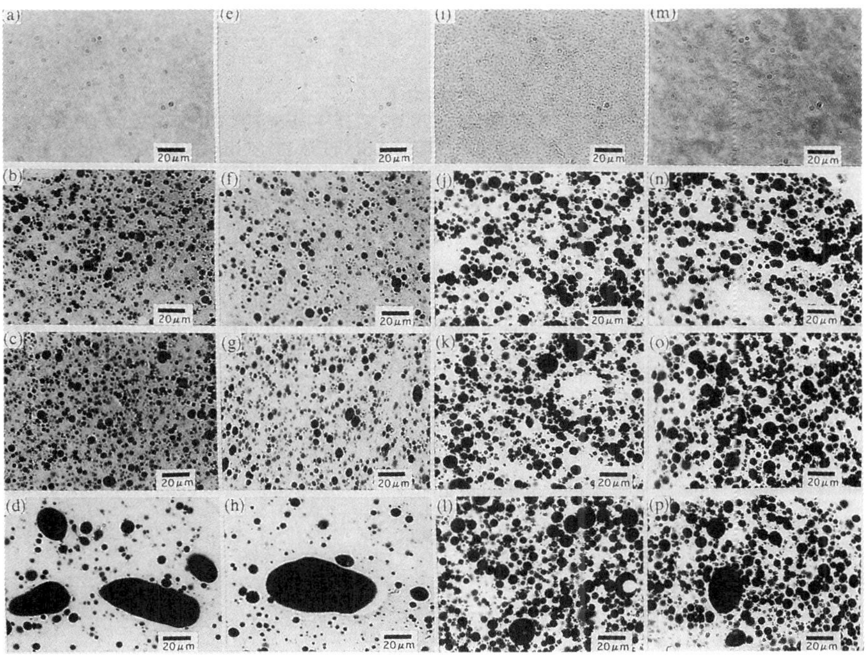

FIG. 3. LIPID DROPLETS IN PRESSURE-INDUCED, HEATED GELS OBSERVED BY MICROSCOPY

Protein conc., 130 mg/100 g (a, b, c, d, e, f, g, h), 70 mg/100 g (i, j, k, l, m, n, o, p). Lipid content, 0% (a, e, i, m), 5% (b, f), 10% (c, g, j, n), 15% (d, h, k, o) and 20% (l, p). Salt-ground meat upon grinding, (a, b, c, d, i, j, k, l). Pressure-induced, heated gel after being stored for 2 days at 5°C, (e, f, g, h, m, n, o, p). Bar, 20 μm.

Evaluation of Lipid Droplets Distributed in Gels

The length and width of lipid droplets in the above mentioned gels are shown in Table 1. At high protein concentration, the mean length and width of lipid droplets in the salt-ground meats containing 5% lipid were 3.0 and 2.4 μm, respectively, whereas those containing 10% lipid were 3.0 and 2.3 μm, respectively. However, the values for the droplets in meats containing 15% lipid were 5.4 and 3.4 μm, respectively, reflecting the inclusion of larger droplets in the analysis. The mean length (L) and width (W), and W/L, of lipid droplets of pressure-induced, heated gels were almost the same as those for salt-ground meats. At low protein concentration, the mean length and width of lipid droplets of the salt-ground meat containing 10% lipid were 3.7 and 3.0 μm, respectively, and those of meat containing 15% lipid were 3.8 and 2.9 μm, respectively. However, for meats containing 20% lipid, the values were 5.0 and 4.0 μm, respectively. In spite of the lipid contents, mean length and width of pressure-induced gels were between 4.3-4.8 μm and 3.4-3.8 μm, respectively. Under these conditions, most of the shapes of the droplets dispersed in the gels were egg-shaped or oval rather than globular because the

TABLE 1.
LENGTH AND WIDTH OF LIPID DROPLETS IN THE PRESSURE-INDUCED, HEATED GELS MEASURED BY COMPUTER ASSISTED IMAGE ANALYSIS

Lipid content			Length (L)[1] (μm)	Width (W)[1] (μm)	W/L[1] value
High protein conc.					
	HO[2]	0%	ND	ND	ND
		5%	3.0 ± 1.00	2.4 ± 0.96	0.8 ± 0.14
		10%	3.0 ± 1.18	2.3 ± 1.00	0.8 ± 0.15
		15%	5.4 ± 9.61	3.4 ± 3.97	0.7 ± 0.17
	HPH[3]	0%	ND	ND	ND
		5%	2.8 ± 1.01	2.2 ± 0.96	0.8 ± 0.16
		10%	3.1 ± 1.29	2.2 ± 0.95	0.7 ± 0.13
		15%	4.3 ± 9.50	2.9 ± 4.73	0.8 ± 0.18
Low protein conc.					
	LO[2]	0%	ND	ND	ND
		10%	3.7 ± 1.65	3.0 ± 1.52	0.8 ± 0.12
		15%	3.8 ± 2.00	2.9 ± 1.88	0.8 ± 0.17
		20%	5.0 ± 2.82	4.0 ± 2.52	0.8 ± 0.14
	LPH[3]	0%	ND	ND	ND
		10%	4.3 ± 2.04	3.4 ± 1.82	0.8 ± 0.16
		15%	4.7 ± 2.08	3.8 ± 1.84	0.8 ± 0.13
		20%	4.8 ± 3.14	3.8 ± 2.24	0.8 ± 0.14

[1]Mean ± standard deviation
[2]HO and LO, salt-ground meat on grinding
[3]HPH and LPH, pressure-induced, heated gel after storage for 2 days
ND = not detected

mean W/L was about 0.8 notwithstanding the lipid content and protein concentration in the gels. Further, at the protein concentrations studied, it was found that the size but not the shape of lipid droplets was changed significantly during preparation of the gels. At high protein concentration (Table 1), an increase in the lipid content in the salt-ground meat being ground was accompanied by an increase in the standard deviation of the length and width of the lipid droplets, i.e., 1.01 → 9.61 for length and 0.96 → 3.97 for width, whereas at low protein concentration (Table 1), the standard deviations of the length and width of the lipid droplets containing 20% lipid in the salt-ground meat were larger than for those of containing 10% and 15% lipid. Similarly, the results for the pressure-induced, heated gels were about the same as for the salt-ground meat. The results, therefore, suggest that the scattering of lipid droplets in the gels appear to be nearly the same whether the process is carried out under conditions of high pressure, heating and storage or by grinding at high or low protein concentrations.

In summary, it is considered necessary to control closely the size and distribution of the lipid droplets in the salt-ground meat during grinding to texturization with frozen surimi and sardine lipid to obtain the desired results. Thus, in order to make good surimi-based products, the length and width of the lipid droplets should be controlled to within about 3.0 ± 1.00 μm and 2.4 ± 0.96 μm, respectively, in preparing hard type gel (at high protein concentration), and to within about 4.7 ± 2.08 μm and 3.8 ± 1.84 μm, respectively, in preparing soft type gel (at low protein concentration).

ACKNOWLEDGMENTS

We are grateful to Mr. Kenji Yoneda, Mr. Masahiko Kawahara, Mr.Noboru Nakura and Mr.Tougo Miyazaki for their encouragement and support.

REFERENCES

DYERBERG, J., BANG, H.O. and STOFFERSEN, E. 1978. Eicosapentaenoic acid and prevention of thrombosis and atherosclerosis. Lancet *11*, 117–119.

FOLCH, J., LEES, M. and SLOANE-STANLEY, G.A. 1957. A simple method for the isolation and purification of total lipid from animal tissue. J. Biol. Chem. *226*, 497–509.

GOHTANI, S., ARIUCHI, N., KAWASOME, S. and YAMANO, Y. 1992. Computer image analysis of Sudachi (gas cell distribution) of baked cereal products. Nippon Shokuhin Kogyo Gakkaishi *39*, 749–754 (in Japanese).

HASHIMOTO, A. and OKUYAMA, H. 1987. Re-evaluation of essential polyunsaturated fatty acid. Seikagaku *59*, 1233–1238 (in Japanese).

HAYASHI, R. 1989. Food making under high pressure. Sanei, Kyoto (in Japanese).

IKEUCHI, Y., TANJI, H., KIM, K. and SUZUKI, A. 1992. Dynamic rheological measurements on heat-induced pressurized actomyosin gels. J. Agric. Food Chem. *40*, 1751–1755.

KAWASAKI, K., FUNATSU, Y. and ITO, Y. 1996. Texturization with frozen surimi and sardine lipid by high pressure treatment. Nippon Shokuhin Kagaku Kogaku Kaishi *2*, 146–156 (in Japanese).

KOBATAKE, Y., KURODA, K., JUNNOUCHI, H., NISHIDA, E. and INNAMI, S. 1984. Differential effects of dietary eicosapentaenoic and dokosahexaenoic fatty acids on lowering of triglyceride and cholesterol levels in the serum of rats on hypercholesterolemic diet. J. Nutr. Sci. Vitaminol. *30*, 357–372.

MALLORY, F.B. 1938. Pathological Technique. W.B. Saunders Co. Philadelphia, Pennsylvania.

SHOJI, T., SAEKI, H., WAKAMEDA, A., NAKANURA, M. and NONAKA, M. 1990. Gelation of salted paste of Alaska pollack by high hydrostatic pressure and change in myofibrillar protein in it. Nippon Suisan Gakkaishi *56*, 2069–2076 (in Japanese).

YAMAMOTO, N., SAITOH, M., MORIUCHI, A., NOMURA, M. and OKUYAMA, H. 1987. Effect of dietary-linolenate/linoleate balance on brain lipid compositions and learning ability of rats. J. Lipid Res. *28*, 144–151.

RHEOLOGICAL PROPERTIES AND MICROSTRUCTURE OF MONODISPERSED O/W EMULSION GEL

S. GOHTANI, K.H. KIM and Y. YAMANO

Department of Bioresource Science
Kagawa University
Miki, Kagawa 761-07, Japan

ABSTRACT

Effect of oil droplet size on the rheological properties and microstructure of monodispersed O/W emulsion agar gel prepared by membrane emulsification technique was investigated by mechanical measurements and SEM observation. The compressive gel strength of emulsion gel decreased with an increase in oil droplet size, while that of emulsion gel determined by puncture test showed almost no change. Cryo-SEM observation revealed that oil droplets aggregated in the emulsion gel and that the gel had some void spaces between gel network and the oil droplet aggregate.

INTRODUCTION

An emulsion gel containing oil droplets is a good food model. Oil droplet size and oil volume fraction have important effects on the texture and rheological properties of the emulsion gel (Kinsella 1984; Langley and Green 1989; McClements *et al.* 1993; Matsumura *et al.* 1993; Rohm and Kovac 1994; Yang and Chen 1994). Most studies, however, have reported on the behavior of polydispersed emulsions. It is necessary to use an emulsion gel containing the monodispersed emulsion for rheological discussion of the emulsion gel.

The objectives of this study are to investigate the filler effects of oil droplet size and volume fraction on the rheological properties and to observe microstructure of emulsion agar gel.

MATERIALS AND METHODS

Commercial corn oil of food grade quality (Ajinomoto Co. Inc., Tokyo) and reagent grade agar powder (Daishin Co., Tokyo) were used for gel preparation. Emulsifier (polyglycerolesters of fatty acid) was purchased from Sakamoto Co. Ltd., Osaka.

Emulsion Preparation

The aqueous phase was prepared by dissolving 1% emulsifier in distilled water. Emulsions of different droplet sizes were produced by using different pore size porous glass membranes (Chen *et al.* 1993). The emulsions with mean drop diameters of 1.5, 3.3, 6.5 and 12.2 μm were prepared. An Image-Analyzer was used to measure the distributions of oil droplets in o/w emulsions (Yamano *et al.* 1984) and the mean number diameter was calculated. The photographed oil droplets of the emulsions are shown in Fig. 1.

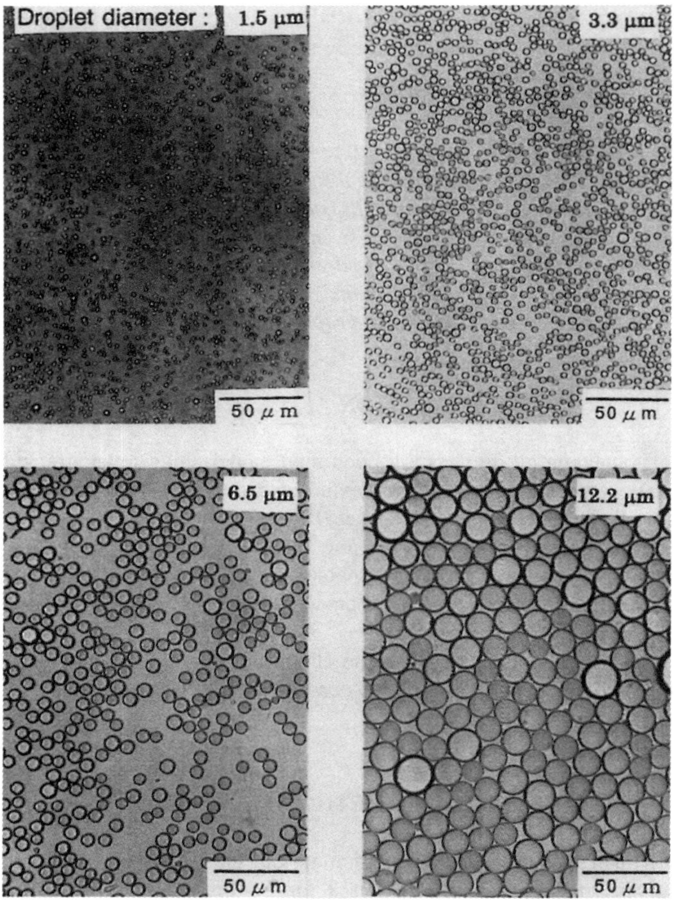

FIG. 1. MICROPHOTOGRAPHS OF EMULSION PREPARED BY MEMBRANE EMULSIFICATION
Each number (mm) shows the mean oil droplet size.

Gel Formation

Agar powder (1%) was dispersed in the emulsions containing 0.1, 0.2 and 0.3 volume fractions of oil, after which these agar emulsion dispersions were stirred gently for 60 min at 20 C, heated for 30 min at 70 C and then heated again for 30 min at 90

C during swelling. After being degassed, these sols were poured into cylindrical glass containers (inside diameter 24 mm, height 38 mm). These glass containers were held for 1 h at room temperature and then held in a water bath for 24 h at 25 C before measurements. In each gel, the uniformity of dispersibility of emulsion droplets was confirmed by determining droplet number and diameter at top, center and bottom of emulsion gel as described by Yamano *et al.* (1996).

Mechanical Analysis

Gel samples used for determining gel strength by Rheolometer (RE-33005, Yamaden Co., Tokyo) at 25 C were cut into sections 20 mm in height and 24 mm in diameter. For determining compression gel strength, the gels were compressed to 80% deformation with a 2 kg compression load cell by a plunger with a diameter of 40 mm at a cross head speed of 0.5 mm/s. For puncture test, the gels were punctured at 1 mm/s to a depth of 16 mm by a flat plunger with a diameter of 5 mm. The results for compressive and puncture properties were expressed in terms of relative values: R = Se/So, where Se and So are the data of the filled gel and the droplet free gel, respectively (McClements *et al.* 1993).

Cryo-Scanning Electron Microscopy (Cryo-SEM)

The center of the gels were cut into cubes (approx. 3 × 3 × 3 mm) and were dehydrated in a 50% ethanol for 2 min. After being frozen by immersing in liquid nitrogen, the specimens were fractured in liquid nitrogen. After the ice on the specimens was sublimed, the specimens were coated with gold and observed in a Cryo-SEM (S-800, Hitachi Co., Ltd., Tokyo) at -120 C.

RESULTS AND DISCUSSION

Effect of Oil Droplets on Compression of Emulsion Gel

The compressive properties of emulsion gels containing different sizes of oil droplets are shown in terms of relative values in Fig. 2. The change in compressive stress of emulsion gels decreased as the oil volume fraction increased (Fig. 2A). The compressive stress showed a much greater difference between the gels of oil volume fractions 0.1 and 0.2 than between those of oil volume fractions 0.2 and 0.3. For each oil volume fraction gel, the change in compressive stress decreased as the oil droplet size increased. Little difference in compressive strain with the oil volume fraction was found in Fig. 2B. For each oil volume fraction gel, the decrease in compressive strain of the gels was significant with increasing oil droplet size. As shown in Fig. 2C, the compressive energy of the emulsion gels decreased with increasing oil volume fraction. The compressive energy of the emulsion gel with oil volume fraction 0.1 decreased remarkably up to 6.5 μm but only gradually thereafter, while those of 0.2 and 0.3 oil volume fractions decreased linearly.

Effect of Oil Droplets on Puncture of Emulsion Gel

The puncture properties of emulsion gels containing different sizes of oil droplets are shown in terms of relative values in Fig. 3. The changes in puncture values of emulsion gels with oil droplets were very small in comparison with the changes in compressive values (Fig. 2) and puncture test is not available to compare mechanical properties for the emulsion gels with different size oil droplets. Thus, compressive measurement is more useful to investigate the effect of oil droplet size on the physical properties of the emulsion gel than puncture measurement.

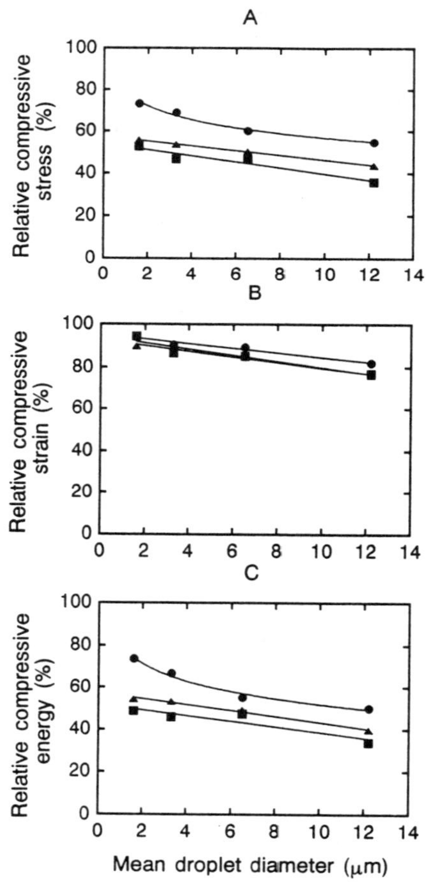

FIG. 2. THE EFFECTS OF DROPLET SIZES ON COMPRESSIVE PROPERTIES OF EMULSION GELS

A, B and C show the relations of mean droplet diameter and the relative compressive stress, strain and energy, respectively. The symbols represent the gels of oil volume fractions 0.1(●), 0.2(▲) and 0.3(■), respectively.

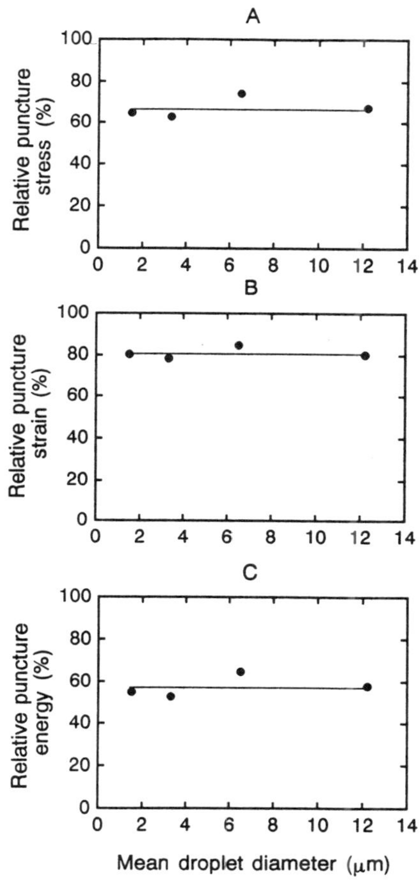

FIG. 3. THE EFFECTS OF DROPLET SIZES ON PUNCTURE PROPERTIES OF EMULSION GELS OF OIL VOLUME FRACTION 0.1

A, B and C show the relations of mean droplet diameter and the relative puncture stress, strain and energy, respectively.

Microstructure of Emulsion Agar Gel

The oil droplets in the gel network are not separately dispersed but tend to aggregate. And emulsion gel had some void spaces between the gel networks and the oil droplets aggregate, and gel strands of the emulsion gel did not cover the oil droplets completely.

REFERENCES

CHEN, E.S., GOHTANI, S., NAKASHIMA, T. and YAMANO, Y. 1993. Creaming rate of o/w emulsion. J. Jpn. Oil Chem. Soc. (Yukagaku) *42*, 972–977.

KINSELLA, J.E. 1984. Milk proteins: Physicochemical and functional properties. Crit. Rev. Food Sci. Nutr. *21*, 197–262.

KOBAYASHI, M. and NAKAHAMA, N. 1986. Rheological properties of mixed gels. J. Texture Studies *17*, 161–173.

LANGLEY, K.R. and GREEN, M.L. 1989. Compression strength and fracture properties of model particulate food composites in relation to their micro-structure and particle-matrix interaction. J. Texture Studies *20*, 191–297.

MATSUMURA, Y., KANG, I.-J., SAKAMOTO, H., MOTOKI, M. and MORI, T. 1993. Filler effects of oil droplets on the viscoelastic properties of emulsion gels. Food Hydrocolloids *7*, 227–240.

McCLEMENTS, D.J., MONAHAN, F.J. and KINSELLA, J.E. 1993. Effect of emulsion droplets on the rheology of whey protein isolate gels. J. Texture Studies *24*, 411–422.

ROHM, H. and KOVAC, A. 1994. Effects of starter cultures on linear viscoelastic and physical properties of yogurt gels. J. Texture Studies *25*, 311–329.

YAMANO, Y., GOHTANI, S. and NAKAYAMA, S. 1984. Foaming power and emulsifying properties of gypsophila paniculata L. saponin. Nippon Nogeikagaku Kaishi *58*, 161–168.

YAMANO, Y., KAGAWA, Y., KIM, K.H. and GOHTANI, S. 1996. Stability and uniformity of oil droplets in preparation of o/w emulsion agar gel. Food Sci. Technol. Int. *2*, 16–18.

YANG, B.K. and CHEN, J.P. 1994. Gel matrix influence on hydrolysis of triglycerides by immobilized lipases. J. Food Sci. *59*, 424–427.

STUDY OF PRESERVING SELENIUM IN SEVERAL VEGETABLES UNDER VARIOUS DEHYDRATING METHODS

M. ZHANG[1], X.L. DING[1], P.H. LU[2], H.K. ZHU[2] and J.M.CHEN[2]

[1]School of Food Science and Technology
Wuxi University of Light Industry
Wuxi 214036, China

[2]Science Association at Liyuan Township of Wuxi City
Wuxi 214074, China

ABSTRACT

The tests of preserving selenium (Se) on sweet pepper, eggplant and cucumber rich in Se by means of four dehydrating methods of the microwave, low-vacuum, heated air, and freezing-vacuum were made. The affected curves were obtained under different dehydrating temperatures. The effects of the dehydrating methods, initial Se concentrations, sample moisture contents and blanching time on the Se preserving ratio of sweet pepper enriched with Se are discussed.

INTRODUCTION

It is well known that Se is the main active part of glutathione peroxidase(GSH-Px) in human body. Each adult needs about 0.2 mg every day (Wang and Wang 1996). Lack of Se in diet can lead to several diseases (Xu 1983). In many Se lacking areas of China, famous endemic diseases are prevalent, for example, Keshan disease found in the northeastern areas of China (Keshan county) and stomach cancer found in the northern central areas of China (Linxian county). In China, each person only obtains less than 0.06 mg Se from his diet on an average, which belongs to a slight Se deficient state. It is also reported that organic Se is superior to inorganic Se needed for human body (Xia and Zhao 1993), especially in the process of biological anti-oxidation (Xue and Hou 1993). The recent study by American scientists found that proteins enriched with Se have the function of inhibition of AIDS virus. So developing an effective food enriched with Se, especially organic Se, for Chinese is necessary and very significant to our society today. Selenium in plant is one of main resources for mankind and animals to acquire Se, some forms of which has the characteristic of less toxification (Wang 1991). It is very expensive to synthesize the organic Se. So almost all studies on the botanical foods enriched with organic Se focus to translation from the inorganic form to the organic one. It is a hopeful direction to obtain some proportion of organic Se through spraying the flower of the fruit-type vegetables with inorganic Se(SFI) before harvest (Shi 1992). In this study, some vegetables with different initial Se contents were obtained by means of SFI for the dehydrating tests.

The dehydrated vegetable is important to many occasions, such as: tourism, navigation, geological prospecting, military needs in some remote areas, snack, etc.

(Zhang *et al* 1992a). Sweet pepper (*Copsicum annum* L), eggplant (*Solanum melongena* L) and cucumber (*Cucumis sativus* L), which are very popular in the Chinese dining tables, are three fruit-type vegetables suitable for both Se absorption before harvest and dehydration after harvest. In this study, four common dehydration methods were chosen in the tests for comparing the effects of preserving Se in the four vegetables.

EQUIPMENT AND METHODS

Equipment

The EB-330 MOC moisture determining balance (Japan) was selected for determining the moisture contents of the samples. The wet basis was adopted in it as the expression of moisture content. The Sartorius microbalance (Germany) was used for weighing the sample during the fluorescent analysis, with accuracy of $\pm$ 0.1 mg. The HITACHI 650-60 Fluorescence Spectrophotometer was used for determining the Se contents in the samples, sensitivity of 0.01 g/g.

The Consol 24 freeze dryer (USA) was used as the dehydrating device of freezing-vacuum, or high vacuum after freezing. Its vacuum pressure was regulated to 37.8 Pa. The Shangling microwave oven (China), output 1.25 kw, was chosen for microwave dehydration. There are nine levels of heating temperatures on it, with accuracy of 0.5 C. The airflow dryer NC101-2 (China) was used for heated-air dehydration, with accuracy of 1 C. The vacuum dryer DZ-88 (China) was used for the low-vacuum dehydration, the vacuum pressure was adjusted to 1.2×10^4 Pa.

Indices of Experiments

1. The total Se content, S_z (g/g), and its preserving ratio, K_z(%)

$$K_z = 100a.S_{z1}/S_{z0} \quad (1)$$

Where a is the conversion coefficient from the dried samples to the fresh of the same variety; S_{z1} and S_{z0} are the total Se contents of the dried and the fresh, respectively. The aim of conversion is to eliminate the enriched effect after dehydration.

2. The organic Se percentage of total Se contents, S_o(%), and its keeping ratio, K_o(%)

$$K_o = 100S_{o1} / S_{o0} \quad (2)$$

Where S_{o1}, S_{o0} are the organic Se percentages of the dried and the fresh, respectively. When the moisture contents of samples are definite, the Se preserving ratio of the samples depends on the amount of the S_z and S_o.

Steps of Experiments and Measuring Methods

Three kinds of vegetable samples with different initial Se concentrations were obtained from the testing fields for vegetables enriched with Se at Liyuan Township in Wuxi City. The samples were cut into slices of 6 mm width before dehydration, then weighed 100 g for dehydration. Except for the special explanation, the dehydrating conditions in the tests will be as follows: 1) dehydrating temperature, T=60 C; 2) moisture content, M=8.9%; 3) initial total Se contents and organic Se percentages of sweet pepper, eggplant and cucumber: 0.096 g/g, 54.3%; 0.181 g/g, 60.3% and 0.184 g/g, 65.2%, respectively.

The determination of S_z basically depends on the steps of examining Se in plant (Xia 1991). During the determination, the overlapping phenomenon of the fluorescent peaks of impurity and examined Se was found, which made the measuring results higher. A graphics using one-level derivative for eliminating the interference by Hu and Su (1996) has been successfully applied to the determination of Se in tea. But it is found in the study that a graphics using two-level derivative is needed in vegetables.

The extracting method using cyclohexane has been applied to the determination of organic Se in honey (Jiang and Ba 1994). But after the paste from the fresh vegetable sample was made, it is difficult for the layer extracted by cyclohexane to be separated from the layer of the paste. A squeezing method with good separating effect was determined during the measurement. The model is explained in Fig. 1, where an assumption that almost all inorganic Se in the plant after squeeze is still in the juice has been adopted (Xu and Hou 1993). According to the inorganic Se content and S_z, the organic Se percentage could be easily calculated. The organic Se of the dehydrated sample can be determined after rehydration in the deionized water of fixed quantity.

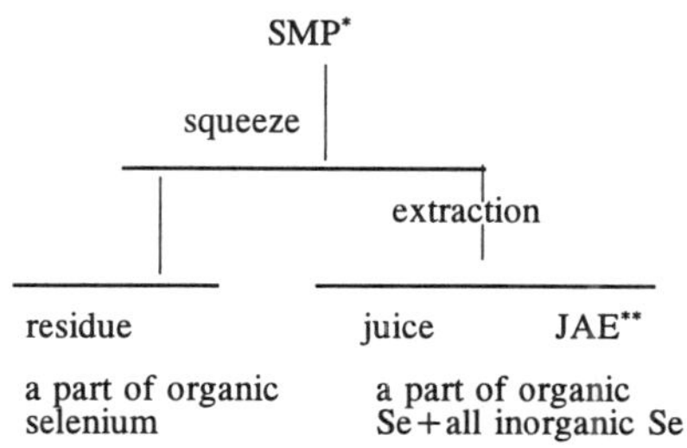

FIG. 1. THE FRACTIONATING MODEL OF INORGANIC SELENIUM FROM VEGETABLE SAMPLES

*SMP means sample after making paste. **JAE means juice after extraction.

RESULTS AND ANALYSIS

Effects of the Dehydrating Temperatures on the Se Contents in the Dehydrated Vegetables Enriched With Se Under the Microwave Dehydrator

The microwave dehydration can make the moisture in vegetables vibrate fiercely after absorbing microwave, then evaporate the moisture owing to the large amount of heat produced inside the vegetables. So it has characteristic of high dehydrating efficiency which has some applications in the dehydration of fruits and vegetables at present (Luh and Woodroof 1975). The microwave drying tests on the samples of sweet pepper, eggplant, and cucumber were made under four temperatures suitable for dehydration. The measuring results after dehydration are shown in Fig. 2. Both S_z and

S_0 values of three vegetables decreased with the increase of dehydrating temperature. The S_z values decreased very little, while the S_0 decreased more obviously. The higher the dehydrating temperature is, the more seriously the dissolution of organic Se is. So under the circumstances of permitting the low drying speed, the lower drying temperature (60 C) is recommended for the sake of keeping the organic Se in the samples. The reason why total Se contents slightly decreased with the increase of temperature is the evaporation of selenium above a certain point of temperature. The dissolution of organic Se affected by temperature can be explained by the fact that some organic structures can be denatured after heated.

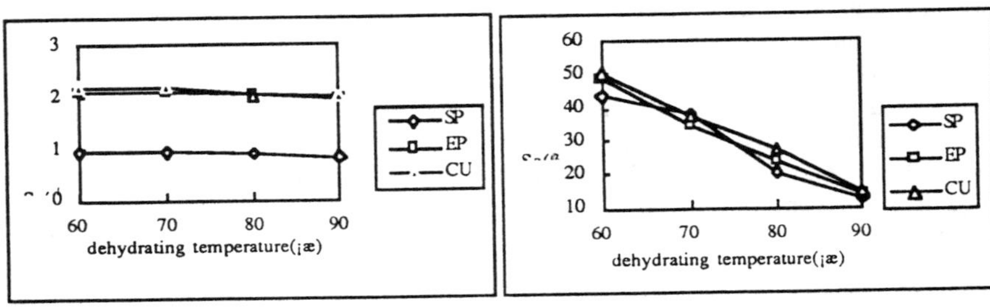

a. on S_z b. on S_0

FIG. 2. THE EFFECTS OF DEHYDRATING TEMPERATURE ON THE SELENIUM CONTENTS IN DEHYDRATED VEGETABLES UNDER MICROWAVE (M = 10.8%)
SP = sweet pepper, EP = eggplant, CU = cucumber, M = moisture content

Effects of the Dehydrating Temperatures on the Se Contents of the Dehydrated Vegetables Enriched with Se under the Low-vacuum Dehydrator

The low-vacuum dehydration is a dehydrating way with low cost and energy consumption in the range of vacuum pressure of $1.010^4 \sim 9.610^4$ Pa (Zhang *et al.* 1992b). Figure 3 shows the dehydrating tests under the vacuum pressure of 1.210^4 Pa. Both S_z and S_0 values of three vegetables decreased very little with the increase of dehydrating temperature. Therefore, the temperature during the low-vacuum dehydration can be determined mainly according to the needed drying time.

Effects of the Dehydrating Temperatures on the Se Contents of the Dehydrated Vegetables Enriched with Se under the Heated Air Dehydrator

The heated airflow dehydration is a widely used drying way in China at present (Zhang *et al.* 1992a). The measuring results of the heated airflow dehydrating tests are shown in Fig. 4. Both S_z and S_0 values of three vegetables decreased with an increase in dehydrating temperature. But S_z decreased less than S_0. The S_0 values above 70 C decreased considerably. Therefore, it is suitable to select the temperature of 60-70 C for the heated air dehydration.

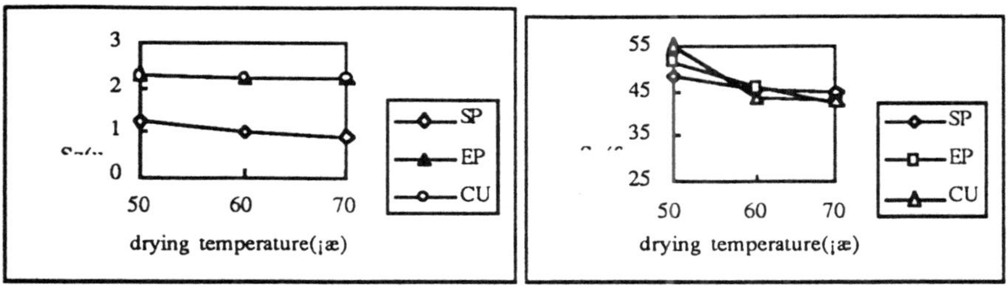

a. on S_z b. on S_o

FIG. 3. THE EFFECTS OF DEHYDRATING TEMPERATURE ON THE SELENIUM CONTENTS IN DEHYDRATED VEGETABLES UNDER LOW VACUUM (M = 11.6%)

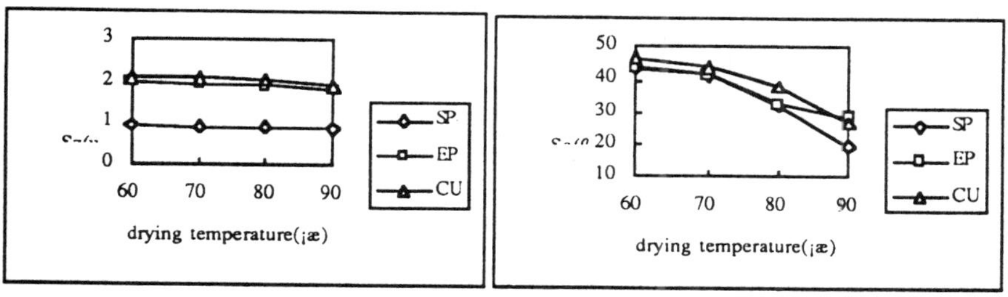

a. on S_z b. on S_o

FIG. 4. THE EFFECTS OF DEHYDRATING TEMPERATURE ON THE SELENIUM CONTENTS IN DEHYDRATED VEGETABLES UNDER HEATED AIRFLOW (M = 9.7%)

Effects of the Dehydrating Temperatures on the Se Contents of the Dehydrated Sweet Peppers, Enriched with Se, in a Freeze-vacuum Dehydrator

The freeze-vacuum dehydration, or high vacuum dehydration after freezing, is a drying method with high quality of the products (Luh and Woodroof 1975). Table 1 shows the measuring results of the samples during freeze-vacuum dehydration. Both S_z and S_o values of sweet pepper decreased with an increase in dehydrating temperature. The S_z values decreased very slowly, while the S_o decreased obviously. So the drying temperature of 35 C is recommended for the sake of preserving the organic Se in the samples.

DISCUSSION

Effects of Different Dehydrating Methods and Initial Se Concentration on the Se Contents of the Dehydrated Sweet Peppers Enriched With Selenium

The dehydrating tests of sweet peppers with three initial Se concentrations under four dehydrating methods were carried out. Table 2 shows the effects of dehydrating methods and initial Se concentrations on the Se contents in dehydrated sweet peppers. The total Se contents under all four dehydrating methods increased with an increase of the initial Se concentrations, while there is little difference among their organic Se percentages. It possibly refers to the enriched effect of total Se after dehydration and combining way of organic Se in vegetable. Generally, the freeze-vacuum dehydration can preserve the highest organic Se value, followed by the low-vacuum, the microwave, and the heated air, respectively. The reason why the freezing-vacuum dehydration has high organic Se preservation can be explained by the high-vacuum dehydration after quick freezing can keep the cellular structure unchanged, thus reducing the dissolution of the organic Se.

TABLE 1.
THE EFFECTS OF DEHYDRATING TEMPERATURE ON THE SELENIUM CONTENTS IN DEHYDRATED SWEET PEPPERS UNDER VACUUM AFTER FREEZING (M=8.9%)

indexes / T(C)	S_z(g/g)	S_o (%)
35	1.32	58.9
45	1.26	54.6
55	1.23	50.7

TABLE 2.
THE EFFECTS OF DEHYDRATING METHODS (DM) AND INITIAL SE CONCENTRATIONS (ISC) ON THE SELENIUM CONTENTS IN DEHYDRATED SWEET PEPPER

ISC / indexes / DM	0.096g/g, 54.3%		0.209g/g, 56.8%		0.511g/g, 55.4%	
	Sz(g/g)	So(%)	Sz (g/g)	So(%)	Sz(g/g)	So(%)
MW(M=10.8%)	0.93	43.5	2.54	45.3	6.86	45.6
LV(M=11.6%)	0.99	45.3	2.76	45.7	6.85	45.9
HA(M=9.7%)	0.95	43.5	2.62	42.5	6.91	40.3
FV(M=8.9%)	1.23	50.7	2.94	50.7	7.01	51.2

MW=microwave, LV=low vacuum, HA=heated air, FV=freezing vacuum

Effects of Different Moisture Contents on the Se Preserving Ratio of Dehydrated Sweet Peppers Enriched with Se

In order to understand the loss of Se contents during different dehydrating periods, measurement of the Se preserving ratio of dehydrated sweet peppers enriched with selenium under different moisture contents (representing different dehydrating periods) were made (Fig. 5). Under four dehydrating methods, the declining range of the K_z and K_o is large between the moistures of 93.5-43.5% during previous dehydrating stage, but narrow between the moistures of 43.5-8.9% during later dehydrating period.

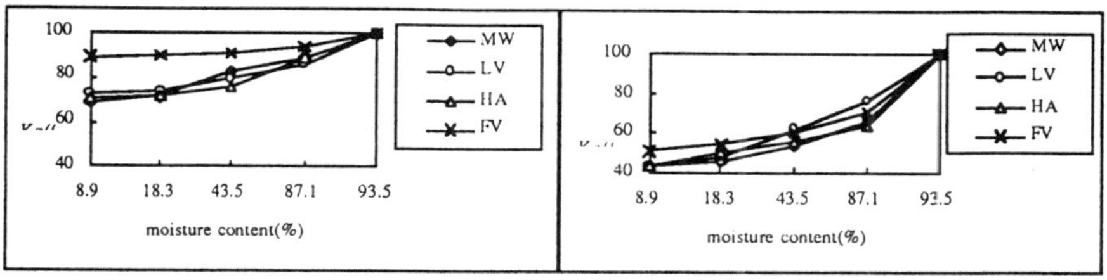

a. on K_z b. on K_o

FIG. 5. THE CHANGE OF THE SELENIUM KEEPING RATES IN SWEET PEPPER UNDER DIFFERENT MOISTURE CONTENTS

Effects of Different Blanching Times on the Se Contents of Dehydrated Sweet Peppers Enriched with Se

In order to preserve the pigment, most dehydrated vegetables should be blanched before processing. Table 3 shows the comparison of sweet peppers with different initial Se contents for three blanching times. Both S_z and S_o values of sweet pepper decreased with an increase of blanching time. The greatest reduction took place in the range of 6-10 min. Therefore, the recommended blanching time is 6 min for sweet pepper.

TABLE 3.
THE EFFECTS OF BLANCHING ON THE SELENIUM CONTENTS IN SWEET PEPPER

ISC indexes BT	0.096g/g, 54.3%		0.209g/g, 56.8%		0.511g/g, 55.4%	
	Sz(g/g)	So(%)	Sz(g/g)	So(%)	Sz(g/g)	So(%)
6min	0.093	41.6	0.198	51.2	0.411	51.3
10min	0.082	38.7	0.186	43.9	0.399	40.7
15min	0.081	31.6	0.183	42.5	0.397	40.3

BT=blanching time, ISC=initial Se concentration.
*Here the blanching means the process of soaking in 1%$NaHCO_3$ concentration at 100 C.

CONCLUSIONS

1. Under low drying speed, the lower drying temperature is recommended for the sake of preserving the organic Se in the samples during both microwave and freezing-vacuum dehydration; during the low-vacuum dehydration the temperature can be determined mainly according to the required drying time; it is suitable to select the temperature of 60-70 C for the heated air dehydration.

2. The total Se contents under all four dehydrating methods increased with the increase of the initial Se concentrations, while there is little difference among their organic Se percentages; the freeze-vacuum dehydration preserved the highest organic Se

value, followed by the low-vacuum, the microwave, and the heated air, respectively.

3. Under four dehydrating methods, the declining range of the K_z and K_0 is large between the moistures of 93.5-43.5% during earlier dehydrating stage, but narrow between the moistures of 43.5-8.9% during later dehydrating period.

4. Both S_z and S_0 values of sweet pepper decreased with the increase of blanching time. The greatest reduction took place in the range of 6-10 min; the recommended blanching time is 6 min for sweet pepper.

ACKNOWLEDGMENTS

The authors thank Dr. Richard Fuchs and members of Appraisal Committee of the International Foundation for Science (IFS) at Stockholm for supporting the presentation in the conference. Also they gratefully acknowledge financial support from IFS under contract No. E/2467-1 to Dr. Zhang Min.

REFERENCES

HU, Y.S. and SU, W.Z. 1996. Measuring the Se contents in tea by means of the one-scale derivative fluoroscope. Chinese Journal of Analytical Chemistry *24*(3), 371.

JIANG, L.K. and BA, Y.Q. 1994. Effects of synthetic organic selenium on honey. Food Science *7*, 45.

LUH, B.S. and WOODROOF, J.G. 1975. Commercial vegetable processing. The Avi Publishing Co., Inc. USA, p. 53.

SHI, H.P. 1992. ^{75}Se absorption by leaves, its distribution and transformation in tomato seedlings. Acta Agriculturae Nucleatae Sinica *6*(3), 190–192.

WANG, L. 1991. Trace elements in life science. Beijing: China Metrology Press, pp. 189–248.

WANG, Y.Y. and WANG, H.Q. 1996. Comparison of effects among three additives with Se. Food Science *17*(1), 52.

XIA, J.Y. 1991. Practical fluoroscope. Beijing: Press of Chinese University of Public Security, pp. 320–322.

XIA, Y.M. and ZHAO, X.E. 1993. Effects of chemical structures of selenium on composition with Se in human blood. Acta Nutrimenta Sinica *15*(2), 157.

XU, H.B. 1983. Biological trace element: selenium. Wuhan: Press of Engineering College of Central China, p. 58.

XUE, T.L. and HOU, S.F. 1993. Anti-oxidation of Se in higher plants. Chinese Science Bulletin *38*(4), 356.

ZHANG, M., WANG, C.Z. *et al.* 1992a. Thin-layer airflow drying of sword bean after pretreatment, Proceedings of the 9th Drying '92, Canada, pp. 1544–1548.

ZHANG, M., WANG, C.Z. *et al.* 1992b. Study of carrot and sword bean on thin-layer low vacuum drying, J. Northeast Agricultural College (4), 384–388.

RHEOLOGY OF CLARIFIED KIWIFRUIT JUICES

YANQUN LI and SHIWANG SHE

Food Engineering Department of Sino-German Joint Institute (Jiangxi-OAI)
No.17 Nanjingdong Road, Nanchang 330047, P. R. China

ABSTRACT

The rheological behavior of the depectinized and clarified kiwifruit juice was studied in this paper. The results indicated that this juice behaved as a Newtonian fluid. The effects of temperature and concentration on the viscosity of this juice were determined. The temperature effect was studied at 7 different temperatures between 5 and 60 °C. The concentration effect was studied at 7 different concentrations from 11.0 to 64.5 °Brix. Finally, an equation expressing the combined effect of temperature and concentration on the viscosity was given.

INTRODUCTION

Kiwifruit (*Adinidia chinensis*), also known as Chinese gooseberry, is a nutritional fruit. It was mostly used as fresh fruit until recent years; more recently kiwifruit juice has become an important product.

In the processing of kiwifruit juice, reverse osmosis and evaporation are often used to concentrate the clarified juice. The flow characteristics or rheology are important properties in designing pumping, especially in the processing by reverse osmosis.

Different equations are available for the description of rheological behavior of fruit juice (Saravacos 1970; Holdsworth 1971; Rao 1977; Rao *et al.* 1984; Rao and Rizvi 1986; Ibarz and Pagan 1987). Generally, the rheological behavior of a clarified juice can be described by a power-law relationship (Rao 1977; Rao and Rizvi 1986; Ibarz and Pagan 1987):

$$\tau = K (\gamma)^n \tag{1}$$

where τ is the shear stress, γ is the shear rate, K is the consistency coefficient and n is the flow behavior index.

However, if the clarified juice has been depectinized, the flow behavior index n in equation (1) would become 1 and the juice will be Newtonian (Saravacos 1970; Rao and Rizvi 1986; Ibarz *et al.* 1987; Ibarz *et al.* 1992). That is:

$$\tau = \eta (\gamma) \tag{2}$$

where η is the coefficient of viscosity.

In this research the rheological behavior of kiwifruit juice was studied. The results may be useful in the production of clarified kiwifruit juice and concentrated clarified kiwifruit juice.

EXPERIMENTAL

Kiwifruit Juice Preparation

The kiwifruit used in the experiment was produced in Fengxin County of Jiangxi province of the People's Republic of China. After paring the skin away, the fruit was pulped. The kiwifruit pulp was added with 0.5% (w/w) pectinase and agitated for 4 hours at the temperature of 40°C, and then the clarified juice was obtained through filtration of the pulp.

The soluble solids in the clarified juice were determined by refractometry using an Abbe-Zeiss refractometer at a temperature of 25°C. The measured concentration of soluble solids in the clarified kiwifruit juice was 11.0 °Brix.

The pH value of the clarified kiwifruit juice was measured with a pH-meter and the result was 3.50. The acidity of the clarified kiwifruit juice was measured by titration with 0.1 M NaOH solution using a phenolphthalein indicator. The acidity of the juice was 0.24 eq. of acid/liter.

Then the juice was concentrated to 64.5 °Brix by evaporation. Distilled water was used to dilute the concentrated juice to make the samples of 58.1, 49.6, 36.5, 29.5 and 20.0 °Brix for measurement of rheological behavior at the different concentrations.

Rheological Measurements

Rheological measurements were carried out on a Brookfield LVDV-II+ viscometer which can transmit a maximum torque of 673.7 dyne-cm using an UL coaxial cylinders adapter. Circulating water flowing through the sleeve of the adapter column from the thermostatic bath controlled the test temperature (± 0.1 °C). Rotor speeds were variable in the range 0.5-100 rpm.

RESULTS

Rheological Behavior

The rheological behavior of kiwifruit juice was studied at different temperatures within the range of 5 ~ 60 °C and different concentrations over the 11.0 ~ 64.5 °Brix. Figures 1 and 2 show the experimental results of shear stress (τ) and shear rate (γ) of kiwifruit juice obtained at 64.5 and 11.0 °Brix at different temperatures. The viscosity coefficients of the juices in different concentrations and different temperatures are given in Table 1 which were obtained by fitting the experimental results to Eq. (2) with the least squares method. All the correlation coefficients were higher than 0.99, except one was 0.9641. The degree of fit and the estimates of the viscosity coefficient were significant at the 95% probability level. The results indicated that the clarified depectinized kiwifruit juice was Newtonian. It also can be seen that the viscosity of kiwifruit juice was smaller at higher temperature and larger at higher soluble solids contents.

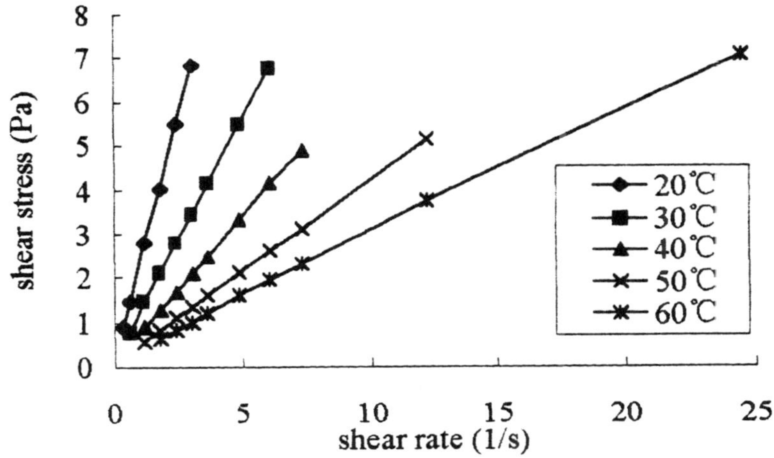

FIG. 1. THE RHEOGRAM OF KIWIFRUIT JUICE OF 64.5 °BRIX AT DIFFERENT TEMPERATURES

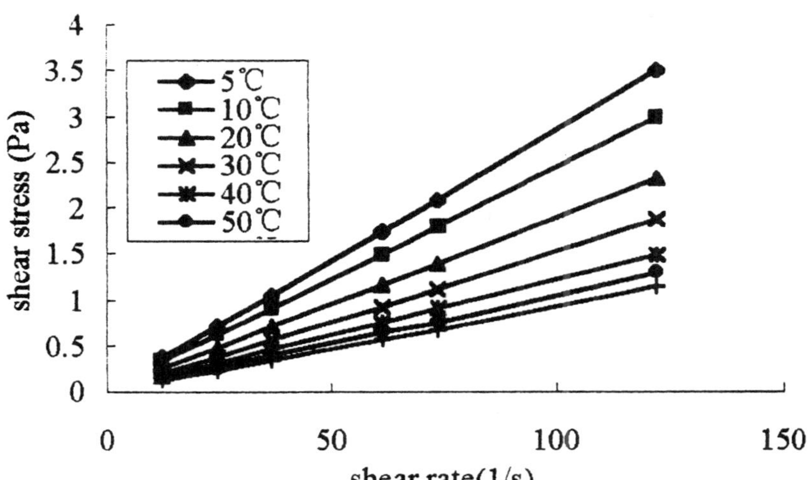

FIG. 2. THE RHEOGRAM OF THE KIWIFRUIT JUICE OF 11.0 °BRIX AT DIFFERENT TEMPERATURES

TABLE 1.
VISCOSITIES OF KIWIFRUIT JUICES AT DIFFERENT TEMPERATURES AND SOLUBLE SOLIDS CONTENT

T (°C)	C(°Brix)	η(Pa·S)	r	T(°C)	C(°Brix)	η(Pa·S)	r
5	11.0	0.0286	0.9999	40	11.0	0.0138	0.9922
	20.0	0.0433	0.9999		20.0	0.0173	0.9996
	29.5	0.0808	0.9999		29.5	0.0286	0.9999
	36.5	0.1487	0.9999		36.5	0.0448	0.9999
	49.6	0.6510	0.9995		49.6	0.1322	0.9998
10	11.0	0.0245	0.9999		58.1	0.3429	0.9996
	20.0	0.0378	0.9999		64.5	0.6727	0.9998
	29.5	0.0682	0.9999	50	11.0	0.0126	0.9824
	36.5	0.1231	0.9999		20.0	0.0144	0.9998
	49.6	0.4923	0.9998		29.5	0.0236	0.9999
	58.1	1.9186	0.9944		36.5	0.0351	0.9999
20	11.0	0.0191	0.9999		49.6	0.0942	0.9998
	20.0	0.0279	0.9999		58.1	0.2366	0.9996
	29.5	0.0488	0.9999		64.5	0.4239	0.9999
	36.5	0.0834	0.9998	60	11.0	0.0114	0.9781
	49.6	0.2944	0.9995		20.0	0.0123	0.9999
	58.1	0.8985	0.9996		29.5	0.0197	0.9998
	64.5	2.2389	0.9997		36.5	0.0289	0.9998
30	11.0	0.0153	0.9997		49.6	0.0715	0.9998
	20.0	0.0215	0.9998		58.1	0.1697	0.9997
	29.5	0.0370	0.9999		64.5	0.2961	0.9995
	36.5	0.0594	0.9641				
	49.6	0.1918	0.9998				
	58.1	0.5262	0.9998				
	64.5	1.1199	0.9999				

Effect of Temperature

The effect of temperature on the fruit juice can be described by the Arrhenius equation (Saravacos 1970; Rao *et al.* 1984):

$$\eta = K_0 \exp(Ea/RT) \tag{3}$$

where η is the viscosity, K_0 is a constant, Ea is the activation energy of flow, R is the gas constant, and T is the absolute temperature in K.

Figure 3 is the logarithm of the experimental viscosity plotted against 1/T. The values of the constants K_0 and Ea, and the correlation coefficient of each concentration are given in Table 2. Activation energies for each concentration were obtained from the results of multiplying the gas constant R by the slope of the corresponding straight lines. The values of the constants K_0 are the experimental function values of the intersection on viscosity axis by the straight lines.

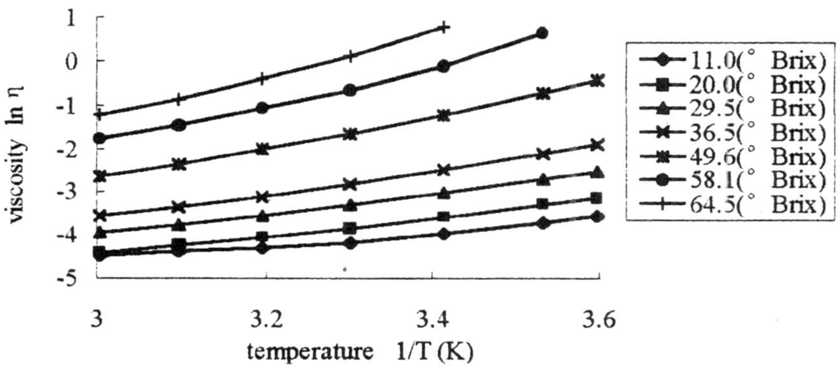

FIG. 3. EFFECTS OF TEMPERATURE ON THE VISCOSITY OF KIWIFRUIT JUICE

In Table 2, it can be observed that the activation energies of kiwifruit clarified juice increased with the soluble solids content.

TABLE 2.
VALUES OF FLOW ACTIVATION ENERGY Ea AND CONSTANT K_0 FOR KIWIFRUIT JUICES AT DIFFERENT SOLUBLE SOLIDS CONTENT

C (°Brix)	Ea(kcal mol^{-1})	K_0 (Pa · S)	corr. coeff.
11.0	3.7830	2.9310^{-5}	0.9971
20.0	4.2771	1.8410^{-5}	0.9980
29.5	4.7635	1.4010^{-5}	0.9979
36.5	5.5635	6.0610-6	0.9978
49.6	7.4169	9.0510-7	0.9982
58.5	8.9115	2.1810-7	0.9938
64.5	9.7671	1.0710-7	0.9965

Effect of Concentration

Increase of concentration increases the viscosity of a fluid food. Variation of viscosity with soluble-solids content can generally be described by the power-law type or the exponential type expression (Vitali and Rao 1982; Rao *et al.* 1984; Ibarz *et al.* 1987; Ibarz *et al.* 1992):

$$\eta = K_1(C)^{b1} \tag{4}$$

$$\eta = K_2\exp(b_2C) \tag{5}$$

In both equations, η and bi are constants and C is the concentration in °Brix.

The parameters of these equations were calculated by fitting the values of viscosity in Table 1 to the linear forms of the equations obtained by expressing them in a logarithmic form. These fits were made with least squares method, and the fit and the estimates of parameters were significant at a probability level of 95%. The values of the parameters of the power-law (Eq. (4)) and the exponential (Eq. (5)) relations are in Table 3.

TABLE 3.
EFFECT OF CONCENTRATION AND TEMPERATURE ON THE VISCOSITY OF KIWIFRUIT JUICE

T(°C)	η_1	b_1	r_1	η_2	b_2	r_2
5	1.87710^{-4}	1.926	0.9177	9.29810^{-3}	0.08080	0.9832
10	3.59010^{-5}	2.438	0.9069	6.16310^{-3}	0.09142	0.9797
20	1.61910^{-5}	2.597	0.9109	4.60310^{-3}	0.08953	0.9830
30	2.45110^{-5}	2.366	0.9149	4.24810^{-3}	0.08139	0.9850
40	3.05010^{-5}	2.211	0.9174	3.78410^{-3}	0.07591	0.9860
50	4.10310^{-5}	2.047	0.9181	3.56610^{-3}	0.07024	0.9862
60	5.12810^{-5}	1.917	0.9180	3.35610^{-3}	0.06578	0.9862

From the values of the regression coefficient obtained, it can be seen that the exponential model seems to describe better the effect of the soluble solids on the viscosity of the kiwifruit juice.

Combined Effect of Temperature and Concentration

A simple equation containing the parameters of temperature and concentration is useful to describe the combined effect of temperature and concentration on kiwifruit juice viscosity in practical engineering applications.

Different expressions can describe the combined effect of temperature and concentration. From the results obtained in the proceeding, the following equation was proposed:

$$\eta = K_3 \exp(Ea/RT + b_3C) \tag{6}$$

where η_3 and b_3 are constants.

Fitting the viscosity values given in Table 1 to the equation by multilinear regression, the values of the constants were obtained. The fit and the estimates of the constants are significant at a probability level of 95%. In the range of concentrations and temperatures used, a simple equation is proposed to describe the viscosity of clarified and depectinized kiwifruit juice:

$$\eta = 4.006 \times 10^{-7} \exp(2.839 \times 10^3/T + 0.0787C)$$

in which C is the concentration in °Brix, T the temperature in Kelvin and η the viscosity in PaS.

NOMENCLATURE

b_1	Constant of Eq. (4) (dimensionless)
b_2	Constant of Eq. (5) (°$Brix^{-1}$)
b_3	Constant of Eq. (6) (°$Brix^{-1}$)
C	Soluble solids content (°Brix)
Ea	Activation energy of flow (kcal mol^{-1} or cal mol^{-1})
K	Constant of Eq. (1) ($Pa \cdot S^n$)
K_0	Constant of Eq. (3) (PaS)
K_1	Constant of Eq. (4) (PaS °$Brix^{-b1}$)
K_2	Constant of Eq. (5) (PaS)
K3	Constant of Eq. (6) (PaS)
n	Flow behavior index (dimensionless)
R	Gas constant (cal mol^{-1} K^{-1})
T	Temperature (K or °C)
τ	Shear stress (Pa)
η	Viscosity (PaS)
γ	Shear rate (S^{-1})

REFERENCES

HOLDSWORTH, S.D. 1971. Applicability of rheological models to the interpretation of flow and processing behaviour of fluid food products. J. Texture Studies *2*, 393–418.

IBARZ, A. and PAGAN, J. 1987. Rheology of raspberry juices. J. Food Eng. *6*, 269–289.

IBARZ, A., VICENTE, M. and GREALL, J. 1987. Rheological behaviour of apple juice and pear juice and their concentrates. J. Food Eng. *6*, 257–267.

IBARZ, A., PAGAN, J. and MIGUELSANZ, R. 1992. Rheology of clarified fruit juices. II: Blackcurrant juices. J. Food Eng. *15*, 49–61.

RAO, M.A. 1977. Rheology of liquid foods – a review. J. Texture Studies *8*, 135–168.

RAO, M.A. and RIZVI, S.S.H. (eds) 1986. Engineering Properties of Foods, Marcel Dekker, Inc., New York.

RAO, M.A., COOLEY, M.J. and VITALI, A.A. 1984. Flow properties of concentrated juices at low temperatures. Food Technol. *38* (3), 113–119.

SARAVACOS, G.D. 1970. Effect of temperature on viscosity of fruit juices and purees. J. Food Sci. *35*, 122–125.

VITALI, A.A. and RAO, M.A. 1982. Flow behaviour of guava as a function of temperature and concentration. J. Texture Studies *13*, 275–289.

FERMENTATION TECHNOLOGY FOR THE PRODUCTION OF HIGH-VALUE FOOD ADDITIVES

FENG CHEN

Department of Botany
The University of Hong Kong
Pokfulam Road, Hong Kong

ABSTRACT

*Fermentation technology has been widely used for the production of various food products such as alcohol, amino acids, organic acids and fermented foods. The current trend in fermentation biotechnology is toward the development of processes for high-value products including high-value food additives. In this paper, the use of fermentation technology for the production of high-value food additives such as algal biomass (*Spirulina, Chlorella*, etc.), food pigments (phycocyanin, lutein, β-carotene, astaxanthin, etc.) and polyunsaturated fatty acids (eicosapentaenoic acid, docosahexaenoic acid, γ-linolenic acid, etc.) is reported with emphasis on the employment of microalgae as the producing organisms. Also the various high cell density fermentation strategies (i.e. fed-batch, chemostat and membrane cell recycle systems) which can be used to enhance the product yields are discussed.*

INTRODUCTION

Fermentation technology is one of the oldest technologies employed in the food processing industry. Conventionally, fermentation technology is used to manufacture various food products such as alcohol, amino acids, organic acids, and fermented foods, most of which are of relatively low-value (Knorr and Sinskey 1985). More recently, the development of fermentation biotechnology has been mainly focused on the production of high-value foods including nutrient foods, functional foods, and high-value food additives (Bell and White 1989; Gudin and Chaumont 1991). New sources of organisms such as genetic engineered organisms and newly exploited organisms are being investigated to establish novel fermentation processes for production of various high-value products. The present paper reports on the use of fermentation technology and microalgae (the largely untapped biological resources) for the production of various high-value food additives including microalgal biomass (i.e. *Spirulina*, *Chlorella*, etc.), food pigments (i.e., phycocyanin, lutein, β-carotene, astaxanthin, etc.) and polyunsaturated fatty acids (i.e. eicosapentaenoic acid, docosahexaenoic acid, γ-linolenic acid, etc.).

MATERIALS AND METHODS

Microorganisms

The microalgae used in this work include *Chlorella prothothecoides* CS-41 (the CSIRO Marine Laboratory, Hobart, Australia), *Spirulina platensis* UTEX 1926

(University of Texas Culture Collection), *Crypthecodinium cohnii* UTEX L1649 (University of Texas Culture Collection), and *Haematococcus lacustris* UTEX 16 (University of Texas Culture Collection).

Media and Cultivation

The media used for the cultivation are Basal medium (pH 6.1) for *C. prothothecoides* (Shi *et al.* 1997), Zarouk medium (pH 9.5) for *S. platensis* (Chen *et al.* 1996), Porphyridium medium (pH 8.5) for *C. cohnii* (Starr and Zeikus 1993), and MCM medium (pH 7.0) for *H. lacustris* (Yuan *et al.* 1996).

C. prothothecoides was grown heterotrophically with 9 g/l glucose in a 3.7-liter fermenter (Bioengineering AG, Switzerland) at 26°C, and the dissolved oxygen concentration was maintained at 50% saturation. *C. cohnii* was grown heterotrophically with 10 g/l glucose in a 16-liter fermenter (Bioengineering AG) at 25°C, and the dissolved oxygen concentration was kept at 50% saturation. *S. platensis* (at 30°C) and *H. lacustris* (at 25°C) were grown mixotrophically in 3.7-liter fermenters (Bioengineering AG) at a light intensity of 80 $\mu E/m^2s$ (90-190 $\mu E/m^2s$ for *H. lacustris*) and an aeration rate of 100 l/h. The media were supplemented with 2 g/l glucose for *S. platensis* and 1 g/l acetate for *H. lacustris*, respectively.

Analytical Methods

Cell concentrations were determined according to the procedure of Chen *et al.* (1996). The glucose and acetate concentrations were determined by HPLC according to Shi *et al.* (1997), and Chen and Johns (1994), respectively.

Phycocyanin concentration was determined according to the method reported by Boussiba and Richmond (1980).

Other pigments including chlorophylls, β-carotene, astaxanthin, canthaxanthin and lutein were determined by HPLC according to Yuan *et al.* (1997).

Fatty acids were determined by GC according to the method reported by Vazhappilly and Chen (submitted for publication).

RESULTS AND DISCUSSION

Production of Biomass and Phycocyanin by *S. platensis*

The time course for a typical batch culture of *S. platensis* grown with 2 g/l glucose in a 3.7-liter fermenter under mixotrophic conditions is given in Fig. 1. After a 24-h lag, the microalga grew exponentially and entered the stationary phase at the 120th h as a result of glucose exhaustion (Fig. 1). The maximum cell concentration obtained was approximately 2.4 g/l (dry weight). The cellular phycocyanin content increased continuously during the course of cultivation, and the final phycocyanin content obtained was about 110 mg/g (Fig. 1). The cell concentration achieved using a fermenter is much higher than that obtained in commercial pond photoautotrophic culture where typical cell concentrations were between 0.4-0.8 g/l, whereas the phycocyanin content was comparable to that obtained in pond culture (Richmond 1988). The use of *Spirulina* as food has a long history. *Spirulina* biomass is now widely used as health food and food additives (Yamaguchi 1997). A bright blue water soluble pigment, phycocyanin from *Spirulina* is used as food additives in a wide variety of foods such as ice cream, chewing gum, jelly, candy and yogurt (Yamaguchi 1997). The addition of *Spirulina* biomass as a health promoting stuff to cereal products such as noodles and breads have recently been attempted (Kato 1992).

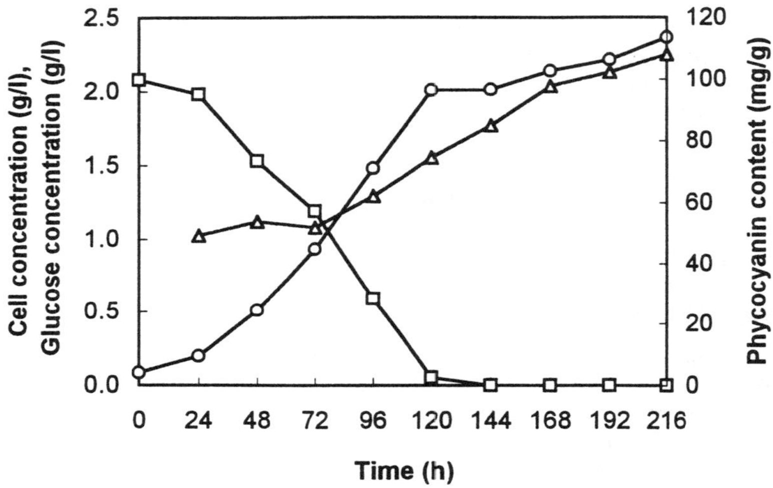

FIG. 1. THE TIME COURSE OF A TYPICAL BATCH CULTURE OF *S. PLATENSIS* GROWN MIXOTROPHICALLY WITH 2 G/L GLUCOSE IN A 3.7-LITER FERMENTER

Cell concentration, ○; phycocyanin content, Δ; glucose concentration, □.

Production of Biomass and Lutein by *C. prothothecoides*

Results of biomass and lutein production by *C. prothothecoides* in a 3.7-liter fermenter are shown in Fig. 2. As can be seen from the Figure, the maximum biomass concentration (4.6 g/l, dry weight) was obtained on the third day, and the maximum lutein content (4.6 mg/g dry cells) and yield (16 mg/l) were achieved on the 8th and 6th day, respectively. The cell growth yield and lutein yield on the carbon source, glucose, were 0.48 g/g and 1.73 mg/g, respectively. The consumption of carbon source by *C. prothothecoides* responded well to the growth of the alga. Glucose was found to be completely exhausted on the third day when the alga started to enter the stationary phase (data not shown). This cell concentration was very high compared to that generally achieved in pond systems (typically less than 1 g/l).

Chlorella health food products are now available in the form of tablets, powders and drinks. Many companies are producing and marketing *Chlorella* products worldwide. In Japan, more than 70 companies have registered their *Chlorella* products which represent the annual sales of above 40 billion yen (Yamaguchi 1997). Lutein is one of the most important carotenoids. Lutein has been used for the pigmentation of animal tissues and products, as well as for the coloration of foods, drugs and cosmetics (Klaui 1982). In the USA, two lutein-containing products, Aztec Marigold and Tagets have recently been commercialized (Rayner 1993). *Chlorella* is one of the most important sources of naturally occurring lutein (Goodwin 1980).

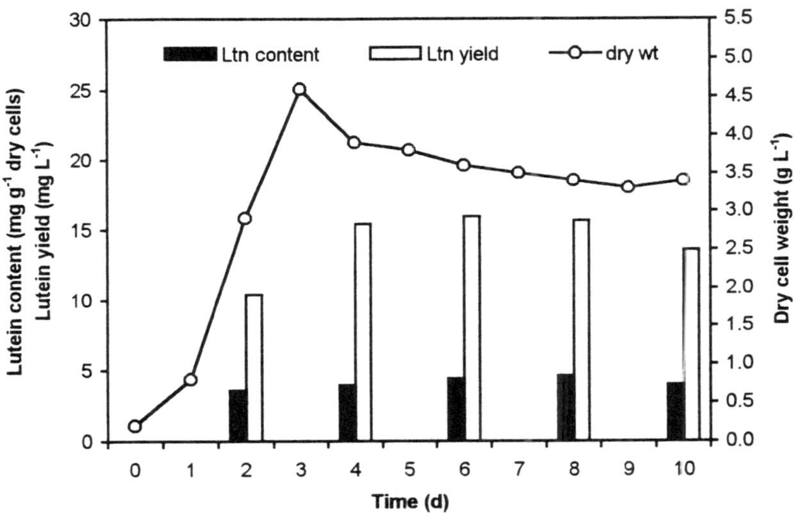

FIG. 2. BIOMASS AND LUTEIN PRODUCTION BY *C. PROTHOTHECOIDES* GROWN HETEROTROPHICALLY WITH G/L GLUCOSE IN A 3.7-LITER FERMENTER

Production of Carotenoids by *H. lacustris*

H. lacustris is a potential natural source of food pigments, particular carotenoids. Figure 3 shows the growth of *H. lacustris* cells in batch culture in a 3.7-liter fermenter. The final cell concentrations were similar for both cultures in which the light intensity was raised from 90 to 190 μE/m^{2}s after 4 d and 8 d of cultivation respectively. The highest cell concentration achieved was approximately 2 g/l (dry weight). The cellular pigment production is summarized in Table 1. It is clear that astaxanthin is the major pigment in the cells of the microalga. Astaxanthin is an important carotenoid widely used as pigmentation source in the poultry and aquaculture industries (Johnson and An 1991). Due to its biological functions as vitamin A precursor, and the higher antioxidative activity than β-carotene and vitamin E, astaxanthin can also be used as food colorant and in medicine (Johnson and An 1991). The current market price of astaxanthin is above US $2,000 per kg. Relatively the algal cells contained smaller quantities of β-carotene which is commercially produced by another microalga, *Dunalialla* (Chen 1996).

Production of Polyunsaturated Fatty Acids by *C. cohnii*

The fatty acid composition of *Crypthecodinium cohnii* grown on glucose (10 g/l) in a 16-liter fermenter under heterotrophic conditions is shown in Table 2. The microalga contained significant amounts of polyunsaturated fatty acids, particularly docosahexaenoic acid (DHA). The heterotrophic production of DHA in batch culture in a 16-liter fermenter is tabulated in Table 3. Results clearly demonstrate that the microalga has great potential to be employed for commercial production. Polyunsaturated fatty acids, particularly eicosapentaenoic acid, docosahexaenoic acid and gamma-linolenic acid, have been recognized as essential dietary compounds, which are useful for the prevention and treatment of a number of diseases including cardiovascular diseases (Drevon *et al.* 1993). Research is continuing in our laboratory to further screen microalgae for their polyunsaturated fatty acid production potential, and develop optimal large scale fermentation processes for the production of the products.

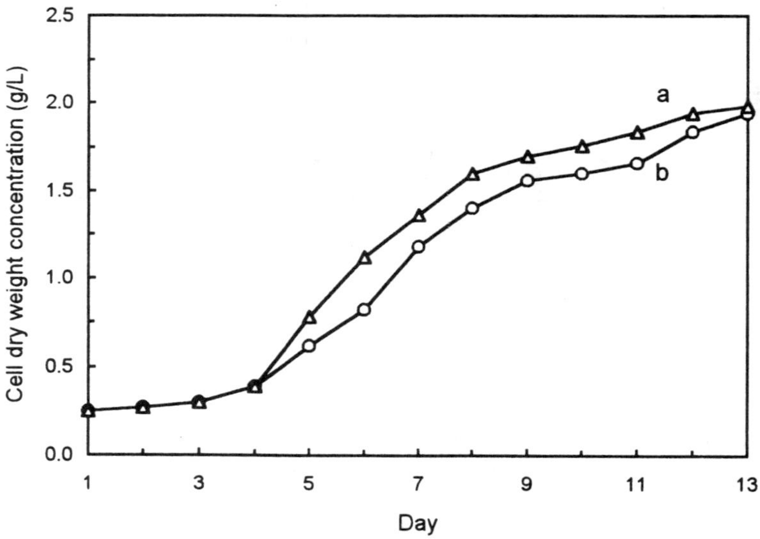

FIG. 3. GROWTH OF *H. LACUSTRIS* CELLS IN MIXOTROPHIC BATCH CULTURE WITH 1 G/L ACETATE IN A 3.7-LITER FERMENTER. THE LIGHT INTENSITY WAS RAISED FROM 90 TO 190 $\mu E/M^2S$ AFTER 4 DAYS OF CULTIVATION (a) OR 8 DAYS OF CULTIVATION (b).

High Cell Density Strategies

One of the major advantages for the use of fermentation technology and facilities to produce high value food additives is that we can easily modify the fermentation processes so as to improve the cell densities and yields. In another

TABLE 1.
PRODUCTION OF CHLOROPHYLLS AND CAROTENOIDS BY *H. LACUSTRIS* IN A 3.7-LITER FERMENTER AT 2°C ON DAY 13[1]

Pigment	Cellular pigment content (mg/g cell dry weight)
Total astaxanthin esters	6.8
Chlorophyll a	5.5
Chlorophyll b	2.5
lutein	1.9
canthaxanthin	0.4
β-carotene	0.4

[1] The cell dry weight concentration was 2.0 g/l at day 13.

TABLE 2.
FATTY ACID COMPOSITION OF *CRYPTHECODINIUM COHNII* GROWN IN A 16-LITER FERMENTOR UNDER HETEROTROPHIC CONDITIONS (IN EARLY STATIONARY PHASE, 60 H)

Fatty acid	% of total fatty acids
14:0	7.4
14:1	2.3
16:0	11.2
16:1	2.9
18:0	2.6
18:1	12.6
18:2	9.0
18:3	4.4
20:4	0.0
20:5	0.0
22:5	17.0
22:6 (ω-3, DHA)	30.6

TABLE 3.
PRODUCTION OF DHA BY *CRYPTHECODINIUM COHNII* GROWN IN A 16-LITER FERMENTER UNDER HETEROTROPHIC CONDITIONS (IN EARLY STATIONARY PHASE, 60 H)

Biomass concentration (g/l)	DHA % of biomass (w/w)	DHA yield (mg/l)	Productivity (mg/l/day)
4.5	1.2	54	22

experiment, we have been able to raise the cell concentration of *Spirulina platensis* to 10 g/l (compared to 2.4 g/l in batch culture) by using fed-batch culture techniques (Chen and Zhang 1997). Similarly, the cell concentration of *C. prothothecoides* has recently been enhanced to 45 g/l in the same fermenter (3.7-liter) using fed-batch techniques (data not shown). Other potential microalgae such as *H. lacustris* and *C. cohnii* are being investigated using high cell density techniques such as fed-batch, chemostat and membrane cell recycle systems. We have previously demonstrated the possibility of employing these high cell density culture strategies for other microalgae, *Chlamydomonas reinhardtii* (Chen and Johns 1995).

CONCLUSIONS

The results demonstrate that microalgae are potential sources of high value food additives. Fermentation technology which is frequently used in the food processing industry can be employed to improve and manipulate the product yields.

ACKNOWLEDGMENTS

The author gratefully acknowledges the support of the Hong Kong Research Grants Council, University of Hong Kong Committee on Research and Conference Grants, and Industry Department of Hong Kong Government for this work and the technical assistance provided by X.M. Shi, R. Vazhappilly, Y.M. Zhang, X.D. Gong and J.P. Yuan.

REFERENCES

BELL, E.R.J. and WHITE, E.B. 1989. The potential of biotechnology for the production of flavours and colours for the food industry. Intl. Ind. Biotechnol. *9*, 20–26.

BOUSSIBA, S. and RICHMOND, A.E. 1980. C-phycocyanin as a storage protein in the blue-green alga *Spirulina platensis*. Arch. Microbiol. *125*, 143–147.

CHEN, F. 1996. High cell density culture of microalgae in heterotrophic growth. Trends Biotechnol. *14*, 421–426.

CHEN, F. and JOHNS, M.R. 1994. Substrate inhibition of *Chlamydomonas reinhardtii* by acetate in heterotrophic culture. Process Biochem. *29*, 245–252.

CHEN, F. and JOHNS, M.R. 1995. A strategy for high cell density culture of heterotrophic microalgae with inhibitory substrates. J. Appl. Phycol. *7*, 43–46.

CHEN, F. and ZHANG, Y.M. 1997. High cell density mixotrophic culture of *Spirulina platensis* on glucose for phycocyanin production using a fed-batch system. Enzyme Microbial Technol. *20*, 221–224.

CHEN, F., ZHANG, Y.M. and GUO, S.Y. 1996. Growth and phycocyanin formation of *Spirulina platensis* in photoheterotrophic culture. Biotechnol. Lett. *18*, 603–608.

DREVON, C.A., BAKSAAS, I. and KROKAN, H.E. 1993. Omega-3 Fatty Acids: Metabolism and Biological Effects. Birkhauser Verlag, Basel, Switzerland.

GOODWIN, T.W. 1980. The Chemistry of the Carotenoids, Vol. 1, Plants. Chapman and Hall, London.

GUDIN, C. and CHAUMONT, D. 1991. Microalgae, new sources of metabolites. Biofutur *106*, 27–30.

JOHNSON, E.A. and AN, G.H. 1991. Astaxanthin from microbial sources. Crit. Rev. Biotechnol. *11*, 297–326.

KATO, T. 1992. *Spirulina*. *In* Utilization of Microalgae, K. Yamaguchi (ed.). Koseisha-Koseikaku, Tokyo.

KLAUI, H. 1982. Industrial and commercial uses of carotenoids. *In* Carotenoid Chemistry and Biochemistry, G. Britton and T.W. Goodwin (eds.). Pergamon Press, Oxford.

KNORR, D. and SINSKEY, A.J. 1985. Biotechnology in food production and processing. Science USA *229*, 1224–1229.

RAYNER, P.B. 1993. Food & drink colors from natural sources. Food Marketing Technol.-Intl. *7*, 9–10.

RICHMOND, A. 1988. *Spirulina*. *In* Micro-algal Biotechnology, M.A. Borowitzka and L.J. Borowitzka (eds.). Cambridge University Press, Cambridge.

SHI, X.M., CHEN, F., YUAN, J.P. and CHEN, H. 1997. Heterotrophic production of lutein by selected *Chlorella* strains. J. Appl. Phycol. (In press).

STARR, R.C. and ZEIKUS, J.A. 1993. The culture collection of algae at the University of Texas at Austin. J. Phycol. *29* (Suppl.), 90–95.

VAZHAPPILLY, R. and CHEN, F. 19--. Eicosapentaenoic acid and docosahexaenoic acid production potential of microalgae and their heterotrophic growth. (submitted).

YAMAGUCHI, K. 1997. Recent advances in microalgal bioscience in Japan, with special reference to utilization of biomass and metabolites: a review. J. Appl. Phycol. *8*, 487–502.

YUAN, J.P., GONG, X.D. and CHEN, F. 1996. Separation and identification of astaxanthin esters and chlorophylls in *Haematococcus lacustris* by HPLC. Biotechnol. Tech. *10*, 655–660.

YUAN, J.P., GONG, X.D. and CHEN, F. 1997. Separation and analysis of carotenoids and chlorophylls in *Haematococcus lacustris* by high-performance liquid chromatography photodiode array detection. J. Agric. Food Chem. *45*, 1952–1956.

STUDIES ON BIOACTIVE COMPOUNDS PRODUCTION BY SUBMERGED FERMENTATION OF *GANODERMA LUCIDUM*

PINGZUO LI, ROU XU and KECHANG ZHANG

School of Biotechnology
Wuxi University of Light Industry
Wuxi, 214036, P.R. China

ABSTRACT

A 25L laboratory fermentor was used to produce a water soluble, antitumor polysaccharide and ganoderic acids by submerged fermentation of G.lucidum. *An optimum medium was obtained through orthogonal test, $L_9(3^4)$, which contained 80 g/l distilled grain (contained 75% water), 10 g/l glucose, 10 g/l corn powder and 5 g/l wheat bran, and the maximum polysaccharide yield was about 2.25 g/l.*

Three ganoderic acids were isolated from the culture of G.lucidum by the methanol-ether-n-butanol extraction system, and Rf value was 0.56, 0.49 and 0.17 respectively. The antimicrobial test showed the compounds could inhibit growth of Shigella dysenteriae, Pseudomonas pyocyanea, Staphylococcus aureus, Escherichia coli *and* Bacillus subtilis.

INTRODUCTION

Since the earliest times, mushrooms have been treated as a special food. They have been widely consumed not only for their taste, texture, and nutritious composition, but also for their claimed therapeutic value. The practice of using fungi as medicines was found in the traditions of many cultures, past and present. In Chinese folklore the fruit body of *Ganoderma* has been regarded as a panacea for all types of diseases. This is probably due to its demonstrated efficacy as a popular remedy to treat hepatopathy, chronic hepatitis, nephritis, hypertension, hyperlipemia, leukopenia, immunocompetence and antitumor activity (Liu *et al.* 1979; Kabir *et al.* 1988; Willard 1990). Recent findings (Nishitoba *et al.* 1985; Su 1991) that certain types of fungal β-1,3-D-glucans have antitumor activity have attracted attention toward the polysaccharide components and ganoderic acids have been regarded as the main bioactive compounds of *Ganoderma lucidum.* We (Zhang *et al.* 1994) have reported on the antitumor activity of polysaccharides produced by submerged fermentation of *Ganoderma lucidum*, and confirmed the structure is β-1,3-D-glucans. It is known that polysaccharides and ganoderic acids were usually produced by solid culture method; the yield is very low, and method of submerged fermentation has many advantages, for example, large scale, low labor intensity, high efficiency and high quality control.

MATERIALS AND METHODS

Organism

The fungus *Ganoderma lucidum* is maintained in our laboratory.

The test bacteria *Shigella dysenteriae, Pseudomonas pyocyanea, Staphylococcus aureus, Escherichia coli* and *Bacillus subtilis* are also maintained in our laboratory.

Fermentation

Medium. For slants: PDA. For seed culturing (500 ml shaking flasks): 2% glucose, 1% corn powder, 0.5% wheat bran, 0.2% $(NH_4)_2SO_4$ and $MgSO_4 \cdot 7H_2O$. The initial pH was 5.5 and the medium was autoclaved at 121°C for 45 min.

Fermentation Conditions

The fermentation broth was agitated at 150 rpm, the temperature was controlled at 30°C, the oxygen was provided by sparging an air stream through the fermentor at a rate of 1 vvm, and the fermentation period was 72-96 h.

Isolation and Purification of Polysaccharides (Miyazaki *et al.* 1981)

The fermentation broth was centrifuged at 6000 rpm, the supernant was added to the ethanol at 30% and 60%, respectively, then deproteined by pronase and Savag method. Each precipitate as crude polysaccharides was collected by centrifugation and dried in a vacuum.

Extraction and Isolation of Ganoderic Acids (Nishitoba *et al.* 1987)

The fermented mash were concentrated in vacuum, and blended with a blender, defatted with ether, then extracted with methanol and n-butanol. The methanol extractable matter was further purified through Silica gel column chromatography (C-200), analyzed by pre-coated TLC plates of silica gel F254 (0.2 mm thick), plates developed with hexane-ethyl acetate (1:1, v/v) and spots were detected by use of methanol-sulfuric acid (1:1, v/v) regent.

Analytical Methods

Assay of biomass: The fermentation broth was centrifuged at 6000 rpm, the precipitate was collected, washed with water and dried in the oven at 80°C for 24 h, then weighed.

Assay of polysaccharides (Dubois *et al.* 1956): Phenol-Sulfuric acid method.

Antimicrobial Test (Pereira *et al.* 1996)

Antimicrobial activity was determined by the conventional paper disk diffusion method using the following nutrient media: 0.4% beef extract, 0.1% yeast extract, 0.4% peptone, 1% dextrose, 0.25% NaCl, 2% agar, pH 7.0. Growth inhibition was examined after 24 h incubation at 37°C. Crude methanol-extractable matter was dissolved in methanol and a paper disk containing each of the products was placed on agar plates.

RESULTS AND DISCUSSION

Fermentation

Selection of Fermentation Medium

Figure 1 shows the effects of different carbon and nitrogen sources on the yield of extracellular polysaccharides. From this result, distilled grain, glucose, corn powder and wheat bran were used for the fermentation medium optimization. Table 1, Table 2, and Table 3 show the result of orthogonal test (Montgomery 1976), $L_9(3^4)$; as can be seen from Table 3, factor A (distilled grain) has significant effect at 1 percent, factor B and D has significant effect at 5 percent. Therefore, a suitable medium was determined as, A3B2C2D3, namely, 80 g/l distilled grain (containing 75% water), 10 g/l glucose, 10 g/l corn powder and 5 g/l wheat bran. The maximum yield of polysaccharide was about 2.25 g/l, which was verified in a 25 L fermentor (see Fig. 2). Additionally, as distilled grain contains monosaccharide, semicellulose and cellulose, these compounds may promote the formation of exopolysaccharide. Especially, it is very important for the antitumor activity of the polysaccharide to have various monosaccharides, such as D-galactose, D-mannose, D-arabinose, D-xylose (Sone *et al.* 1985).

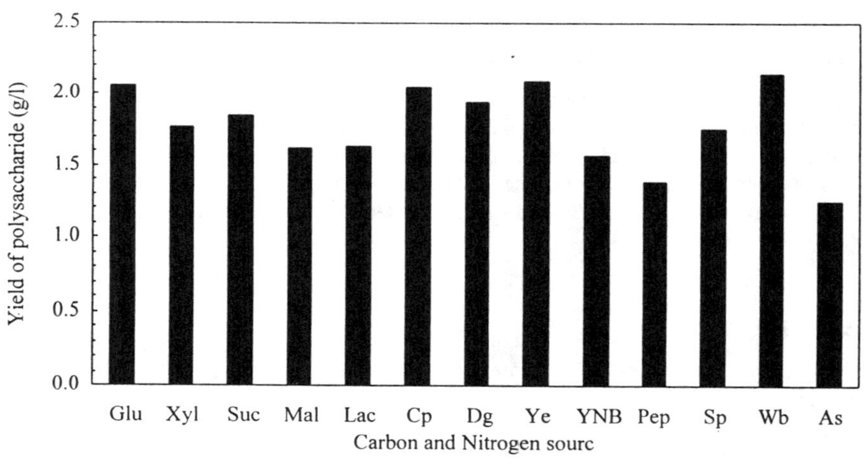

FIG. 1. EFFECTS OF CARBON AND NITROGEN SOURCES ON POLYSACCHARIDE PRODUCTION OF *G. LUCIDUM*

Glu-glucose, Xyl-xylose, Suc-sucrose, Mal-maltose, Lac-lactose, Cp-corn powder, As-ammonium sulfate, Dg-distilled grain, Ye-yeast extract, YNB-yeast nitrogen base, Pep-peptone, Wb-wheat bran

As can be seen from Fig. 2, the start of polysaccharide formation occurred approximately 48 h after the exponential growth phase, which indicates that polysaccharide of *G. lucidum* is a secondary metabolite which has been noted for other fungal glucans, such as pullulan (Heald 1985), but not reported as polysaccharide of *G. lucidum*. The maximum yield of polysaccharide increased to 2.25 g/l; it is 1.5 times that of the former report.

TABLE 1.
FACTORS AND LEVELS OF ORTHOGONAL TEST

factors level	A (g/l) distilled grain	B corn powder	C glucose	D wheat bran
1	50	0.5	1.5	1
2	65	1.0	1.0	0.75
3	80	1.5	0.5	0.5

TABLE 2.
RESULT OF ORTHOGONAL TEST $L_9(3^4)$

No. of experiment	A	B	C	D	Polysaccharide (y)	Sum
1	1	1	1	1	1.95 1.80 2.10	5.85
2	1	2	2	2	2.10 1.95 2.55	6.60
3	1	3	3	3	1.95 2.10 2.40	6.45
4	2	1	2	3	1.65 1.80 2.40	5.85
5	2	2	3	1	1.50 1.35 2.10	4.95
6	2	3	1	2	1.20 1.14 1.26	3.60
7	3	1	3	2	2.10 2.10 1.95	6.75
8	3	2	1	3	2.55 2.55 2.40	7.50
9	3	3	2	1	1.50 1.95 1.95	5.40
Ij	18.9	18.45	16.95	16.20		
IIj	14.4	19.05	17.85	16.95	T=52.95	
IIIj	19.65	15.45	18.15	19.80	y=1.96	
Sj	1.793	0.826	0.087	0.801	SSt=4.95	

TABLE 3.
ANALYSIS OF VARIANCE FOR ORTHOGONAL TEST $L_9(3^4)$

Source of Variation	Sum of Squares	Degree of Freedom	Mean Square	F	Significant
A	1.793	2	0.8965	11.73	**
B	0.826	2	0.413	5.41	*
C•	0.087	2	0.0435		
D	0.801	2	0.4005	5.24	*
Error	1.44	18	0.08		
Error•	1.527	20	0.0764		

$F_{0.95}(2, 20)=3.49$, $F_{0.99}(2, 20)=5.85$; $\text{Sum Square}_{\text{Error}}{}^{\bullet}=\text{Sum Square}_{\text{Error}}+\text{Sum Square}^{\bullet}$

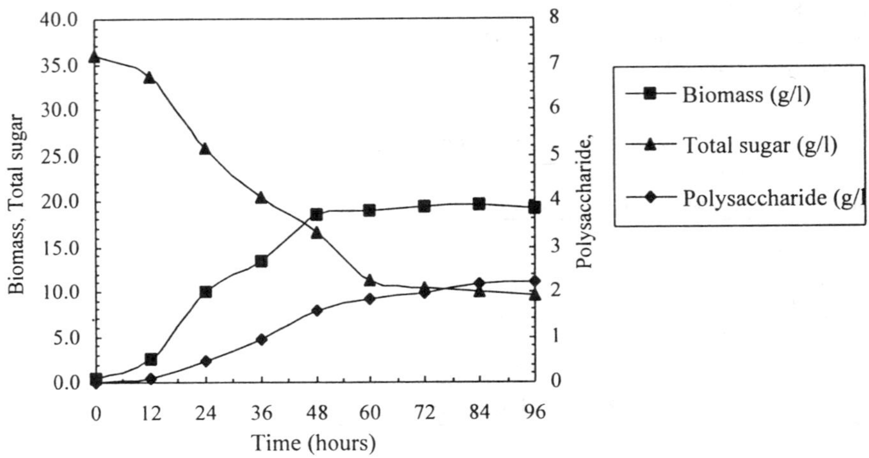

FIG. 2. FERMENTATION PROCESS CURVE

Ganoderic Acids Isolation and Purification

Data in Table 4 show that three ganoderic acids m1, m2, and m3 were isolated from the culture of *G. lucidum*; m1 and m2 eluted with CH_3OH:$CHCl_3$=3:97 were less polar than m3 eluted with CH_3OH:$CHCl_3$=1:9. These three compounds have absorption in the range 1200-1400 cm^{-1} of I.R, and maximum absorption at 253 nm, 241 nm and 223 nm of UV spectrum, which can preliminarily confirm that m1, m2 and m3 belong to triterpenoid family (Snatzke *et al.* 1962; Nishitoba *et al.* 1988).

TABLE 4.
RESULTS OF GANODERIC ACIDS ISOLATION AND PURIFICATION

Elute (CH_3OH: $CHCl_3$)	R_f	Elute rate (ml/min)	Maximum absorption of UV (nm)	IR spectrum (cm^{-1})
3:97	0.56	2.0	253	1220, 1360
3:97	0.49	2.0	241	1255, 1360
1:9	0.17	2.0	223	1230, 1349

Antitumor Activity (Zhang *et al.* 1994)

The antitumor test showed that crude polysaccharides precipitated by 30% and 60% ethanol had antitumor activity; its inhibition ratio to human tumor K562 was about 60%.

Antimicrobial Activity

The results in Table 5 show that the activity observed against tested organisms is different. The inhibition activity of m3 was stronger than that of m1 and m2, which may be caused by their differences of structure, but there is no published report on it.

TABLE 5.
GROWTH INHIBITORY EFFECT AGAINST DIFFERENT MICROORGANISMS

Compound	*Shigella dysenteriae*	*Pseudomonas pyocyanea*	*Staphylococcus aureus*	*Escherichia coli*	*Bacillus subtilis*
m1	++	+	+	++	-
m2	++	+	+	++	-
m3	+++	++	+	+++	+

-, +, ++, +++ mean inhibition growth activity, no, weak, medium and strong.
The size of zones of growth inhibition was 12-15 mm(+++), 10-12 mm(++), 7-9 mm(+).

CONCLUSION

The optimum fermentation medium was obtained through orthogonal test $L_9(3^4)$, and the maximum yield of polysaccharide in 25L fermentor was 2.25 g/l using that medium; it is 1.5 times the former report. Especially, distilled grain has significant effect on the production of polysaccharide, as distilled grain contains monosaccharides, semicellulose and cellulose.

Polysaccharides produced by submerged fermentation is a secondary metabolite. Reasonable fermentation process control needs to be continued to improve the formation of polysaccharide.

Three ganoderic acids isolated from the culture of *G. lucidum* have antimicrobial activity; especially m3 can inhibit the growth of every tested microorganism. The structures of ganoderic acids present in crude mixture will be further investigated by NMR and GC-MS.

In order to increase the antitumor activity, the polysaccharide isolation by DEAE-cellulose column chromatography and Sepharose Cl-6B gel filtration is being studied.

The culture of *G. lucidum* has been added to a food product to enhance the nutritional value, a subject of a future publication.

REFERENCES

DUBOIS, M., GILLES, K.A., HAMILTON, J.K., REBERS, P.A. and SMITH, F. 1956. Colorimetric determination of sugars and related substances. Anal. Chem. *28*, 350–356.

HEALD, P.J. and KRISTIANSEN, B. 1985. Synthesis of polysaccharides by yeast-like forms of *Aureobasidium pullulans*. Biotechnol. Bioeng. *27*, 1516–1519.

KABIR, Y., KIMURA, S. and TAMURA, T. 1988. Dietary effect of *Ganoderma lucidum* mushroom on blood pressure and lipid levels in spontaneously hypertensive rats (SHR). J. Nutri. Sci. Vitaminol. *34*, 433–438.

LIU, G.-T., BAO, T.-T., NIU, X.-Y., LI, S.-Z. and SONG, Z.-Y. 1979. Some pharmacological actions of the spores of *Ganoderma lucidum* and the mycelium of *Ganoderma capense* (Lloyd) Teng cultivated by submerged fermentation. Chin. Med. J. *92*, 496–500.

MIYAZAKI, T. and NISHIJIMA, M. 1981. Studies on fungal polysaccharides. XXVII. Chem. Pharm. Bull. V *29*(12), 3611–3616.

MONTGOMERY, D.C., ed. 1976. Design and Analysis of Experiments. John Wiley and Sons, New York, London, Sydney, Toronto.

NISHITOBA, T., SATO, H., KASAI, T., KAWAGISHI, H. and SAKAMURA, S. 1985. New bitter C27 and C30 terpenoids from the fungus *Ganoderma lucidum* (Reishi). Agric. Biol. Chem. *49*, 1793–1798.

NISHITOBA, T., SATO, H., SHIRASU, S. and SAKAMURA, S. 1987. Novel triterpenoids from the mycelial mat at the previous stage of fruiting of *Ganoderma lucidum*. Agric. Biol. Chem. *51*, 619–622.

NISHITOBA, T., ODA, K., SATO, H. and SAKAMURA, S. 1988. Novel triterpenoids from the fungus *Ganoderma lucidum*. Agric. Biol. Chem. *52*(2), 367–372.

PEREIRA, E.R., SANCELME, M., TOWA, J.J., PRUDHOMME, M., ARTRE, A., MOUSSET, G. and RAPP, M. 1996. Syntheses and antimicrobial activities of five membered ring heterocycles coupled to *Indoe moietieds*. J. Antibiotics, *49*(4), 380–385.

SNATZKE, G., LAMPERT, F. and TSCHESCHE, R. 1962. Triterpenes VIII. Assignment of triterpenes to fundamental types by infrared spectroscopy. Tetrahedon, *18*, 1417–1431.

SONE, Y., OKUDA, R., WADA, N., KISHIDA, E. and MISAKI, A. 1985. Structures and antitumor activities of the polysaccharides isolated from fruiting body and the growing culture of mycelium of *Ganoderma lucidum*. Agric. Biol. Chem. *49*(9), 2641–2653.

SU, C.-H. 1991. Taxonomy and physiologically active compounds of *Ganoderma* - A review. Bull. Taipei Med. Coll. *20*, 1–6.

WILLARD, T. 1990. Reishi Mushroom-herb of Spiritual Potency and Medical Wonder. Sylvan Press, Issaquah, Washington.

ZHANG, K., WU, X., XU, R. and ZHANG, T. 1994. Proceedings of The Third Asia-Pacific Biochemical Engineering Conference, Singapore, 1994, pp. 117–121.

PIGMENTAL IMPROVEMENT OF GREEN VEGETABLES BY CONTROLLING FREE RADICALS DURING HEAT DEHYDRATION

MIN ZHANG, XIAOLIN DING, ZHENGBIAO GU and CHUNLI LI

School of Food Science and Technology
Wuxi University of Light Industry
Wuxi 214036, P.R. China

ABSTRACT

Electron spin resonance (ESR) and chemiluminescent method (CLM) were used for establishing a relationship between the increase of free radical concentration produced by heat dehydration and respective changes of chlorophyll preservation ratio (K_b) during heat dehydration.The results show that the free radicals are the main reason for the K_b degradation. Kidney beans enriched with different selenium concentrations were chosen in the tests for controlling free radicals. The suitable selenium concentration of 0.45-1.30 μg Se/g was obtained.

INTRODUCTION

Traditional theories on free radicals mainly focus on their effect on the human body, so studies on the mechanism of senility and cancerology are available (Ni 1992). But in recent years, the research range of free radicals has been extended into many other fields. One of them is an area of improving the biochemical quality of food (Zhao 1992). The reasons for free radical formation in organisms generally depend on the stimulating factors of physics, chemistry and biochemistry (Zheng 1995). According to some reports, heat stimulation (physical factor) has been found to be responsible for free radicals in some processed plants, such as tea (Zhao *et al.* 1993).

Many measurements and analyses have shown that selenium (Se), especially organic Se, can be used to eliminate free radicals in some simulated organisms, as determined by electron spin resonance (ESR) (Wang 1991). But a biological system of vegetables during dehydration in our study is different from other simple systems because cells of the vegetables undergo a process from life to death.

The phenomenon of chemiluminescent method (CLM) appears when stimulated energies are released during the molecular transition from excited state to ground state (Hu and Ding 1996). So a process in which free radicals transit from excited state to ground state will surely create the phenomenon of CLM. In our study, ESR was used for calibrating the values of free radical concentration determined by CLM. The restraining effect on free radicals was studied by means of different Se concentrations.

MATERIALS AND METHODS

Procedures for ESR Measurement of Free Radicals

Three green vegetables (sweet pepper, kidney bean and Chinese onion), at maturity for processing, were obtained from the testing vegetable fields at Liyuan Township in

Wuxi City. Preliminary ESR measurements showed that using vegetable samples with high moisture (more than 85%, w.b.) did not give satisfactory peaks for calculating the concentration of free radicals. So a Consol 24 freeze dryer made in USA was used as the pre-dehydration device for acquiring the needed samples with lower moistures. Its vacuum pressure and temperature were regulated to 37.8 Pa and 25°C, respectively.

About 100 mg sliced sample after pre-dehydration was transferred to a 10 ml quartz tube carefully, then moved into the microwave cavity of the ESR device for measuring both h and A values in ESR signals. The Mn^{2+} calibrating method was used for measuring the g factor, which determines the source of the measured free radicals. Finally the concentration of free radicals were calculated by formula (1) (See below). Sample weight was determined on an analytical balance to an accuracy of 0.1 mg. A JES-FEIXG ESR device made in Japan was chosen for measuring the free radical parameters. The following parameters of the device were kept constant throughout the study: central magnetic field, 336 mT ±50 mT; modulation, 100 KHz; amplified times 10 × 100; frequency of microwave, 9.227 GHz.

Procedures for CLM Measurement

Chemiluminescent values of samples were measured by a SH6-1 Chemiluminescent Measuring System for organisms connected with a 386 personal computer. About 2.00 g pre-dehydrated samples were weighed and moved into a rectangular tube, then the reaction procedure was started automatically after the sample was put into the device. Time recording began in first 15 s. The preliminary test showed that most fresh vegetables contain some natural chemiluminescent materials which can greatly affect the measured index, while pre-dehydration can eliminate the phenomenon caused by these materials.

Heat Dehydration and Determination of Pigment

The chlorophyll content was generally used for appraisal of pigment in both green vegetables and their dehydrated products (Zhang and Ding 1996). So the chlorophyll preservation ratio (K_b) used in the study can be easily calculated by formula (2) (see below) (Central China College). Drying time was measured with a stopwatch. The heat dehydration was conducted by means of a blast heat dryer. Its controlling precision for temperature was ±1°C.

The Testing Indices

Concentration of free radical, n (spin/g), can be calculated by:

$$n=(N_0h_0/A_0)[A/(hm)] \tag{1}$$

where N_0 is spin number of the standard sample, A and A_0 are areas under the absorptive curves of the measured and standard samples, respectively, h and h_0 are signal strength of recording using stable inner calibration and measured samples with the standard sample, respectively, m is weight of the measured samples.

Chemiluminescent intensity of samples in the first 6 sec period from start, Cp_{6s}, was chosen as the testing index.

Total chlorophyll preservation ratio, K_b (%), can be determined by:

$$K_b = K_{y2}/K_{y1} \times a \times 100(\%) \qquad (2)$$

Where a is moisture conversion coefficient from the pre-dehydrated sample to the fresh, K_{y1} and K_{y2} are total chlorophyll contents of the fresh and the pre-dehydrated samples, respectively.

RESULTS AND ANALYSIS

Variation of Free Radical Concentration in Samples During Heat Dehydration

The heat drying temperatures at 70-100°C were set up according to the practical drying technology (Central China College 1980). The chemiluminescent intensity curves at four drying temperatures under different drying time are shown in Fig. 1. There is an obvious peak value at t=15-35 min in the curves of three higher temperatures (Fig.1b,c and d), while it is not clear at 40°C (Fig. 1a). A shorter drying time at the peak value of the drying temperature of 85 and 100°C is needed than under that of 70°C.

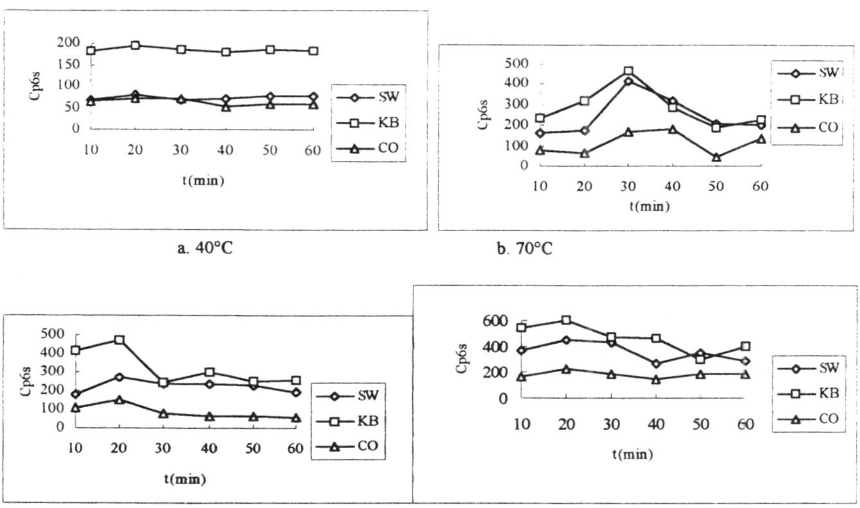

FIG. 1. THE CHEMILUMINESCENT STRENGTH CURVES AT FOUR DRYING TEMPERATURES UNDER DIFFERENT DRYING TIME MOISTURE CONTENT 47.7% w.b. (sweet pepper), 54.4% w.b. (kidney bean), 46.9% w.b. (Chinese onion); SW, sweet pepper; KB, kidney bean; CO, Chinese onion.

In order to observe whether or not the chemiluminescent phenomenon was caused by free radicals, a series of ESR tests on kidney bean at 70°C were made. Figure 2 shows that the concentration of free radicals (CFR) varies in the same way with the CL values shown in Fig.1b, which indicates CL values can be used as a tool for analyzing the CFR variation qualitatively.

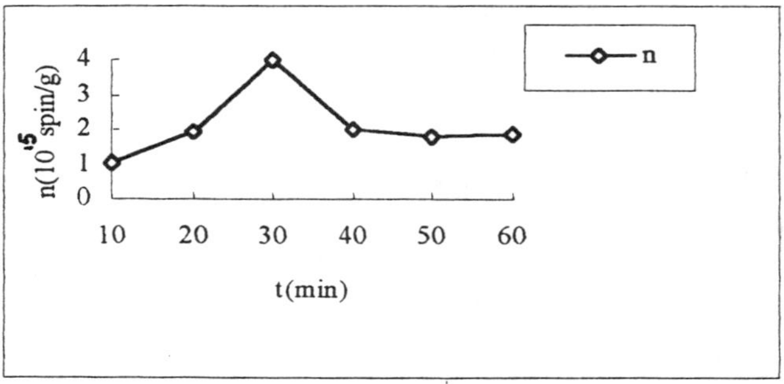

FIG. 2. THE CFR CHANGE OF KIDNEY BEAN UNDER DIFFERENT DRYING TIMES
CFR, concentration of free radicals

Since the g factor in the ESR spectrum is considered as the characteristic factor of molecules which include the non-paired electrons, the source of free radicals can be determined according to the peak signal of the spectrum (Zhao 1992). Zhao (1992) found that the organic free radicals added by the processing (in dried teas) have the same g values as ones in fresh teas, but the CFR varies obviously.

It was found that the g factor of dried kidney bean, between 2.0025~2.0028, is similar to that of the fresh-like tea. On the basis of the g value table with the biological meaning (Zhao 1992), the signals of the organic free radicals in the study belong to some material related with chlorophyll. Figure 1 also shows that the highest CL value, which represents the organic free radicals qualitatively, was for kidney bean, the middle one for sweet pepper, and the lowest one for Chinese onion. The measurement for chlorophyll contents of the three vegetables indicated that the higher the chlorophyll contents in the samples, the greater the CL values are relevantly, which also indicated the organic free radical in the study comes from materials related to chlorophyll.

Effect of Free Radical on Pigment in Kidney Bean

Some reports concluded that bruising of some fruits, such as apple, pear etc., can cause an increase of free radicals which speed up the browning process (Zhao *et al.* 1993). To observe the effect of three drying temperatures, which affect the free radicals greatly, on pigment of kidney bean, some experiments of K_b versus drying time have been made at the same conditions as in Fig. 1 and 2. The results are shown in Fig. 3. The greatest decreasing points of the three curves appear in the range of 15-35 min, which is consistent with the variation of CFR. Therefore, the free radicals in kidney bean are possibly responsible for the degradation of chlorophyll.

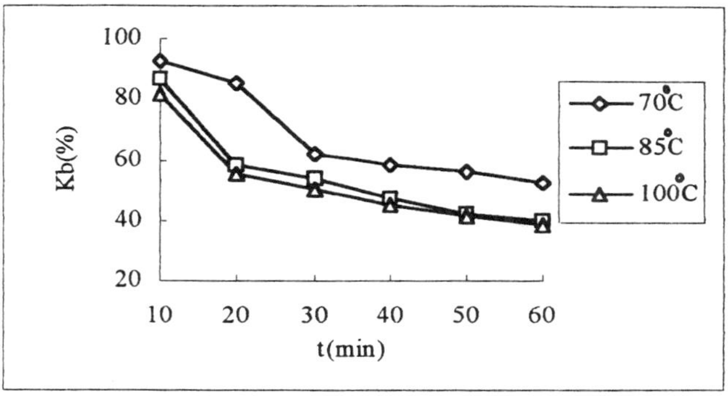

FIG. 3. THE K_b CHANGE OF KIDNEY BEAN UNDER DIFFERENT DRYING TIME

Effect of Selenium (Se) Content in Kidney Bean on Both CFR and Pigment

Many researchers reported that micro-Se can eliminate the free radicals in organisms (Zheng 1995; Wang 1991; Chen and Xu 1996). However, it still is not clear about the ability of eliminating free radicals in processed higher plants (such as vegetable) by Se, especially organic Se. At present, two main methods for improving the pigment in dehydrated green vegetables are to adjust the pH of blanching solution or to replace the magnesium by other metal ions, such as zinc (Zhang *et al.* 1991). However, the former method is often harmful to other quality aspects of dehydrated vegetables. The latter method is usually difficult to control in practice. For the sake of finding a new pigmental controlling resource for dehydrated green vegetables, the effect of different Se concentrations on CL value has been investigated. Figure 4 shows that the ability for eliminating free radicals mainly depends on the content of organic Se. Except for the concentration of 2.31 μgSe/g, the CL values, which represent the free radicals, decreased obviously with increase of the organic Se content. The conclusion that the high concentration (generally higher than 2.00 μgSe/g) led to increase of free radicals (Xue and Hou 1993) can explain the exception of concentration of 2.31 μgSe/g here. So the suitable enriching Se range for kidney bean is recommended to be between 0.45-1.30 μgSe/g. Three Se contents from this range were selected for dehydrating tests. The results of K_b after measurement are shown in Fig. 5. It seems that the rate of pigment degradation slows down at the drying time of 15-35 min at which the degradation rate of pigment reached the greatest in normal kidney bean.

CONCLUSIONS

1. The free radicals are possibly the main cause for pigmental change of kidney bean.
2. The CL values can be used as a tool for analyzing the CFR change qualitatively. The CL peak value means the greatest increasing speed of free radical formation.
3. Both drying temperature and drying time have great effect on peak values. The greatest affecting ranges for drying temperature and drying time are at t=15-35 min and 40-85°C, respectively.

4. The organic free radicals in the study come from materials related with chlorophyll.
5. For inhibition of free radicals and avoidance of pigmental degradation, the suitable enriching Se range in kidney bean is 0.45-1.30 μgSe/g.

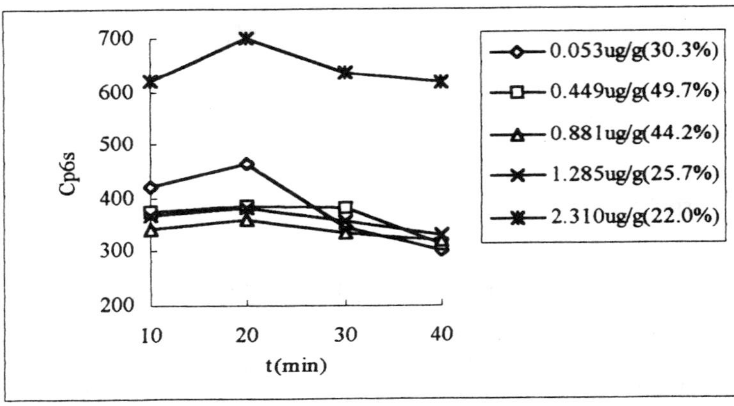

FIG. 4. THE Cp_{6s} VALUE CHANGE OF KIDNEY BEAN WITH FIVE SE CONCENTRATIONS UNDER DIFFERENT DRYING TIME (85°C)
*Total Se concentration and organic Se proportion, respectively, so it is in Fig. 5.

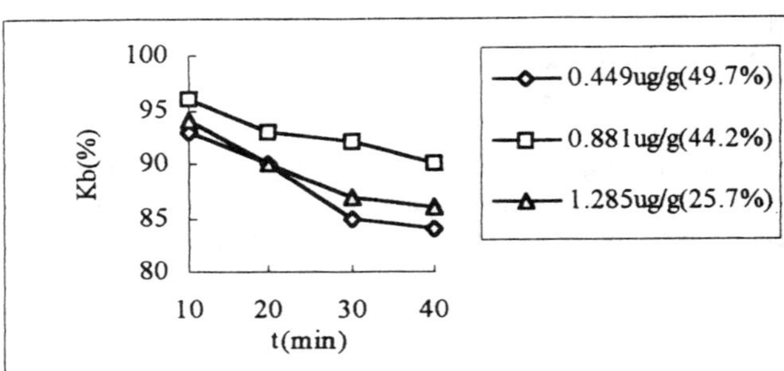

FIG. 5. THE K_b VALUES FOR KIDNEY BEAN WITH THREE SE CONCENTRATIONS

ACKNOWLEDGMENTS

The authors thank the International Foundation for Science (IFS) for financial support under contract No. E/2467-1 to Dr. Zhang Min.

REFERENCES

CENTRAL CHINA COLLEGE, 1980. Storage and Processing on Vegetables. Agricultural Press, Beijing, China.

CHEN, C.Y. and XU, H.B. 1996. Study on the relationship of concentration of selenium biological effect and oxygen free radical by chemical system. Acta Nutrimenta Sinica, *18*(1), 57.

HU, C. and DING, X.L. 1996. Research of the scavenging capacities of flavonoid on superoxide radical and hydroxy radical by chemiluminescent method. J. Wuxi Univ. Light Industry, *15*(3), 194.

NI, J.A. 1992. Relationship among selenium, free radicals and health. J. Wuxi Inst. Light Industry, *11*(3), 274.

WANG, L. 1991. Trace Elements in Life Science. Beijing, China Metrology Press, pp. 189–248.

XUE, T.L. and HOU, S.F. 1993. Anti-oxidation of Se in higher plants. Chinese Sci. Bull. *38*(4), 356.

ZHANG, M. and DING, X.L. 1996. Effects of pretreatments on the pigments of several dehydrated vegetables. J. Wuxi Univ. Light Industry, *15*(3), 205.

ZHANG, M. *et al.* 1991. A summary of pretreatment of vegetables before drying at home and abroad, Machinery for Agriculture, Animal Husbandry and Food Processing *3*, 53.

ZHAO, Z.H. 1992. Activated Intermediate During the Electron's Transfer in the Processed Tea and Their Positive Function in Formation and Regulation of the Tea Quality Involved. Ph.D. thesis, Zhejiang Agricultural University, Hangzhou, China.

ZHAO, Z.H. *et al.* 1993. Study of free radicals in natural foods. Proceedings First Chinese Postdoc. Researcher's Symp., Beijing, pp. 687–691.

ZHENG, J.X. 1995. Functional Foods. China Light Industry Press, Beijing, China.

APPLICATION OF ULTRASONICATION TO SPEED UP PROCESS OF SALTED DUCK EGG PRODUCTION

JIN-MING GUO, SHU-TAO LIU, YU-QIANG ZHENG, RONG-ZHEN ZHANG, JIAN-CAI LI, RU-MING CHEN, LONG LI, BI-HONG SHI, WEN-HONG GAO, GONG-RUI CHEN and PING-FAN RAO

Institute of Biotechnology
Fuzhou University
Fuzhou, Fujian, 350002, P.R. China

ABSTRACT

Salted duck egg is a traditional Chinese egg product. It is an effective way to preserve duck egg in which fresh shelled duck eggs are soaked in saturated salt brine at room temperature for about 25 days to obtain eggs with gelled yolks and salty egg white. It is very much favored by Chinese as a side dish with its gelled yolk which has a nice flavor and pleasant texture, and as a food decoration material with its gelled yolk's bright color.

In the first effort to elucidate traditional technology of egg salting, the NaCl concentration inside the shelled egg was determined by an ion meter with a chloride-ion electrode over the whole period of time of salting. An abrupt increase in salting speed was observed when the NaCl concentration of the egg white reached 1 M, corresponding exactly to the point where egg white viscosity decreased due to the increase of NaCl concentration. Importance of egg white viscosity to the salting process was thus understood, and ultrasonification treatment of whole egg before salting was tested as an alternative method of lowering the egg white viscosity. Minutes of ultrasonic treatment of duck egg prior to salting lowered the egg white viscosity to the point which takes more than 10 days for natural salting to occur. NaCl diffusion and osmosis was thus greatly enhanced, and yolk "elation was obtained in 10 days rather than about 25 days by the traditional method."

Ultrasonic treatment of egg prior to the salting not only greatly shortens the salting time but also remarkably lowers NaCl concentration in the final products. It is a very promising technology to reform the traditional egg salting industry.

INTRODUCTION

Salted duck egg is a traditional Chinese egg product. It is an effective way to preserve duck egg. There are many kinds of salted eggs in different parts of China according to the different ways of processing and seasoning, but the principal process remains basically the same, in which fresh whole duck eggs (in shell) are soaked in saturated salt brine at room temperature for about 25 days to obtain eggs with gelled yolks and salty egg whites. It is very much favored by Chinese as a side dish for its gelled yolk which has a nice flavor and pleasant texture, and as a food decoration material for the bright color of gelled yolk (Gao 1992).

The traditional procedure for salted egg production is very simple. This makes salted egg production an easy family business, but also primitive, leaving great room for modern technology to improve on quality control, production scale and efficiency. A few researchs have been done to investigate this traditional food, mostly focusing on the properties of salted eggs, and surprisingly, the production process in these days remains not much different from what it was at the very beginning. Apparently, a sound understanding of the salting process is the basis for further ideas to improve the traditional process. In this work, salt concentration changes were investigated over the whole process of salting, and factors influencing salting velocity were studied. On the basis of these results, the possibility of application of ultrasonication treatment to the salted egg processing was explored.

EXPERIMENTAL

Salting of Eggs

Fresh duck eggs were purchased from the market; salt was analytical grade NaCl. Intact eggs with similar size and shape were selected for the experiment. Eggs were washed and put into a container. Brine of 17.8% NaCl was poured into the container to cover the eggs, and a cover was used to prevent the eggs from floating to the surface. The eggs in brine were then incubated at 40°C.

Determination of NaCl Concentration

A calibration curve for chloride ion concentration was determined according to a reported method (Zhang *et al.* 1989) with a P^H S-3C ion meter (Shanghai, China). Two eggs were picked out of the brine, broken and egg white and egg yolk were carefully separated, and each homogenized by ultrasonication. Electric voltages of the both homogenized egg white and egg yolk were determined by the same method to determine the calibration curve. Chloride ion concentration was obtained from the calibration curve, and sodium chloride concentration was calculated accordingly.

Viscometric Determination

Viscometry was carried out on an NDJ-1 rotary viscometer (Shanghai, China) in a water incubator at 40°C. The rotor used was #0 and the speed was set to be 6 rpm.

Ultrasonication Treatment

Ultrasonication treatment of duck egg was carried out with a CQ-50 ultrasonication cleaner (Shanghai, China) with an output of 50 W and a fixed frequency of 33 KHz.

RESULTS AND DISCUSSION

Change of NaCl concentration in egg white with salting time is shown in curve A of Fig. 1. NaCl concentration increased smoothly until it reached about 2%, at about 12 days 1.6%, then the concentration continued to increase with salting time at much lower rate and eventually leveled off, illustrating the changing pattern in a more explicit manner.

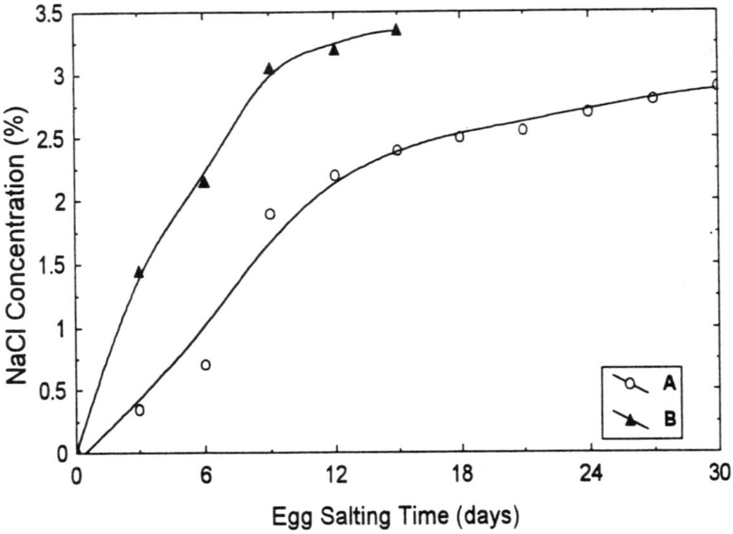

FIG. 1. COMPARISON OF EGG WHITE NACL CONCENTRATION CHANGE IN THE COURSE OF EGG SALTING OF DUCK EGGS WITHOUT (A) AND WITH (B) ULTRASONICATION TREATMENT

The egg salting process can be considered as diffusion of NaCl into the whole egg, hence diffusion velocity of NaCl at a point with a distance of X from the surface can be expressed with the following diffusion equation:

$$V = -D(dC/dX) \quad (1)$$

where D is the diffusion constant, dC/dX is the solute concentration gradient at X.

According to Equation (1), NaCl diffusion velocity can only become smaller and smaller since the NaCl concentration gradient can only monotonously decrease in the course of salting unless the diffusion constant D varies. The factors that determine D can be expressed by the following equation:

$$D = -RT/6\pi Nr\eta \quad (2)$$

where R is the gas constant, T is the absolute temperature, N is Avogadro constant, r is the diameter of the solute molecule, and η is the media viscosity. Apparently, the media viscosity η is the only factor in Equation (2) that is variable in the course of salting.

Influence of NaCl concentration on the egg white viscosity was investigated and the results are shown in Fig. 2. Increase of NaCl concentration in the egg white resulted in decrease of the egg white viscosity, which is a typical "salting in" phenomena of proteins (Wood *et al.* 1981). The viscosity decrease was drastic before the NaCl concentration increased to about 1.5%, and then became more modest. The turning point of the different patterns almost corresponds to that of the diffusion velocity. It can be concluded that the increase of NaCl diffusion velocity was due to the egg white viscosity decrease, which was so drastic that the effect of decrease of NaCl concentration gradient was offset. When η decrease became less dramatic, the effect of narrowing difference in NaCl concentrations of the salting brine and the egg white led to the decrease of NaCl diffusion velocity.

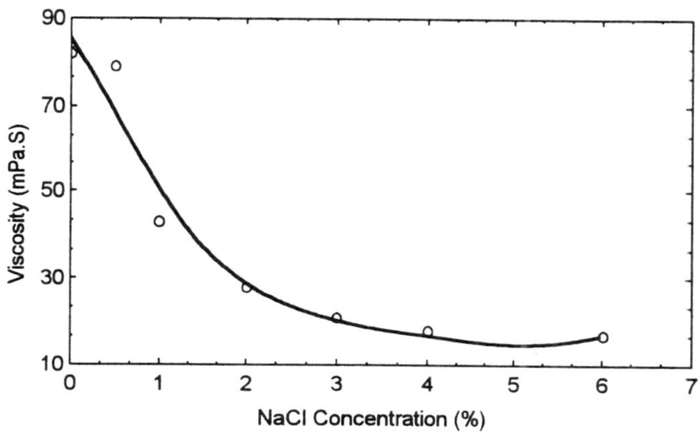

FIG. 2. EFFECT OF NACL CONCENTRATION ON EGG WHITE VISCOSITY (η)

It is the decreased egg white viscosity because of natural diffusion of NaCl that in turn greatly enhanced the diffusion velocity of NaCl in the egg white, hence accelerated the salting process. Salting in of proteins, however, is not the only possible method to thin the egg white. Ultrasonication can be a very useful process to homogenize a system or to lower the viscosity of a system. Primitive pre-salting treatment of duck eggs by ultrasonication has shown encouraging results.

Fresh and intact duck eggs soaked in distilled water were subjected to 10 min ultrasonication treatment. Effect of ultrasonication treatment time on the egg white viscosity is shown in Fig. 3. With 10 min treatment by ultrasonication egg white viscosity was only 0.02 Pa.S, corresponding to the final egg white viscosity, which required almost 20 days to achieve by the natural "salting in" process.

As shown in curves A and B in Fig. 1, NaCl diffusion and osmosis in egg white were much faster with sonification than the untreated egg. Egg yolk gelation of sonification-treated eggs was completed in just 12 days in comparison with 20 days for the untreated eggs. The processing time was shortened by 40%, implying improvement of this ultrasonication processing in the egg salting industry.

When duck eggs were subjected to ultrasonication in the salting brine for an extensive period of time, yolk gelation was not accelerated but totally inhibited. In salted eggs, yolk forms gel because of de-emulsification due to the increase of NaCl in the yolk. Ultrasonication treatment, however, effectively enhances emulsification. Therefore, it is concluded that ultrasonication should be only applied to the eggs before the salting process for a limited period of time. Further investigation on the influence of the frequency and intensity of the treatment needs to be carried out.

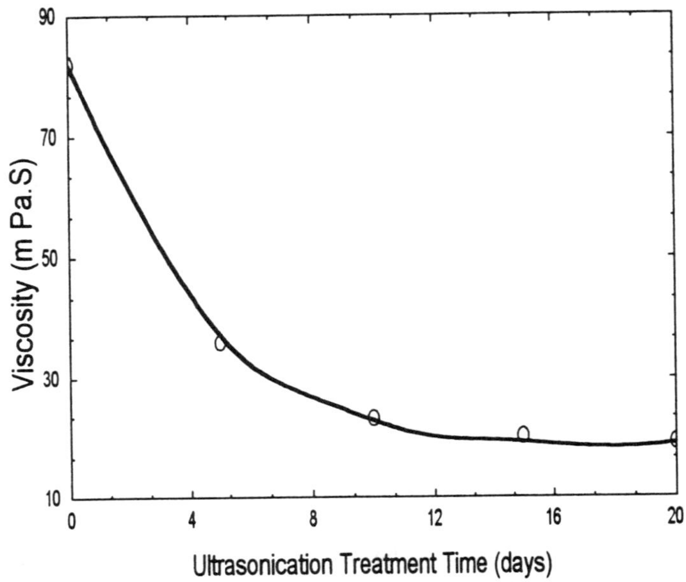

FIG. 3. EFFECT OF ULTRASONICATION TREATMENT TIME ON EGG WHITE VISCOSITY

SUMMARY

Egg white viscosity was found to be the most important factor determining the salting process, and ultrasonication treatment of whole egg before salting was found to be an effective alternative method of lowering the egg white viscosity. Ten minutes of ultrasonic treatment of duck egg prior to salting lowered the egg white viscosity to the point which takes more than 12 days for natural salting to reach NaCl diffusion and osmosis were thus greatly enhanced, and yolk gelation was obtained in 12 days rather than about 20 days by the traditional method. Ultrasonic treatment of egg prior to the salting shortens the salting. It is a very promising technology to reform the traditional egg salting industry.

REFERENCES

GAO, Z. 1992. Egg Product Technology. Commercial Publication Company, Beijing, P. R. China.

WOOD, W.B., WILSON, J.H., BENBOW, R.M. and HOOD, L.E. 1981. Biochemistry: A Problem Approach. Second Edition, The Benjamin/Cummings Publishing Company, California, USA.

ZHANG, J.-X., ZHOU Y.-L. and FANG, X.-H. 1989. Experiments in Analytical Chemistry. Publication Company of Chemical Engineering College in East of China, Shanghai, P. R. China.

AN IMPROVED METHOD OF CHOLESTEROL DETERMINATION IN EGG YOLK BY HPLC

RONG-ZHEN ZHANG, LONG LI, JIAN-CAI LI, SHU-TAO LIU,
RU-MING CHEN, BI-HONG SHI, WEN-HONG GAO, GONG-RUI CHEN,
YU-QIANG ZHENG and PING-FAN RAO

Institute of Biotechnology, Fuzhou University
523 Gong-ye Road, Fuzhou, Fujian, 350002
P.R. China

ABSTRACT

An improved method for cholesterol determination in egg yolk is reported in this paper. Egg yolk was first diluted. Cholesterol was then extracted with ether and petroleum ether, and quantified by reverse phase chromatography on a Zorbax ODS column (0.46 × 15 cm, 5-6 um) using a mobile phase of acetonitrile and 2-propanol (4:1) with a flow rate of 0.6 mL/min. A linear correlation was observed between 0.05-0.40 mg/mL of cholesterol and its peak heights. The determination limit was 0.02 mg/mL. No difference in final results was observed between egg yolk sample with saponification and a sample without saponification. Rapid and reproducible quantification of cholesterol in egg yolk can be obtained with this new method.

INTRODUCTION

Elucidation of the physiological role of cholesteryl esters in genesis of atherosclerosis has resulted in great interest in cholesterol distribution among different foods, and in factors that determine cholesterol concentration. This has led to numerous attempts to develop rapid, accurate and convenient methods for determination of cholesterol.

Egg is one of the most complete foods in nature in terms of nutrition. High cholesterol content in the yolk has, however, caused great concern. The average cholesterol value reported by the USDA Marketing Service is 213 mg per large egg (USDA 1989). There are reported egg yolk cholesterol values varying from 9.21 to 22.8 mg/g of yolk (Cunningham *et al.* 1974; Nix *et al.* 1974; Washburm and Nix 1974; Bar and Marion 1978; Ingr and Simeonova 1983). Enormous efforts have been made to reduce cholesterol levels in foods, requiring a simple, rapid and reproducible method for cholesterol determination.

Various kinds of methods are available for cholesterol determination in foods, including spectrophotometry (Abell *et al.* 1952; Folch *et al.* 1957; Bachman *et al.* 1976; Bohac *et al.* 1988), gas-liquid chromatography (Punwar 1975; Beyer *et al.* 1989; Tsui 1989), high performance liquid chromatography (Newkirk and Sheppard 1981; Carroll and Rudel 1981; Hurst *et al.* 1984; Kou and Holmes 1985; Indyk 1990; Bocos *et al.* 1992; Casiraghi *et al.* 1994) and others (Allain *et al.* 1974; Papastathopoulos and Rechnitz 1975; Shen *et al.* 1982; Contreras *et al.* 1992; Crockett *et al.* 1995). Due to the water-insolubility of cholesterol, its determination is always complicated by the co-existing lipids. Consequently, all reported procedures inevitably include a saponification-extraction step, a multistage solvent extraction followed by purification and concentration. Sample saponification, in particular, is a major cause of operational inconvenience and error.

The objective of the present study was to develop an assay method for cholesterol determination in chicken egg yolk by high performance chromatography without sample pretreatment such as saponification.

MATERIALS AND METHODS

Preparation of Egg Yolk Cholesterol Sample

Approximately 2.00 g of egg yolk separated from the albumin were accurately weighed and diluted to 20 ml with distilled water, then mixed thoroughly. One (1.0) ml of the diluted egg yolk was accurately added into a 15 ml stoppered test-tube, then 1.0 ml of 95% ethanol was added to the sample, and the test-tube was vigorously shaken to prevent aggregation. Ether (2.5 ml) was added to the sample and mixed. Petroleum ether (2.5 ml) was added and the mixture shook adequately. After 30 min, 1.0 ml of the organic phase was accurately measured into an Eppendof tube (1.5 ml) and evaporated to dryness (<45°C). The residue was dissolved in 0.5 ml of ethanol, and 0.010 ml of the solution was applied to a HPLC system.

Saponified samples were also prepared in order to determine the difference in the final results of the samples with different pretreatments. One (1.0) ml of the diluted egg yolk was accurately added directly into a 25 ml test-tube with a stopper. Three (3.0) ml of 95% ethanol was added to the sample and the test tube was vigorously shaken to prevent aggregation. Saponification of the sample was carried out according to Sim and Bragg (1977) by adding 2.0 ml of 50% potassium hydroxide solution immediately to the test tube, and the loosely capped tube was incubated for 60 min at 50°C. During incubation, periodic agitation was done to ensure efficient digestion of lipid. Following cooling, extraction solvent (5.0 ml of hexane) was added and the tubes were stoppered securely and shaken mechanically for 5 min. Distilled water (3.0 ml) was added and the tube was capped and shaken ten times and centrifuged at 1000 × g for 10 min. Then 1.0 ml of the organic phase was accurately removed into an Eppendof tube (1.5 ml) and evaporated to dryness (<45°C). The residue was dissolved in 0.5 ml of ethanol and 0.010 mL of the solution was applied to an HPLC system.

Calibration of Cholesterol Concentration

Cholesterol was purchased from Sigma (St. Louis, MO, USA). All solvents used were HPLC grade or analytical grade purchased from Biological Science and Technology of Shanghai Co. Ltd. (Shanghai, China).

Cholesterol was dissolved in ethanol (1 mg cholesterol /ml) and stored at 20°C as stock standard solution. A series of working standards were obtained by diluting the stock standard solution in the same medium to obtain values ranging from 0, 0.05, 0.10, 0.15, 0.20, 0.25, 0.30, 0.35 to 0.40 mg cholesterol /ml.

HPLC

HPLC analysis was carried out at ambient temperature with a TSK Model CCPD high-speed liquid chromatograph (Tosoh Co. Ltd., Toyo, Japan) using a Zorbax ODS column (0.45 × 15 cm; Dupont Instruments, Wilmington, DE). The eluate was monitored by a TSK Model UV-8000 detector (Tosoh Co. Ltd., Toyo, Japan). The mobile phase was an isocratic mixture of acetonitrile and 2-propanol (3:1) and the flow rate was 0.60 ml/min. Injection volume was 0.010 mL of sample. The eluate was monitored at 208 nm with a Tosoh UV-8000 monitor (Tokyo, Japan).

Cholesterol content of the egg yolk sample could be determined easily by comparing the cholesterol peak height on the chromatograms of the sample with that of the standard cholesterol solution.

Cholesterol Determination by Colorimetry

Egg yolk cholesterol was also determined by colorimetry according to the methods of Abell *et al.* (1952) and Folch *et al.* (1957). Samples of egg yolks were subjected to alcoholic KOH saponification and hexane extraction prior to color reaction with Liebermann-Burchard reagent.

Statistical Analysis

A one-way ANOVA was used to analyze the effect of cholesterol assay methods on egg cholesterol values. Assay methods were the main effects, with the mean square of method by replication as the error term. Duncan's multiple range test (Steel and Torrie 1980) was used to differentiate treatment means.

RESULTS AND DISCUSSION

Calibration of Cholesterol Standard

The reverse phase chromatogram of the cholesterol standard is shown in Fig. 1. The retention time for cholesterol was 19 min. Figure 2 shows the calibration curve of cholesterol concentration against its peak height. Perfect linearity was maintained in a cholesterol concentration range from 0 to 0.40 mg/ml, indicating that no interaction occurred between cholesterol and the column matrix.

Determination of Cholesterol Content in Egg Yolk

Figure 3(A) is the chromatogram for the yolk samples by direct extraction, and Fig. 3(B) for the yolk samples by saponification prior to extraction. In both chromatograms, cholesterol was eluted at the same retention time, indicating saponification resulted in no influence on the cholesterol. Small peaks can be observed in the chromatograms of the direct extraction sample, but disappeared in the chromatograms of the saponification sample together with a large fraction at the beginning. Since egg yolk lipids were completely separated from the cholesterol as is shown in Fig. 3(A), there is no worry that those lipids interfere with cholesterol quantification. As a matter of fact, cholesterol peaks on both chromatograms are basically of similar heights, indicating no serious discrepancy between egg yolk extraction samples with and without saponification. It is clear that with the set of chromatographic conditions adopted in this study, saponification is not a necessary step to obtain reliable results.

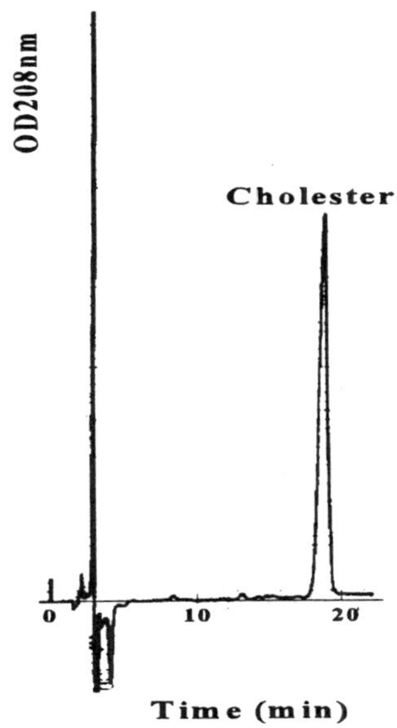

FIG. 1. HPLC SEPARATION OF STANDARD CHOLESTEROL
Conditions: column, Zorbax ODS (0.46 × 15 cm, 5-6 μm); mobile phase, acetonitrile: 2-propanol (V:V = 4:1); flow rate, 0.6 mL/min; detector, UV-208 nm; injection volume, 0.010 mL.

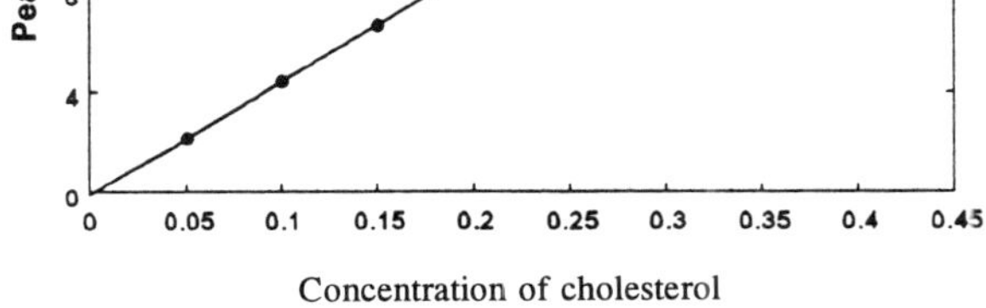

FIG. 2. THE CALIBRATION GRAPH OF CHOLESTEROL

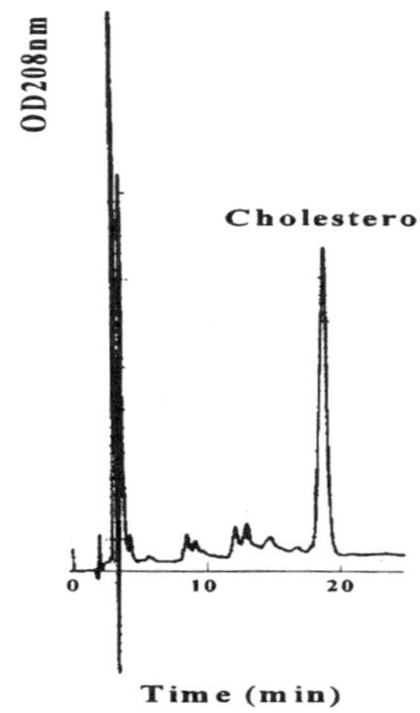

FIG. 3(A). HPLC SEPARATION OF SAMPLE OF DIRECTLY EXTRACTION
Conditions: column, Zorbax ODS (0.46 × 15 cm, 5-6 μm); mobile phase, acetonitrile: 2-propanol (V:V = 4:1); flow rate, 0.6 mL/min; detector, UV-208 nm; injection volume, 0.010 mL.

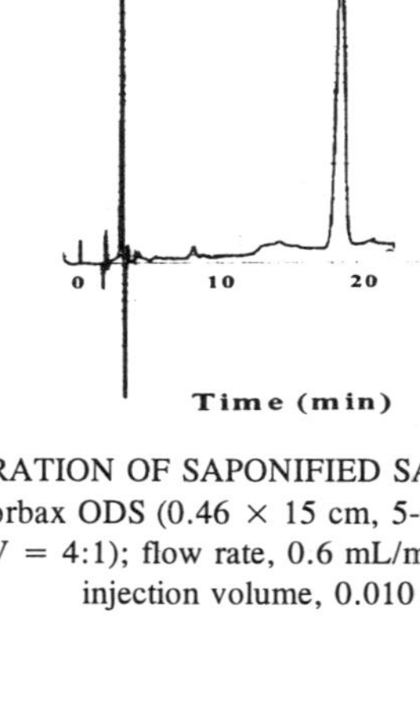

FIG. 3(B). HPLC SEPARATION OF SAPONIFIED SAMPLE PRIOR TO EXTRACTION
Conditions: column, Zorbax ODS (0.46 × 15 cm, 5-6 μm); mobile phase, acetonitrile: 2-propanol (V:V = 4:1); flow rate, 0.6 mL/min; detector, UV-208 nm; injection volume, 0.010 mL.

Listed in Table 1 are results of cholesterol determination of yolk samples pretreated with or without saponification prior to extraction, and by different methods of colorimetry and HPLC (8 replicates). Cholesterol content is expressed as either milligrams per gram of yolk or milligrams per egg. As shown in Table 1, cholesterol values of chicken eggs determined by both colorimetry and HPLC methods agreed with the reported values (9.21 to 22.8 mg/g of yolk).

TABLE 1.
EGG CHOLESTEROL VALUES DETERMINED BY COLORIMETRIC AND HPLC METHODS

Sample	Cholesterol Values[1](n=8)					
			HPLC			
	Colorimetric		Sample of saponification prior to extraction		Sample of directly extraction	
	mg/g yolk	mg/egg	mg/g yolk	mg/egg	mg/g yolk	mg/egg
A (yolk weight =13.70g)	16.16 ±0.26[a]	221.38 ±3.60[a]	15.18 ±0.51[a]	207.93 ±6.98[a]	15.27 ±0.25[a]	209.20 ±3.49[a]
B (yolk weight =13.97g)	12.22 ±0.29[b]	170.71 ±4.01[b]	10.86 ±0.23[b]	151.75 ±3.27[b]	10.94 ±0.34[b]	152.76 ±4.72[b]
C (yolk weight =15.54g)	11.21 ±0.37[b]	171.41 ±5.77[b]	9.57 ±0.35[b]	148.72 ±5.50[b]	9.77 ±0.25[b]	151.79 ±3.88[b]

n = replicates.
a,b Means within the same column with no common superscripts are significantly different ($P < 0.01$).
1, $\bar{x} \pm SD$.

Because of strong interference by co-existing lipids such as triglycerides, which can also be extracted into organic agents, it is impossible to determine egg yolk cholesterol content without saponification of the yolk samples prior to extraction. But even with the same yolk extraction sample with saponification, egg yolk cholesterol content values obtained colorimetrically are still significantly higher ($P < 0.01$) than that by the HPLC method (8 replicates), as shown in Table 1. This result agrees with reported data (Jiang *et al.* 1991), and can be explained by Fig. 3(B). While most fractions other than cholesterol in Fig. 3(A) disappear as the result of saponification, some fractions still chromatograph from the egg yolk hexane extract with saponification prior to extraction;

some remained even after saponification. When those fractions react with the coloring agent in colorimetry, overestimation occurs. Apparently, cholesterol determination by HPLC without saponification is a more reliable method than colorimetric determination with or without saponification.

From Table 1, it is clear that excellent precision and reproducibility can be expected by HPLC determination of cholesterol of yolk samples with or without saponification prior to extraction (8 replicates). Although cholesterol values of yolk samples of direct extraction were slightly higher than those of yolk samples after saponification prior to extraction, the differences were not significant, as is indicated by Fig. 3.

CONCLUSION

This proposed method of HPLC determination of cholesterol in egg yolk without saponification is superior to colorimetric determination on the sample with saponification, and comparable to HPLC determination with saponification of the yolk sample in terms of reliability. Omission of saponification has made this proposed method more convenient than those previously reported, and it can be used in yolk cholesterol studies with greater ease.

REFERENCE

ABELL, L.L., LEVY, B.B., BRODIE, B.B. and KENDALL, F.E. 1952. A simple method for the estimation of total cholesterol in serum and demonstration of its specificity. J. Biol. Chem. *195*, 357–366.

ALLAIN, C.C., POON, L.S., CHAN, C.S.G., RICHMOND, W. and FU, P.C. 1974. Enzymatic determination of total serum cholesterol. Clin. Chem. *20*, 470–475.

BACHMAN, K.C., LIN, J.H. and WILCOX, C.J. 1976. Sensitive colorimetric determination of cholesterol in dairy products. J. Assoc. Off. Anal. Chem. *59*, 1146–1149.

BAR, C.W. and MARION, W.W. 1978. Yolk cholesterol in eggs from avian species. Poultry Sci. *57*, 1260–1265.

BEYER, J.D., MILANI, F.X., DUTELLE, M.J. and BRADLEY, R.L. JR. 1989. Gas chromatographic determination of cholesterol in egg product. J. Assoc. Off. Anal. Chem. *72 (5),* 746–748.

BOCOS, C., CASTRO, M., OROZCO, E., CONTRESRAS, J.A. and HERRERA, E. 1992. A rapid and sensitive method for HPLC cholesterol determination in bile. Rev. Eps. Fisiol. *48 (3),* 211–214.

BOHAC, C.E., RHEE, K.S., CROSS, H.R. and ONO, K. 1988. Assessment of methodologies for colorimetric cholesterol assay of meats. J. Food Sci. *53,* 1642–1644.

CARROLL, R.M. and RUDEL, L.L. 1981. Evaluation of a high performance liquid chromatography method of isolation and quantitation of cholesterol and cholesteryl esters. J. Lipid Res. *22,* 359–363.

CASIRAGHI, E., LUCISANO, M., POMPE, C. and DELLEAL, C. 1994. Cholesterol determination in buffer by high performance liquid chromatography. Milchwissenschaft *49(4),* 194–196.

CONTRERAS, J.A., CASTRO, M., BOCOS, C., HERRERA, E. and LASUNCION, M.A. 1992. Combination of an enzymatic method and HPLC for the quantitation of cholesterol in cultured cells. J. Lipid Res. *33*, 931–936.

CROCKETT, E.L. and HAZEL, J.R. 1995. Sensitive assay for cholesterol in biological membranes reveals membrane-specific differences in kinetics of cholesterol oxidase. J. Exp. Zool. *271 (3),* 190–195.

CUNNINGHAM, D.L., KRUEGER, W.F., FANGUY, R.C. and BRADLEY, J.W. 1974. Preliminary results of bidirectional selection for yolk cholesterol level in laying hens. Poultry Sci. *53*, 384–391.

FOLCH J., LEES, M. and SLOANE STANLEY, G.H. 1957. A simplified method for the isolation and purification of total lipids from animal tissues. J. Biol. Chem. *226*, 497–509.

HURST, W.J., ALEO, M.D. and MARTIN, R.A. 1984. Nonaqueous reverse phase liquid chromatographic analysis for cholesterol in milk chocolate. J. Assoc. Off. Anal. Chem. *67,* 698–700.

INDYK, H.E. 1990. Simultaneous liquid chromatographic determination of cholesterol, phytosterols and tocopherols in foods. Analyst. *115,* 1525–1530.

INGR, I. and SIMEONOVA, J. 1983. A rapid determination of cholesterol in egg yolks using the Bio-La-Test. Vet. Med. (Praha) *28,* 97–104.

JIANG, Z.R., FENTON, M. and SIM, J.S. 1991. Comparison of four different methods for egg cholesterol determination. Poultry Sci. *70,* 1015–1019.

KOU, I.L. and HOLMES, R.P. 1985. The analysis of 25-hydroxycholesterol in plasma and cholesterol-containing foods by high-performance liquid chromatography. J. Chromatogr. *330*, 339–346.

NEWKIRK, D.R. and SHEPPARD, A.J. 1981. High pressure liquid chromatographic determination of cholesterol in foods. J. Assoc. Off. Anal. Chem. *64,* 1344–1346.

NIX, D.F., THORNTON, E.J., WASHBURN, K.W. and MARKS, H.L. 1974. The influence of molting on yolk cholesterol level. Poultry Sci. *53*, 412–414.

PAPASTATHOPOULOS, D.S. and RECHNITZ, G.A. 1975. Enzymatic cholesterol determination using ion-selective membrane electrodes. J. Assoc. Off. Anal. Chem. *47*, 1792–1796.

PUNWAR, J.K. 1975. Gas-liquid chromatographic determination of total cholesterol in multicomponent foods. J. Assoc. Off. Anal. Chem. *58 (4)*, 804–810.

SHEN, C.S., CHEN, I.S. and SHEPPARD, A.J. 1982. Enzymatic determination of cholesterol in egg yolk. J. Assoc. Off. Anal. Chem. *65 (5)*, 1222–1224.

SIM, J.S. and BRAGG, D.B. 1977. Effect of dietary factors on serum and egg yolk cholesterol levels of laying hens. Poultry Sci. *56*, 1616–1621.

STEEL, R.G.D. and TORRIE, J.H. 1980. Principles and Procedures of Statistics: A Biometrical Approach. *2nd ed.* McGraw-Hill, New York, NY.

TSUI, I.C. 1989. Rapid determination of total cholesterol in homogenized milk. J. Assoc. Off. Anal. Chem. *72 (3),* 421–424.

USDA. 1989. Composition of foods, dairy and egg products, raw-processed-prepared. USDA Agriculture Handbook 8-1. USDA, Washington, DC.

WASHBURM, K.W. and NIX, D.F. 1974. Genetic basis of yolk cholesterol content. Poultry Sci. *53*, 109–115.

PURIFICATION OF PEROXIDASE FROM FROZEN VEGETABLE PLANT WASTES AND REGIONAL VEGETABLES USING REVERSE MICELLES

OFELIA PÉREZ ARVIZU, BLANCA E. GARCÍA and CARLOS REGALADO

Dept. of Food Research and Postgraduate Studies
Universidad Autónoma de Querétaro
Querétaro, 76010 Qro., México

ABSTRACT

Peroxidase is widely used in kits for clinical analyses, and as a marker for enzyme immunoassays. Its world annual production [30 × 10^9 ABTS {2,2′-azino-di-(3-ethyl-benzthiazoline-6-sulfonic acid}units] indicates a good market potential. Therefore, it is important to look for peroxidase alternative sources and methods of purification. Reverse micelles are thermodynamically stable w/o dispersions containing spheroidal aggregates stabilized by a surfactant. They can be economically used as a liquid extraction technology for bioseparations, with a potential for continuous operation. México exported in 1995 more than 10^4 tons of frozen vegetables; however, at least 10% of this production is waste. A higher added value of these wastes was sought as well as an alternative source of peroxidase from vegetables grown in the Bajío region, using reverse micelles of the anionic surfactant aerosol-OT in isooctane.

Crude extracts from 8 Brassicaceae *vegetables (turnip, broccoli, etc.) were assessed for protein content (Bradford), while the chromogen ABTS was used to assay peroxidase activity. Reverse micelles were used in a two step process on the dialyzed extracts. The first step reduced contaminant protein (pH 4.5), while peroxidase isoenzymes were selectively extracted in the second stage (pH 3.2). Purity and isoelectric points of peroxidases were conducted using SDS-PAGE and IEF.*

Crude extract activities ranged from 1.8 (cauliflower) to 15 (turnip) ABTS units (U)/g of fresh material. After the two step purification process, turnip purification factor was 5.3 (308 U/mg protein), but yield was low (20%). This was attributed to the small pH difference (and hence electrostatic interaction) between the main isoenzyme pI (6.9) and the pH values (3.5-5.0) used for extraction. Broccoli (major waste) showed three main isoenzymes (pI's: > 9.3, 9.3, 6.9), with good activity (39.0 U/mg) and better extraction yields (60%). It is concluded that broccoli may be an inexpensive source of this enzyme and further work is under way to optimize the process.

INTRODUCTION

The impressive advances in genetic engineering have made it possible to produce proteins important for research, pharmaceutical and industrial purposes. However, the technology for separating and purifying proteins has not advanced at the same pace. It has been estimated that up to 90% of new product costs are attributable to downstream processing (Sadana and Raju 1990). Generally protein purification techniques should be simple, easily scalable, continuous, low cost and should not inactivate the protein. Liquid-liquid extraction using reverse micelles may well be adapted, with economic advantage, to the purification of biopolymers at early stages of purification (Asenjo and Patrick 1990). The relative simplicity of the process involved and the low cost of the solvent/surfactant system provide fewer drawbacks than many other processes, especially if high aqueous:organic volume phase ratios are used (Rahaman *et al.* 1988).

Reverse micelles are thermodynamically stable, optically transparent, isotropic dispersions of water in oil (w/o) stabilized by a surfactant. Surfactants that may be used to produce reverse micelles can be charged (anionic, cationic and zwitter-ionic) or uncharged (non-ionic). Hydrophilic molecules can be solubilized in the aqueous core of reverse micelles, with little or no damage to their biological activity. In the phase transfer method an aqueous phase containing the protein of interest is contacted with a reverse micellar organic phase, and under proper conditions a protein may selectively partition to the organic phase. Electrostatic interactions have been identified as the main driving force towards equilibrium. However, hydrophobic interactions have also been shown to be one of the factors responsible for solubilization of hydrophobic amino acids and proteins, probably in the surfactant shell of the reverse micelles. The anionic surfactant AOT {aerosol-OT [sodium bis(2-ethyl-hexyl) sulfosuccinate]} is very efficient in reducing the interfacial free energy (Eicke and Kvita 1984), shows a good water solubilization capacity, and can be obtained in high purities (Adachi and Harada 1994). Thus, AOT has been widely used for solubilization of proteins with relatively high isoelectric points (pI > 6). When the protein's pI is low, a cationic surfactant [e.g. CTAB (hexadecyl trimethyl ammonium bromide)] can be used for solubilization into a reverse micellar phase. Castro and Cabral (1988) provide examples of systems (surfactant, cosurfactant, solvent) forming reverse micelles.

The size of the aqueous core of reverse micelle aggregates, which ranges from 1 to about 10 nm, is approximately proportional to the Wo (molar ratio of water to surfactant) values, as checked by small angle neutron scattering (SANS) (Robinson *et al.* 1984). The size of AOT reverse micelles in equilibrium with a bulk aqueous phase is a strong function of both cation concentration and type, while for CTAB the aggregate's size depends on anion concentration and type. The main factors affecting protein solubilization are pH, ionic strength, types of solvent and surfactant, temperature and the presence of ligands (Goklen and Hatton 1987). Matzke *et al.* (1992) have shown that surfactant concentration affects protein extraction capacity, but not the size of reverse micelles. Ionic surfactants can generally solubilize globular proteins up to a size equivalent to 100 kDa (Krei and Hustedt 1992).

Peroxidase is a glycoprotein which has a heme prosthetic group, catalyzes redox reactions and is ubiquitous in the plant and animal kingdoms, the richest source being horseradish root. As many as 40 isoenzymes have been reported from crude preparations. This is because of slightly different carbohydrate compositions which are normally added to the enzyme by post-translational modifications. Plant peroxidases play an active role in lignin synthesis and plant hormone metabolism, and could be part of a first line of plant defense. Although peroxidase isoenzymes appear to catalyze the same reaction, individual isoenzymes differ markedly in physicochemical properties, amino acid composition and catalytic properties (Dunford 1991). Peroxidase is used to produce test kits for the determination of glucose, cholesterol, etc., and is probably the most popular of the enzymes used as a label for immunoassays and immunohistochemistry.

Most of the frozen vegetable products, such as broccoli, cauliflower, etc., which are exported by Mexico come from the central part of the country known as "El Bajío".

This work has been carried out to purify peroxidase from different plant materials common in this area, as well as to determine the feasibility of obtaining this enzyme from the huge amount of waste vegetables (which for broccoli is calculated as 20% of the 7,200 tons exported in 1990) produced by the frozen food companies. There are no reports of peroxidase characterization from these vegetables, and work conducted for that purpose is reported here. Here we also compare the yield by traditional peroxidase purification methods with the liquid-liquid extraction method of reverse micelles.

MATERIALS AND METHODS

Materials

The vegetables tested were purchased fresh from the local market and kept in the cold room before use. AOT (99%), analytical grade *n*-pentanol, DEAE-cellulose, Sephadex G-100, concanavalin A-Sepharose affinity resin, 12 kDa molecular weight cut off dialysis membranes, and isooctane (99%) were purchased from Sigma. CTAB (>99 %) was purchased from Fluka. De-ionized water (Milli-Q) was used to prepare all aqueous solutions. All other reagents used were of analytical grade and obtained from commercial suppliers.

Methods

Crude extracts of 8 vegetables (turnip, broccoli, radish, Brussels sprouts, pineapple, cauliflower, spinach, cabbage, watercress) were obtained by homogenizing, keeping a constant extractant:tissue ratio in all cases, at 4°C using a laboratory blender and separating the insoluble material by centrifuging 15 min at 10,000 rpm (4°C). Protein was determined according to the BCA method (Smith *et al.* 1985), while activity was tested using ABTS as the chromogen, reading the absorbance of the oxidation products at 414 nm (Childs and Bardsley 1975). The amount of substrate (mg) consumed per min was defined as an activity unit (U). A screening test was conducted to select the materials having a compromise between high peroxidase activity and availability.

Ammonium sulfate was used to precipitate the protein, followed by dialysis at 4°C for 48 h. Cold acetone (-20°C) was used to further purify peroxidase, using two stages: one volume acetone to one volume enzyme solution was used in the first followed by centrifugation, while the supernatant was mixed with three volumes of acetone in the second stage. The solution was centrifuged and the precipitate was dialyzed against a 50 mM Tris-HCl buffer, pH 7.0.

The extract was subjected to anion-exchange chromatography at pH 7.0, using a linear gradient of 0.5 M NaCl. A Bio-Rad fraction collector was used to separate fractions of 4 mL, and those having peroxidase activity were pooled and subjected to affinity chromatography (concanavalin A-Sepharose), using mannose as eluent to recover the separated glycoproteins. Finally, the extract was passed through a Sephadex G-100 gel filtration column equilibrated with Tris-HCl buffer, pH 7.0.

The final extract was subjected to molecular weight determination under denaturing (SDS-PAGE) and non-denaturing (native-PAGE) electrophoresis (Gersten 1996) using a

Hoeffer Mini Protean vertical chamber, while the isoelectric point was measured using the Phast-System (Pharmacia).

Reverse Micelles

Two ionic surfactants were tested to extract peroxidase using reverse micelles. When AOT (0.1 M) in isooctane was used, the dialyzed extract was contacted using a two step reverse micellar extraction process (Fig. 1) as depicted by Regalado *et al.* (1996) for horseradish peroxidase extraction. CTAB (0.2 M) reverse micelles in isooctane/*n*-pentanol (95:5) were used for peroxidase extraction at higher pH (7 to 11), at varying ionic strength (0.1 to 0.6 M KCl). Forward and backward transfer for both surfactants were conducted using equal volumes of aqueous and organic phases in a well stirred vessel for 5 and 10 min, respectively, at room temperature, and the phases were separated by centrifugation at 2000 rpm for 2 min. A 2 M KCl solution, pH 4.0, was used for peroxidase re-extraction from CTAB reverse micelles.

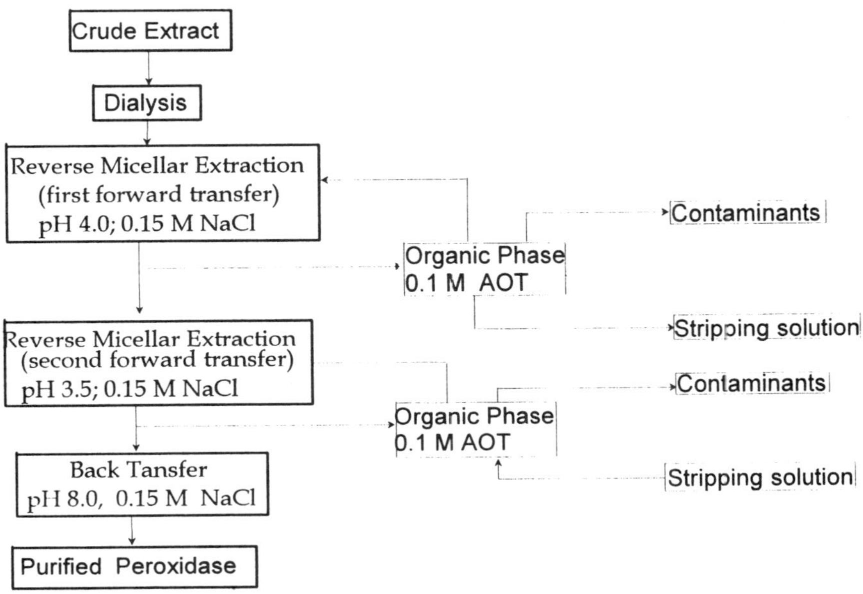

FIG. 1. FLOW DIAGRAM OF THE TWO STAGE REVERSE MICELLAR EXTRACTION OF PEROXIDASE

RESULTS

From the screening tests of peroxidase activity, only three vegetables were chosen to carry out studies on peroxidase characterization and extraction with reverse micelles.

This was because of the massive availability of broccoli as a waste material and the good activity shown by Brussels sprouts (12.40 U/g fresh material) and radish (6.6 U/g fresh material). Broccoli was divided in two parts: one included the florets (11.0 U/g fresh material), while the stems (10.0 U/g fresh material) comprised the other part.

A test of ammonium sulfate precipitation (Fig. 2) indicated that most of the peroxidase activity could be separated by using the precipitated protein in the range of 35% to 90% saturation. This was done because well defined peaks could not be obtained. Acetone precipitation was conducted as a further step because peroxidase purification is well improved and color precipitation on the ion-exchange resin was difficult to remove and caused major blocking of the ion-exchange column.

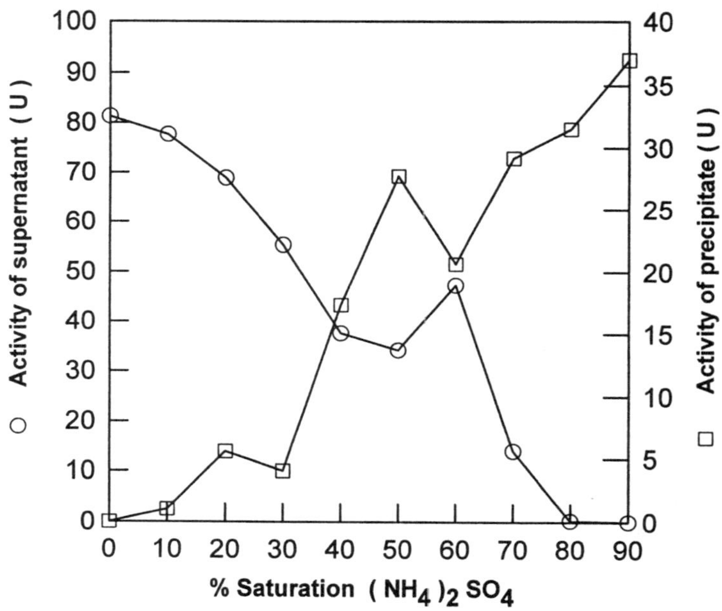

FIG. 2. PRECIPITATION CURVE OF BRUSSELS SPROUTS PEROXIDASE USING AMMONIUM SULFATE

Table 1 shows the results of traditional purification steps on Brussels sprouts. The first two steps involving precipitation with ammonium sulfate and acetone gave a 58% loss of total activity, while the purification factor increased about 10 times, suggesting that these batch processes have little efficiency but involve high consumption of valuable chemicals and are time consuming.

The anion-exchange chromatogram (Fig. 3) showed two peaks, corresponding to acid (non retained) and basic (eluted with the salt gradient) proteins, having peroxidase activity. This type of chromatography gave a great improvement in specific activity and purification factor.

TABLE 1.
RESULTS OF TRADITIONAL PURIFICATION STEPS OF PEROXIDASE FROM BRUSSELS SPROUTS

Purification step	Protein (mg)	Activity (U)	Specific activity (U/mg)	Purification factor	Yield %
Crude extract	17778	6686	0.38	1	100
Precipitation (35-90%) ammonium sulfate	8482	4293	0.50	1.3	64.2
Precipitation (1:3) with acetone	735	2830	3.85	10.4	42.0
Anion exchange (DEAE-cellulose)	30	2393	80.0	212.0	36.0
Gel filtration (Sephadex G-100)	10	1700	170.0	452.0	25.0

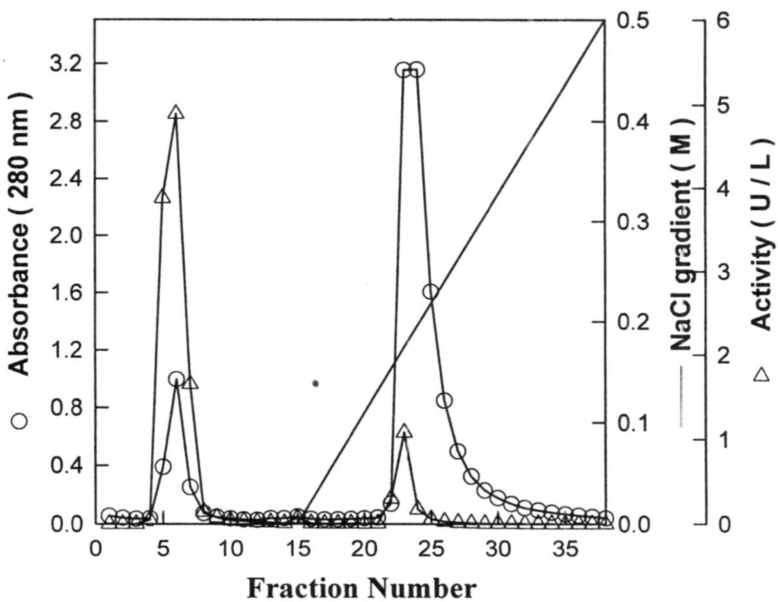

FIG. 3. ANION EXCHANGE (DEAE-CELLULOSE) OF BRUSSELS SPROUT EXTRACT PRECIPITATED WITH ACETONE (3:1)
Flow rate 1.45 mL/min. Buffer A: Tris 20 mM, pH 7.0; Buffer B: A+0.5 M NaCl)

The pooled fractions of each peak were subjected to affinity chromatography, but the separated protein had a low activity yield. This was attributed to contaminant glycoproteins which saturated the affinity sites of the column and therefore this purification step was not effective. Gel filtration chromatography of each peak separated by ion exchange gave further separation of mixed proteins. Figure 4 shows a chromatogram of a Brussels sprouts pooled extract eluted with the salt gradient during ion-exchange chromatography. Essentially two peaks appear, one with a relatively high molecular weight having high activity, and the other with lower molecular weight showing no activity. Specific activities and yield factors were approximately doubled (see Table 1). From the elution volume compared with molecular weight standards, the peroxidase activity peak had a molecular weight of about 90 kDa.

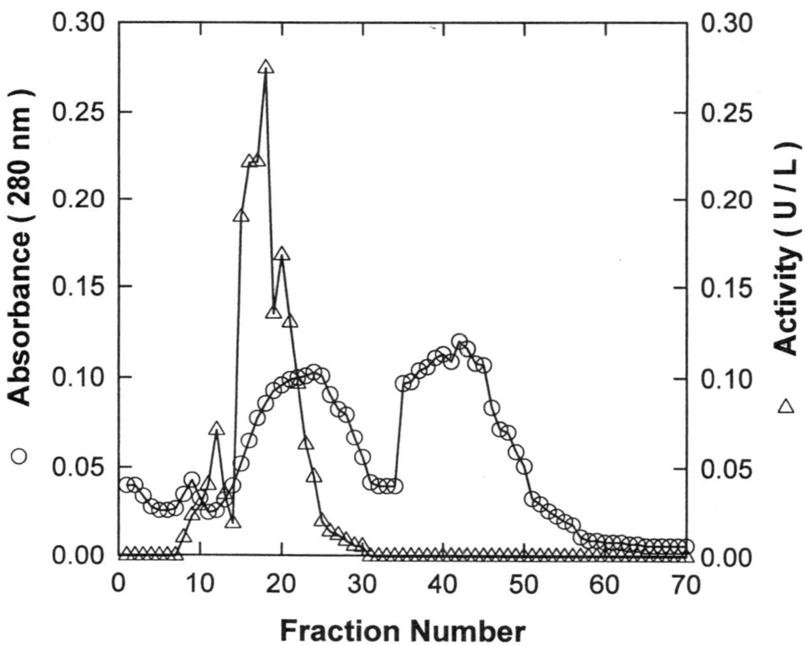

FIG. 4. GEL FILTRATION (SEPHADEX G-100) OF BRUSSELS SPROUTS EXTRACT (FRACTION WITH PEROXIDASE ACTIVITY ELUTED WITH NaCl FROM IEC).
Flow rate: 1.2 mL/min, buffer: Tris 50 mM, pH 7.0, 0.2 M NaCl

SDS-PAGE gave a molecular weight of the purified samples between 45 and 50 kDa depending on the extract, while electrophoresis conducted on the native protein gave values between 85 and 90 kDa. This indicates that this protein contains two subunits. From preliminary results of isoelectric focusing gels, the broccoli extract showed three different isoenzymes with isoelectric points (pI's) of >9.3, 9.3 and 6.9, while the Brussels sprouts had pI's of about 5 and 8.

Preliminary tests using reverse micellar peroxidase extraction from the crude extract gave low activity yields. Results using the two step extraction of AOT reverse micelles on radish extract showed a 40% activity yield, with a purification factor of 3. Similar data were found for the other extracts. For example, turnip purification factor after the two step process was 5.3 (308 U/mg protein), while a 20% activity yield was obtained. Most of the enzyme activity was lost as a precipitate at the aqueous:organic interface. However, using CTAB reverse micelles on an extract of broccoli stems, activity yield could be improved up to 60% (Fig. 5). Based on conditions of extraction at pH 8.0, 0.1 M KCl, the purification factor and activity yields are similar to those obtained after differential precipitation with ammonium sulfate and acetone (see Table 2). These results are encouraging since in a single operation, amenable to scaling up, good activity yields are obtained. However, it must be realized that perhaps the type of extract might influence the purification results. More experiments are needed to test the effect of different types of anions and co-solvents on extraction yields, as well as the possibility of a cascade extraction to check activity yield improvements.

CONCLUSIONS

Peroxidase pre-purification using reverse micelles produced similar activity yields and purification factors as the traditional differential precipitation methods. However, reverse micellar extraction can be done faster and, if liquid-liquid extraction equipment is adapted to this technology, it can be done in a continuous way.

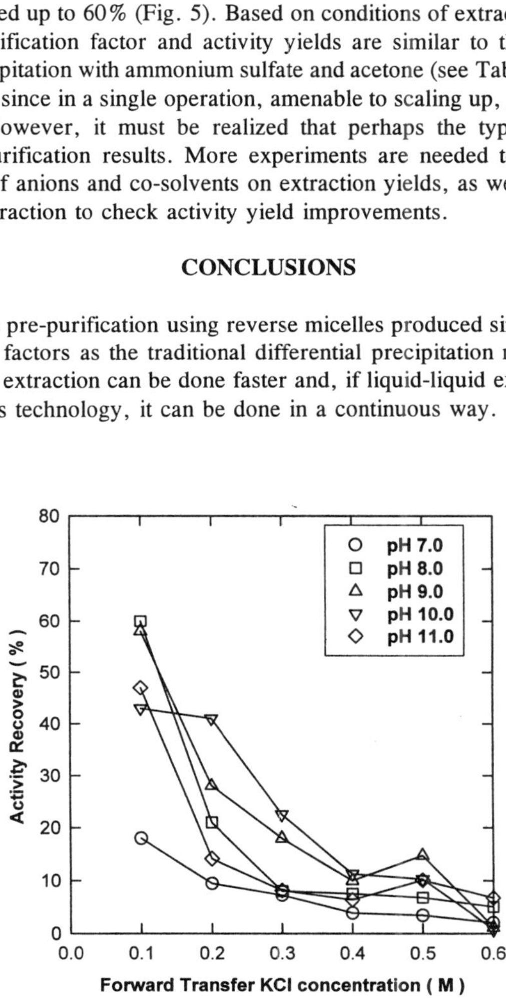

FIG. 5. PEROXIDASE RE-EXTRACTION AS A FUNCTION OF pH AND [KCl] USING 0.2 M CTAB REVERSE MICELLES IN ISOOCTANE/PENTANOL (95:5)
Conditions of back extraction: 2 M KCl, pH 4

TABLE 2.
RESULTS OF REVERSE MICELLAR PRE-PURIFICATION OF PEROXIDASE FROM BROCCOLI STEMS USING 0.2 M CTAB IN ISOOCTANE/*N*-PENTANOL (95:5)

Purification Stage	Protein (mg)	Activity (U)	Specific activity (U/mg)	Purification Factor	Yield %
Crude extract	0.75	4.4	5.8	1	100
Re-extraction	0.07	2.6	39.0	6.7	60

Forward transfer: 0.1 M KCl, pH 8.0
Back extraction: 2 M KCl, pH 4.

Brussels sprouts and the large amounts of waste products from broccoli processing plants can be used to extract peroxidase, which may constitute an alternative source of this enzyme which is not produced in Mexico.

Peroxidase from broccoli and Brussels sprouts seem to be composed of two subunits in their native state, since the molecular weight using native-PAGE was about twice the one observed using SDS-PAGE.

The isoelectric points of the different isoenzymes found for broccoli were 6.9, 9.3 and > 9.3, while those found in Brussels sprouts had pI's of 5 and 8.

Preliminary results with reverse micellar extraction of peroxidase from the crude extracts suggest that the best conditions of forward extraction are 0.2 M CTAB in isooctane/*n*-pentanol (95:5), 0.1 M KCl, pH 8.0. Optimum back transfer conditions were 2 M KCl, pH 4.0. However other factors not considered in these experiments may produce better results.

REFERENCES

ADACHI, M. and ARADA, M. 1994. Time dependence of the solubilization state of cytochrome c in AOT water-in-oil microemulsion. *J. Colloid Interface Sci. 165*, 229–235.

ASENJO, J.A. and PATRICK, I. 1990. Large-scale protein purification. In E.L.V. Harris and S. Angal (eds.). *Protein Purification Applications. A Practical Approach*. Chapter 1. IRL Press. Oxford. Ch. 1. pp. 14–15.

CASTRO, M.J.M. and CABRAL, J.M.S. 1988. Reversed micelles in biotechnological processes. *Biotech. Adv. 6*, 151–167.

CHILDS, R.E. and BARDSLEY, W.G. 1975. The steady-state kinetics of peroxidase with 2,2′-azino-di-(3-ethyl-benzthiazoline-6-sulphonic acid) as chromogen. Biochem. J. *145*, 93–103.

DUNFORD, H.B. 1991. Horseradish peroxidase: structure and kinetic properties. In J. Everse, K.E. Everse and M.B. Grisham (eds.). *Peroxidases in Chemistry and Biology*. Chapter 1. Vol. II. CRC Press. Boca Raton. pp. 1–24.

EICKE, H.F. and KVITA, P. 1984. Reverse micelles and aqueous microphases. In P.L. Luisis and B.E. Straub (eds.). *Reverse Micelles. Biological and Technological Relevance of Amphiphilic Structures in Apolar Media.* Plenum Press. New York. pp. 21–35.

GERSTEN, D.M. 1996. *Gel Electrophoresis: Proteins. Essential Techniques.* John Wiley & Sons. Chichester. pp. 54–61.

GOKLEN, K.E. and HATTON, T.A. 1987. Liquid-liquid extraction of low molecular weight proteins by selective solubilization in reversed micelles. Sep. Sci. Technol. *22*, 831–841.

KREI, G.A. and HUSTEDT, H. 1992. Extraction of enzymes by reverse micelles. Chem. Eng. Sci. *47*, 99–111.

MATZKE, S.F., CREAGH, A.L., HAYNES, C.A., PRAUSNITZ, J.M. and BLANCH, H.W. 1992. Mechanisms of protein solubilization in reverse micelles. Biotechnol. Bioeng. *40*, 91–102.

RAHAMAN, R.S., CHEE, J.Y., CABRAL, J.M.S. and HATTON, T.A. 1988. Recovery of extracellular alkaline protease from whole fermentation broth using reverse micelles. Biotechnol. Prog. *4*, 218–224.

REGALADO, C., ASENJO, J.A. and PYLE, D.L. 1996. Studies on the purification of peroxidase from horseradish roots using reverse micelles. Enzyme Microb. Technol. *18*, 332–339.

ROBINSON, B.H., TOPRAKCIOGLU, C., DORE, J.C. and CHIEUX, P. 1984. Small-angle neutron-scattering study of microemulsions stabilized by aerosol-OT. Part 1. Solvent and concentration variation. J. Chem. Soc. Faraday Trans. I. *80*, 13–27.

SADANA, A. and RAJU, R.R. 1990. Bioseparation and purification of proteins. BioPharm. May, 53–60.

SMITH, P.K., KROHN, R.I., HERMANSON, G.T., MALLIA, A.K., GARTNER, F.H., PROVENZANO, M.D., FUJIMOTO, E.K., GOEKE, N.M., OLSON, B.J. and KLENK, D.C. 1985. Measurement of protein using bicinchoninic acid. Anal. Biochem. *150*:76–85.

PREPARATION OF BREADCRUMB BY EXTRUSION

Z.Y. JIN and X.M. XU

School of Food Science and Technology
Wuxi University of Light Industry
Wuxi 214036, China

and

B. CLOUGH, A. FULLER and S. ALCOCK

British Sugar Technical Centre
Norwich NR4 7UB, England

ABSTRACT

Breadcrumb is a product made from dried and crushed bread products mainly for coating meat or fish. An extruded superbake breadcrumb has been made on the BC-45 twin-screw extruder, which performs as well as the traditional crumb from Mortons Company (England). An optimized formulation and extrusion process were found to develop a cost effective superbake breadcrumb with better functionality by extrusion. An acceptability test of two extruded breadcrumbs against Mortons was determined in application on chicken nuggets. A significant difference was found between the acceptability of the breadcrumbs with one of the extruded sample (42810) being preferred.

INTRODUCTION

Coatings are typically used in the food industry to form a seal against moisture loss during frozen storage and consumer reheating. During reheating, coatings can absorb the natural juices of a food product while maintaining a desirable, crisp outer surface and thereby conserve and retain the natural flavor and nutritive value of the food. The texture and flavoring of the coating can be adjusted to meet or create consumer demand. Coatings can also give a more pleasing appearance, both in a food product's frozen, storage form and also when it is reheated and served by the consumer.

Consumers typically enjoy food with a fried-like taste and texture. However, consumers also typically prefer the ease and simplicity of baking or cooking as an alternative to frying. Consequently, the food industry has responded by developing products which, upon conventional oven reheating, result in food with a fried-like texture and flavor. Bread crumb-like products are often used in the food industry to enhance the fried-like texture (Rosenthal 1990).

Conventional Breadcrumbs

Breadcrumb is a product made from dried and crushed (<2 mm) bread products mainly for coating meat or fish so that roasting or frying rapidly forms a tasty brown crust while reduces loss of juice from the product (Nestl and Seibel 1990). Breadcrumb should therefore adhere well to the food product, give a low fat absorption and a crunchy "bite".

The traditional method for the production of breadcrumb comprises production of dough, short fermentation, and baking, followed by precrush drying, milling, sieving to the required particle size distribution, and packaging. According to the conventional yeast leavening procedure, the time required for staling is normally about 1 to 3 days, necessitating a large space for the loaving while staling occurs, and the rehandling of the same, with interrupted unit process thus being involved (Pyson *et al.* 1982).

Extrusion of Breadcrumb

Because of the time required and the number of steps needed to make conventional breadcrumb, several attempts were made to streamline the process making it less time consuming and more economical.

The use of gaseous materials such as carbon dioxide for leaving of bread has also been suggested. U.S. Patent No. 3,041,176 by Baker discloses the use of continuous mixers in combination with added gaseous materials. The introduction of gas as disclosed by Baker is used to raise the dough in subsequent baking to avoid the use of any yeast or fermentation.

Extrusion technology offers the possibility of producing a wide range of breadcrumb products based on different recipes, with rapidly adjustable extrusion. U.S. Patent No. 4,364,961 by Darley *et al.* (1982) discloses a continuous process for manufacturing a bread crumb-like product wherein the farinaceous product-forming components are mixed in an extruder with carbon dioxide to form a gas-leavened dough. The extruded dough is then comminuted to form discrete dough particles which are exposed to hot air to dry the surface of the particles and to stabilize the structure, and then dried to the desired moisture content.

U.S. Patent No. 4,218,480 by Pyson *et al.* (1982) discloses baking and expanding the gas-leavened dough to form a baked bread product which has characteristics of stale bread. The overall procedure in the above references requires only a short period of time compared with conventional baking processes and staling procedure.

U.S. Patent No. 4,440,793 by Seki (1984) discloses a method for producing breadcrumbs forming an essentially yeast-free mixture obtained by adding 0.5-6.0% soybean protein to wheat flour and mixing with salt, fats, emulsifier, pH adjustment, coloring and flavoring materials as secondary, adding alpha-converted starch to the mixture from a die into a rope-like configuration. The rope-like material is drawn from the die of the extruder at a speed greater than the extrusion speed to produce bubbles in the rope-like material. The material is then flattened, cut and crushed, and dried. The above reference produces a bread crumb-like product within 8 h compared with the conventional process which would have taken up to 36 h.

Superbake Breadcrumb

A cost effective superbake breadcrumb has been developed by Mortons Company (UK) for the chilled and frozen markets. The crumb is produced by a conventional method rather than by extrusion. The final coated substrate is flash fried by the producer, chilled or frozen, and baked by the consumer.

Superbake breadcrumb has a crisp but "melts in the mouth" texture. This characteristic is a key parameter for us to develop an extruded breadcrumb. Of equal importance are: The crumb must sink. If the crumb floats then eventually the crumb will carbonize and give the coated substrate an unacceptable appearance. The crumb must absorb a limited amount of oil during frying. If the fat absorption is too large, then the oil cost to the manufacture is prohibitive, and the increased amount of oil consumed by the consumer is not good for their health.

Our objective was to produce a cost effective superbake breadcrumb with excellent characteristics by extrusion.

MATERIALS AND METHODS

Extrusion Facilities

A French Clextral BC-45 co-rotating twin-screw extruder was used throughout the research project. The operation parameters and the screw configuration of the extruder are shown in Tables 1 and 2. A belt conveyor was employed for stretching the rope-like extrudate coming out from the die to get a more porous structure. The belt speed can be adjusted, as shown in Table 3. The extrudates (rope-like or pellet) were dried in a steam heated Tek-Dryer with an exhaust fan at 100°C for 35 min.

TABLE 1.
PARAMETERS OF EXTRUDERS

PARAMETERS	BC-45
type	twin screw, co-rotating
barrel length (mm)	650
screw diameter (mm)	50
length/diameter	13
barrel sections	2
heater	1
motor power (kw)	14.7
highest throughput (rice powder)	100 kg/hr
highest screw speed (r.p.m.)	300
highest die temperature (°C)	120
die in diameter (circle, mm)	4.5

TABLE 2.
SCREW CONFIGURATION

BC-45
100 × 50
100 × 35
100 × 25
50 × 20
50 × 15
2 × mixing disc
50 × 15
100 × 15
50 × reverse pitch

TABLE 3.
CONVEYOR BELT SPEED

Scale in Conveyor	Belt Speed (m/min)
4	0.60
5	0.76
6	0.91
7	1.02
8	1.15
9	1.28
10	1.39

Raw Material and Formulation

Basic formulation of Superbake Breadcrumb is shown in Table 4. All the ingredients were mixed in a mixer for 20 min. A 20% glycerol solution was injected into the barrel during extrusion in some cases.

Assessments

Moisture content: 105 °C, standard method

Bulk density measurement:

* Place a 50 ml clear plastic graduated measuring cylinder on 2 d.p. balance and tare
* Pour sample particles into cylinder up to 50 ml mark
* Place on balance and record weight
* Multiply weight by 2, this gives bulk density in g/100 ml
* Repeat and get an average result

TABLE 4.
BASIC FORMULATION OF SUPERBAKE BREADCRUMB

Ingredients	Percentage(%)
Wheat Flour	74
Defatted Soya Flour	5
Salt	2
Emulsifier*	0.3
Baking Powder**	2.8
Pregelled Starch	7.5
Sugar	3.4
Glycerol	5

*Monoglyceryl fatty acid ester
**A mixture of disodium hydrogen phosphate, sodium bicarbonate and wheat flour

Fat uptake measurement (use Fraction 1.4-2.0 mm)

* Switch on deep fat fryer and allow to heat up to 190 °C
* Weigh exactly 10 g of sample and place into a clear, dry sieve
* Lower sieve and sample into fat and fry for 2 min, agitating half way through
* After 2 min, estimate float sink ratio, raise sample from fat and allow to drain for 1 min, agitating half way through
* Place fried sample on absorbent paper and leave for 5 min
* When this time has elapsed, weigh paper and sample to 2 d.p. (A)
* Remove crumb from paper and weigh paper alone to 2 d.p. (B)
* Perform the following calculation to determine the amount of fat soaked up by the sample:

  Calculation: $A - B - 10$

Sink Float ratio

This can be estimated during the fat uptake test. After 1.5 min frying note the approximate percentage of the sample which has sunk to the base of the sieve.

Coating application (use Superbake blend such as Morton's Foods)

* Fresh chicken breast cut into small pieces (20-30 g)
* Chicken put into batter for approximately 10 s
* Battered chicken placed into bowl of crumb sample and crumb gently pressed onto substrate
* The coated chicken pieces were then flash fried for 1 min at 190 °C then placed in the chiller at about 0-4 °C or frozen
* The nuggets were baked for 20 min at 200C after being chilled or frozen

Product Acceptability Test

Objective

To determine the acceptability of two of the extruded breadcrumb samples against a control of the market leader (Morton's Foods)

Material

* The three breadcrumbs were: Morton's Foods, Tech Centre 42810, and Tech Centre 30111

* The chicken was Asda Chicken Breast Fillets BBF 9th and 11th November,1996

* Batter mix: ABR Goldfield 0020w (pregelled wheat flour) 70%, maize flour 25%, wheat flour 5%. The dry blend was mixed with water at a ratio of 1:1

Preparation of samples

Approximately even sized pieces of chicken were dipped into the batter for about 5 s. The excess batter was shaken off, and the nugget lightly pressed into the crumb to give a total weight of about 20-25g per nugget.

The nuggets were then fried for one min, at 190 °C, in fresh vegetable oil in a Lincat double fryer. The nuggets were then frozen for four days, when they were heated in the Hobart oven at 200 °C for 20 min, being turned once after 10 min. The position of the samples in the oven was rotated between batches in order to minimize oven temperature variations. The samples were served at 85-90 °C.

Sensory method and data analysis

The sensory test took place at British Sugar Technical Centre on 11th November, 1996. The acceptability test was performed by 43 tasters. Each taster was presented with one each of the three nuggets on coded paper plates with plastic knives and forks. The serving order was balanced and randomized over panelists. The panelists were told to concentrate on the coating rather than the chicken. They were also asked about their frequency of consumption of breaded fish and chicken (more/less than once a month) and to explain what they particularly liked or disliked about each coating.

Each breadcrumb was scored from 1 (dislike extremely) to 9 (like extremely). An analysis of variance was performed on the acceptability scores to determine if a statistically significant difference exists. And also, the Least Significant Difference was calculated to determine the relationship among the three breadcrumbs.

RESULTS AND DISCUSSION

Experimental data on extrusion parameters and functionality is shown in Table 5.

TABLE 5.
EXPERIMENTAL DATA ON EXTRUSION PARAMETERS AND FUNCTIONALITY

No.	Moisture %	Density g/100ml	Barrel T °C	Flow Rate kg/hr	Die Pres. psi	Stretching Yes/No
1	33.3	29.8	90	51.1	953	Y
2	32.8	27	91	50.3	1110	Y
3	30	28	92	50.5	1200	Y
4	36.82	31	90	50.6	905	Y
5	33.1	23.4	90	50.6	1070	Y
6	30.3	25	92	50.7	1179	Y
7	36.3	30.4	90	50.8	913	Y
8	32.8	26.8	90	50.5	1050	N
9	33.5	24.2	89	50	970	N
10	32.8	26.8	90	50.5	1050	N
11	33.5	25.6	89	50	970	N
12	30.4	24	93	50.1	1003	Y
13	30.35	27	92	49.9	1003	N
14	30	26	93	67.75	1170	N
15	32.66	28	91	67.6	1030	N
16	32.7	28	89	50.6	950	N
17	30.35	29	92	66.65	1220	N
18	27.1	28	95	66.6	1350	N
19	32.8	29	93	66.75	1040	N
20	30.3	23.8	94	51.2	1070	Y
21	30.2	23.7	95	67.5	1190	Y
22	27.5	28.4	92	67.6	1350	N
23	27.4	28	91	67	1375	N
24	27.3	27.9	91	67.7	1270	N
25	27.3	29.3	91	67.6	1240	N
26	27.5	31.1	91	67.5	1300	N
27	27.2	27.2	91	67.1	1320	N
28	25	23	93	67.1	1480	N
29	27.29	30.7	90	50.9	1084	N
30	29.72	30.7	90	50.4	971	N
31	33.36	34	90	51	809	N
32	27.22	29.7	90	50.4	1132	N
33	30.19	29.6	90	50.9	965	N
34	33	34	88	50.9	841	N
35	26.61	31	90	50.6	1042	N
36	30.11	25	90	51.3	907	N
37	33.04	35	90	51	777	N
38	27.61	35	96	68.3	1270	N
39	27.61	27	96	68.3	1270	N

Effect of Extrusion Parameters on Functionality

Barrel moisture. Barrel moisture is a key factor to get a good result. With the decrease of moisture content, the torque and the die temperature increased, respectively, showing that more energy was consumed, and higher pressure was set up to give the extrudate lower density. Good scores in taste test are usually from those with lower density. But when the moisture was adjusted to 25%, the density of the extrudate was too low to sink during the frying, and frosting (white spots on the fried particles) appeared.

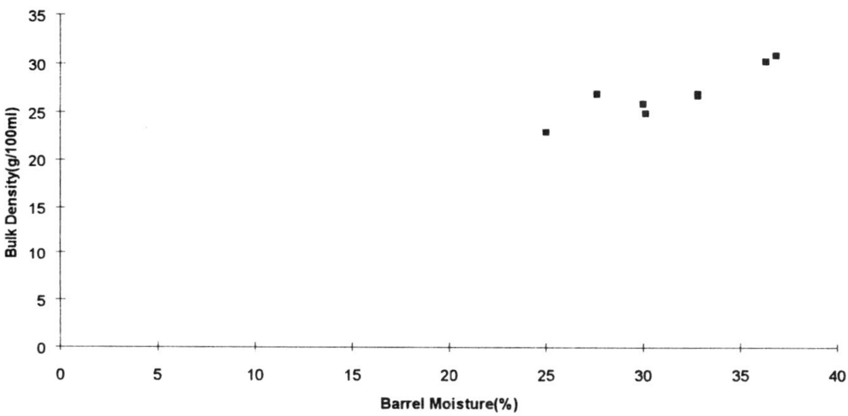

FIG. 1. EFFECT OF BARREL MOISTURE ON THE BULK DENSITY

Screw speed. Higher screw speed gave the extrudates higher expansion in a certain range (100-150 rpm), because more shear action was involved. But with an increase in screw speed, the residence time of the material inside the extruder became shorter. So, too high a screw speed is not suitable to make an extrudate with good functionality.

Barrel temperature. Normally the barrel temperature was controlled at about 90 °C. Very high temperature was not available because only one heater was working on the BC-45. But other extrusion parameters (barrel moisture, flow rate) could affect the barrel temperature and finally affect the functionality of the extrudate.

For example, when we separated the available 39 experimental point population into two groups according to whether the barrel temperature was higher than 90 °C, we found that the average bulk density of the extrudate (27.4) in the higher barrel temperature group was lower than that in the lower barrel temperature. This difference is statistically significant at low level (shown in Table 6).

Flow rate. Usually we ran the extruder at about 50 or 67 kg/h separately. At higher flow rate, a higher pressure was built up behind the die because higher energy was consumed by friction. This made a significant difference ($P<0.01$) in die pressure between two different flow rate groups (shown in Table 7).

Even when there was a very significant changes in die pressure with different flow rate, there was no significant difference in bulk density between the two flow rate groups, although the average bulk density in the higher flow rate group (28.35) is higher than that in the lower flow rate group (28.04), as shown in Table 8.

TABLE 6.
COMPARISON OF BULK DENSITY IN DIFFERENT BARREL TEMPERATURE GROUPS

Avova Summary: Single-Factor

Barrel Temperature	Groups	Count	Sum	Average	Variance
< =90 °C	Column 1			27.4	7.434
>90 °C	Column 2	19	525.7	29.20	11.477

Source of Variance

	SS	df	MS	F	P-value	F-crit
Between	31.59722	1	31.59722	3.40062	0.073191	4.105459
Within Gro	343.7894	37	9.291607			
Total	375.3867	38				

TABLE 7.
COMPARISON OF DIE PRESSURE IN DIFFERENT FLOW RATE GROUPS

Avova Summary: Single-Factor

Flow Rate	Groups	Count	Sum	Average	Variance
>55 kg/hr	Column 1	15	18875	1258.333	14255.95
<55 kg/hr	Column 2	24	23924	996.8333	11750.93

Source of Variance

	SS	df	MS	F	P-value	F-crit
Between	631220.8	1	631220.8	49.70722	2.43E-08	4.105459
Within Gro	469854.7	37	12698.77			
Total	1101075	38				

TABLE 8.
COMPARISON OF BULK DENSITY IN DIFFERENT FLOW RATE GROUPS

Avova Summary: Single-Factor

Flow Rate	Groups	Count	Sum	Average	Variance
>55 kg/hr	Column 1	15	420.6	28.04	7.9697
<55 kg/hr	Column 2	24	680.5	28.35	11.430

Source of Variance

	SS	df	MS	F	P-value	F-crit
Between	631220.8	1	631220.8	49.70722	2.43E-08	4.105459
Within Gro	469854.7	37	12698.77			
Total	1101075	38				

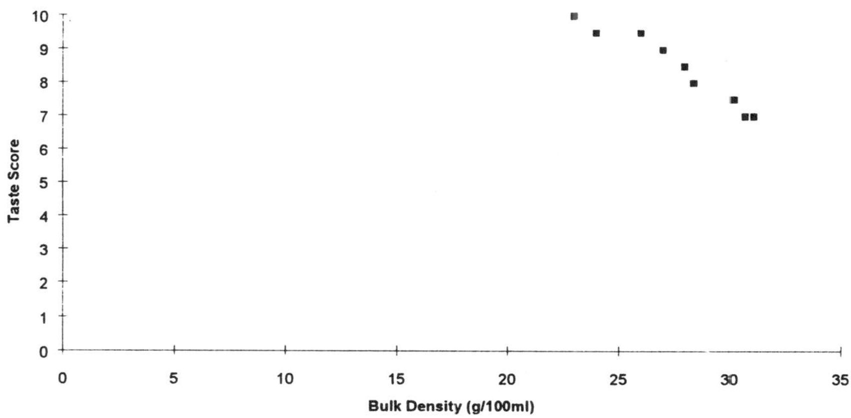

FIG. 2. RELATIONSHIP BETWEEN THE TASTE SCORE AND THE BULK DENSITY

Stretching. A belt conveyor was employed to draw the rope-like extrudate coming out of the die at a speed greater than the extrusion speed to produce more porous structure (shown in Table 9).

There was a low level difference in bulk density of the extrudate with or without stretching. The stretched one was better in relatively low bulk density, but the rope-like extrudate was very difficult to cut into pieces especially in a production scale. We prefer to cut the extrudate at the die face (without stretching), because the change with or without stretching was not very significant.

So far, an optimized process was found to develop a cost effective superbake breadcrumb with better functionality by extrusion. The preferable parameters are: barrel moisture content 27-33%; screw speed 150 rpm; barrel temperature 90-95 °C; flow rate (BC-45) 50-67 kg/hr; cut at die face.

TABLE 9.
COMPARISON OF BULK DENSITY WITH OR WITHOUT STRETCHING

Avova Summary: Single-Factor

Stretching	Groups	Count	Sum	Average	Variance
No	Column 1	10	266.1	26.61	9.107667
Yes	Column 2	29	835	28.79	9.213522

Source of Variance

	SS	df	MS	F	P-value	F-crit
Between	35.43905	1	35.43905	3.857196	0.057079	4.105459
Within Gro	339.9476	37	9.187774			
Total	375.3867	38				

Effect of Ingredients on Functionality

Basic formulation is shown in Table 10.

TABLE 10.
BASIC FORMULATION (%):

Ingredients	F1	F2*	F3	F4	F5	F6	F7	F8
Wheat Flour	81.5	74	79	81.5	84	86.5	76.5	89
Defatted Soya Flour	2.5	5	5	5	2.5	5	2.5	2.5
Salt	2	2	2	2	2	2	2	2
Emulsifier*	0.3	0.3	0.3	0.3	0.3	0.3	0.3	0.3
Baking Powder**	2.8	2.8	2.8	2.8	2.8	2.8	2.8	2.8
Pregelled Starch	7.5	7.5	7.5	0	0	0	7.5	0
Sugar	3.4	3.4	3.4	3.4	3.4	3.4	3.4	3.4
Glycerol	0	5	0	5	5	0	5	0

Ingredients	F9	F10	F11	F12	F13	F15	F16	F17
Wheat Flour	84	77	79	79.8	77.8	88.7	90.7	89.7
Defatted Soya Flour	5	5	5	5	5	5	5	5
Salt	2	2	2	2	2	2	2	2
Emulsifier*	0.3	0.3	0.3	0.3	0.3	0.3	0.3	0.3
Baking Powder**	2.8	2.8	2.8	2	4	4	2	2
Pregelled Starch	0	7.5	7.5	0	0	0	0	0
Sugar	3.4	3.4	3.4	3.4	3.4	0	0	0
Fat		2					0	1
Glycerol	2.5	0	0	0	5	0	0	0

Glycerol, pregelled starch and soya flour. As shown in Table 11, the most important factor on the texture of the extrudate was the addition level of soya flour, compared with the ingredients of glycerol and pregelled starch. High level of soya flour (5%) preferred.

Although the addition of glycerol could contribute a good texture to the extruded breadcrumb, the difference was not significant. A lower level of pregelled starch even gave a better result in taste. Both of them can be taken out of the formulation to get a more economical and simple recipe.

Baking powder and sugar. Two different addition levels of baking powder in the formulation (F12 2% and F13 4%) were compared in a designed experiment with different barrel moisture content. As shown in Fig. 3, there was a significant change in bulk density between two different addition level of baking powder. High level of baking powder gave lower bulk density associated with better texture in taste. The baking powder was added at 4% to give the required bulk density. From the results, reducing the baking powder increased the density making the crumbs too dense.

TABLE 11.
EFFECT OF GLYCEROL, PREGELLED STARCH, AND SOYA FLOUR ON THE TEXTURE OF EXTRUDED BREADCRUMB

Formu	Des. No.	Run No.	Glycerol(%)	Prestarch(%)	Soyflour(%)	Texture score
F8	1	8	0	0	2.5	7
F5	2	5	5	0	2.5	9
F1	3	1	0	7.5	2.5	6
F7	4	7	5	7.5	2.5	6.5
F6	5	6	0	0	5	7.5
F5	6	5	5	0	5	8.5
F3	7	3	0	7.5	5	8.5
F2	8	2	5	7.5	5	7.5

Average Score	Glycerol	Prestarch	Soya Flour
Low Level	7.25	8.00	7.13
High Level	7.88	7.13	8.00
Difference	0.63	0.87	0.87
Difference per 2.5% change	0.315	0.29	0.87

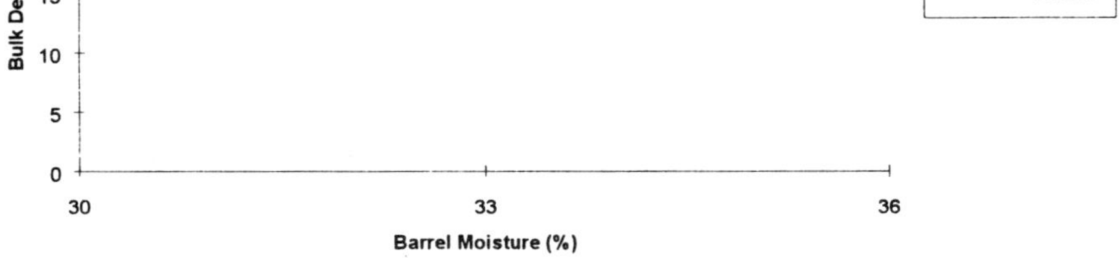

FIG. 3. EFFECT OF BAKING POWDER LEVEL ON THE BULK DENSITY OF EXTRUDED BREADCRUMB

At last, we took the sugar out of the formulation, which did not affect the functionality of the extruded breadcrumb.

So far, we got a cost effective formulation for the extrusion of superbake breadcrumb. It consists of:

Ingredients	Percentage (%)
Wheat Flour	88.7
Defatted Soya Flour	5
Salt	2
Emulsifier	0.3
Baking Powder	4

Taste Acceptability

Characteristics of tasted samples. Characteristics of tasted samples are shown in Table 12.

TABLE 12.
CHARACTERISTICS OF TASTED SAMPLES

Sample No.	Morton's	42810	30111
Extruder		BC-45	BC-45
Die Hole in diameter (mm)		4.5	4.5
Screw Speed (rpm)		150	152
Barrel Moisture (%)		27.2	27.0
Barrel Temperature (°C)		90	96
Flow Rate (kg/hr)		50.4	61.0
Stretching		No	No
Cut at die face		Yes	Yes
Drying		100 °C for 35 min	100 °C for 35 min
Formulation		F15	F15
Moisture of final particle (%)	8	3.89	2.5
Bulk Density (g/100ml)	24	29.7	35
Sink (%)	95	95	90
Fat uptake (g/10g)	4.8	4.4	5.4

Taste score. Only 41 tasters were available. When the data were examined, approximately half the tasters were regular consumers of breaded products. The data were therefore additionally split into the two groups and an analysis of variance was performed on the separate groups. All breadcrumbs scored "like slightly/moderately" (1 = dislike extremely; 9 = like extremely). The mean scores were shown in Table 13.

TABLE 13.
TASTE SCORE

Samples	Morton's	Tech Centre 30111	Tech Centre 42810
All Tasters	6.0	6.4	6.6
Frequent Consumers	6.0	6.6	6.8

Sensory statistics. No significant difference was found between the acceptability of the samples at the 90% confidence level when all tasters were included. However when only the data for frequent consumers was included, a statistically significant difference at the 90% confidence level was apparent. The averages and Least Significant Difference groups are displayed in Fig. 4 (groups with different subscripts are significantly different from each other). When the extruded samples were compared against the Morton's separately, there was a very significant difference (at a 99.9% confidential level) between every extruded sample and the Morton's Foods even when all the tasters were included. There was no significant difference between the two extruded samples (246 and 678) whatever the statistics were from the frequent consumers or the total.

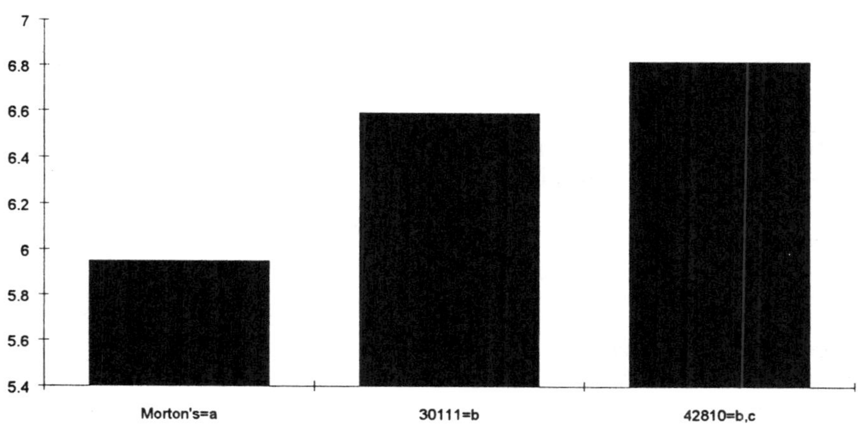

FIG. 4. ACCEPTABILITY OF BREADCRUMBS: FREQUENT CONSUMERS

The reasons given for liking and disliking the samples

The reasons given for liking and disliking the samples are shown in Table 14. There were very few adverse comments about any of the samples. The extruded samples were generally commented on as being 'crispier/harder' than the Morton's Foods sample, and whether people preferred the crisper sample determined their acceptability score.

There were some general comments that the Tech Centre samples had a bigger particle size than the Morton's Foods crumb, despite all the crumbs having been sieved to be the same size. Possibly the extruded samples absorbed more oil on cooking.

TABLE 14.
THE REASONS GIVEN FOR LIKING AND DISLIKING THE SAMPLES

		Morton's	Tech Centre 42810	Tech Centre 30111
Frequent Consumers	Why Liked	Crispy	Crunchy/ crispy	Crunchy/ crispy
	Why Disliked	Bland Not as crispy	Hard Dry	Hard
Infrequent Consumers	Why Liked	Crispy	Crunchy/ crispy	Crunchy/ crispy
	Why Disliked	Bland Not as crispy	Hard	Hard

Some information from the taste test

All the samples were rated as "like slightly/moderately". The extruded samples both scored higher than the Morton's Foods sample. There was a very significant difference between all extruded samples and the Morton's Foods sample whatever the scores were from the frequent tasters or from the total tasters. There was no significant difference between the two extruded samples whatever the scores were from the frequent tasters or from the total tasters, which means that some of changes in extrusion parameters (barrel temperature 90-96 °C; flow rate 50-61 kg/hr) did not affect the texture of the final products significantly.

One of the extruded crumb samples (42810) was significantly preferred, at the 90% confidence level, for 'frequent consumers' of breadcrumb coated products.

CONCLUSIONS

Barrel moisture is a key factor to get good results. With decrease of moisture content, the torque and the die temperature increased respectively, showing that more energy was consumed, and higher pressure was set up to give the extrudates lower density. Good scores in taste test usually are from those with lower density. But when the moisture was adjusted to 25%, the density of the extrudate was too low to sink during the frying, and frosting appeared.

An optimized process was found to develop a cost effective superbake breadcrumb with better functionality by extrusion. The preferable parameters are: Barrel moisture content 27-33%; screw speed 150 rpm; barrel temperature 90-95 °C; flow rate (BC-45) 50-67 kg/hr; cut at die face.

There was a significant change in bulk density between two different addition levels of baking powder. High level of baking powder gave lower bulk density associated with better texture in taste. The baking powder was added at 4% to give the required bulk density. From the results, reducing the baking powder increased the density making the crumbs too dense.

A cost effective and optimized formulation for extrusion of superbake breadcrumb has been developed. It consists of: wheat flour 88.7%; soya flour 5%; emulsifier 0.3%; salt 2%; baking powder 4%.

An acceptability test of two extruded breadcrumbs against a leading product (Mortons Foods) in the present market was determined in application on chicken nuggets. A significant difference was found between the acceptability of the breadcrumbs with one of the extruded samples (42810) being preferred.

REFERENCES

DARLEY, K.S., FENN, M.A.F. and PYSON, D.V. 1982. Manufacture of Bread Crumb-like Product, U.S. Patent 4,364,961.

NESTL, B. and SEIBEL, W. 1990. Analytical characterisation of domestic breadcrumbs. Lebensmitteltehnik (6), 312–319.

PYSON, D.V., DARLEY, K.S. and FENN, M.A.F. 1982. Manufacture of Bread Crumb-like Product, UK Patent Application, GB2,095,529A.

ROSENTHAL, S.W. 1990. Bread Crumb Coating Composition and Process for Imparting Fried-like Texture and Flavour to Food Products. U.S. Patent 4,943,438.

SEKI, M. 1984. Method for Producing Breadcrumbs. U.S. Patent 4,440,793.

ANTIOXIDANT ACTIVITY OF NORTH AMERICAN GINSENG

DAVID D. KITTS, CHUN HU and AROSHA N. WIJEWICKREME

Department of Food Science
University of British Columbia
Vancouver, B.C. V6T-1Z4

ABSTRACT

North American ginseng was assayed for antioxidant activity using a battery of chemical and biological test methods. Samples of crude ginseng extract were diluted 100 to 1000 fold with 50 mM phosphate buffered saline solution (pH 7.4) and assayed for scavenging activity against superoxide anion ($O_2^{\bullet-}$) and hydroxyl ($OH^{\bullet}$) radicals. Relative scavenging affinity of 400- and 600-fold dilutions of ginseng extract against $O_2^{\bullet-}$ was 30% and 25%, respectively. At similar dilutions, $OH^{\bullet}$ scavenging activity of ginseng extract was 53% and 41%, respectively. The inhibition of lipid peroxidation in a linoleic acid emulsion by ginseng extract (0.01 - 0.1%; w/v) using the ammonium thiocyanate assay was dramatic and characterized by a significant prolongation in the initiation phase. Ginseng extract was also shown to effectively protect phage DNA strand scissions induced by 10 - 70 μmol of Fe^{2+} and Cu^{2+} ions. These results corresponded to a marked chelating power of ginseng against both Cu^{2+} and Fe^{2+} transition metals.

INTRODUCTION

Ginseng is a term that refers to any of 22 different plants usually derived from the genus *Panax*. The three primary medicinal species of ginseng are *Panex ginseng* (Chinese or Korean ginseng), *Panex pseudo-ginseng* (Japanese ginseng) and *Panex quinqueofolium* (North American ginseng). Ginseng is used as a general tonic for its claimed efficacy to improve physical and mental performance. It has many forms such as traditional herbal teas and more contemporary products, which include ginseng tablets and capsules, the contents of which are derived from extracts of whole roots and root fibers. Due to its role in traditional Chinese medicine, an aura of mystery has surrounded the diverse pharmacological effects claimed to exist with ginseng. A number of studies conducted with ginseng have reported evidence for bioactivity towards enhanced carbohydrate and lipid intermediatory metabolism (Samira *et al.* 1985), immunoenhancement (Scaglione *et al.* 1990), and learning and memory capabilities (Petkor and Mosharrof 1987). There are also reports for potential antioxidant activity of ginseng (Zhang *et al.* 1996) which could represent one, if not the primary underlying mechanism(s) for the observed bioactivity of ginseng reported by others.

Studies conducted in our laboratory have demonstrated that free radical oxygen species including singlet oxygen, superoxide anion ($O_2^{\bullet-}$), and hydroxyl radical ($OH^{\bullet}$), despite being products of normal cellular respiration, also represent a potential toxic hazard to various biomembranes containing susceptible lipids or proteins (Yuan and Kitts 1997). Antioxidants retard the process of lipid peroxidation and formation of secondary lipid oxidation products such as malondialdehyde (MDA), which binds nonspecifically to biomacromolecules causing membrane damage, cell injury, or death, and may lead to an increased susceptibility to certain chronic and acute diseases. The purpose of the present study was to characterize the antioxidant activity of a ginseng extract (CNT - 2000), derived from North American ginseng, by employing a number of *in vitro* tests which would demonstrate the antioxidant efficacy of the ginseng extract in both lipid and non-lipid model systems.

MATERIALS

All chemicals and reagents used were of highest purity. $CuSO_4.5H_2O$, $FeSO_4$, $Fe_2(SO_4)_3$, potassium chloride, ferrous chloride, ferric chloride, mono basic and dibasic hydrogen orthophosphate, ferrous sulfate, tetramethyl murexide (TMM), hexamine, linoleic acid, ammonium thiocyanate, Tween-20, haemoglobin, L-ascorbic acid, potassium ferricyanide, ethylenediaminetetraacetic acid (EDTA), ethidium bromide, electrophoresis grade agarose, Chelex-100, pBR322 plasmid DNA, bromophenol blue, xylene cyanol FF, ficoll, and molecular biology grade Trizma base were purchased from Sigma Chemical Co. (St. Louis, MO). Metal free micro-centrifuge tubes and polaroid type 665 positive films were obtained from BioRad Laboratories (Richmond, CA). Hydrochloric acid and ethanol were obtained from BDH Chemical Co. (Toronto, ON). North American ginseng CNT 2000 (ultra concentrate) was obtained from Cha-Na-Ta Corporation (Abbotsford, Canada).

METHODS

Biochemical Analysis

Total Phenolic Acid Content. The Folin-Ciocalteu method of Shahidi and Naczk (1995) was used to evaluate the total phenolic acid content of crude ginseng extract. Rutin was used as the phenolic acid standard.

Metal Chelating Activity of Ginseng. Solutions consisting of 0.05 to 0.4 mmol $CuSO_4$, $FeSO_4$, $Fe_2(SO_4)_3$, crude ginseng extract (300 μg/mL), and TMM (1 mM) were prepared in 10 mM hexamine·HCl buffer (pH 5.0) containing 10 mM KCl. The ginseng extracts (1 mL) were individually incubated with 1 mL of 0.05 to 0.4 mM $CuSO_4$, $FeSO_4$, or $Fe_2(SO_4)_3$ and 100 μL of TMM reagent for 10 min at room temperature and the absorbance was read at 460 and 530 nm. The amount of free cupric, ferric, or ferrous ions in the samples were read from a standard curve where the absorbance ratio (A_{460}/A_{530}) in a solution of 1 mL $CuSO_4$, $FeSO_4$, or $Fe_2(SO_4)_3$ (0.05-0.4 mM), 1 mL of hexamine HCl·buffer, and 0.1 mL TMM was plotted against the amount of total cupric, ferric, or ferrous ions added. The difference between the absorbance ratio of the control metal solutions and the ginseng added metal solutions indicated the concentration of metal bound to ginseng extract.

Ammonium Thiocyanate Assay. The method used is a modification of the procedure of Ramarathnam *et al.* (1988) and Asamari *et al.* (1996). A linoleic acid pre-emulsion was made by vortexing 3 mL of linoleic acid with 3 mL of Tween 20 and 200 mL of 30% (v/v) ethanol. One mL of crude ginseng extract in water (0.01%-1%; v/v) was added to 10 mL of pre-emulsion, and the total volume was brought to 25 mL with potassium phosphate buffer (pH 7.4). The prepared solutions were incubated in conical flasks at 40°C for three days. Aliquots (100 μL) from the incubated mixture were withdrawn at several intervals and tested for lipid peroxidation by adding 5 mL of ethanol (75%), 0.1 mL of ammonium thiocyanate (30%; w/v), and 0.1 mL of ferrous chloride (0.1%; w/v). The absorbance of the reaction mixture was measured at 500 nm against ethanol.

Oxygen Consumption Measurements. The method of Lingert *et al.* (1979) was adopted for oxygen depletion measurements. Rate of oxygen consumption in a linoleic acid emulsion with added Fe^{2+} ions was measured in the presence of ginseng extract using a YSI model 5300 biological oxygen electrode (Yellow Springs, OH). A pre-emulsion for the studies was prepared by sonicating 1.5 g of linoleic acid and 0.4 g Tween-20 with 40 mL of potassium phosphate buffer (0.1 M, pH 7.0). The working solution consisted of 1.5 mL of pre-emulsion, 15 mL of phosphate buffer, 600 μL of Fe^{2+} (10 μM), and 600 μL of ginseng (0.01% to 1%; v/v). Soon after adding the hemin solution to the emulsion, the emulsion was injected into a jacketed reaction vessel (volume = 600 μL) connected to an oxygen electrode. The percentage of oxygen remaining in the chamber was recorded every 30 sec. Oxygen depletion rate in an emulsion devoid of ginseng was used as the control.

Reducing Activity. Reducing activity of ginseng extract (0.001 - 0.1%; w/v) was assessed by the method of Yen and Chen (1995).

DNA Nicking Assay. pBR322 plasmid DNA from *Escherichia coli* strain RRI was used for studying the modulation of metal induced DNA strand scissions by ginseng extracts. All experiments were conducted in potassium phosphate buffer (pH 7.4, 50 mM) under ambient oxygen pressure. All glassware used were washed with 2 N HCl and the water and buffers used were treated with Chelex 100 before use to remove metal contaminants. 2 μL each of ginseng (0.005%; w/v), ferrous sulfate (10, 50, 70 μM), buffer, and DNA (0.1 μg/mL) were mixed in a 500 μL microcentrifuge tube. The final volume of the reaction mixture was brought to 10 μL with deionized distilled water and incubated for 1 h at 37°C. Following incubation, 2 μL of loading dye (0.25% bromophenol blue, 0.25% xylene cyanol FF, and 15% ficoll in water) was added to the incubated mixture and 10 μL was loaded onto an agarose gel well. Electrophoresis was conducted at 60 volts in Tris acetate ethylenediaminetetraacetic acid (TAE) buffer (0.04 M Tris acetate and 0.001 M EDTA, pH 7.4). The agarose gel was stained with ethidium bromide (0.5 μg/mL deionized distilled water) for 20 min. DNA bands were visualized under illumination of UV light and photographed with a Bio-Rad polaroid camera using type 665 positive films.

Non-site Specific OH$^\bullet$ Radical Scavenging Activity. Non-site specific OH$^\bullet$ radical scavenging activity of ginseng extracts was measured according to the method given by Halliwell *et al.* (1987). Solutions of $FeCl_3$ and ascorbate were made up in deaerated water immediately before use and the concentrated ginseng extract was diluted two times with 50 mM potassium phosphate buffer (pH 7.4) for conducting the assay. One mL of the final reaction solution consisted of aliquots (0 - 200 μL) of diluted ginseng extract, $FeCl_3$ (100 μmol), EDTA (100 μmol), H_2O_2 (1 mmol), deoxyribose (3.6 mmol), and L-ascorbic acid (100 μmol) in potassium phosphate buffer. The reaction mixture was incubated for 1 h at 37°C. Following incubation, 1 mL of TCA (10%) and 1 mL of TBA (0.5% 2-TBA in 0.025 M NaOH containing 0.02% BHA) were finally added to the reaction mixtures and they were heated in a boiling water bath for 15 min. After cooling, color development was measured at 532 nm.

Superoxide Radical Scavenging Activity. The final reaction mixture (3 mL) consisted of 200 to 1000 times dilutions of concentrated ginseng extract (500 μL), 30 mM EDTA.2Na (100 μL), 30 mM xanthine (10 μL) in 50 mM NaOH, 1.42 mM NBT (200 μL), and 1.8 mL of phosphate buffer (pH 7.4). The reaction was started by adding 100 μL of xanthine oxidase (0.5 unit/mL) and the incubation was conducted at room temperature for 10 min. The color development in the reaction was measured at 560 nm against a blank (without xanthine oxidase).

RESULTS AND DISCUSSION

The concentration dependent effect of ginseng in decreasing oxygen depletion in a model linoleic acid emulsion using an oxygen electrode is shown in Fig. 1. The efficacy of ginseng to inhibit lipid oxidation, as measured by the oxygen depletion assay, represents an outcome to retard the initiation phase of lipid peroxidation, in particular. The characteristic inhibition of oxygen depletion by ginseng CNT 2000 ginseng extract was evidenced by a reduced slope of the oxygen depletion curve which occurred at both very low (0.001% ginseng; w/v) and high (0.01% ginseng; w/v) ginseng extract concentrations. The oxygen depletion assay procedure represents a sensitive method for evaluating antioxidant potential since the results correspond directly to the inhibition of lipid oxidation, compared to other measurements of lipid oxidation which use primary or secondary products of oxidation as endpoint measurements. For example, while the consumption of oxygen is an absolute indicator of total activity of reactive oxygen species, the commonly used thiobarbituric acid (TBA) method which measures malonaldehyde has limitations in precisely estimating free radical reactions (Draper and Handley 1990).

The antioxidant activity of the ginseng extract was further characterized by the ammonium thiocyanate assay which employed a similar linoleic acid emulsion system used in the oxygen depletion test but without hemin (Fig. 2). Ginseng extract at both 0.001 and 0.01% (w/v) concentrations effectively decreased the generation of peroxyl radicals. Peroxyl radicals are generated in response to a multitude of actions including those generated from metabolic reactions and certain xenobiotic agents. These agents are known to contribute to lipid peroxidation reactions *in vivo* which can potentiate damage to proteins, nucleic acids, and membranes and result in the development of human diseases as well as ageing. Thus, the results of the present study are tempting to suggest that the ginseng extract used herein could be potentially effective in minimizing the biological damage caused by products of lipid peroxidation reactions. Further studies are required to confirm this suggestion.

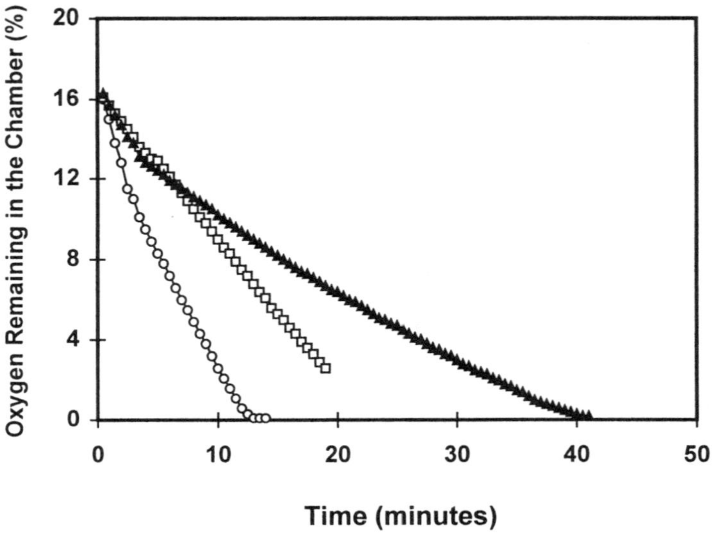

FIG. 1. PERCENT OXYGEN DEPLETION IN A MODEL LINOLEIC ACID EMULSION (MLE) IN THE PRESENCE OF CRUDE GINSENG EXTRACT AND Fe^{2+} CATALYST
o = Control (MLE without ginseng), □ = MLE + 0.001% (w/v) ginseng,
▲ = MLE + 0.01% (w/v) ginseng.

In addition to suppressing the generation of peroxyl radicals, the crude ginseng extract was also found to be effective at reducing the generation of superoxide radical (Fig. 3A) and hydroxyl radical (Fig. 3B). The affinity of crude ginseng extract to inhibit superoxide radical ranged from 18% at 1/1000 dilution to 35% at 1/200 dilution of the crude extract. Generation of superoxide radical occurs naturally as a result of normal oxidative metabolism which involves numerous enzyme complexes, and cellular metabolic functions (Yuan and Kitts 1997). Damage from reactive oxygen species can be prevented by dietary consumption of antioxidants such as α-tocopherol, β-carotene, and ascorbic acid (Byers and Perry 1992). Although superoxide radical is not a relatively strong oxidant it can nevertheless be the source of oxidative injury, as evidenced by its role in the inactivation of iron-sulfur centers of some enzymes (Kuo *et al.* 1987). Moreover, the reactions of superoxide are particularly important from the standpoint that superoxide can react with nitric oxide to produce peroxynitrite, a strong oxidant implicated in cardiovascular disease (Beckman *et al.* 1990). A relatively greater quenching of the hydroxyl radical was also observed with the different dilutions of ginseng extract. This highly electrophilic hydroxyl radical which is predominately generated from the Fenton reaction, not only reacts both with biological membranes by abstracting hydrogen atoms, but is also involved in oxidative damage *in vivo* by initiating the generation of lipid peroxyl radicals.

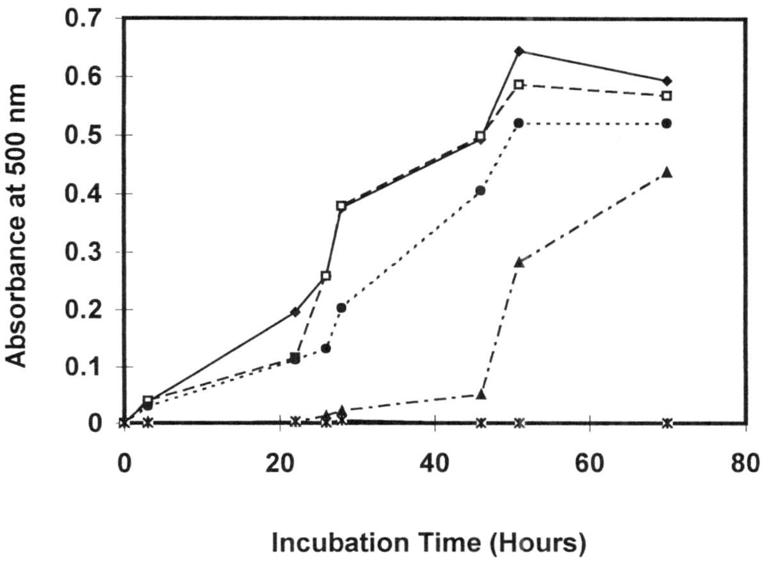

FIG. 2. ASSESSMENT OF RATE OF LIPID OXIDATION IN A METAL FREE MODEL LINOLEIC ACID EMULSION (MLE) IN THE PRESENCE OF CRUDE GINSENG EXTRACT

◆ = MLE without ginseng, □ = MLE + 0.001% (w/v) ginseng, ● = MLE + 0.01% (w/v) ginseng, ▲ = MLE + 0.1% (w/v) ginseng, * = MLE + 1% (w/v) ginseng.

The ability of plant constituents to inhibit the generation of peroxyl radicals has been reported extensively and in a number of different fruit and vegetable sources (Foti *et al.* 1996; Cao *et al.* 1996; Guo *et al.* 1997). In many instances the reported antioxidant activity of plant material has been attributed to the presence of flavonoids and other simpler phenolic acids (Larson 1988). In the present study, although the concentration of total phenolics relative to the concentration of total ginsenosides is fairly low, we are not able to ascertain the contribution of ginsenosides to the observed antioxidant activity relative to the activity of other phenols present in the ginseng extract. Further work is required to characterize the source of the ginseng constituents that contribute either individually or collectively towards the total antioxidant activity observed herein.

The reducing potential of ginseng, relative to ascorbic acid, is shown in Fig. 4. Ginseng, at a wide range of concentrations, was found to possess a relatively small amount of reducing activity, compared to ascorbic acid. The significance of this finding is associated with the apparent lower affinity of ginseng constituents to promote prooxidant reactions which will result in the reduction of Fe^{3+} to Fe^{2+} and subsequent catalysis of the Fenton reaction to produce hydroxyl radicals. The prooxidant character of known antioxidant compounds in the presence of polyvalent metal ions, namely ascorbic acid and α-tocopherol, and a number of plant flavonoids has been reported (Mahoney and Graf 1986; Laughton *et al.* 1989).

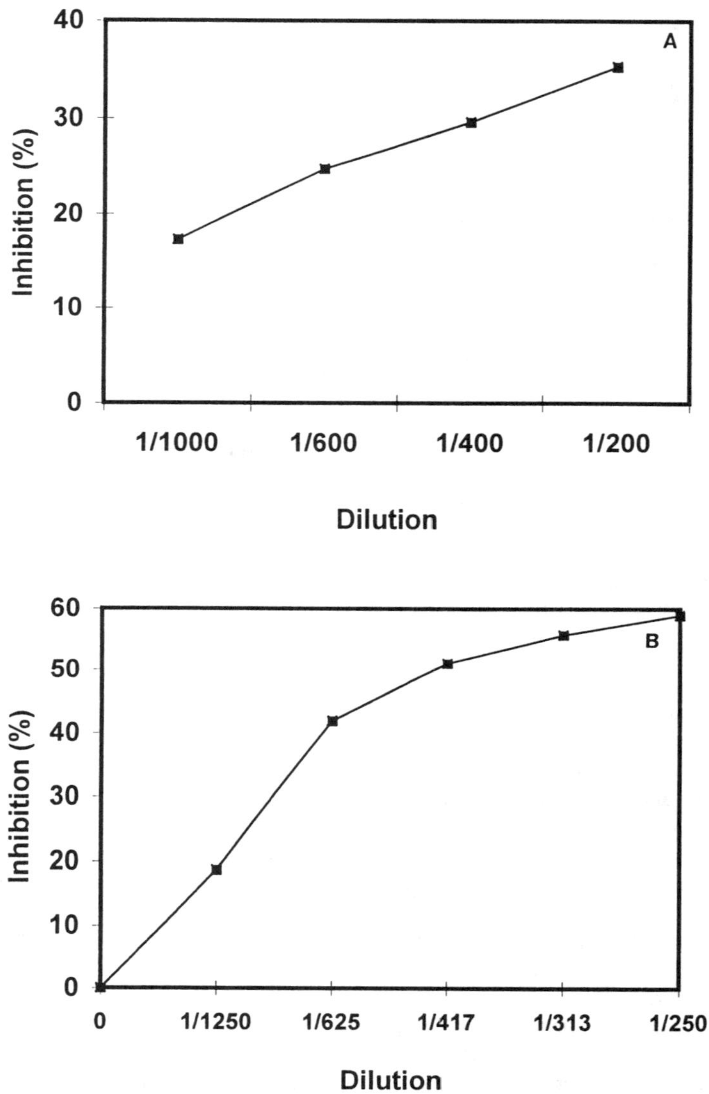

FIG. 3. SUPEROXIDE ANION ($O_2^{\bullet -}$) AND HYDROXYL RADICAL ($OH^{\bullet}$) SCAVENGING ACTIVITY OF CRUDE GINSENG EXTRACT
A: Scavenging of superoxide radical,
B: Scavenging of hydroxyl radical.

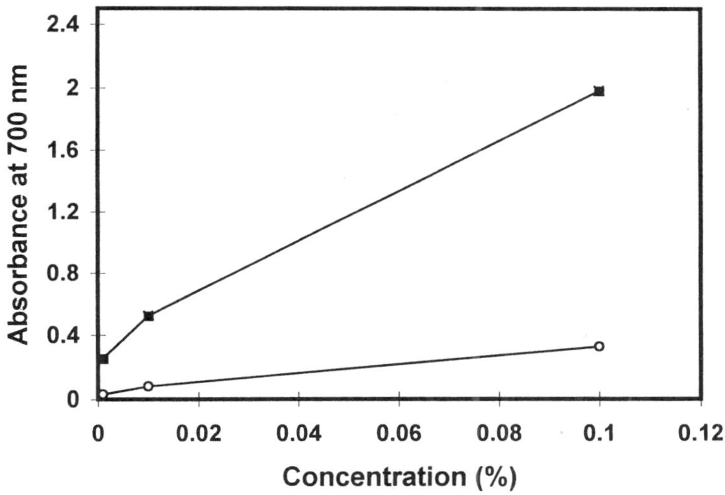

FIG. 4. REDUCING ACTIVITY OF CRUDE GINSENG EXTRACT AND L-ASCORBIC ACID

■ = L-ascorbic acid, o = crude ginseng extract

The presence of antioxidant and the absence of a prooxidant actions of the ginseng extract in a non-lipid model system (e.g. plasmid bacterial DNA) in the presence of divalent metal ions is shown in Fig. 5. Ginseng was found to effectively inhibit the dose-dependent Fe^{2+} catalyzed DNA strand scissions over a range of 10-70 μM Fe^{2+} *in vitro*. In this study, damage to DNA caused by metal ions was assessed by visualizing the degree of supercoiled (S), nicked circular (NC), and linear (L) forms of DNA left following incubation of various concentrations of metal ions and ginseng with supercoiled plasmid DNA. Strand scissions in DNA molecules result from the oxidation of nucleic acid by free radicals produced through the metal driven Fenton reaction. According to Fig. 5B, failure of Fe^{3+} to induce strand scissions in the presence of ginseng, can be attributed in part to the low reducing activity of ginseng extract. Unlike various tea extracts which have been shown to possess both antioxidant and prooxidant actions (Yen *et al.* 1997), there is evidence from the experimental methods used in the present study to suggest that ginseng does not readily promote prooxidant activity. Further studies however, are required to confirm this conclusion.

An additional potential explanation for the observed apparent antioxidant activity and the absence of prooxidant activity of ginseng also involves the strong metal chelation activity of ginseng extract shown in Table 1. The results demonstrate that ginseng extract was effective at chelating both cupric and ferric ions, while having a relatively low affinity for ferrous ion. The chelation of transition metals that otherwise contribute to catalysis of oxidation reactions is a significant characteristic of some plant derived compounds with noted antioxidant activity (e.g., phytic acid; Mahoney and Graf 1986). Graf *et al.* (1984) have demonstrated the importance of the availability of co-ordination sites in determining the ability of chelating compounds to produce hydroxy-radicals.

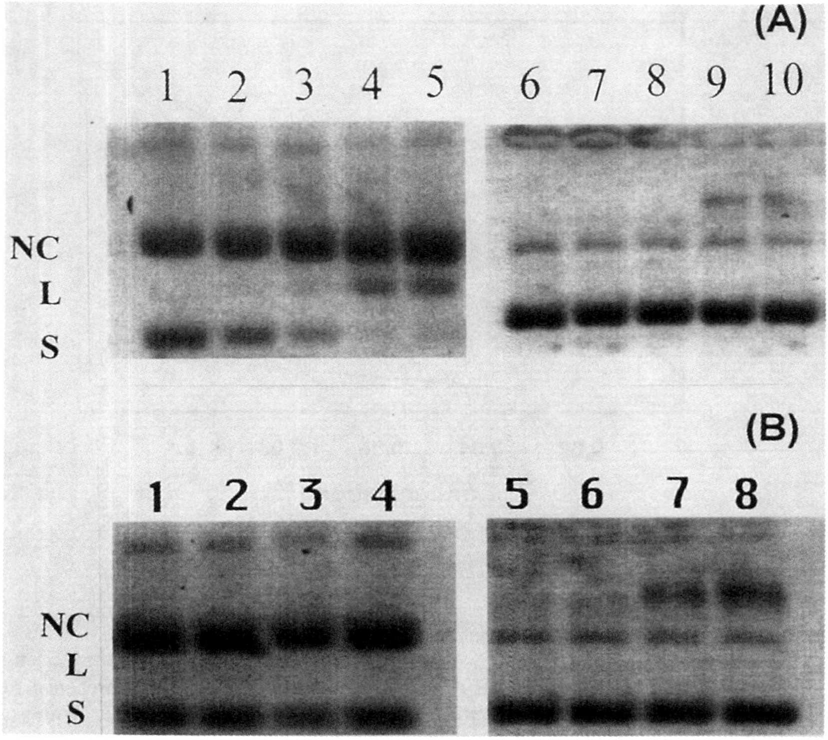

FIG. 5: MODULATION OF DNA STRAND SCISSIONS CAUSED BY Fe^{2+} AND Fe^{3+} IONS BY CRUDE GINSENG EXTRACT.

A: DNA strand scissions caused by Fe^{2+}, B: DNA strand scissions caused by Fe^{3+}.

S = supercoiled DNA, NC = nicked circular DNA, L = linear DNA.

Fig. 5A: Lane 1 = Original supercoiled plasmid DNA, Lane 2- 5 = DNA + 5, 10, 50, or 70 μM of Fe^{2+}, respectively, Lane 6 -10 = DNA + ginseng (0.5 g/mL) + 5, 10, 50, or 70 μM of Fe^{2+}, respectively.

Fig. 5B: Lane 1 = Original supercoiled plasmid DNA, Lane 2-4 = DNA + 10, 50, or 70 μM of Fe^{3+}, respectively, Lane 5-8 = DNA + ginseng (0.5 g/mL) + 10, 50, or 70 μM of Fe^{3+}, respectively.

CONCLUSION

The use of a battery of methods to test the characteristic antioxidant potential of a ginseng extract obtained from North American ginseng provided strong evidence to conclude that North American ginseng has a number of important antioxidant activities. Further characterization of the CNT-2000 ginseng extract is needed to define the contribution of ginsenosides and other plant phenolics to the observed antioxidant activity. Moreover, more studies are required to evaluate the apparent low prooxidant activity of the ginseng extract.

TABLE 1.
CUPRIC [CU(II)], FERRIC [FE(III)], AND FERROUS [FE(II)] ION CHELATING ACTIVITY OF GINSENG EXTRACT

Concentration of Total Metal[1] (μmol)	Bound Cu(II) μmol Cu(II)/ μg ginseng	Bound Fe(III) μmol Fe(III)/ μg ginseng	Bound Fe(II) μmol Fe(II)/ μg ginseng
10	0.0013	0.0017	0.00015
50	0.0039	0.0042	0.00011
100	0.0054	0.0047	0.00010

[1] = Amount of total Cu(II) or Fe(III) or Fe(II) added

ACKNOWLEDGMENTS

The authors thank CHAI-NA-TA for donation of the ginseng CNT-2000 extract. This study was funded by a industry-partnership grant from British Columbia, Agriculture, Fisheries and Food.

REFERENCES

ARUOMA, O.I., HALLIWELL, B., HOEY, B.M. and BUTLER, J. 1988. The antioxidant action of taurine, hypotaurine and their metabolic precursors. Biochem. J. *256*, 251–255.

ASAMARI, A.M., ADDIS, P.B., EPLEY, R.J. and KRICK, T.P. 1996. Wild rice hull antioxidants. J. Agric. Food Chem. *44*, 126–130.

BECKMAN, J.S., BECKMAN, T.W., CHEN, J., MARSHALL, P.A. and FREEMAN, B.A. 1990. Apparent hydoxyl radical production by peroxinitrite: Implications for endothelial injury from nitric oxide and superoxide. Proc. Natl. Acad. Sci. USA. *87*, 1620–1624.

BRAND-WILLIAMS, W., CUVELIER, M.E. and BERSET, C. 1995. Use of a free radical method to evaluate antioxidant activity. Lebensmittel-Wissenschaft-und-Technologie *28*, 25–30.

BYERS, T. and PERRY, G. 1992. Dietary carotenes, vitamin C, and vitamin E as protecting antioxidants in human cancers. Annu. Rev. Nutr. *12*, 139–159.

CAO, G., SOFIC, E. and PRIOR, R.L. 1996. Antioxidant capacity of tea and common vegetables. J. Agric. Food Chem. *44*: 3426–3431.

DRAPER, H.H. and HANDLEY, M. 1990. Malonaldehyde determination as an index of lipid peroxidation methods. Methods Enzymol. *186*, 421–431.

GRAF, E., MAHONEY, J.R., BRYANT, R.G. and EATON, J.W. 1984. Iron catalyzed hydroxyl radical formation: Stringent requirement for free ion coordination site. J. Biol. Chem. *259*, 3620–3624.

GUO, C., CAO, G., SOFIC, E. and PRIOR, R.L. 1997. High performance liquid chromatography coupled with coulometric array detection of electroactive components in fruits and vegetables: Relationship to oxygen radical absorbance. J. Agric. Food Chem. *45*; 1787–1796.

HALLIWELL, B. and GROOTVELD, M. 1987. Methods for the measurement of hydroxyl radicals in biochemical systems. Deoxyribose degradation and aromatic hydroxylation. Methods Biochem. Analysis *30*, 59–90.

HOMMA, S., AIDA, K. and FUJIMAKI, M. 1988. Chelation of metal with brown pigments of coffee. *In* Amino Carbonyl Reactions in Foods and Biological Systems. Fujimaki, M., Namiki, M. and Kato, H., eds. Elsevier, Amsterdam, Netherlands. p. 165.

KUO, C.F., MASHINO, T. and FRIDOVICH, I. 1987. Dihydroxyisovalerate dehydratase. A superoxide sensitive enzyme. J. Biol. Chem. *262*, 4724–4727.

LARSON, R.A. 1988. Review article number 30: The antioxidants of higher plants. Phytochemistry *27*, 969–978.

LAUGHTON, M.J., HALLIWELL, B., EVANS, P.J. and HOULT, J.R.S. 1989. Antioxidant and pro-oxidant actions of the plant phenolics quercetin, gossypol and myricetin. Biochem. Pharmacol. *38*, 859–865.

LINGERT, H., VALLETIN, K. and ERIKSSON, C.E. 1979. Measurement of antioxidant effect in model system. J. Food Process. Preserv. *3*, 87–103.

MAHONEY, J.R. and GRAF, E. 1986. Role of α-tocopherol, ascorbic acid and EDTA as oxidants in model systems. J. Food Sci. *51*, 1293–1296.

PETKOR, V.D. and MOSHARROF, A.H. 1987. Effects of standardized ginseng extract on learning, memory, and physical capabilities. Am. J. Chinese Med. *15*, 19–29.

RAMARATHNAM, N., OSAWA, T., NAMIKI, M. and KAWAKISHI, S. 1988. Chemical studies on novel rice hull antioxidants. I. Isolation, fractionation, partial characterization. J. Agric. Food Chem. *36*, 732–737.

SAMIRA, M.M.H., ATTIA, M.A., ALLAM, M. and ELWAN, O. 1985. Effects of the standardized ginseng extract G 115® on the metabolism and electrical activity of the rabbit brain. J. Int. Med. *13*, 342–347.

SCAGLIONE, F., FERRARA, F., DUGNANI, S., FALCHI, M., SANTROTO, G. and FRASCHINI, F. 1990. Immunomodulatory effects of two extracts of *Panax ginseng* C.A. Meyer. Drugs Exptl. Clin. Res. *16*, 537–542.

SHAHIDI, F. and NAZCK, M. 1995. *In* Food Phenolics: Sources, Chemistry, Effects and Applications. Lancaster Technomic Pub. Co. pp. 292–293.

YEN, G.C. and CHEN, H.Y. 1995. Antioxidant activity of various tea extracts in relation to their antimutagenicity. J. Agri. Food Chem. *43*, 27–30.

YUAN, Y.V. and KITTS, D.D. 1997. Endogenous antioxidants: Role of antioxidant enzymes in biological systems. *In* Natural Antioxidants: Chemistry, Health Effects and Applications F. Shahidi, (ed.). AOAC Press, Champaign, IL. pp. 258–270.

ZHANG, D., YASUDA, T., YU, Y., ZHENG, P., KAWABATA, T., MA, Y. and OKADA, S. 1996. Ginseng extract scavenges hydroxyl radical and protects unsaturated fatty acids from decomposition caused by iron-mediated lipid peroxidation. Free Rad. Biol. Med. *20*, 145–150.

ANTIOXIDATIVE ACTIVITY AND MECHANISM OF ISOLATED COMPONENTS FROM FLOWERS OF *DELONIX REGIA*

JENG-DE SU and CHANG-TENG FAN

Department of Food Science
Tunghai University
Taichung, Taiwan 407, R.O.C.

ABSTRACT

The purpose of this study was to isolate and identify the major antioxidative components from the flowers of Delonix regia. *The antioxidative mechanisms of the isolated components were also studied.*

The antioxidative ethyl acetate extract of flowers of Delonix regia *was fractionated and purified by various chromatographies to obtain four isolated components which were identified as 2'-(3",4",5"-trihydroxyphenyl)-ethyl-margarate (**1**), isorhamnetin 3-0-β-D-glucopyranoside (**2**), quercetin-3-0-β-D-xylopyranoside (**3**) and quercetin (**4**). The antioxidative efficiency of the isolated components found was in the order of BHA=**1**>**3**->**4**>α-tocopherol >**2**>control by using the thiocyanate method.*

*The results from antioxidative mechanism studies showed that **1** had strong activity in hydrogen peroxide scavenging effect. It also showed good activity on hydrogen-donating and superoxide anion scavenging effect, and inhibition on DEMP-OH formation, but had poor activity on singlet oxygen scavenging and metal chelating effects. Both **3** and **4** not only had equal activity to BHA on hydrogen donating and hydrogen peroxide scavenging effects, but also had good activity on superoxide anion scavenging. In spite of their metal chelating ability they were not as good as EDTA; they exhibited the better activity on metal chelating, hydroxy radical-scavenging and singlet oxygen scavenging effects than the others. **2** didn't show any good activity in all antioxidative mechanism tests.*

INTRODUCTION

The flower of *Delonix regia* (Boj.) Rof., which exhibits a bright red color, is also called the peacock flower because of its shape (Hu 1982). *D. regia* grows in the central and southern part of Taiwan, especially on all school campuses. The flower stands for graduation in Taiwan because when it's in full bloom in June, school graduations are coming soon. The red color of the flower lasts throughout the whole summer even if the flower falls down. This stimulated us to investigate whether it contains antioxidants against photo-oxidation (Barber 1965; Kano and Miyakashi 1976).

In the previous paper, the isolation and identification of two antioxidant anthocyanins, cyanindin-3-0-β-rutinoside and cyanidin-3-0-β-glucoside, from the flowers of *D. regia* were reported (Fan and Su 1996). In this study, we investigated the separation, isolation, and identification of the four phenolic components of these flowers. In addition, we studied the antioxidative mechanisms of the isolated components by means of determination of the inhibitory effects on reactive oxygens.

MATERIALS AND METHODS

Material

The flowers of *D. regia* were picked and collected from the plants growing in the campus of Tunghai University, Taichung, Taiwan, R.O.C. The weight of the decalyxed flowers was six kg.

Extraction, Separation and Isolation Procedure

The decalyxed flowers were extracted with methanol. The methanol extract was then extracted with *n*-hexane, ethyl acetate, and *n*-butanol successively. The ethyl acetate extract was separated and the phenolic compounds isolated by silica gel, thin layer, gel filtration and high performance liquid chromatographies to obtain the isolated components **1**, **2**, **3** and **4**. 1, 2′-(3″,4″,5″-trihydroxyphenyl)-ethyl-margarate; 2, isorhamnetin 3-O-β-D-glucopranoside. R_1 = Me, R_2 = glycosyl; 3, Quercetin-3-O-β-D-xylopyranoside. R_1 = H, R_2 = xylosyl; and 4, Quercetin. R_1 = H, R_2 = H.

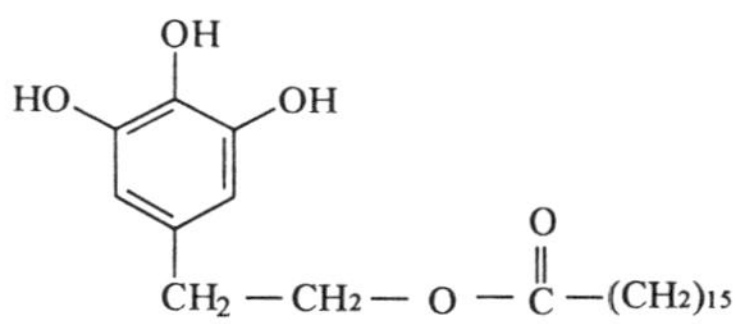

1

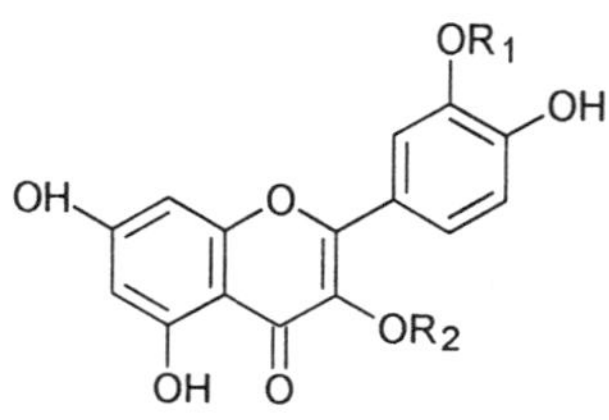

2	R_1=Me ,	R_2=glucosyl
3	R_1=H ,	R_2=xylosyl
4	R_1=H ,	R_2=H

Antioxidative Activity Determination

The antioxidative activity of extracts and isolated components were measured by the thiocyanate method (Osawa and Namiki 1985). 200 μl of sample solution (mg/ml) was added to a solution of linoleic acid (0.13 ml) in 99.0% ethanol (10 ml) and 0.2 M phosphate buffer (pH 7.0, 10 ml) and the volume was made up to 25 ml with distilled water. The mixed solution was incubated in a conical flask at 40°C. At regular intervals, the extent of peroxidation was determined with 9.6 ml of ethanol (75%), 0.2 ml of an aqueous solution of ammonium thiocyanate (30%) and 0.2 ml of ferrous chloride solution (20 mM in 3.5% HCl) being added sequentially. After stirring for 3 min, the absorbance of the mixture measured at 500 nm was used as the peroxide value. Chloroform was used as control.

Hydrogen Donating Activity Determination

A volume of 0.08% 1,1-diphenyl-2-picrylhydrazyl (DPPH) in 50% methanol solution, freshly prepared, was added to the isolated component solution (1 ml). After mixing, the absorbance of the mixture was measured at 528 nm (Shimada *et al.* 1992) BHA was used as a reference standard.

Fe^{2+} Binding Activity Determination

Each 1.0 ml of hexamine (30 mM), potassium chloride (30 mM) and ferrous sulfate (9 mM) and 0.2 ml of tetramethyl murexide (TMM,1 mM) were added to 2 ml of the isolated component solution. The absorbance of the mixed solution was measured at 485 nm after reaction for 3 min at the room temperature (Shimada *et al.* 1992). Ethylene diaminetetraacetic acid (EDTA) was used as reference standard.

Hydrogen Peroxide Scavenging Activity

4 mM H_2O_2 solution was prepared in phosphate buffer-saline (pH 7.4). The solution (3 ml) was added to the isolated component solution (2 ml). After thorough mixing for 10 min, the absorbance of the mixture was measured at 230 nm (Ruch *et al.* 1989; Wu 1995).

Measurement of Superoxide Anion Scavenging Activity

40 μM phenazinemethosulfate (PMS), 312 μM dihydronicotinamide adenine dinucleotide (NADH) and 100 μM nitroblue tetrazolium (NBT) were prepared in 0.1 M phosphate buffer (pH 7.4). Each one ml of PMS, NADH and NBT solution was added to one ml of the isolated component solution. The absorbance of the mixture produced at room temperature in 5 min was measured at 560 nm (Robak and Gryglewski 1988).

Hydroxy Radical Scavenging Activity

A 0.1 ml of the isolated component solution was added to 0.5 ml of potassium phosphate buffer (pH 7), and then 0.01 ml of EDTA (166 mM), 0.1 ml of hydrogen peroxide (0.62 mM), 0.1 ml of 22.4 mM 5,5′-dimethyl-1-pyrroline N-oxide (DMPO) and 0.2 ml of ferric sulfate solution (0.04 mM) were added successively. The reaction solution was analyzed by ESR spectrometry (Kumuda and Hara 1992).

Singlet Oxygen Scavenging Activity

1.6 ml of potassium phosphate buffer (pH 7) was added to a mixture containing 0.1 ml of the isolated component, 0.2 ml of 2,2,6,6-tetramethyl-piperidine (TEMP) and 0.1

ml of rose bengal solutions. After irradiation under strong light, the reaction solution was analyzed by ESR spectrometry (Kumuda and Hara 1992).

Analyses of the Phenols

2′-(3″,4″,5″-Trihydroxyphenyl)-ethyl-margarate (1). Formula: $C_{25}H_{42}O_5$; UV-visible λ_{max}nm: in (MeOH) 278 and 283 nm; FAB-MS (*m/z*): 422[M^+]; ^{1}H-NMR($CDCl_3$ at 300M*Hz*) δ: 0.88, 1.28, 1.42 (31H, alkyl protons), 2.58 (2H, t, *J*=7.2*Hz*, H-2), 2.83 (2H, t, *J*=7.2*Hz*, H-2′), 4.08 (2H, t, *J*=7.2*Hz*, H-1′), 6.99 (2H, s, H-2″ and H-6″); ^{13}C-NMR($CDC1_3$ at 75M*Hz*) δ: 14.09-36.50 (17C, alkyl carbons), 64.63 (C-1′), 124.79 (C-2″ and C-6″), 131.18 (C-4″), 135.89 (C-1″), 152.20 (C-3″, C-5″), 173.80 (C-1).

Isorhamnetin-3-O-β-D-glucopyranoside (2). Formula: $C_{22}H_{22}O_{12}$; UV-visible λmax nm: (MeOH) 254 and 355 nm, (NaOMe) 272, 330, and 413, ($AlCl_3$) 254 and 356, (NaOAc) 274, 324, and 404, (NaOAc/H_3BO_3), 361; FAB-MS (*m/z*): 479 $[M+1]^+$, 317 [M-glucose+H_2O+1]$^+$; NMR($CDCl_3$ at 300M*Hz*) δ: 3.23-3.78 (5H, sugar protons), 3.94 (3H, m, OCH_3), 5.40 (1H, d, *J*=7.5*Hz*, H-1″), 6.19 (1H, d, *J*=1.8*Hz*, H-6), 6.39 (1H, d, *J*=1.8*Hz*, H-8), 6.89 (1H, d, *J*=8.4*Hz*, H-5′), 7.58 (1H, dd, *J*=1.8*Hz* & 8.4*Hz*, H-6′), 7.93 (1H, d, *J*=1.8*Hz*, H-2′); ^{13}C-NMR($CDCl_3$ at 75M*Hz*) δ: 56.75 (3′-OCH_3), 62.51 (C-6″), 71.48(C-4″), 75.93 (C-2″), 78.08 (C-5″), 78.59 (C-3″), 94.86 (C-8), 100.08 (C-6), 103.60(C-1″), 105.65 (C-10), 114.47 (C-5′), 116.03 (C-2′), 123.15 (C-1′), 123.82 (C-6′), 135.32 (C-3), 148.46 (C-4′), 150.90 (C-3′), 157.48 (C-9), 158.65 (C-2), 163.16 (C-5), 166.66 (C-7), 179.45 (C-4).

Quercetin-3-O-β-D-xylopyranoside (3). Formula: $C_{20}H_{18}O_{11}$; UV-visible λmax nm: (MeOH) 256 and 358, (NaOMe) 271, 327 and 407, ($AlCl_3$) 265 and 391, ($AlCl_3$/HCl) 268 and 364, (NaOAc) 273, 324 and 400, (NaOAc/H_3BO_3) 262 and 380; FAB-MS (*m/z*): 435 $[M+1]^+$, 303 [M-xylose+H_2O+1]$^+$; ^{1}H-NMR($CDC1_3$ at 300M*Hz*) δ: 3.09-3.91 (6H, sugar protons), 5.15 (1H, d, *J*=6.6*Hz*, H-1″), 6.18 (1H, d, *J*=2.4*Hz*, H-6), 6.37 (1H, d, *J*=2.4*Hz*, H-8), 6.86 (1H, d, *J*=8.4*Hz*, H-5′), 7.58 (1H, dd, *J*=2.4*Hz* & 8.4*Hz*, H-6′), 7.74 (1H, d, *J*=2.4*Hz*, H-2′); ^{13}C-NMR($CDCl_3$ at 75M*Hz*) δ: 66.98 (C-5″), 71.01 (C-4″), 75.29 (C-2″), 77.57 (C-3″), 94.87 (C-8), 100.12 (C-6), 104.68 (C-1″), 105.483 (C-10), 116.21 (C-5′), 117.46 (C-2′), 122.92 (C-5′) 123.31 (C-6′), 135.66 (C-3), 146.04 (C-3′), 150.02 (C-4′), 158.54 (C-9), 158.67 (C-2), 163.07 (C-5), 166.75 (C-7), 179.48 (C-4).

Quercetin (4). Formula: $C_{15}H_{10}O_7$; UV-visible λmax nm (MeOH) 255 and 370, (NaOMe) 279, 324 and 418, ($AlCl_3$) 266 and 430, ($AlCl_3$/HCl) 267, 374 and 431, (NaOAc) 275, 322 and 398, (NaOAc/H_3BO_3) 259 and 386; FAB-MS (*m/z*): 303 $[M+1]^+$; ^{1}H-NMR($CDCl_3$ at 300M*Hz*) δ: 6.17 (1H, d, *J*=2.1*Hz*, H-6), 6.37 (1H, d, *J*=2.1*Hz*, H-8), 6.88 (1H, d, *J*=8.7*Hz*, H-5′), 7.62 (1H, dd, *J*=2.1 *Hz* & 8.7*Hz*, H-6′), 7.73 (1 H, d, *J*=2.1*Hz*, H-2′); ^{13}C-NMR($CDCl_3$ at 75M*Hz*) δ: 94.46 (C-8), 99.31 (C-6), 104.51 (C-10), 116.02 (C-2′), 116.27 (C-5′), 121.70 (C-6′), 124.19 (C-1′), 137.28 (C-3), 146.29 (C-3′), 148.03 (C-2), 148.84 (C-4′), 158.31 (C-9), 162.58 (C-5), 165.80 (C-7), 177.40 (C-4).

RESULTS AND DISCUSSION

Identification of Antioxidative Components

The extraction, separation and isolation of the antioxidative components from the flowers of *D. regia* are shown in Fig. 1. The ethyl acetate extract of the flowers was chromatographed on the silica gel column to give thirteen fractions. Fraction (I) was purified on preparative HPLC and TLC chromatographies to give **1**. Then fraction (XII) was purified on HPLC and Toyo Pearl HW-40F column chromatographies to give 2-**4**. The isolated components **1-4** were identified as 2′, (3″,4″,5″-trihydroxyphenyl)-ethyl-margarate, isorhamnetin-3-O-β-D-glucopyranoside, quercetin-3-O-β-D-xylopyranoside and quercetin, respectively, by the published data on MS, UV, ^{1}H-NMR and ^{13}C NMR spectra.

The calculated yield of isolated components were **1**, 0.008%; **2**, 0.00073%; **3**, 0.000175%; and **4**, 0.0013% by means of HPLC co-chromatography.

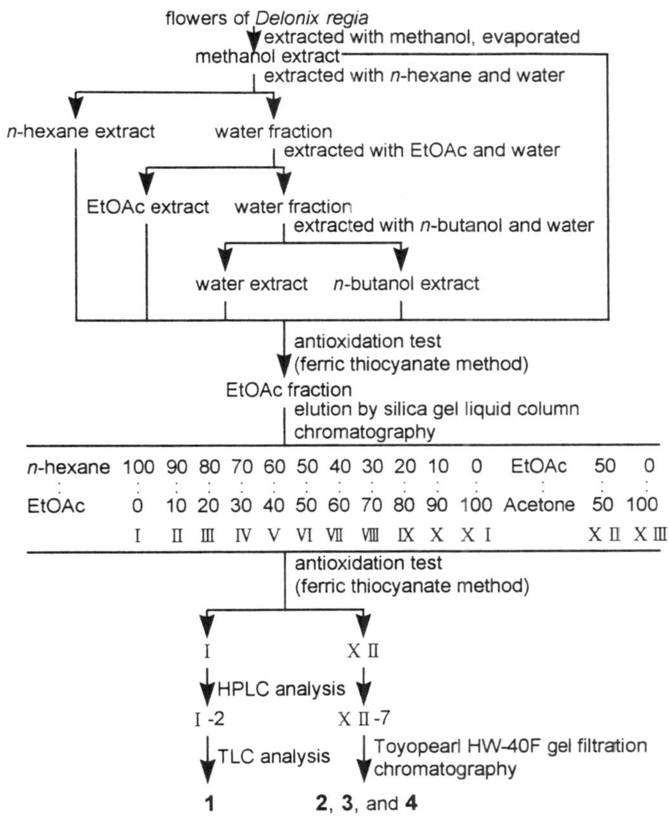

FIG. 1. SCHEME OF SEPARATION AND ISOLATION OF TYPICAL ANTIOXIDANTS FROM FLOWERS OF *DELONIX REGIA*

Effect on Autoxidation of Linoleic Acid in Alcohol-Water System

The inhibitory effect on oxidation of the isolated phenolic components was examined in the alcohol-water model system with the thiocyanate method (Osawa and Su 1996). Each sample (0.2 mg), α-tocopherol and BHA were used as references in the assay. As shown in Fig. 2, **1** markedly inhibited the formation of linoleic acid hydroperoxides, more than that of BHA. **3** and **4** exhibited stronger activities than that of α-tocopherol. The antioxidative efficiency increased in the order of control **2** < α-tocopherol < **4** < **3** < BHA < **1** (Fig. 2).

Hydrogen Donating Activity

The primary antioxidants, such as ascorbic acid and triose reductone, mean that they can donate a proton to the alkyl peroxyl radical formed by lipid autoxidation in order to break the chain reaction (Shimada *et al.* 1992). As shown in Table 1, the hydrogen donating activities of **3** and **4** were similar to that of BHA on stabilizing the DDPH radical, and **1** and **2** exhibited weaker activity. The results show that the isolated components of the flowers also belong to the primary antioxidants which can donate a proton to the alkyl peroxyl radicals.

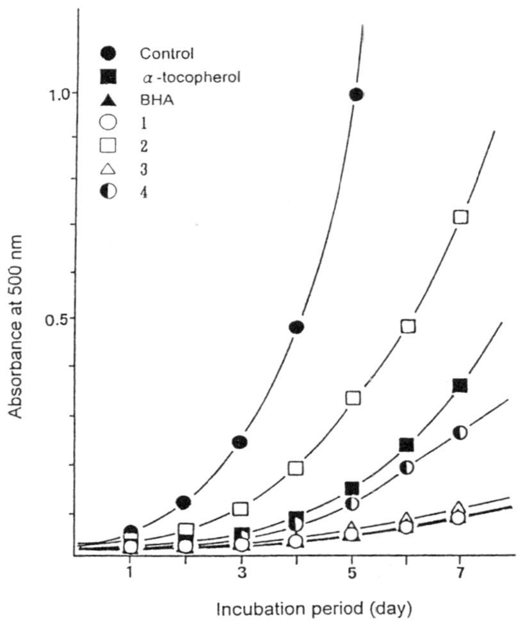

FIG. 2. ANTIOXIDATIVE ACTIVITY OF THE ISOLATED COMPONENTS FROM THE ETHYL ACETATE EXTRACT OF FLOWERS OF *DELONIX REGIA*

0.2 mg of each sample, α-tocopherol and BHA, were used for the assay. ●, 2′-(3″, 4″, 5″-trihydroxyphenyl)-ethyl-margarate (**1**) □, isorhamnetin-3-O-β-D-glucopyranoside (**2**); Δ, quercetin-3-O-β-D-xylopyranoside (**3**) and ◐, quercetin (**4**)

TABLE 1.
THE EFFECT OF THE ISOLATED COMPONENTS FROM FLOWERS OF *DELONIX REGIA* ON 50% DPPH RADICAL SCAVENGING ACTIVITY

sample	50% reduction (mg/ml)
BHA	0.0251
1	0.0551
2	0.0632
3	0.0252
4	0.0277

1, 2′-(3″,4″, 5″-trihydroxyphenyl)-ethyl-margarate; **2**, isorhamnetin-3-O-β-D-glucopyranoside; **3**, quercetin-3-O-β-D-xylopyranoside; and **4**, quercetin.

Fe^{2+} Binding Activity

The transition metals (eg. copper and iron) are major pro-oxidants that can decrease the length of the induction period and increase the rate of oxidation even at low concentrations such as 0.1 ppm. As shown in Table 2, the concentration of **3** and **4** were 3.177 and 3.439 mg/ml, respectively, and exhibited markedly weaker activity than that of EDTA in chelating 50% Fe^{2+}. The Fe^{2+} chelating activity of flavonoids is due to 3-hydroxy-4-keto or 5-hydroxy-4-keto structures (Hudson and Lewis 1983). Although **2**, **3** and **4** exist in both structures they don't show good chelating activity.

TABLE 2.
THE EFFECT OF THE ISOLATED COMPONENTS FROM FLOWERS OF *DELONIX REGIA* ON 50% Fe^{2+} CHELATING ACTIVITY

sample	50% reduction (mg/ml)
BHA	0.121
1	not calculated
2	not detected
3	3.177
4	3.439

1, 2′-(3″,4″, 5″-trihydroxyphenyl)-ethyl-margarate; **2**, isorhamnetin-3-O-β-D-glucopyranoside; **3**, quercetin-3-O-β-D-xylopyranoside; and **4**, quercetin.

Hydrogen Peroxide Scavenging Activity

Hydrogen peroxide doesn't have a direct influence on lipid autoxidation, but hydroxy radical formed by the reaction of Fe^{2+} and hydrogen peroxide is a stronger pro-oxidant (Namiki 1990). The hydrogen peroxide scavenging activity of **1** is similar to that of BHA, and **3** and **4** showed a medium activity (Table 3).

TABLE 3.
THE EFFECT OF THE ISOLATED COMPONENTS FROM FLOWERS OF *DELONIX REGIA* ON 50% REDUCTION OF HYDROGEN PEROXIDE SCAVENGING ACTIVITY

sample	50% reduction (mg/ml)
BHA	0.029
1	0.030
2	not detected
3	0.049
4	0.045

1, 2′-(3″,4″, 5″-trihydroxyphenyl)-ethyl-margarate; **2**, isorhamnetin-3-O-β-D-glucopyranoside; **3**, quercetin-3-O-β-D-xylopyranoside; and **4**, quercetin.

Superoxide Anion Scavenging Activity

Robak and Grayglewsk (1988) indicated that some flavonoids are capable of scavenging superoxide anions formed by both the enzymatic and nonenzymatic systems. The isolated flavonols **3** and **4** showed strong scavenging activity on superoxide anion, and **1** and **2** had medium activity (Table 4). BHA had no activity on scavenging superoxide anion.

TABLE 4.
THE EFFECT OF THE ISOLATED COMPONENTS FROM FLOWERS OF *DELONIX REGIA* ON 50% SUPEROXIDE ANION SCAVENGING ACTIVITY

sample	50% reduction (mg/ml)
BHA	0.029
1	0.030
2	not detected
3	0.049
4	0.045

1, 2′-(3″,4″, 5″-trihydroxyphenyl)-ethyl-margarate; **2**, isorhamnetin-3-O-β-D-glucopyranoside; **3**, quercetin-3-O-β-D-xylopyranoside; and **4**, quercetin.

Hydroxy Radical Scavenging Activity

Namiki (1990) indicated that the hydroxy radical is the most important pro-oxidant of reactive oxygen which causes lipid peroxidation (Namiki 1990). Hydroxy radical occurring in biological cells also attacks and damages the important compounds such as DNA, phospholipid and protein (Gutteridge and Halliwel 1994). The scavenging activity of **1**, **2**, **3** and **4** at the concentration of 0.5 mg/ml on hydroxy radical was 94.8%, 53.4%, 84.7% and 81.5%, respectively (Table 5). The results indicate that the hydroxy radical scavenging activity of the isolated components from the flowers is an important inhibitory factor on lipid peroxidation.

TABLE 5.
INHIBITION OF THE ISOLATED COMPONENTS FROM FLOWERS OF *DELONIX REGIA* ON THE FORMATION OF DMPO-OH ADDUCTS

Sample (mg/ml)	1	2	3	4
0.00	100	100	100	100
0.05	87.5	99.7	97.6	94.1
0.10	38.5	69.2	57.1	42.3
0.50	5.2	47.6	15.3	18.5

Singlet Oxygen Scavenging Activity

Singlet oxygen can be generated in a variety of ways. Probably the most important way is via photosensitization by the natural pigments in foods. The pro-oxidant rate of singlet oxygen is ~ 1500 times faster than that of triplet oxygen. The singlet oxygen scavenging activity of the isolated components was in the order of **4** > **3** > 2 > **1**, as shown in Table 6. Components **4** and **3** showed good activity.

The qualitative analysis of carotenoids was also carried out by thin layer chromatography. The results showed that α-, β- and γ-carotene, which exhibited singlet oxygen quenching activity, were found in the flowers (data not shown). From the previous and current studies, it can be concluded that all these antioxidants, such as anthocyanins, carotenoids, flavonoids and polyphenolic compounds, play an important role against photooxidation in the flower of *D. regia*.

TABLE 6.
INHIBITION OF THE ISOLATED COMPONENTS FROM FLOWERS OF *DELONIX REGIA* ON THE FORMATION OF TEMP-$^1O_2$ ADDUCTS

Sample (mg\ml)	1	2	3	4
0.000	100	100	100	100
0.025	100	98.2	82.4	78.1
0.05	94.1	96.4	79.8	72.3
0.25	89.5	83.8	49.4	43.7

REFERENCES

BARBER, H.N. 1965. Selection in natural populations. Heredity *20*, 551–559.

FAN, C.-T. and SU, J.-D. (1996). Anthocyanins of the flowers of *Delonix regia*. Tunghai J. *37*, 35–54.

GUTTERIDGE, J.M.C. and HALLIWELL, B. 1994. Antioxidants in nutrition, health and disease. Oxford University Press, Oxford.

HU, D.-W. 1982. Garden Vegetation(II), p. 59. Jeou-Jeou Ltd.,Taipei.

HUDSON, B.J.F. and LEWIS. J.I. 1983. Polyhydroxy flavonoid antioxidants for edible oils; Structural criteria for activity. Food Chem. *10*, 47–55.

IGARASHI, K., TAKANASHI, K., MAKINO, M. and YASUI, T. 1989. Antioxidative activity of major anthocyanin isolated from wild grapes (*Vitis coignetiae*). Nippon Shokuhin Kogyo Gakkaishi *36*, 852–856.

KANO, E. and MIYAKOSHI, J. 1976. UV protection effect of keracyanin and anthocyanin derivatives on cultured mouse fibroblast L cells. J. Radiat. Res. *17*, 55–61.

KUMUDA, C.D. and HARA, P.M. 1992. Lidocaine: a hydroxyl radical scavenger and singlet oxygen quencher. Mol Cell. Biochem. *115*, 179–185.

NAMIKI, M. 1990. Antioxidant/antimutagens in foods. Crit. Rev. Food Sci. Nutr. *29*, 281-300.

OSAWA, T. and NAMIKI, M. 1985. A novel type of antioxidants isolated from leaf waxes of *Eucalyptus* leaves. J. Agric. Food Chem. *33*,777–780.

ROBAK, J. and GRYGLEWSKI, R.J. 1988. Flavonoids are scavengers of superoxide anions. Biochem. Pharm. *37*, 837–841.

RUCH, R.J., CHEMG, S.-J. and KLAUNING, J.E. 1989. Prevention of cytotoxicity and inhibition of intercellular communication by antioxidant catechins isolated from Chinese green tea. Carcinogenesis *10*, 1003–1008.

SHIMADA, K., FUJIKAWA, K., YAHARA, K. and NAKAMURA, T. 1992. Antioxidative properties of xanthan on the autoxidation of soybean oil in cyclodextrin emulsion. J. Agric. Food Chem. *40*, 945–948.

WU, S.-J. 1995. Antioxidative components of Mulberry (*Morus alba L.*) leaves. Master's Dissertation of Chung Hsing University, Taichung, Taiwan.

ABSORPTION, METABOLISM AND ANTIOXIDANT EFFECTS OF TEA CATECHIN IN HUMANS

TERUO MIYAZAWA and KIYOTAKA NAKAGAWA

Food Chemistry Laboratory
Department of Applied Biological Chemistry
Tohoku University
Sendai 981, Japan

ABSTRACT

To investigate its absorption and metabolism, we established a chemiluminescence detection-high performance liquid chromatography (CL-HPLC) method to measure plasma (-)-epigallocatechin-3-gallate (EGCg). In humans, the EGCg concentration in fasted plasma was initially below 0.002 nmol/ml (0.9 ng/ml), but dose-dependently increased to 0.65-4.4 nmol/ml (300 - 2020 ng/ml) at 90 min after a single oral intake of 225-525 mg EGCg (corresponded to 2-6 cups of green tea drink). On the other hand, the EGCg levels in rats reached 12.3 nmol/ml in plasma, 48.4 nmol/g in liver, 0.5 nmol/g in brain, 565 nmol/g in small intestinal mucosa and 68.6 nmol/g in colon mucosa at 60 min after an oral ingestion (500 mg EGCg/kg body weight). These findings suggested that tea catechin, EGCg, is absorbed from the digestive tract into blood plasma and tissue organelles in humans, with the intestinal mucosa the most enriched of the organelles. Our recent finding that colon mucosal phospholipid hydroperoxidation in the colon carcinogenic rats is effectively prevented by oral EGCg and the marked accumulation of EGCg in intestinal mucosa and in plasma suggest that the ingested EGCg acts as an effective antioxidative nutrient in preventing intestinal carcinogenesis and atherosclerosis in humans.

INTRODUCTION

(-)-Epigallocatechin-3-gallate (EGCg; Fig. 1) is a tea catechin and is consumed as a popular beverage in Japan and other Asian countries. In recent years, several epidemiologic studies have suggested a lower risk of gastric cancer for green tea drinkers (Kono *et al.* 1988). Tea catechins have been reported to act as water-soluble antioxidants *in vitro* by scavenging oxygen radicals and by chelating metal ions (Rice-Evans 1995; Morel *et al.* 1994). Of these, EGCg has the most effective antioxidant activity (Katiyar *et al.* 1994). If EGCg could be efficiently incorporated into the tissue organelles and blood plasma, its antioxidant activity may provide a beneficial effect in cases involving membrane phospholipid peroxidation, such as development of colon cancer and atherosclerosis (Matsumoto *et al.* 1996). The substantial incorporation of EGCg into tissue organelles of mammals has never been fully confirmed. It is therefore of interest to examine whether EGCg orally ingested is absorbed and incorporated directly in the free form into intestinal mucosa, liver and other tissues.

Recently, we established a chemiluminescence detection-high performance liquid chromatography (CL-HPLC) method for the sensitive and selective assay of EGCg

(Nakagawa and Miyazawa 1997a). This method enables EGCg to be determined in the free form at picomole levels in rat and human plasma. In this study, we employed the CL-HPLC method and confirmed the absorption of EGCg in the free form into human plasma and also investigated EGCg in small intestinal mucosa, colon mucosa, liver and brain of the rat after oral ingestion.

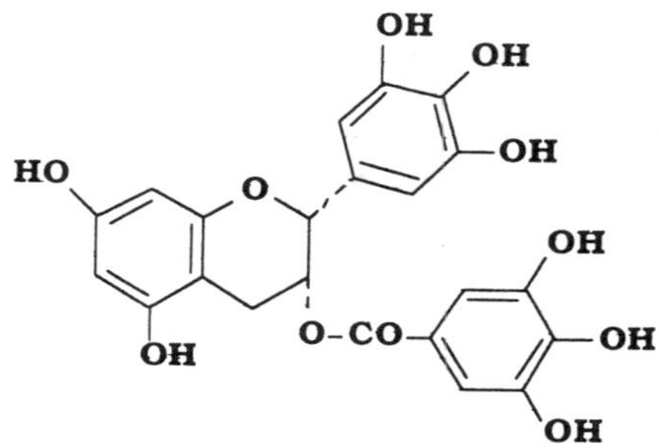

FIG. 1. STRUCTURE OF (-)-EPIGALLOCATECHIN-3-GALLATE (EGCg)

MATERIALS AND METHODS

CL-HPLC

The CL-HPLC system (Fig. 2) used in the EGCg assay was the same as that reported in the methods paper (Nakagawa and Miyazawa 1997a). Briefly, the CL-HPLC system consisted of reversed phase HPLC and chemiluminescence detector, in which separated EGCg generates chemiluminescence after post column modification, successively reacting with the following two chemiluminescence cocktails; 8.2 M acetaldehyde in 50 mM phosphate buffer (pH 7.4, containing 108 mg horseradish peroxidase/L) and 8.8 M hydrogen peroxide aqueous solution. The standard EGCg solution was made by dissolving authentic EGCg in a Vc-EDTA solution which consisted of 2% ascorbic acid and 0.1% ethylenediamine tetraacetic acid disodium salt (EDTA) in 0.4 M NaH_2PO_4 buffer, pH 3.9. The concentrations of EGCg in the sample solutions were determined from a calibration curve made with standard EGCg solution.

Human Study

Two female and one male adult volunteers (21-23 years old, non-smokers) participated in this study. After fasting for 12 h, each volunteer orally ingested 3, 5 or 7 capsules of green tea extract (Sunphenon DCF-1®, Taiyo Kagaku Co., Yokkaichi, Japan; corresponding, respectively, to 225, 375 and 525 mg EGCg/subject) (Nakagawa *et al.* 1997). Blood from the subjects was collected into heparinized tubes before and at 90 min after the ingestion and submitted to EGCg assay by CL-HPLC.

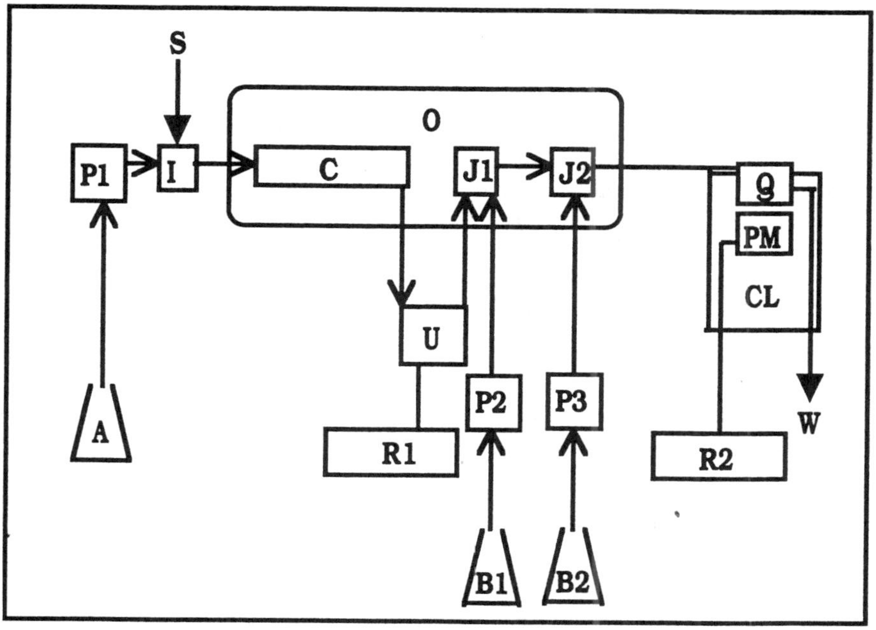

FIG. 2. SCHEMATIC DIAGRAM OF CL-HPLC FOR EGCG ASSAY
A=mobile phase, methanol-water (2:8, v/v, containing 0.1% phosphoric acid, 1.0 ml/min flow rate); P1, P2 and P3 = pumps (Jasco PU-980); I=sample injection valve (Rheodyne Model 7125, 100 μl); O = column oven (Jasco CO-963, at 40°C); S=sample; C=ODS column (Merck Lichrospher RP-18(e), 4250 mm, in a column oven at 40°C); U=UV detector (Jasco UV-980, at 280 nm); J1 and J2 = mixing joints (Kyowa Seimitsu Y type, in a column oven at 40°C); B1 = chemiluminescence reagent B (8.8 M hydrogen peroxide aqueous solution) at a 1.0 ml/min flow rate; B2 = chemiluminescence reagent A (8.2 M acetaldehyde in 50 mM phosphate buffer at pH 7.4, containing 108 mg HRP (horseradish peroxidase)/L) at a 3.0 ml/min flow rate; Q=flow cell; PM = photomultiplier; CL=chemiluminescence detector (CLD-100); R1 and R2 = integrators; W=waste.

Rat Study

Male Sprague-Dawley rats (9-weeks old, 290-300 g body wt, n=12) were unfed for 24 h, and six of the rats received once by stomach tube the EGCg (500 mg/kg body weight) dissolved in 2.5 ml distilled water (Nakagawa and Miyazawa 1997b). The other six rats (control rats) were not treated with EGCg. The EGCg (above 95 % purity) was provided from Taiyo Kagaku Co. After 60 min of EGCg administration, blood was collected from the abdominal artery with a heparinized syringe. Then the liver and brain were perfused *in situ* with ice-cold 0.15 M saline, and the liver, brain, small intestinal mucosa and colon mucosa were excised.

Extraction and Determination of EGCg

Plasma was prepared by centrifuging the heparinized blood at 1000 × g for 15 min at 4°C. Rat liver, brain, small intestinal mucosa and colon mucosa (500 mg of each) was minced and homogenized in 2.5 ml of Vc-EDTA solution with a Teflon-glass homogenizer. For the EGCg determination, plasma (250 μl, diluted with the same volume of Vc-EDTA solution) and tissue homogenates (500 μl, 20% w/w) were used. To each sample, 500 μl of acetonitrile was added, and the mixture was vortexed for 5 min, after which 3 ml of ethyl acetate was added (Nakagawa *et al.* 1997; Nakagawa and Miyazawa 1997b). This mixture was vortexed again vigorously for 4 min and centrifuged (1000×g) at 4°C for 15 min. The supernatant ethyl acetate layer was collected. This ethyl acetate extraction was repeated three times. The combined ethyl acetate layer was evaporated to dryness with a rotary evaporator. The dried extract was redissolved in 900 μl of methanol/water (8:1, v/v) and passed through a HPLC chromatodisc with 4 ml of methanol as eluant to exclude contaminated cell debris. The methanol filtrate was evaporated to dryness and dissolved in an appropriate amount of 10% acetonitrile aqueous solution. An aliquot of this acetonitrile aqueous solution was injected into the CL-HPLC system to determine the EGCg concentration. The EGCg peak on the chemiluminescence chromatogram was identified by comparing its retention time with that of standard EGCg. The EGCg recovery was 84% for human plasma, 86% for rat plasma, 70% for rat liver, 65% for rat brain, 70% for rat intestinal mucosa and 74% for rat colon mucosa.

RESULTS AND DISCUSSION

CL-HPLC Chromatogram of EGCg

No chemiluminescence peak was detected in the control human plasma. The plasma from the subject who received catechin capsules (equivalent to 525 mg EGCg/subject) gave an intense chemiluminescence peak ascribed to EGCg (Fig. 3). This EGCg peak (10.7 min retention time) was identical in its retention time to that of standard EGCg. When human plasma obtained after EGCg ingestion was treated with tannase, which is capable of hydrolyzing the galloyl ester of EGCg, the EGCg peak in the plasma extract disappeared (data not shown). No interference peaks were observed on the chemiluminescence chromatograms of the human plasma extracts. The results indicated that a substantial amount of EGCg in the free form is absorbed and is present in human plasma after the EGCg ingestion.

Distribution of EGCg in Human Plasma and Rat Tissues

Figure 4 shows plasma EGCg concentrations at 90 min after a single oral administration of 3, 5 or 7 capsules of green tea extract (Sunphenon DCF-1, corresponded, respectively, to 225, 375 and 525 mg EGCg) to the healthy volunteers. Plasma EGCg level before the administration was below the detection limit (< 0.002 nmol/ml). Ninety min after a single oral intake, EGCg was significantly increased to 0.65, 4.3 and 4.4 nmol/ml (300, 1970 and 2020 ng/ml) in the subjects who received 3, 5 and 7 capsules, respectively. The results suggested a dose-dependent incorporation of EGCg in the free form into human plasma (Nakagawa *et al.* 1997). The total amount of EGCg in the blood mass was calculated to be 450-7500 μg/subject, accounting for 0.2%-2.0% of ingested EGCg, when the whole blood mass was estimated to be 4 L/subject. The catechin supplementation had no effect on the basal levels of human plasma endogenous antioxidants, i.e. ß-carotene, lycopene and α-tocopherol. No significant influences with the catechin supplementation were also observed on the levels of total-cholesterol, free-cholesterol, cholesterol ester, HDL-cholesterol, triacylglycerol and phospholipids in human plasma.

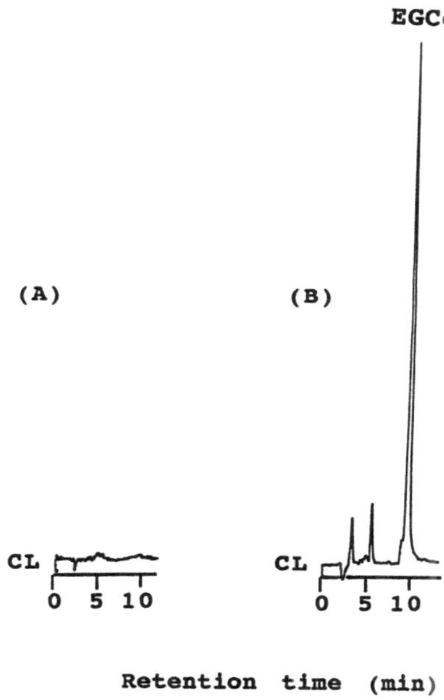

FIG. 3. CL-HPLC CHROMATOGRAMS OF HUMAN PLASMA EGCg
The plasma extract (B) from a healthy subject 90 min after a single oral administration of seven capsules of green tea extract (Sunphenon DCF-1, equivalent to 525 mg EGCg/subject) and (A) from the same subject before catechin ingestion, were analyzed by CL-HPLC as given in Fig. 2

Table 1 shows the EGCg concentrations in blood plasma and tissues of the rat after 60 min of EGCg administration (500 mg/kg body weight). Although the tissue EGCg levels before the administration were below the detection limit (< 0.002 nmol/ml plasma and < 0.002 nmol/g tissues), substantial amounts of EGCg in the free form were detected in all tissue samples examined for the EGCg-treated rats. The total amount of EGCg in the rat blood mass was calculated to be 37 μg/rat, accounting for 0.024% of ingested EGCg (500 mg/kg body weight); the whole blood mass was estimated provisionally to be 15 ml (corresponding to 6.5 ml plasma) per rat. Therefore, 0.0003%-

0.45% of the ingested EGCg was recognized to be present in the free form in the tissues, among which the small intestinal mucosa was the most enriched (Nakagawa and Miyazawa 1997b).

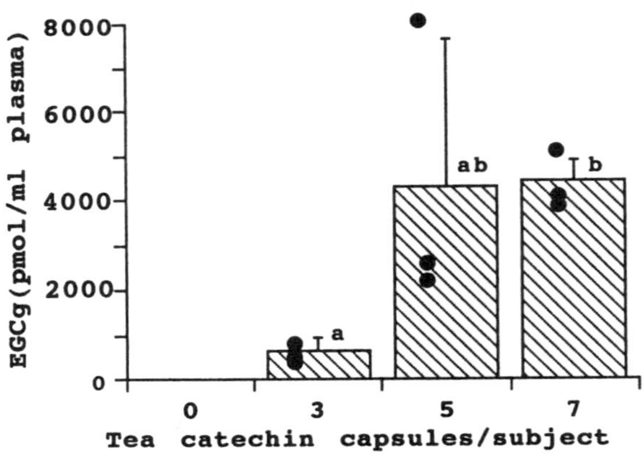

FIG. 4. HUMAN PLASMA EGCG CONCENTRATIONS BEFORE AND AFTER SUPPLEMENTATION OF GREEN TEA EXTRACT

Each subject received 0, 3, 5 or 7 capsules of green tea extract (corresponding, respectively, to 0, 225, 375 and 525 mg EGCg/subject) with a single oral supplementation after 12 h of fasting, and the plasma EGCg levels were analyzed 90 min after the oral intake. Values are Mean±SD (n = 3 subjects). [a,b]Values with different superscript letters are significantly different at $p<0.05$.

In terms of possible therapeutic use of EGCg against digestive cancer, we recently reported that green tea extract, mainly consisting of EGCg, clearly prevents 1,2-dimethylhydrazine-induced colonic carcinogenesis in rats, in which the levels of phospholipid hydroperoxide as a peroxidized membrane lipid marker is significantly and dose-dependently lowered in colon mucosal cells compared to control rats (Matsumoto *et al.* 1996). As shown here, since relatively high concentrations of EGCg were found in the intestinal mucosa in the EGCg-supplemented rats, the ingestion of EGCg as an antioxidative nutrient to prevent intestinal carcinogenesis may be recommended.

Several epidemiological studies (Weisburger 1996) have shown that individuals who consume four or more cups of green tea drink daily have a lower risk of atherosclerosis. The amount of tea catechins in four cups of green tea is roughly comparable to the EGCg concentration provided by five capsules of Sunphenon DCF-1 used in the present study. Since ingestion of five capsules of Sunphenon DCF-1 resulted in plasma EGCg concentration of 4.3 nmol/ml (Fig. 4), drinking four or more cups of green tea daily would maintain plasma levels of catechin high enough to be of therapeutic benefit against atherosclerosis other than colon carcinogenesis.

TABLE 1.
EGCG DETECTED IN BLOOD PLASMA AND TISSUE ORGANELLES OF THE RAT

Tissue	Before administration	After 60 min of administration[a]	EGCg detected (%)
Plasma (nmol/ml)	< 0.002[b]	12.3 ± 6.2	(0.024 ± 0.012)[c,d]
Liver (nmol/g)	< 0.002	48.4 ± 19.7	(0.19 ± 0.09)[c,d]
Brain (nmol/g)	< 0.002	0.5 ± 0.3	(0.0003 ± 0.0002)[c,d]
Small intestinal mucosa (nmol/g)	< 0.002	565 ± 153	(0.45 ± 0.14)[c,d]
Colon mucosa (nmol/g)	< 0.002	68.6 ± 40.4	(0.013 ± 0.008)[c,d]

The data are expressed as the mean ± SD of six rats.

[a] Rats received a single oral administration of EGCg (500 mg/kg body weight) after 24 h of food deprivation.

[b] Below the detection limit (<0.002 nmol).

[c] Percentage against ingested EGCg.

[d] Calculated from the blood mass to be 15 ml/rat and from the tissue weights (liver, 13.0 ± 1.7 g/rat; brain, 2.6±0.5 g/rat; small intestinal mucosa, 1.9 ± 0.2 g/rat; colon mucosa, 0.6 ± 0.2 g/rat for mean ± SD of six rats).

In the present study, the plasma EGCg in the free form was first demonstrated to be profoundly increased following the increase of catechin ingestion (Fig. 4), indicating dose-dependent incorporation of tea catechins into human plasma. The present study also first demonstrated the incorporation of EGCg in free form into the liver, brain, small intestinal mucosa and colon mucosa of the rat (Table 1). It was confirmed that relatively high levels of EGCg are retained in alimentary tract tissues such as the small intestinal mucosa and colon mucosa. These findings suggest that tea catechin, EGCg, is absorbed from the digestive tract into blood plasma and tissue organelles in humans, with the intestinal mucosa the most enriched of the organelles. The marked accumulation of EGCg in intestinal mucosa and in plasma suggest that the ingested EGCg can act as an effective antioxidant in preventing intestinal carcinogenesis and atherosclerosis in humans.

ACKNOWLEDGMENTS

The gift of EGCg and green tea extract (Sunphenon DCF-1®) from Taiyo Kagaku Co. (Yokkaichi, Japan) is gratefully acknowledged.

REFERENCES

KATIYAR, S.K., AGARWAL, R. and MUKHTAR, H. 1994. Inhibition of spontaneous and photo-enhanced lipid peroxidation in mouse epidermal microsomes by epicatechin derivatives from green tea. Cancer Lett. *79*, 61–66.

KONO, S., IKEDA, M., TOKUDOME, S. and KARATSUNE, M. 1988. A case-control study of gastric cancer and diet in northern Kyushu. Jpn. J. Cancer Res. *79*, 1067–1074.

MATSUMOTO, H., YAMANE, T., INAGAKE, M., NAKATANI, H., IWATA, Y., TAKAHASHI, T., NISHIMURA, H., NISHINO, H., NAKAGAWA, K. and MIYAZAWA, T. 1996. Inhibition of mucosal lipid hyperoxidation by green tea extract in 1,2-dimethylhydrazine-induced rat colonic carcinogenesis. Cancer Lett. *104*, 205–209.

MOREL, I., LESCOAT, G., CILLARD, P. and CILLARD, J. 1994. Role of flavonoids and iron chelation in antioxidant action. Methods Enzymol. *234*, 437–443.

NAKAGAWA, K. and MIYAZAWA, T. 1997a. Chemiluminescence-high performance liquid chromatographic determination of tea catechin, (-)-epigallocatechin-3-gallate, at picomole levels in rat and human plasma. Anal. Biochem. *248*, 41–49.

NAKAGAWA, K. and MIYAZAWA, T. 1997b. Absorption and distribution of anticarcinogenic tea catechin, (-)-epigallocatechin-3-gallate, in the rat. J. Nutr. Sci. Vitaminol. (In press).

NAKAGAWA, K., OKUDA, S. and MIYAZAWA, T. 1997. Dose-dependent incorporation of tea catechins, (-)-epigallocatechin-3-gallate and (-)-epigallocatechin, into human plasma. Biosci. Biotech. Biochem. (In press).

RICE-EVANS, C. 1995. Plant polyphenols: free radical scavengers or chain-breaking antioxidants? Biochem. Soc. Symposia *61*, 103–116.

WEISBURGER, J.H. 1996. Tea antioxidants and health. *In* Antioxidants: E. Cadenas and L. Packer (eds.). Marcel Dekker Inc., New York.

STUDIES ON THE ANTIOXIDATIVE ACTIVITY OF TEA SEED OIL

ZHENG HUI ZHAO, XIUPING QIAN and HONG JIANG WANG

Laboratory of Natural Product Research
Department of Tea Science
Zhejiang Agriculture University
Hangzhou 310029, P.R. China

ABSTRACT

Comparative investigation on the antioxidative activity of roasted sesame, virgin and partially refined tea seed oil was carried out under incubation at 60°C for 48 h by the Rapid Oxidation Salad Oil model system. The antioxidative activity decreased in the order of roasted sesame oil, virgin tea seed oil, bleached-, degummed- tea seed oil and deastringent tea seed oil. Numerous phenolic substances were successfully separated by HPLC from deastringent ethanolic extractives of tea seed oil. These extractives play important roles as antioxidants and influence the flavor of the oil.

INTRODUCTION

Tea (*Camellia sinensis*) seed oil has been traditionally considered to be a valuable edible oil and is recently produced on a commercial scale in China. It is estimated that China produces about 125,000 tons of tea seed and about 18,750 tons of oil as a by-product of tea annually (Xia and Zhu 1986). The fundamental interest in the nutritional and pharmacological properties of the oil rich in monounsaturated fatty acids (MUFA) (Zhu and Tian 1985) has enhanced further research prospects in this direction (Zhang and Zhou 1995; Chen and Gu 1996). Chen and Gu found that tea seed oil could inhibit atheromatic formation by lowering liver and blood lipids increasing the antioxidative enzymes SOD and GSH-Px activities. Zhang and Zhou (1995) further postulated that the significant tea seed oil reduction of free oxygen radicals with subsequent promotion of SOD activity in the liver of rats was related to new types of unknown antioxidants as well as the fatty acid composition. But the new types of unknown antioxidants have not yet been clearly elucidated in recent research.

Our laboratory is focusing on screening the new types of natural antioxidants in tea seed oil based on its high resistance to oxidation. Through comparative investigation on the antioxidative activity of partially refined tea seed oil using the Rapid Oxidation Salad Oil model system, the natural phenolic antioxidants from deastringent ethanolic extract of tea seed oil were successfully separated by HPLC.

MATERIALS AND METHODS

Sample Preparation

Virgin Tea Seed Oil. The oil, donated by Zhejiang Heng Fa Company, was processed by the hot pressing method.

Degummed Tea Seed Oil. Degumming was carried out on the virgin tea seed oil by adding 2% water to the oil. The water and oil were agitated for 30 min to 1 h at 60° to 80°C and hydrated gums were then removed by centrifugation.

Bleached Tea Seed Oil. Bleaching was carried out on the virgin tea seed oil by adding 10% activated charcoal followed by heating and filtration to remove the adsorbent along with the pigment in the activated charcoal.

Deastringent Tea Seed Oil. Deastringent removal was carried out on virgin tea seed oil by adding EtOH to the oil at room temperature with agitation for 15 min, followed by removal of the EtOH layer.

Roasted Sesame Oil and Common Salad Oil. These were purchased from a supermarket in Hangzhou and used in the experiment as controls.

Antioxidative Assay

Stabilization assays were made with 20-ml aliquots of the oil placed in 100 × 20 mm petri dishes for 48 h under air in the dark at 60°C. Five partially refined treatments were compared to the control under the same experimental procedure.

Peroxidation was monitored for peroxide content (expressed as meq/kg oil) according to the analytical procedure in the Association of Analytical Chemists (13th Edn. 1980).

Separation of Deastringent Extractives by HPLC

Deastringent extractives (i.e. EtOH extractives) of virgin tea seed oil were brought to dryness in a vacuum rotary evaporator at 40°C, defatting residue was dissolved in methanol and stored at -10°C until it was separated by HPLC.

The MeOH solution was separated by HPLC using a 3 Ãm C18 column (150 mm × 4.6 mm i.d.). The mobile phase (flow rate 1 ml/min) consisted of 0.1% formic acid (solvent A) and 80% methanol +0.1% formic acid (solvent B). The best separation was obtained at 35°C by the following gradient: at 0 min, 0% B; at 5 min, 0% B; at 65 min, 100% B; at 80 min, 100%B; at 85 min, 0%B. UV wavelength = 280 nm.

RESULTS AND DISCUSSION

Oxidative Stability of Virgin Tea Seed Oil

The high resistance of virgin tea seed oil to oxidation is known from our previous investigation (Zhao 1997, in press), but has not been compared with other vegetable oils in detail. Roasted sesame oil (with high stability against autoxidation; Namiki 1990), common salad oil (a mixture of soybean and rapeseed oils) and virgin tea seed oil were rapidly oxidized after 2 days of incubation at 60°C, as summarized in Table 1. The results show that sesame and tea seed oils have markedly higher stability against oxidation than salad oil and the tea seed oil has almost the same stability as the sesame oil. Results presented here demonstrate a clear oxidative stability of virgin tea seed oil.

TABLE 1.
COMPARISON OF THE OXIDATIVE STABILITY OF COMMON SALAD OIL, ROASTED SESAME OIL AND VIRGIN TEA SEED OIL

Oil Type	Peroxide values after incubation (2 days at 60°C) 0 h (meq/kg oil)	48 h	pv*	(Δpv/pv) × 100
Common salad oil	25.59	46.63	21.04	82.22
Roasted sesame oil	3.50	3.80	0.30	8.57
Virgin tea seed oil	3.60	4.01	0.41	11.39

ΔPV = change in peroxide values

Antioxidative Activity of Partially Refined Tea Seed Oil

It is reported that numerous natural antioxidants in other vegetable crude oils are usually removed in the various refining stages (Weiss 1983), remarkably reducing the oxidative stability. The antioxidative activity of the five treatments of partially refined tea seed oil was measured by incubation at 60°C in the salad oil model system. As shown in Fig. 1, all of the refined oils were less active than virgin tea seed and roasted sesame oil. Among them, deastringent tea seed oil gave the lowest activity compared to degummed- and bleached-tea seed oil.

Further investigation was carried out to verify the oxidation stability before and after deastringent treatment as shown in Table 2. It is noteworthy that deastringent ethanolic extractives are strong natural antioxidants for stability of virgin tea seed oil.

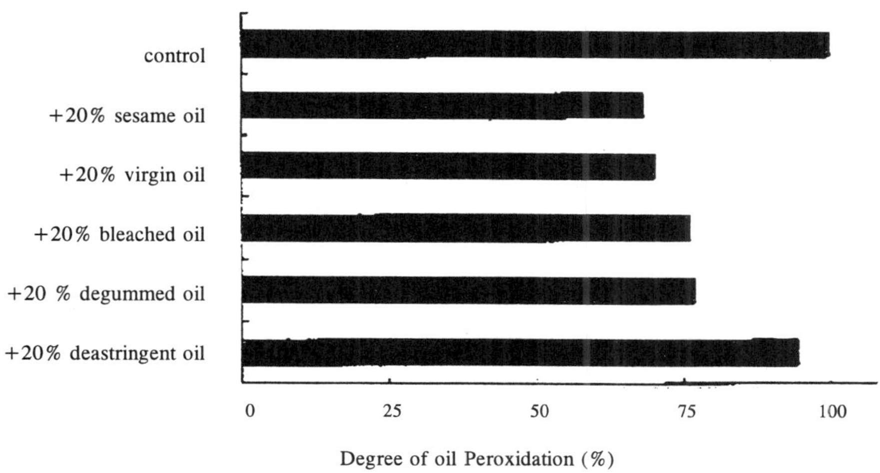

FIG. 1. ANTIOXIDATIVE ACTIVITY OF PARTIALLY REFINED TEA SEED OIL IN SALAD OIL MODEL SYSTEM AFTER 2 DAYS OF INCUBATION AT 60°C

TABLE 2.
OXIDATIVE STABILITY BEFORE AND AFTER DEASTRINGENT REFINING FOR SEVERAL TEA SEED OILS

Peroxide values after 2 days incubation at 60°C (meq/kg oil)	sample number No. 5	No. 8	No. 10	No. 12
Before deastringent treatment	4.10	3.9	2.08	2.74
After deastringent treatment	49.14	48.75	51.32	53.90

Natural Phenolic Antioxidants Separation from Deastringent Ethanolic Extractives by HPLC

Compared to other vegetable oils, tea seed oils contain small amounts of tocopherols (28, 60 and 92 mg/100 g of oil in tea seed, rapeseed and soybean oil, respectively) (National Institute of Nutrition and Food Hygiene 1991), the main natural antioxidants for stability of vegetable oils. It is therefore important to investigate the presence of other natural antioxidants that induce high oxidative stability of virgin tea seed oil and the low antioxidative activity of deastringent tea seed oil. The phenolic substances, rich in secondary metabolism of *Thea sinensis* with a strong influence on flavor of tea and a significant biochemical role as antioxidants (Wang 1992; Cheng and Ho 1986), were then examined by qualitative reaction with $FeCl_3$ in tea seed oil. By visual inspection, it was observed that the addition of $FeCl_3$ to ethanol extractives formed characteristic colors of phenolic substances in the extract. Further separation was done by HPLC using a C18 column. The chromatogram at UV = 280 nm shown in Fig. 2 substantially confirmed that the virgin tea seed oil contained relatively high phenolic components in Peaks 21 and

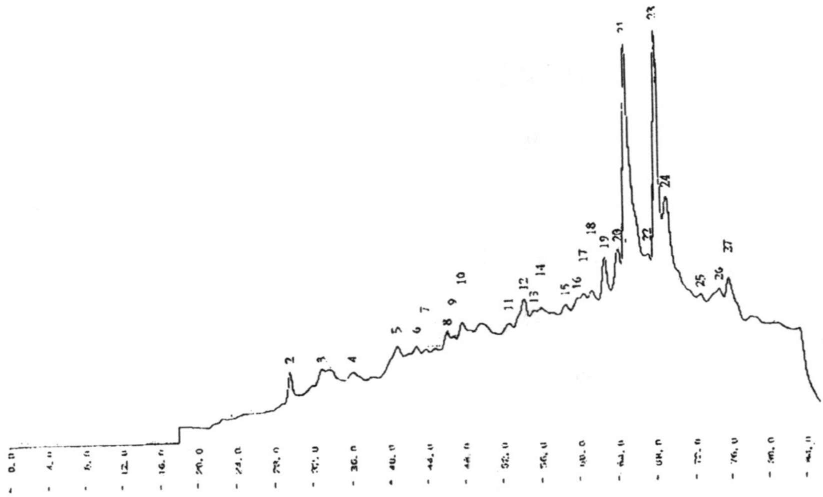

FIG. 2. NATURAL PHENOLIC ANTIOXIDANTS SEPARATION FROM DEASTRINGENT ETHANOLIC EXTRACTIVES BP HPLC

23. The phenomenon of these high peaks is yet unclear, but further research is anticipated to identify the phenolic substances in these high peaks.

CONCLUSION

Virgin tea seed oil has high resistance to oxidation. Addition of perennial tea xylophyta plant seed oil can obviously improve the oxidative stability of vegetable oils. Phenolic substances play important roles as natural antioxidants and influence the flavor of tea seed oil.

ACKNOWLEDGMENTS

The authors thank Prof. Z.C. Wang, Dr. Bashirn Mohamed Koroma and graduate student,L. Liu for their valuable discussions, and Zhejiang Heng Fa Co. for supplying the materials.

REFERENCES

CHENG, S.J. and HO, C.T. 1986. A preliminary study on the antimutagenicity of green tea antioxidant. Acta Biol. Exp. Sinica *19*, 427.

CHEN, M.F. and GU, J.F. 1996. Effect of tea-seed oil on the atheromatic formation and its mechanism. Acta. Nutr. Sinica *18*(1), 13–19.

HUDSON, B.J.F. 1990. Food Antioxidants. Elsevier Applied Science, London and New York.

NATIONAL INSTITUTE OF NUTRITION AND FOOD HYGIENE. 1991. Food Constitution. Peoples Hygiene Press, China.

NAMIKI, M. 1990. Antioxidants/Antimutagens in Food. Crit. Revs. Food Sci. Nutr. pp. 273–300.

OFFICIAL METHODS OF ANALYSIS. 1980. Association of Official Analytical Chemists, 13th edn. Washington, D.C. pp. 440–441.

WEISS, T.J. 1983. Food Oils and Their Uses. 2nd. Edn., AVI Publishing Company, Inc., Westport, Connecticut.

WANG, Z.N. 1992. Tea Biochemistry. 2nd Edn. Agriculture Press.

XIA, C.H. and ZHU, Q.F. 1986. Outlook of tea seed edible oil production. J. Tea Sci. *6*(1), 15–20.

ZHANG, B. and ZHOU, Y.Z. 1995. Effects of tea seed oil and soybean oil on free oxygen radical and activities of antioxidative enzymes in rats. Acta. Nutr. Sinica. *17*(2), 199–203.

ZHAO, Z.H. 1997. In Press.

ZHU, Q.F. and TIAN, J.H. 1985. Study on the fatty acid composition in tea seed oils of main tea varieties in China. Tea Sci. Res. J. pp. 104–113.

THE BIO-ANTIOXIDATIVE ACTIVITY OF FUNCTIONAL FACTORS IN BAMBOO LEAVES

YING ZHANG[1] and XIAOLIN DING[2]

[1]Department of Food Science and Technology
Zhejiang Agricultural University
Hangzhou 310029, P.R. China

[2]School of Food Science and Technology
Wuxi University of Light Industry
Jiangsu, Wuxi 214036, P.R. China

ABSTRACT

The effective scavenging concentration of bamboo-leaf-total-flavonoids (BLTF) on active oxygen radicals was investigated using a Chemiluminescence(CL) method, which determined $O_2^{\cdot-}$ *in the range of 0.1 mg/L and 10 μg to 1g/L of* $\cdot OH$*, respectively. In the X-XOD-Luminol model, when the concentration of BLTF reached 5g/L, which was equal to 6300 times,* IC_{50} *,* $O_2^{\cdot-}$ *was still scavenged entirely; and in the* $Vc\text{-}Cu^{2+}\text{-}H_2O_2$*-yeast polysaccharide system, high BLTF concentration also did not contribute to pro-oxidative effect. This evidence suggested that effective fractions in bamboo leaves have excellent and stable anti-radicals activity, especially to* $O_2^{\cdot-}$ *. Pyrogallol (PR) auto-oxidation and ESR methods proved further this SOD-like activity. In order to determine the biological effect of the effective fraction of bamboo leaf in vivo, feeding tests of bamboo leaf-crude extract (BLCE) were done using aged mice as targets and pure bee-pollen as a positive control. After 35 days, the activities of SOD and GSH-Px in the blood, and the contents of LPO in plasma and LF in liver tissue were measured, respectively. Results showed that BLCE could induce the activities of endo-antioxidases, inhibit the post-oxidation of lipid and scavenge post-oxidized products in experimental mice. It is concluded that bamboo leaves contain a functional factor which has bio-antioxidative action.*

INTRODUCTION

Recently, there is considerable interest in the fields of food industry and preventive medicine in the development of "natural antioxidants" from plant material. A lot of investigations have been done with various vegetables, fruits, seaweeds, tree leaves and herbs. Among these, traditional Chinese herbs have received much more attention as sources of bio-active substances including antioxidants, antimutagens, and anticarcinogens.

Most natural antioxidants are scavengers of active oxygen species which have been proposed to be agents that attack polyunsaturated fatty acids in cell membranes giving rise to lipid peroxidation (Aust and Sringen 1982). Lipid peroxidation is strongly associated with aging and carcinogenesis (Yagi 1987; Haman 1982; Cutler 1984). Even though living cells are generally protected from active oxygen species by endo-antioxidases, e.g. SOD and SHG-Px, dietary antioxidants such as α-tocopherol, ascorbic acid and flavonoids may be effective in protection from peroxidative damage, especially in aged and/or injured cells.

Flavonoids and other plant phenolics have been reported to have multiple biological effects such as anti-inflammatory, anti-allergic and anti-viral activities (Havsteen 1983), and inhibiting tumor promotion (Nakamura *et al.* 1985). Many flavonoids are also found to be strong free radical scavengers and antioxidants (Scott and Slater 1981; Robak and Gryglewski 1988; Rafat *et al.* 1987; Chen *et al.* 1989; Chen *et al.* 1990).

China possesses abundant resources of bamboo leaf, which is a traditional Chinese herb. It has been reported in our prior study (Zhang and Ding 1994) that the extracts made from bamboo leaves contain valuable flavonoid and phenolic acid compounds, of strong scavenging capacity on oxygen radicals and inhibiting activity on nitrosation. This paper determined the effective scavenging concentration of the functional factors in bamboo leaves on $O_2^{\cdot-}$ and ·OH using a chemiluminescence method (CL), and determined further their SOD-like activity by spectrophotometry and ESR. At the same time, feeding tests were done using aged mice as experimental targets and bee-pollen as a positive control; the bio-antioxidative action of BLCE in vivo was studied.

MATERIALS AND METHODS

Chemical

X (xanthine) and Luminol were obtained from Sigma Chemical Co., XOD (xanthine oxidase), SOD (superoxide dismutase), GSH and DTNB [5,5'-dithiobis (2-nitrobenzic acid)] were purchased from Shanghai Dongfeng Biochemicals Shop. Other chemicals and reagents were all AR grade. Pure bee-pollen was produced by Huifeng Nutritional Food Factory of Wuxi. The water used in CL was of high purity.

Bamboo Leaves

The leaves of 17 species of bamboo such as *Ph. bambusoides Sieb.* Et Zucc and *Ph. nigra* var. *henonis* were collected at Hangzhou Botanical Garden in autumn seasons of 1992 to 1994. The sampling information was presented by Zhang and Ding (1994). Green leaves were washed after picking, and dried for 2 to 3 days under sunlight. The dried leaves were subsequently ground into fine and uniform powders for extraction with a mill equipped with a 20-mesh-sieve to form 17 varieties. The moisture of powders was determined individually by a Moisture Balance 330 MOC (made in Japan).

Sample Preparation

The extracts of bamboo leaves were divided into two groups: bamboo leaf-crude extract (BLCE) including $BLCE_1$ and $BLCE_2$ and bamboo leaf-total flavonoid (BLTF) including $BLTF_1$, $BLTF_2$ and $BLTF_3$. The extracting procedures are as follows.

The powder of *Ph. bambusoides* (100 g) was packed into a glass column (6.5 $\times$ 60 cm), and 1000 ml of petroleum benzine (60 to 90 °C) was passed through the column at a rate of 10 ml/min to remove most of lipid-soluble components. Subsequently, the column was eluted with 70% ethanol (150 ml) at the same rate. After the ethanol was removed in vacuo using a rotary flash evaporator, the water phase was extracted by 1:1

(v/v) ethylacetate ester twice. The phase of ethylacetate ester was concentrated and dried in vacuum, and approximately 1.25 g of green-yellow powder was obtained (recorded as $BLTF_2$). The residual water phase was extracted further by 1:1 (v/v) *n*-butanol twice; 2.4 g of yellow powder ($BLTF_1$) was obtained.

The powder of *Ph. nigra* (100 g) was put into a 2000-ml distilling bottle, 30% ethanol (1500 ml) added, refluxed 1.5 h in a boiling water base, and subsequently filtered and concentrated in vacuo, then 100 ml of extract liquid ($BLCE_1$) was obtained. Half of $BLCE_1$ was extracted by 1:1 (v/v) *n*-butanol three times; 3.5 g of yellow powder ($BLTF_3$) was obtained after removing the solvent.

The dried powders from 17 bamboo species were mixed, 100 g was removed, distilled water (1500 ml)) added, boiled 1.5 h, and 100 ml extract liquid ($BLCE_2$) was obtained after filtering, concentrating and centrifuging.

Measurement Of Scavenging Capacity On Active Oxygen Radicals

Chemiluminescence (CL). The superoxide anion ($O_2^{\cdot-}$) was produced by the X-XOD-Luminol model; hydroxyl radical (·OH) was produced by Vc-Cu^{2+}-H_2O_2-yeast polysaccharides system, and the scavenging activities of samples on $O_2^{\cdot-}$ and ·OH were monitored using the SHG-I Biochemical Luminometer (made in Shanghai). The results are expressed by inhibition effect (I%) or half inhibiting concentration (IC_{50}) (Zhang and Ding 1994).

Pyrogallol (PR) Autooxidation. PR autooxidizes in an alkaline solution to release $O_2^{\cdot-}$ and form colored intermediate compounds, which can be monitored by a spectrophotometer. The measurement parameters were as follows: wavelength 320 nm, PR concentration of 0.1 mmol/L, temperature 25°C, incubation time 10 min, pH 8.2 $\pm$ 0.01, reaction time 4 min + lag of 30 s, using SOD as control (Zhang 1997).

Electron Spin Resonance (ESR). $O_2^{\cdot-}$ was formed by the Na_2O_2-DMSO system and determined with a JES-FEIXG ESR METER (JEOL, Japan) at -120°C (Feng *et al.* 1995). The concentration of $O_2^{\cdot-}$ is represented by the height of signal peak, and the inhibition effect of sample on $O_2^{\cdot-}$ was obtained by comparing with the control (distilled water).

Animal Test

Six-month-old mice (Kunming species), weights of 35 $\pm$ 5 g, were purchased from the Medicine Institute of Suzhou. After qualified tests, the mice were divided into 5 groups at 1:1 ratio of male to female and lodged individually; free intake of feed and water was given. The samples and controls were drenched at the same volume to each experimental mouse one time a day. The experimental groups were follows:

a. negative control group: drenched with physiological saline
b. low dosage group: drenched with $BLCE_1$ at 0.25 $g \cdot kg^{-1} \cdot d^{-1}$
c. middle dosage group: drenched with $BLCE_1$ at 0.50 $g \cdot kg^{-1} \cdot d^{-1}$
d. high dosage group: drenched with $BLCE_1$ at 1.00 $g \cdot kg^{-1} \cdot d^{-1}$
e. positive control group: drenched with pure bee-pollen at 1.00 $g \cdot kg^{-1} \cdot d^{-1}$.

After 35 days of continuous feeding, the activities of SOD and GSH-Px in the blood of the experimental mice were estimated using CL and DTNB methods. The contents of

LPO in plasma and LF in liver tissue were measured by MDA-TBA colorimetry and micro-fluorescence analysis method, respectively (Chen 1993). At the same time, the same analysis was carried out on some young mice, 3 to 4 weeks old and weights of 20 $\pm$ 5 g. The measured data were recorded as youth reference.

RESULTS AND DISCUSSION

Effective Concentration of BLTF on $O_2^{\cdot-}$ and ·OH

The scavenging capacity of $BLTF_1$ and $BLTF_2$, both at final concentrations of 1×10^{-3} to 5×10^3 mg/L, on $O_2^{\cdot-}$ and ·OH, was investigated by CL, as shown in Fig. 1a,b.

In the X-XOD-Luminol model, $BLTF_1$ and $BLTF_2$ showed the same pattern. The effective scavenging concentration on $O_2^{\cdot-}$ was determined in the range of 0.1 to 10 mg/L; and in the Vc-Cu^{2+}-H_2O_2-yeast polysaccharide system, the concentration range of ·OH was 1×10^{-3} to 1×10^3 mg/L. Results showed that the functional factors in bamboo leaves have excellent anti-radical activity, especially for $O_2^{\cdot-}$. The inhibiting activity of BLTF to $O_2^{\cdot-}$ was about 400 to 600 times as strong as to ·OH calculated from the IC_{50} value.

Some natural products which have been used as antioxidants appear to have prooxidative effect under certain conditions. Using tea polyphenol (TP) as an example, some experiments showed (Shen *et al.* 1992a) that TP only had anti-radical activity at certain concentration ranges and would promote oxidation at higher concentrations. Shen *et al.* (1992b) studied the anti- and pro-oxidation effect of TP by ESR, using the same systems as we report to produce $O_2^{\cdot-}$ and ·OH; the results showed that TP at high concentrations did not appear to have antioxidative activity; on the contrary, it displayed a strong pro-oxidative effect, which may be the reason that TP caused toxicological effects at high dosage. But in our study using CL, when the concentration of BLTF reached 5 g/L, which was equal to 6300 times of its IC_{50} , $O_2^{\cdot-}$ was still scavenged entirely (Fig. 1a,b). In the Vc-Cu^{2+}-H_2O_2-yeast polysaccharide system, high BLTF concentrations also did not contribute to pro-oxidative effect (Fig. 1 a,b). These results show primarily that BLTF has anti-oxidative effects.

The SOD-like Activity of BLCE and BLTF

The SOD-like activity (i.e. dismutating ability on $O_2^{\cdot-}$) has been taken as a very important index for some functional foods and health drugs. Besides the CL, PR auto-oxidation and ESR also were used to investigate the SOD-like activity of the functional factors in bamboo leaves, and the results are listed in Tables 1 and 2, respectively.

The scavenging capacity of BLCE and BLTF on $O_2^{\cdot-}$ was determined in this study by several systems, they support strongly the prior study by CL and increase our understanding of their activity as well. Table 2 shows that the SOD-like activity of BLTF is far higher than that of BLCE.

Anti-aging Effect of BLCE

Inducing Effect on Endo-antioxidases. SOD and GSH-Px are the most important enzymes of the antioxidative preventive system *in vivo*. The analytical results of 5 tested

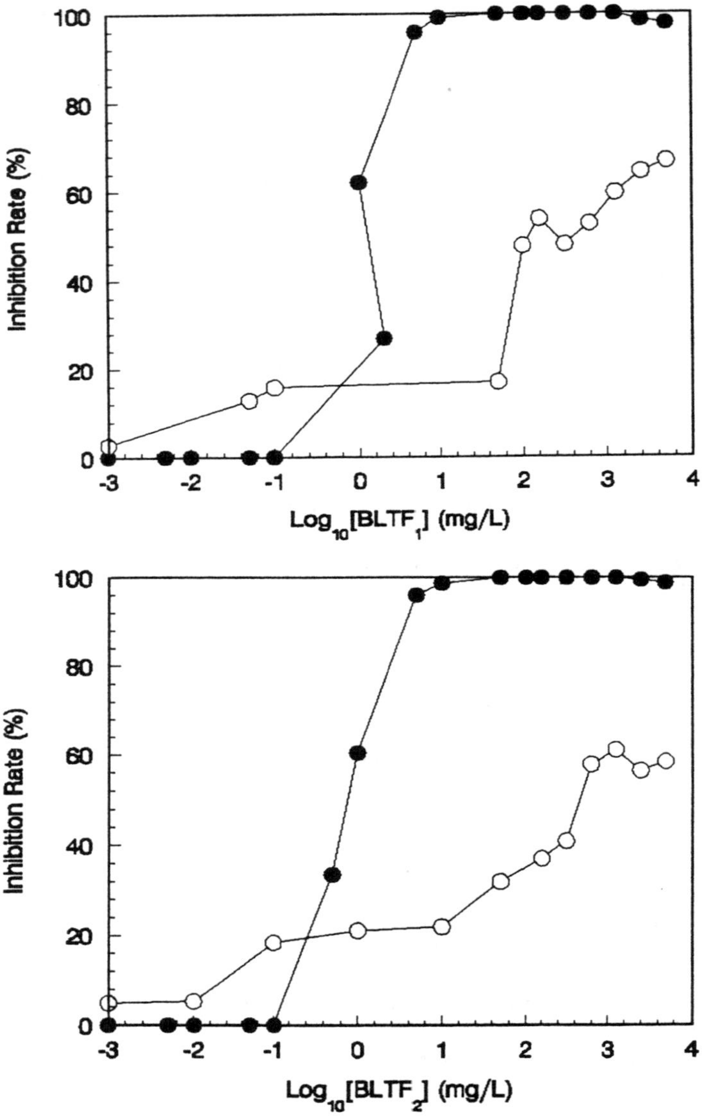

FIG. 1. SCAVENGING EFFECT OF BLTF ON $O_2^{\cdot-}$ AND ·OH

(a)--- $BLTF_1$ (b)---$BLTF_2$

● --- Inhibition effect on $O_2^{\cdot-}$; O --- Inhibition effect on ·OH

(Chemiluminescence method; X-XOD-Luminol For $O_2^{\cdot-}$, pH 10.0; Vc-Cu^{2+}-H_2O_2-yeast polysaccharide for ·OH, pH 7.8)

TABLE 1.
SCAVENGING CAPACITY OF BLCE ON $O_2^{\cdot-}$ PRODUCED BY PR AUTO-OXIDATION (n=3)

Groups	Dosage of sample (final concentration)	OD320 nm (at 2 min)	Inhibition rate I(%)
Control	0	0.104 ± 0.001	0
$BLCE_1$	0.33 g/L	0.099 ± 0.002	4.8
	0.67 g/L	0.083 ± 0.001	20.2
	1.00 g/L	0.071 ± 0.003	31.7
$BLCE_2$	0.33 g/L	0.094 ± 0.004	9.6
	1.00 g/L	0.083 ± 0.001	20.2
	1.67 g/L	0.073 ± 0.002	29.8
SOD	710 U/L	0.070 ± 0 003	32.7
	1410 U/L	0.041 ± 0.002	60.6
	2100 U/L	0.022 ± 0.001	78.8

TABLE 2.
SCAVENGING CAPACITY OF BLCE AND BLTF ON $O_2^{\cdot-}$ MEASURED BY ESR (n=3)

Sample	Final conc. (mg/L)	Signal Strength (mm)	Inhibition rate I(%)
Control	0	41.5 ± 2.12	0
$BLCE_1$	35	32.2 ± 1.11	22.5
	117	23.7 ± 0.35	42.5
	3421	3.1 ± 0.21	92.5
$BLTF_3$	4	8.7 ± 0.31	79.1
	43	2.0 ± 0.18	95.3
	130	0.0 ± 0.00	100.0

TABLE 3.
ACTIVITY COMPARISON OF SOD AND GSH-PX IN THE BLOOD OF TESTED MICE

Groups	n	SOD activity I(%) on $O_2^{\cdot-}$	n	GSH-Px activity U/ml blood
youth reference	11	55.82 ± 6.32	9	35.5 ± 2.61
negative control	9	54.82 ± 8.60	8	19.8 ± 2.23
low dosage	8	60.22 ± 8.82	7	27.0 ± 4.66**
middle dosage	11	64.19 ± 14.18	7	38.1 ± 5.08***
high dosage	9	65.32 ± 11.02*	5	43.0 ± 4.52***
positive control	12	68.33 ± 11.37**	9	32.3 ± 3.30***

*$p < 0.05$; ** $p < 0.01$; *** $p < 0.001$; compared with negative control group

groups of aged mice and 1 youth reference group are given in Table 3. The SOD activity was reflected indirectly by the inhibition rate on $O_2^{\bar{\cdot}}$ measured using CL, and the effect of $BLCE_1$ at high dosage was close to the positive control. The activity unit of GSH-Px per ml blood estimated by the DTNB method showed that $BLCE_1$ gave a promoting effect even at low dosage, and the better effects appeared in middle and high dosage groups. It has been suggested that functional factors in bamboo leaf are capable of inducing the activity of endo-antioxidases of aged mice.

Inhibiting Effect on Lipid Peroxidation. LPO and LF are the products of free radical damage *in vivo* and can be used as indices of aging. Their content indicates the peroxidative level, and further infer the aging extent of a cell. After a 35-day-feeding of $BLCE_1$, the concentration of LOP in plasma and LF in liver tissue decreased significantly (Table 4). Results show that functional factors in bamboo leaf have strong inhibiting effect on lipid peroxidation and scavenging ability to peroxidized products.

TABLE 4.
THE CONTENTS OF LPO AND LF OF EXPERIMENTAL MICE

Groups	n	LPO in plasma nmol/ml	n	LF in liver tissue U/g
youth reference	5	0.85 ± 0.22	10	15.2 ± 5.1
negative control	8	1.07 ± 0.06	5	26.4 ± 4.8
low dosage	8	0.88 ± 0.18*	5	17.3 ± 6.2*
middle dosage	10	0.91 ± 0.19	5	18.6 ± 5.0*
high dosage	9	0.61 ± 0.09**	5	17.6 + 5.1*
positive control	9	0.61 ± 0.13**	7	16.3 ± 3.2**

*$p < 0.05$; ** $p < 0.01$; *** $p < 0.001$; compared with negative control group.

Based on the experimental data both *in vitro* and *in vivo*, it is concluded that bamboo leaves contain a class of functional factors which have bio-antioxidative activity.

REFERENCES

AUST, S.D and SRINGEN, B.A. 1982. The role of iron in enzymatic lipid peroxidation. *In* Free Radicals in Biology, W.A. Pryor (ed.). Academic Press, Orlando.

CHEN, Y., LI, X., ZHAO, B., ZHENG, R. and XIN, W. 1989. Superoxide and hydroxyl radical scavenging activities of rutin and other natural products studied by ESR. Acta Biophys. Sinica *5*, 240–253.

CHEN, Y., ZHENG, R., JIA, Z. and JU, Y. 1990. Flavonoids as superoxide scavengers and antioxidants. Free Radical Biol. Med. *9*, 19–21.

CHEN, Q. 1993. Methodology of Pharmacological Study of Chinese Drugs. People Hygiene Press, Beijing.

CUTLER, G. 1984. Antioxidants, aging, and longevity. *In* Free Radicals in Biology, W. A. Pryor (ed.). Academic Press, Orlando.

FENG, Y., CHEN, D., XU, Y. and HE, L. 1995. ESR study on the formation of superoxide anion by the Na_2O_2-DMSO system. Chinese J. Magnetic Resonance *12*, 185–188.

HAMAN, D. 1982. The free-radical theory of aging. *In* Free Radicals in Biology, Vol. 5, Chapter 8. W.A. Pryor (ed.) Academic Press, Orlando.

HAVSTEEN, B. 1983. Flavonoids, a class of natural products of high pharmacological potency. Biochem. Pharmacol. *32*, 1141–1148.

NAKAMURA, Y., COLBURN, H.N. and GINHART, T.D. 1985. Role of reactive oxygen in tumor promotion: Implication of superoxide anion in promotion of neoplastic transformation in JB-6 cells by TPA. Carcinogenesis *6*, 229–235.

ROBAK, J. and GRYGLEWSKI, R.J. 1988. Flavonoids are scavengers of superoxide anions. Biochem. Pharmacol. *37*, 837–841.

RAFAT, H.S., CILLARD, J. and CILLARD, P 1987. Hydroxyl radical scavenging activity of flavonoids. Phytochemistry *26*, 2489–2491.

SCOTT, R. and SLATER, T.F. 1981. Free radical scavenging activity of (+)-catechin and other flavonoids. *In* Recent Advances in Lipid Peroxidation and Tissue Injury, T.F. Slater and A. Garner (eds.). Brunel University Press, London. pp. 233–244.

SHEN, S., YANG, X., ZHAO, B. and XIN, W. 1992a. Scavenging effects of tea polyphenol compounds and (-)-EGCG on oxygen free radicals. J. Tea Sci. *12*, 59–64.

SHEN, S., YANG, X., ZHAO, B. and XIN, W. 1992b. Radical mechanism of pro-oxidant effect on tea polyphenol *in vitro*. J. Tea Sci. *12*, 145–150.

YAGI, K. 1987. Lipid peroxides and human disease. Chem. Phys. Lipids *45*, 337–341.

ZHANG, Y. and DING, X. 1994. Antioxidative fraction in bamboo leaves and scavenging capacity on oxygen free radicals. Presented at the 2nd International Conference on Food Science and Technology, September 27–30, Wuxi, P.R. China.

ZHANG, Y. 1997. Measurement of SOD-like activity of bamboo leaf extracts by pyrogallol autooxidation. Food Sci. (Chinese) *18*(5), 47–49.

MULTIPLE ANTIOXIDANTS PROTECT AGAINST LIPID PEROXIDATION AND DISEASES

AL TAPPEL

Food Science and Technology
University of California
Davis, California 95616

ABSTRACT

Focussing on experimental results from our laboratory, we find that animal tissue experiments are very valuable. Antioxidant protection by multiantioxygenic agents can be quantitated. The evidence indicates that multiantioxygenic nutrients can achieve maximum protection. Considering the biochemistry of β-carotene and our studies of its activity, apparently the popular β-carotene is a weak antioxidant.

INTRODUCTION

The popular press is focussing on health implications of lipid peroxidation and on nutrient antioxidants to prevent oxidative damage to metabolic processes and oxidative damage to human tissues.

Scientists working in this area have found oxidative lipid damage in aging and exercise and the following chronic diseases: cancer, ischemic heart disease, circulatory conditions, cataracts and air pollution (Davies 1991). Of these conditions, our experience has been mainly with air-pollution damage, oxidative damage caused by ozone, nitrogen dioxide and halogenated hydrocarbons. We found that vitamin E protects experimental animals from oxidative air pollution.

The fields of lipid peroxidation and vitamin E are in explosive growth. There are 1,200 publications per year on lipid peroxidation and 800 on vitamin E. Concerning practical applications of this developing knowledge, there are few overall summaries. Approximately 100 million people in the United States take vitamins, with more than one-third taking vitamin E and over one-third taking vitamin C. Global vitamin E production is estimated at 20 million kg, of which 95% goes into animal feeds. The U.S. market is estimated at \$100 million for β-carotene and over \$300 million for vitamin E. From the above information and present knowledge of beneficial health effects of antioxygenic nutrients, some scientists in this area approximate that millions of person years are being saved. A study by Pracon (Reston, Virginia) suggests that antioxidant vitamin use by the U.S. population could save \$8.7 billion in health-care costs annually by reduction of cardiovascular disease and some cancers.

The knowledge of oxidative damage and antioxidants might be thought of as a pyramid of knowledge with chemistry and biochemistry as the basic information. Most of the biochemical knowledge concerns the effects of disease and the biochemistry of tissues. At the apex of the knowledge pyramid is applications for people. Epidemiologic data of antioxidant protection is the gold standard of the field near the applications-for-people portion of the pyramid. Between the basic information and epidemiologic data, I would put experimental animal studies of oxidant damage and antioxidant protection.

There are certain questions important to the field and related to the research done in our laboratory: (a) the importance of animal testing of the effectiveness of antioxidants; (b) the quantitation of antioxidant protection; (c) the achievement of maximum antioxidant protection; and (d) the antioxidant strength of β-carotene.

In the human situation, there are various dietary intakes of antioxidant nutrients and diverse detrimental consequences of oxidative damage leading to aging and diseases. An animal model of this situation consists of using a refined diet with defined addition of dietary antioxidants. After deposition of the antioxidants in the animal's tissues, perhaps taking several weeks to a month, accelerated oxidation can be induced. The ensuing oxidatively damaged products can be measured by analytical procedures such as the thiobarbituric acid assay (TBARS) and heme protein oxidation.

Work on oxidative damage to living animals and animal tissue has defined lipid peroxidation as a major oxidative and deteriorative process (Davies 1991). In the last 50 years, vitamin E has been found to be the primary lipid antioxidant of nature (Packer and Fuchs 1993), a fact of major importance to the lipid and food biochemist. Other antioxidants of some significance include β-carotene, containing a hydrogen more difficult to extract than that of vitamin E for antioxidant protection. Further, when a hydrogen is abstracted from β-carotene, this antioxidant cannot be functionally regenerated as can vitamin E. Therefore, compared to the activity of vitamin E, β-carotene is a weak antioxidant. Another important antioxidant group is coenzyme Q in the reduced form. Coenzyme Q is not only in the mitochondrial electron transport chain but also in other membranes and lipids of the body and consequently can act as a chain-breaking antioxidant. Another important nutrient for antioxygenic activity is selenium, which becomes incorporated as the active site of the enzyme selenium glutathione peroxidase (Tappel *et al.* 1984). This enzyme reduces and thereby inactivates hydrogen peroxide and lipid peroxides which are oxidative compounds.

In addition to early studies on vitamin E, members of our laboratory have investigated coenzyme Q as an important lipid antioxidant and also selenium's incorporation into animal tissue to form the enzyme selenium glutathione peroxidase.

ANTIOXIDANTS IN TISSUES

In these dietary studies to investigate antioxidant protection against oxidation, control rats and chicks were fed vitamin E- and selenium-deficient diets. The basal diet for the rats contained 10% tocopherol-stripped corn oil, 30% torula yeast, 56% sucrose, and 4% minerals and vitamins. The basal diet for chicks contained 5% tocopherol-stripped corn oil, 20% soy protein, 68% starch, dextrose, etc., and 7% minerals and vitamins. The antioxidants to be tested for protection against oxidative damage were added to the basal diets and fed to the rats or chicks. After the animals have incorporated the elements of the diet and the antioxidants, tissues are taken from the animals and kept in metabolic integrity as they are shaken in air with or without an oxidizing agent. After a period of time, tissues are analyzed by methods such as TBARS, which measures lipid peroxidation products, and a test for oxidized heme proteins.

An example of this type of research addresses the quantifying of antioxidant protection and the question of the strength of β-carotene as an antioxidant (Pellett *et al.*

1994). The protocol is shown in Table 1. The protocol includes 0 IU vitamin E with the addition of increasing amounts of β-carotene fed to chicks. Another part of the experiment uses 50 IU vitamin E per kilogram of diet fed to chicks with increasing doses of β-carotene. Since humans consume daily about one kilogram of food on a dry weight basis, the dietary amount per kilogram of animal diets is similar to the dietary amounts of the constituent antioxidants expressed as units or milligrams per day in the human diet. The analyses of the chick liver show that β-carotene is incorporated as a function of its dietary concentration. However, at the highest amount of β-carotene in the chicks' diet, there is a mutual interference in the hepatic absorption of vitamin E and β-carotene, with both being reduced. Particularly, the poor hepatic absorption of vitamin E results in increased lipid peroxidation in liver as measured by TBARS. Figure 1 records, via decreasing TBARS, the protection to liver slices offered by increased amounts of dietary vitamin E and β-carotene in a biological system wherein iron is used to induce lipid peroxidation. Figure 1 indicates lowered concentration of TBARS in liver when the concentration of vitamin E reaches 25 micrograms per gram of liver. The liver is protected by this amount of vitamin E. The results also show that the interference between elevated amounts of vitamin E and β-carotene in the diet decreases the protection recorded by 50 IU vitamin E/kg diet and 0 or 30 mg β-carotene/kg diet.

QUANTITATION OF ANTIOXIDANT PROTECTION

The quantitation of the effects of multiple antioxidants is a challenge. At a basal level of metabolism, the animal always has some antioxidant activity, and this needs to be measured. In this experiment, vitamin E and β-carotene are two important variables. There is the problem of expressing these values in a way that takes into account all the data in the scientific literature. Simulation modeling develops a more quantitative perspective of the data gathered in many experiments (Tappel *et al.* 1989). Although empirical, models we have made incorporate some of the main parameters and relationships in the scientific literature. Some are dynamic working models of chemical reactions that ensue in tissues.

TABLE 1.
HEPATIC VITAMIN E AND β-CAROTENE CONCENTRATION

	Dietary		Liver	
Diet	Vitamin E (IU/kg)	β-Carotene (mg/kg)	Vitamin E (μg/g liver)	β-Carotene (μg/g liver)
EO, CO	0	0	<4	0.6
EO, C30	0	30	<4	2.4
EO, C100	0	100	<4	7.3
E50, CO	50	0	28	1.1
E50, C30	50	30	25	3.0
E50, C100	50	100	9	3.4

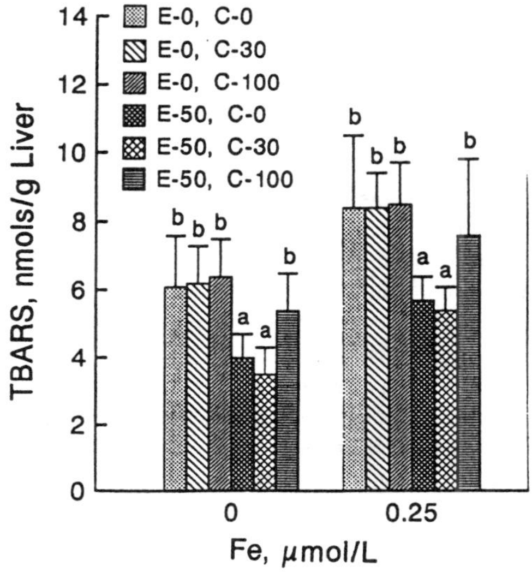

FIG. 1. EFFECT OF DIET AND IRON ON THE TBARS PRODUCED BY LIVER SLICES IN 1 H INCUBATION

(Bars show TBARS means ± standard deviation. TBARS with different letters within the same iron concentration are significantly different at P ≤ 0.05.)

For the experimental results shown in Fig. 1, a simplified model can be developed which presents the main determining parameters of the oxidation reaction, vitamin E and β-carotene:

$$\text{TBARS} = \frac{\text{lipid peroxidation components} \times \log(\text{Fe})}{\text{vitamin E} + 0.5\ \beta\text{-carotene}} + \text{basal lipid peroxidation}$$

"Lipid peroxidation components" is a composite of the factors involved in the reaction which are not otherwise expressed in the equation. In the model, β-carotene is assigned a strength of 0.5 compared to that of vitamin E. However, low concentration of β-carotene in the tissue diminishes its effect as a viable antioxidant. A correlation of the experimental results in a particular study, with the results predicted by a simulation model of the reaction, can test the validity of the simulation model in its highly aggregated form as a good model of the actual experimental results. In this experiment, the correlation between simulated TBARS and experimental TBARS is very good, $R = 0.68$, $P = 0.001$.

HEME PROTEIN OXIDATION AND MULTIANTIOXIDANTS

There is need for new methods of measuring tissue oxidation and the oxidative processes in animals that are being studied. We have developed a new method of measuring heme protein oxidation to delineate tissue oxidation, the Heme Spectral

Analysis Program (HSAP) (North *et al.* 1996). In animal tissue studies, heme proteins are the major chromophoric compounds in the visible region of the spectrum. Heme compounds change from one compound to another upon oxidation. HSAP transmission spectra of tissue slices or homogenates reveal the spectral absorption of all the elements in the tissue and thus have high turbidity. Turbidity is a major problem in the use of the method. On top of the spectrum of the turbidity are the spectra of the heme compounds. To deconvolute the spectra, the literature standard spectra of hemoglobin and its derivatives, deoxyhemoglobin, oxyhemoglobin and methemoglobin are used. We also incorporate the standard spectra of the hemochromes and hemichromes that can be formed as well as minor components, such as the cytochromes of mitochondria and microsomes. Because all these pigments are present in tissue, for example heart tissue, it is a major problem to deconvolute the spectra of the combined absorptions of all pigments into the spectral absorption of each component and thus determine the quantity of each oxidized heme pigment. We have been able to do this. The spectrum of heart homogenate shows in the visible region the major peak of oxyhemoglobin and in the near-ultraviolet region the corresponding γ peak of the heme protein (Fig. 2). After the homogenate is allowed to oxidize, the spectrum indicates principally methemoglobin with the corresponding γ peak in the near ultraviolet region. The spectrum also incorporates the turbidity absorption shown under the spectrum of the major heme proteins which must be subtracted from the absorption of the heme proteins. The study of oxidized heme proteins is useful in experiments of tissues and homogenates being oxidized. Elevated levels of heme protein oxidation correlate with increases in TBARS and enzyme inactivation, another method of measuring oxidative damage.

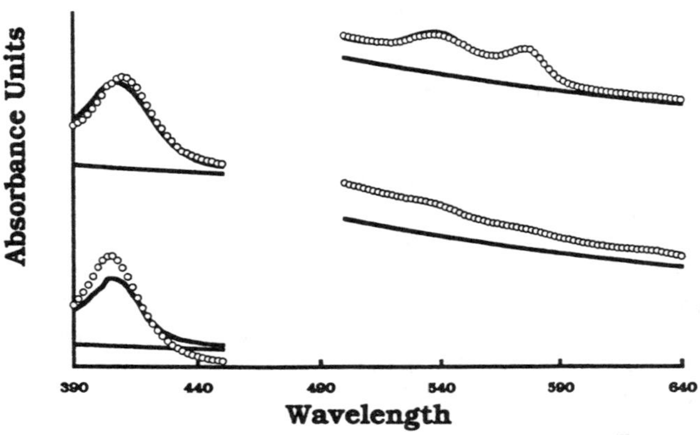

FIG. 2. HEME PROTEIN ANALYSIS

In another experiment (Chen and Tappel 1994), antioxidant nutrients were added to the basal diet (B) to provide maximum protection (Table 2). No antioxidants were added to the control basal diet (B). The second diet (E + Se) contained enough vitamin

E and selenium to offer sufficient protection against normal conditions. For maximum defense against oxidative conditions the third diet (ALL) contained multiantioxidant nutrients including β-carotene, canthaxanthin, coenzyme Q_{10} and coenzyme Q_0 to provide the antioxygenic activity of coenzyme Q, trolox C, a more water soluble model of vitamin E, ascorbyl palmitate as an ascorbic acid antioxygenic agent since the rat makes its own ascorbic acid and (+)-catechin, a polyphenol such as those present in fruits and vegetables. A summary of the results is shown in Fig. 3. Oxidized heme proteins develop

TABLE 2.
ADDITION OF ANTIOXIDANT NUTRIENTS TO BASAL DIET

	Amount of antioxidant (mg/kg)		
		Diet group	
Antioxidant	B	E + Se	ALL
Vitamin E	0	25	25
Selenium	0	0.3	0.3
β-Carotene	0	0	45
Coenzyme Q_{10}	0	0	30
Ascorbic acid 6-Palmitate	0	0	100
Canthaxanthin	0	0	45
Trolox C	0	0	50
Acetylcysteine	0	0	200
Coenzyme Q_0	0	0	100
(+)-Catechin	0	0	100

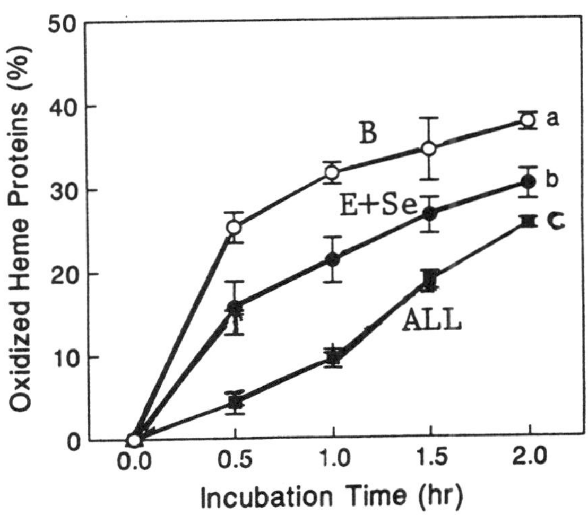

FIG. 3. PRODUCTION OF OXIDIZED HEME PROTEINS DURING THE SPONTANEOUS OXIDATIVE REACTION IN LIVER SLICES

as a function of time with the highest amount forming in the liver of animals on the basal diet. Some protection is given by the vitamin E and selenium diet. Further protection against oxidative damage to the liver is provided by the diet containing multiantioxygenic agents. From a practical standpoint, this is probably maximum protection of tissue. The amounts of antioxygenic nutrients added to the diets are within the range humans can receive from their food supply or supplementary additions to their diets.

REFERENCES

CHEN, H. and TAPPEL, A.L. 1994. Protection by vitamin E, selenium, trolox C, ascorbic acid palmitate, acetylcysteine, coenzyme Q, beta-carotene, canthaxanthin, and (+)-catechin against oxidative damage to liver slices measured by oxidized heme proteins. Free Rad. Biol. Med. *16*, 437–444.

DAVIES, K.J.A. 1991. Oxidative Damage and Repair, Pergamon Press, New York, New York.

NORTH, J.A., REIN, D. and TAPPEL, A.L. 1996. Multicomponent analysis of heme protein spectra in biological materials. Anal. Biochem. *233*, 115–123.

PACKER, L. and FUCHS, J., eds. 1993. Vitamin E in Health and Disease, Marcel Dekker, New York, New York.

PELLET, L.J, ANDERSEN, H.J., CHEN, H. and TAPPEL, A.L. 1994. β-Carotene alters vitamin E protection against heme protein oxidation and lipid peroxidation in chicken liver slices. J. Nutr. Biochem. *5*, 479–484.

TAPPEL, A.L., HAWKES, W.C., WILHELMSEN, E.C. and MOTSENBOCKER, M. A. 1984. Selenocysteine-containing proteins and glutathione peroxidase. Meth. Enzymol. *107*, 602–619.

TAPPEL, A.L., TAPPEL, A.A. and FRAGA, C.B. 1989. Application of simulation modeling to lipid peroxidation processes. Free Rad. Biol. Med. *7*, 361–368.

NUTRITIONAL CHALLENGES AND OPPORTUNITIES FOR IMPROVED HEALTH IN THE PACIFIC RIM

JANET C. KING

Western Human Nutrition Research Center, USDA/ARS
P.O. Box 29997
Presidio of San Francisco, CA 94129

ABSTRACT

Wealth and poverty have profound effects on diet, nutrition, and health. As income rises and populations become more urban, diets high in complex carbohydrate and fiber are generally replaced with diets containing a higher proportion of sugars, fats, and saturated fats. This transition is enhanced by human preferences for dietary sugar and fat, and the change is associated with a higher prevalence of obesity and non-insulin dependent diabetes mellitus (Popkin 1994).

INTRODUCTION

A direct relationship between the gross national product (GNP) per capita and the global diet structure was documented in the early 1960s in studies conducted by the Food and Agriculture Organization of the United Nations (Drewnowski and Popkin 1997). Diets high in fat, especially from animal products such as meat and milk, were tied to a high level of income at both the national and individual level. However, within the past two decades there has been a major shift in the structure of the income - diet relationship. Fat consumption is less dependent on income than ever observed before. Also, the rapid increase in urbanization occurring world-wide is accelerating the transition to a higher fat diet among lower income individuals and nations (Drewnowski and Popkin 1997).

CHEAP VEGETABLE FATS

The marked increase in the availability of cheap vegetable fats in the past 25 years is the primary basis for the uncoupling of the classic relationship between income and fat intake (Drewnowski and Popkin 1997). The production and processing of oilseed-based fats has been enhanced by technological break-throughs. Those break-throughs reduced the cost of margarine, baking, and frying fats in relation to animal fat. Also, a number of economic and political initiatives led to an increase in the development of oil crops around the world. For example, the production of vegetable oils increased four times in the United States between 1945 to 1965. The transition towards an increased intake of vegetable oils was also fueled by health concerns regarding the consumption of animal fat and cholesterol. Soybean oil accounts for the bulk of vegetable oil consumption world-wide; it makes up 70 percent of the edible oils and fats produced in the United States.

DIETARY TRENDS IN ASIA

Economic growth and dietary transition has been particularly evident in the Asian countries. As the economies of these countries have grown over the past 25 years, so has the proportion of energy from fat in the diet. The trend in the Asian countries is towards a diet in which 30-35% of the energy is derived from fat. This is not very different from the fat intakes in the United States.

China, a rapidly-growing world economy, is in the early stages of this diet transition. But, the trend towards a higher intake of vegetable fat and a decline in carbohydrate is already set. As seen elsewhere around the world, this trend is fueled by an increase in oilseed production and imports. China's production of oilseeds increased by 50 percent between 1991 to 1996, and vegetable oil imports more than tripled (Drewnowski and Popkin 1997). Consequently, the percent energy provided by fat in the diet increased several fold in all income groups in China. This increase was most dramatic among the high income groups. The proportion of high income households consuming a high-fat diet (>30% energy as fat) between 1989 and 1993 increased from 22.8 to 66.6%; in low income households, it increased from 19.1 to 26.4% (Campbell and Chen 1994).

Japan is in the later stages of the global dietary transition to a higher fat diet. Japan went through a stage of accelerated economic growth between 1950 and 1970 (Lands *et al.* 1990). During that time, the traditional meal pattern of rice with soybean soup, pickled vegetables, and some fish was replaced by small servings of rice with the addition of meat, fish, vegetables, and milk. Fat intake tripled during the transition with the consumption of vegetable fats and oils rising from 6 to 31 pounds per capita per year (Drewnowski and Popkin 1997).

There also was a marked increase in diet diversity during this transition in Japan. Diet diversity is defined as the number of foods consumed in a day. The intake of animal products rose dramatically and there was a shift from cheap fish sources (i.e. herring, sardines, and mackerel) to expensive sources, such as salmon, tuna, shrimp, and lobster.

Although there is concern that the increase in dietary fat poses a health risk among the Japanese population, others argue that the dietary changes are generally beneficial. The increased intake of animal foods tend to enhance the overall diet quality and may improve the nutritional status of the Japanese people.

These changes in the Japanese diet are especially useful to study because they serve as a model for the dietary transitions occurring in China and other Asian countries. The challenge is to enhance the nutritional benefits of the dietary transition while reducing the negative effects.

INCREASING DIETARY DIVERSITY

As income grows, diets become more diverse as well as higher in fat. People incorporate more meat and fish, milk, eggs, and cheese into their habitual diets. Often the new foods include sweets, which were previously inaccessible to low income populations. Thus, with a rise in income, the intake of sweets and fats increases and places the population at greater risk for obesity and associated chronic diseases (Drewnowski and Popkin 1997).

In China, the mean dietary diversity score, an indicator of the number of different food groups eaten, increased from 5.4 to 6.0 in the four years between 1989 and 1993 among individuals in the low income tertile (Drewnowski and Popkin 1997). More importantly, the number of individuals consuming less than four different food groups decreased from 32.5 to 19.2 percent. During this same period of time the economy of the country increased.

THE GLOBAL DIET TRANSITION: CHALLENGES AND OPPORTUNITIES

The emerging transition in the global diet includes an increased proportion of calories from vegetable fat and, to a lesser extent, sugars, and a rise in diet diversity. Three events account for these trends: 1) the rapid economic growth of developing countries; 2) growing urbanization throughout the world; and 3) the recent availability of cheap vegetable fats.

There is a strong likelihood that a diet containing approximately 30% of the energy from fat will become the global norm. In the United States and other developed countries, high fat diets are generally regarded as unhealthy. However, diets higher in fats are also more varied and may provide improved intakes of vitamins and minerals. One challenge for nutritionists is to develop a tool that evaluates "total" diet quality and healthy eating habits. This tool should assess diet balance and variety as well as the intake of essential nutrients.

Trends towards higher fat diets increase the risk of diet-related chronic diseases such as obesity, cardiovascular diseases, diabetes, and cancer. Health professionals in the developing nations should begin to develop policies for nutrition education and dietary interventions. Such policies should steer the population towards a healthy diet while maintaining diet diversity.

Data from the United States suggest that some success can be achieved at keeping the fat content of the diet around 30 percent. This was largely accomplished with assistance from the food industry. Americans have access to a wide variety of low-fat snack foods or low-fat convenience foods. The addition of those foods to the diet often replaces other more nutrient-dense, low-fat foods such as fruits, vegetables, and selected cuts of meat, fish, and poultry. Nutrition education programs are needed that show the public how to place new food items in the total diet while maintaining overall diet quality.

As food scientists and nutritionists approach these opportunities and challenges, the underlying principles of nutrition interventions need to be kept in mind. First, the vulnerable population groups around the world are not homogeneous, so one remedy will not fit all. The solutions need to be population-specific. Second, to intervene effectively requires that one knows fairly precisely what is lacking or in excess in the diet and why. And, third, the reasons for deviations from a quality diet are complex and multi-disciplinary. Thus, the more varied the talents brought to bear on the problem, the richer the knowledge base and the more secure the design of intervention strategies. It is not too soon for food scientists, nutritionists, economists, policy-makers, and health-care professionals to join forces and develop policies and nutrition intervention programs that promote diet quality and good health.

REFERENCES

CAMPBELL, T.C. and CHEN, J. 1994. Diet and chronic degenerative diseases: Perspectives from China. Am. J. Clin. Nutr. *59* (suppl), 1153S–1161S.

DREWNOWSKI, A. and POPKIN, B.M. 1997. The nutrition transition: New trends in the global diet. Nutr. Rev. *55*, 31–43.

LANDS, W.E.M., HAMAZAKI, T., YAMAZAKI, K., OKUYAMA, H., SAKAI, K., GOTO, Y. and HUBBARD, V.S. 1990. Changing dietary patterns. Am. J. Clin. Nutr. *51*, 991–993.

POPKIN, B.M. 1994. The nutrition transition in low-income countries: An emerging crisis. Nutr. Rev. *52*, 285–298.

NUTRITIONAL ENHANCEMENT OF ASIAN WHEAT PRODUCTS BY STARCH AND PROTEIN SUPPLEMENTATION

HAROLD CORKE, FELICIANO P. BEJOSANO and LILIA S. COLLADO

Cereal Science Laboratory
Department of Botany
University of Hong Kong
Pokfulam Road, Hong Kong

ABSTRACT

Asia is home to a unique cultural history and diversity of wheat flour based products. In much of tropical Asia, such as in the Philippines, wheat is not produced and its importation represents a drain on foreign currency reserves. The utilization of indigenous raw materials (such as sweet potato flour or starch, and various specialty grain products such as amaranth and buckwheat) is being pursued to create wheat-based products with improved nutritional profile and hence consumer appeal. In this paper we will discuss two examples of this approach. In the first case, protein concentrates were made by wet-milling amaranth grain. The protein concentrates showed excellent solubility, foaming and emulsification properties, and had nutritionally desirable quality scores (PDCAAS) with high levels of lysine and other amino acids. The protein concentrates increased the strength of noodle doughs, and somewhat enhanced texture of cooked noodle strands, showing that desirable nutritional and functional properties could be obtained from these materials. In the second study, composite flour noodles were made of 75:25 wheat:sweet potato (SP) flour. Early results indicated that a softer texture resulted from SP flour addition. Further study was conducted to achieve control of high amylase activity which impacted on texture. The addition of novel starches to wheat-based products gives opportunities to provide products with higher levels of resistant starch.

INTRODUCTION

Asian wheat products are extremely diverse, covering a wide range of traditional product types within major classes such as noodles, steamed bread and dough wrapped items. Some of these products have a long history of traditional development and use, and often have specific quality parameters based on exacting consumer demands. Examples include Japanese *udon* (white-salted) noodles, which require wheat starch of particular high-swelling characteristics; and Japanese *soba* or wheat-buckwheat composite flour noodles where there is a long cultural history leading to consumer demand for high-priced premium types. Some products have different characteristics in different regions. For example, we can distinguish Northern-style from Southern-style Chinese steamed bread (Huang and Miskelly 1991), with the latter having a richer formulation with more sugar or fat. Some products have a much more recent history. For example, the common steamed-and-fried instant noodles (*ramen*) were developed in Japan only in the late

1950's but have expanded to a massive industry in Asia and even worldwide. For these recently developed products, we can surmise that consumer demands for specific quality properties are less bound by tradition, and there should potentially be more room for flexibility in developing innovative new variants. There is increasing worldwide concern about the quality of our diet and its impact on health. Reduction in animal fat consumption, increased dietary fiber intake, and a new reliance on plant sources of protein are key elements in some of the dietary trends today.

Grain *Amaranthus* is an emerging specialty grain crop in China. It has long been used as a leafy vegetable and a source of livestock feed in Asia. Since the early 1980's, research and breeding efforts at the Chinese Academy of Agricultural Sciences, Beijing, have resulted in its production as a commercial grain crop on over 40,000 hectares annually in China (Yue *et al.* 1993). *Amaranthus* grain is used in a variety of foods, such as noodles and soy sauce in China (Yue *et al.* 1993), and other products including infant formula in other parts of the world such as Mexico (Breene 1991). *Amaranthus* is known for its unusual starch, in particular the small starch granule size and stable paste properties (Lorenz 1981; Stone and Lorenz 1984; Wu *et al.* 1995; Corke *et al.* 1996). *Amaranthus* starch is effectively purified by alkali wet-milling (Myers and Fox 1994), leaving a protein by-product for which adequate value-added applications have not yet been developed. We are investigating the use of the high-nutritional value protein concentrates of alkali wet-milling of grain *Amaranthus* as functional and nutritive additives to flour-based products such as noodles.

China is the world's largest producer of sweet potato (*Ipomea batatas*) with 85% of the global total of 125 million tons in 1988 (Scott 1992). Production has been declining due to a switch to higher value vegetables, weak demand and lack of alternative markets or value-added uses of sweet potato (Scott 1992). Sweet potato tends to suffer from a negative image of being "a poor man's food" or survival crops in many parts of the world (Collins 1987; Watson 1989).

However, a wide range of food products can be made from sweet potato (reviewed in Collado 1997). The products processed directly from fresh roots are fried chips/strips, flakes, canned roots, frozen cubes/slices, puree/paste alcoholic beverages, vinegar, pickles, candies, jams, sweets, non-alcoholic beverages and catsup. The flour can be further processed into bakery products and noodles while the starch is further processed into noodles, baked products and various industrial products such as sugar syrups, alcohol, citric acid, monosodium glutamate, amino acids and dextrin. In order to change the status of sweet potato from a subsistence to market-oriented commodity, efforts should be devoted to the improvement of present utilization.

Among sweet potato cultivars, starch physical properties (e.g. Shiotani *et al.* 1991; Collado *et al.* 1997) and digestibility (Tsuo and Hong 1989; Zhang *et al.* 1993) vary significantly. The relationship of low starch digestibility to poor cooking quality needs further study (AVRDC 1988). Flatulence factors in sweet potato are due to starch and undigestible fractions as there was no correlation observed between free sugar fractions and flatulence (Tsuo and Yang 1984). Unlike legumes, the concentration of indigestible oligosaccharides in sweet potato are too low for the flatulence that accompanies ingestion of sweet potato (Troung *et al.* 1986). In different circumstances, we may seek low or high starch digestibility for different types of food product development. There is scope for low-digestibility starches in reduced calorie or high-fiber foods. While investigating in more depth the genetic variation in starch digestibility, and the effect of processing variables in modifying it, we should also proceed to select appropriate starch physical properties for favorable textural/sensory outcomes in specific food products.

UTILIZATION OF *AMARANTHUS* PROTEINS

Nutritional Quality

Isoelectric protein concentrates (IPC) were prepared by alkaline wet-milling, acid precipitation and freeze-drying from five varieties of grain *Amaranthus* provided by the Chinese Academy of Agricultural Sciences, Beijing, and agronomically adapted to Chinese conditions. The mean *in vitro* protein digestibility (81%) in the raw IPC was higher than in raw wholemeal flour (74%) (Bejosano and Corke 1997), but the digestibility of IPC unexpectedly decreased on heating. Trypsin inhibitor and polyphenolic compounds were found to be related to *in vitro* digestibility. The amino acid profiles of the five genotypes were similar to each other, and leucine and lysine were slightly inadequate in the IPCs relative to FAO/WHO suggested patterns. The lowest amino acid score in the IPCs was 0.88 for lysine, giving an estimated (based on *in vitro* data) Protein Digestibility-Corrected Amino Acid Score (PDCAAS; Henley and Kuster 1994) of 0.71 (Bejosano and Corke 1997), which is extremely high compared to most cereal-derived proteins.

Functional Properties

IPCs from five *Amaranthus* genotypes were prepared as above, except they were air-dried at 70°C rather than freeze-dried. They were more soluble in water than two soy protein isolate standards over a pH range 3-9, except at pH 9. At all pH levels, most of the *Amaranthus* IPCs had greater foaming stability than the soy proteins. Genotype K350 gave the best result. Similarly, emulsifying ability of *Amaranthus* IPCs exceeded that of soy proteins, and again K350 gave the best result. These results were attributed to the high solubility of *Amaranthus* proteins which led to favorable foam stability and emulsification results.

Effect on Dough and Noodle Rheology

We showed above that *Amaranthus* protein concentrates, normally treated as a waste product of specialty starch wet-milling, are of desirable nutritional quality and also have apparent potential due to their good functional properties. This was further tested by preparation of a specific food product. Freeze-dried IPCs were made from five *Amaranthus* genotypes. Flour dough was made following standard mixograph procedures, supplemented with 4% IPC (flour weight basis), and characterized by dynamic oscillatory rheometry (StressTech, Reologica AB, Sweden) using oscillation frequency sweep at constant stress of 10 pa. Dry noodles were made including 1.5% salt (Rho *et al.* 1988), and the effect of 2% IPC (flour weight basis) was tested.

Added proteins greatly increased elastic modulus (G') of wheat dough (Fig. 1A) and decreased phase degree (δ), the liquid-like behavior (data not shown), showing that the IPCs strengthened dough structure. There were genotypic differences among *Amaranthus* IPCs in their effect, which were highly correlated to the insoluble protein fraction. K112 had the greatest effect. In the case of cooked noodle viscoelastic properties, some of the IPCs especially that of genotype K350 significantly affected G', increasing rigidity (Fig. 1B). Effects on δ were less significant.

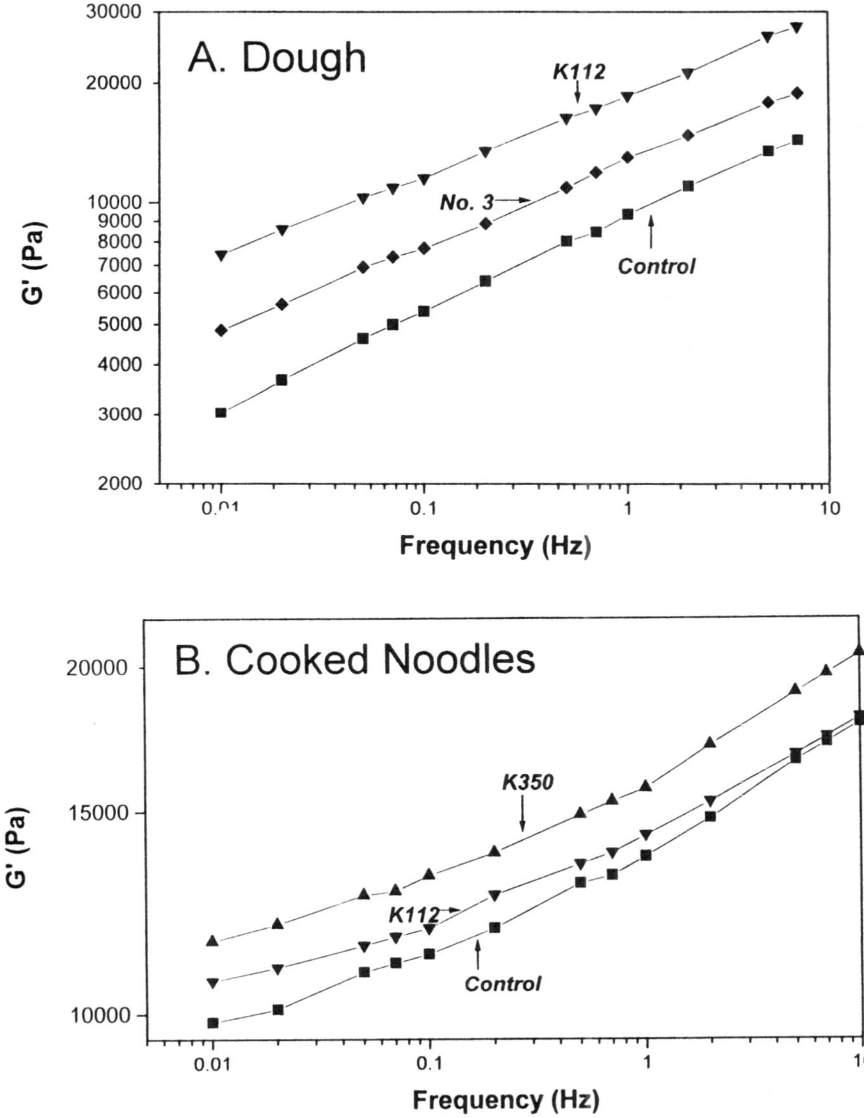

FIG. 1. EFFECT OF ISOELECTRIC PROTEIN CONCENTRATES (IPC) ON ELASTIC MODULUS OF: A. WHEAT FLOUR DOUGH (IPC AT 4% FLOUR WEIGHT BASIS); AND B. COOKED NOODLES (IPC AT 2% FLOUR WEIGHT BASIS).

USE OF SWEET POTATO IN NOODLES

Wheat:Sweet Potato Composite Noodles

In an earlier report (Collado and Corke 1996) we made yellow-alkaline and white-salted noodles from a standard hard red winter wheat flour substituted 25% with each of four genotypes of sweet potato flour. The RVA (Rapid Visco-Analyzer, Newport Instruments, Australia) viscoamylographs were significantly different under 'as-is' or slightly acidic pH (5.7-6.0) (representative of white-salted noodle conditions), but much more similar under alkaline conditions (pH 10) (representative of yellow-alkaline noodle conditions), primarily due to differences in amylase activity. Consistent with this, yellow-alkaline noodles were firmer and showed lower cooking loss than white-salted noodles.

The lower gelatinization temperature and enthalpy of wheat starch compared to sweet potato would explain its susceptibility to sweet potato amylases. Wheat starch granules would be fully gelatinized at the optimum temperature condition for sweet potato diastatic activity (around 70°C) (Collado and Corke 1996; Collado 1997). β-Amylase has little or no effect on intact starch granules, and although α-amylase has some effect it is far more rapid on gelatinized starch (Hoseney 1990). These observations would explain the dramatic effect of sweet potato flour on pasting properties of the composite flours.

pH Dependent Amylase Activity

Clearly, there is a critical interaction between processing condition effects (primarily temperature and pH) and genetic effects on sweet potato amylase activity, and hence the effective use of sweet potato flour in Asian food products. If the amylase activity can be controlled, then there is greater chance of useful manipulation of starch physical properties and starch digestibility by addition of selected genotypes of sweet potato. Figure 2 illustrates the interaction of genotype and pH on peak viscosity of composite flours.

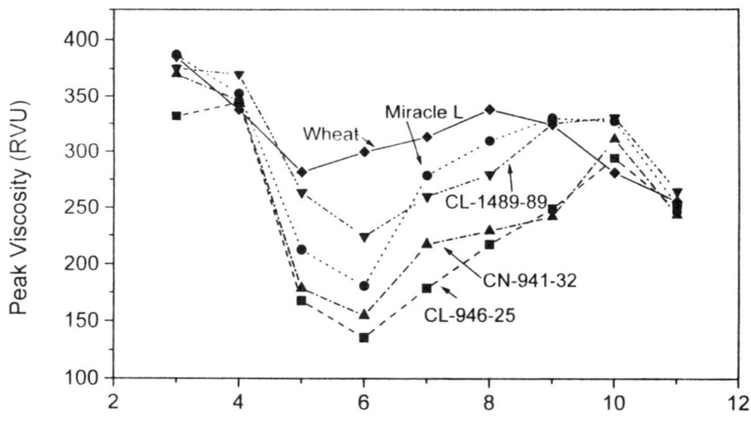

FIG. 2. EFFECT OF PH ON RVA PEAK VISCOSITY OF 25:75 SWEET POTATO: WHEAT FLOUR MADE WITH FOUR DIFFERENT SWEET POTATO GENOTYPES DIFFERING IN AMYLASE ACTIVITY

CONCLUSIONS

Asian cereal/starch based foods are very diverse, and open to new product development for nutritionally improved value-added products. This process can be aided by use of some of the unusual or underutilized raw materials presently available or under development. Nutritional improvement cannot occur independently of physical and sensory quality improvement. There is scope for improvement of Asian-type products for use within Asia, and for products based on traditional Asian foods for increasing development of the "ethnic" foods market in the U.S. and other Western countries.

ACKNOWLEDGMENTS

Financial support was received from the Hong Kong Research Grants Council and the University of Hong Kong Committee on Research and Conference Grants. Continuing collaboration with Profs. S.X. Yue and H.L. Sun (Chinese Academy of Agricultural Sciences, Beijing), on *Amaranthus*; and Dr. Chris Wheatley (CIP, Bogor, Indonesia), on sweet potato is much appreciated.

REFERENCES

AVRDC. 1988. Chemistry - screening for starch digestibility of sweet potato. *In* Progress Report. Asian Vegetable Research and Development Center, Taiwan.

BEJOSANO, F.P. and CORKE, H. 1997. Protein quality evaluation of *Amaranthus* wholemeal flours and protein concentrates. J. Sci. Food Agric. (in press)

BREENE, W.M. 1991. Food uses of grain amaranth. Cereal Foods World *36,* 426–430.

COLLADO, L.S. 1997. Physical Properties and Utilization of Sweetpotato Starch and Flour. Ph.D. dissertation, University of Hong Kong, Hong Kong.

COLLADO, L.S. and CORKE, H. 1996. Use of wheat - sweet potato composite flours for yellow-alkaline and white-salted noodles. Cereal Chem. *73*, 439–444.

COLLINS, W.W. 1987. Improvement of nutritional and edible qualities of sweetpotato for human consumption. *In* Exploration, Maintenance and Utilization of Sweet-potato Genetic Resources. International Potato Center (CIP), Lima, Peru.

CORKE, H., WU, H., YUE, S. and SUN, H. 1996. Developing specialty starches from new crops: A case study using grain amaranth. *In* Cereals: Novel Uses and Processes, G.M. Campbell, C. Webb and S.L. McKee (eds.). Plenum Publishing Corp., New York.

HENLEY, E.C. and KUSTER, J.M. 1994. Protein quality evaluation by protein digestibility-corrected amino acid scoring. Food Technol. *48*(4), 74–77.

HOSENEY, R.C. 1990. Principles of Cereal Science and Technology. American Association of Cereal Chemists, Inc., St. Paul, MN.

HUANG, S. and MISKELLY, D.M. 1994. Steamed bread - a popular food in China. Food Aust. *43*, 346–351.

LORENZ, K. 1981. *Amaranthus hypochondriacus* - characteristics of the starch and baking potential of the flour. Starch/Stärke *33*, 149–153.

MYERS, D.J. and FOX, S.R. 1994. Alkali wet-milling characteristics of pearled and unpearled amaranth seed. Cereal Chem. *71*, 96–99.

RHO, K.L., SEIB, P.A., CHUNG, O.K. and DEYOE, C.W. 1988. Noodles. VII. Investigating the surface firmness of cooked oriental dry noodles made from hard wheat flours. Cereal Chem. *65*, 320–326.

STONE, L.A. and LORENZ, K. 1984. The starch of Amaranthus - physico-chemical properties and functional characteristics. Starch/Stärke *36*, 232–237.

SCOTT, G.J. 1992. Transforming traditional food crops: product development for roots and tubers. *In* Production Development for Root and Tuber Crops. Vol. I, Asia. G.J. Scott, S. Wiersema and P.I. Ferguson (eds.). International Potato Center (CIP), Lima, Peru.

SHIOTANI, I., NISHIMURA, A., YAMANAKA, S., TAKI, M. and YAMADA, T. 1991. Starch properties of the sweet potato, diploid *Ipomea trifida* (H.B.K.) Don and tetraploid hybrids. Starch/Stärke *43*, 133–138.

TSUO, S.C.S. and HONG, T.L. 1989. Digestibility of sweetpotato starch. *In* Improvement of Sweetpotato (*Ipomea batatas*) in Asia. International Potato Center (CIP), Lima, Peru.

TSUO, S.C.S. and YANG, M.H. 1984. Flatulence factors in sweet potato. Acta Hort. *163*, 179–186.

TROUNG, V.D., BIERMANN, C.J. and MARLETT, J.A. 1986. Simple sugars, oligosaccharides and starch concentrations in raw and cooked sweet potato. J. Agric. Food Chem. *34*, 421–425.

WATSON, G.A. 1989. Sweet potato production and consumption surveys: variability and varieties. *In* Improvement of Sweet Potato (*Ipomea batatas*) in Asia. Report of Workshop on Sweet Potato Improvement in Asia. International Potato Center (CIP), Lima, Peru.

WU, H., YUE, S., SUN, H. and CORKE, H. 1995. Physical properties of starch from two genotypes of *Amaranthus cruentus* of agricultural significance in China. Starch/Stärke *47,* 295–297.

YUE, S.X., SUN, H.L. and TANG, F.D. (eds). 1993. The Research and Development of Grain *Amaranthus* in China. Chinese Agricultural Science and Technology Publishing House, Beijing, China.

ZHANG, D., COLLINS, W.W. and SUZANNE, B. 1993. Improving sweet potato starch digestibility for animal feeding. Hort. Sci. *28*, 325–326.

BIOACTIVE PEPTIDES IN MILK AND THEIR BIOLOGICAL AND HEALTH IMPLICATIONS

RUO-JUN XU

Department of Zoology
The University of Hong Kong, Hong Kong

ABSTRACT

Milk contains a large number of bioactive peptides which either exist naturally in milk or derive from milk protein hydrolyses. The natural bioactive peptides found in milk include epidermal growth factor (EGF), transforming growth factor (TGF), nerve growth factor (NGF), insulin, insulin-like growth factor I (IGF-I) and IGF-II. The concentrations of these peptides are generally high in colostrum, and the concentrations are often higher than those found in blood circulation. Animal studies have shown that the natural bioactive peptides in milk may play a role in regulating postnatal gut development in suckling neonates. The second group of bioactive peptides found in milk include casomorphins, immunostimulating peptides and ACE-inhibitory peptides; they are part of the primary structures of milk proteins and can be released by enzymatic hydrolysis. These peptides may act as potential physiological modulators during the gastrointestinal digestion of milk. In addition, they may be a potential source of bioactive ingredients for designing "functional" foods. This review gives a brief summary of various bioactive peptides found in milk and a discussion on biological and health significance of such peptides on consumers.

INTRODUCTION

Milk is not only a source of nutrients but also a carrier of various forms of bioactive compounds. These bioactive compounds are likely to have a significant influence on suckling neonates. Milk-borne immunoglobulins, for example, have long been known to play a significant role in protecting newborn infants from intestinal infections. Various hydrolytic enzymes found in milk are known to facilitate nutrient digestion in the gastrointestinal tract of neonates. More recent studies showed that milk also has a larger number of bioactive peptides. These peptides have a wide range of biological activities, acting in the body either as hormones, growth factors or neurotransmitters. They may exist naturally in milk or derive from milk protein hydrolyses. Their biological significance and their impacts on consumer health are currently under intensive investigation.

NATURAL BIOACTIVE PEPTIDES IN MILK

There are a number of bioactive peptides existing naturally in milk in various species (Koldovsky 1994; Xu 1996). It has been speculated that these milk-borne bioactive peptides may play a functional role in regulating postnatal development in suckling infants, particularly in regulating gastrointestinal development. Animal studies show that the gastrointestinal tract undergoes very rapid maturational changes during the immediate postnatal period (Xu and Cranwell 1990, 1991; Xu *et al.* 1992ab) and that the changes will not occur if animals are prevented from suckling. Oral feeding of colostrum stimulates intestinal and pancreatic tissue growth and enzyme maturation (Wang and Xu 1996; Mubiru and Xu 1997) and the effect diminishes after pretreatment of the colostrum with proteolytic enzymes. These findings indicate that colostrum contains bioactive compounds which stimulate gastrointestinal development in the suckling young. In the following, milk-borne epidermal growth factor (EGF) and insulin-like growth factors I and II (IGF-I & IGF-II) and their possible role in regulating postnatal development in neonates will be discussed in detail.

EGF

Epidermal growth factor (EGF) is a single-chain polypeptide of 53 amino acid residues with a molecular weight of about 6040. EGF is found in various tissues in all mammalian species studied and has a wide range of biological activities, including inhibition of gastric acid secretion and stimulation of epithelial cell proliferation and differentiation (Xu 1996).

It was first shown in 1978 that human milk exhibited mitogenic activity for cultured fibroblasts (Klagsbrun 1978) and the activity could be suppressed by anti-EGF antibodies (Carpenter 1980). Since then EGF has been found in the milk of several species and the concentration is highest in porcine milk, followed by human and mouse milk, and lowest in cattle, horse and rat milk (Read *et al.* 1984; Jaeger *et al.* 1987; Raaberg *et al.* 1990; Iacopetta *et al.* 1992). The concentration of EGF in milk from mothers given premature-birth is higher than that from mothers given term-birth. The concentration is generally higher in colostrum than in milk in most species except tammar wallaby and laboratory rodents, of which milk EGF concentration rises after parturition. EGF concentration in milk increases following exogenous insulin treatment in rats (Thulesen *et al.* 1993).

There is evidence showing that milk-borne EGF can survive the gastrointestinal digestion in neonatal animals. EGF showed little changes in its immunological or receptor binding properties after incubation with gastric intestinal contents of premature human infants (Britton *et al.* 1989), suckling rats (Britton *et al.* 1988), and suckling pigs (Shen and Xu 1996). The binding ability decreased only slightly after incubation with small intestinal contents of suckling rats and piglets, although it decreased to a much greater degree after incubation with the intestinal contents of weaned animals (Britton *et al.* 1988; Shen and Xu 1996; Xu and Shen 1997). Up to 70% of EGF remained intact 30 min after injection into the stomach in suckling rats (Rao 1994). In newborn lambs 60-90% of EGF reached the small intestine in the intact form following orogastric administration. The survival of EGF in the gastrointestinal lumen in neonatal animals has been attributed to the limited proteolytic enzyme secretion in the animals (Shen and Xu 1996). Furthermore, milk of various species contains protease inhibitors which can protect milk-borne EGF from luminal digestion in suckling animals (Xu *et al.* 1996).

Exogenous EGF administered into the gastrointestinal lumen stimulates gastrointestinal tissue growth. Inclusion of EGF in the diet significantly accelerated intestinal growth in normal newborn rats and in weaned rats following 50% removal of the small intestine (Read *et al.* 1986). Administration of EGF through a catheter into the ileum lumen of adult rats significantly increased ileal mucosa DNA synthesis and epithelial cell proliferation (Ulshen *et al.* 1986). In addition to its growth-promoting effect, EGF appears to be able to modulate the enterocyte differentiation. In newborn and weaned piglets, oral or systemic administration of EGF significantly increased jejunal lactase and sucrase activities (James *et al.* 1987; Jaeger *et al.* 1990). Dietary supplementation with a supraphysiological dose of EGF (1.0 mg/L) increased villus height in the proximal and mid small intestine and lactase-specific activity in the mid small intestine in rotavirus-infected pigs (Zijlstra *et al.* 1994). In normal adult rats or adult rats with a damaged intestinal mucosa following methotrexate treatment, dietary supplementation of EGF at 25 or 250 but not at 500 μg/kg body weight per day for 6 to 9 days significantly increased intestinal brush-border aminopeptidase and disaccharidase activities (Petschow *et al.* 1993).

In addition to the action on the gastrointestinal tract, milk-borne EGF may be absorbed into the blood circulation and act at distant targets. Growth-promoting effects following oral administration of EGF have been observed in organs other than the gastrointestinal tract (Xu 1996). It has also been reported that a considerable amount of orally administered EGF was absorbed intact into blood circulation in suckling rats (Thornburg *et al.* 1987). The absorption may be enhanced by milk fat globule membrane emulsification (Adachi *et al.* 1993).

IGF-I and IGF-II

Insulin-like growth factors (IGF-I and IGF-II) are single-chain polypeptides structurally similar to insulin. IGF-I consists of 70 amino acid residues with a molecular weight of about 7600; IGF-II, of 67 amino acid residues, has a molecular weight of about 7500; and insulin, of 51 amino acid residues, has a molecular weight of about 5800. The primary structures of IGF-I and IGF-II are highly conserved across species, and share about 70% and 45% homology with insulin, respectively (Xu 1996). IGF-I and IGF-II stimulate target cell proliferation and differentiation through binding to two types of IGF receptors. The type I receptor binds IGF-I with greater affinity than IGF-II and also binds insulin. The type II receptor binds IGF-II with greater affinity than IGF-I and does not bind insulin (Schober *et al.* 1990).

IGF-I and IGF-II, as well as insulin, have been detected in the mammary secretions of a number of species, including humans (Read *et al.* 1984), pigs (Westrom *et al.* 1987), cattle (Malven *et al.* 1987) and rats (Donovan *et al.* 1990). The concentrations of IGF-I and IGF-II are high in the colostrum and decrease rapidly to a low basal level within a few days of lactation in most species except rats and wallaby. In rats, one study reported a progressive decline of milk concentration of IGF-I during lactation (Donovan *et al.* 1990), while another study reported that the concentration increased during lactation period and peaked at 18 days postpartum (Olanrewaju *et al.* 1996). In wallabies, milk concentration of IGF-I increased during lactation and peaked at 205 days of lactation (Ballard *et al.* 1995). Eriksson *et al.* (1993) reported that at the first day of lactation human colostrum contains 5 times more IGF-I than IGF-II. By day 3 postpartum, IGF-I drops by 80% to a constant level whereas IGF-II increases 3-fold up to day 7. The milk concentration of IGF-I and IGF-II varies widely among species (Xu 1996). The concentration of IGF-I, for example, ranges between 72-541 ng/mL in porcine and bovine colostrum, while in human colostrum it is only 17-30 ng/mL. Similar variations are seen for insulin and IGF-II concentrations. The concentration of IGF-I and IGF-II in milk also vary widely among species. In addition, the concentration of IGF-I in milk may be increased by growth hormone treatment of lactating cows or lactating mothers.

Following oral ingestion, milk-borne IGF-I and IGF-II are likely to survive the gastrointestinal digestion in suckling animals and may even be absorbed into the blood circulation. Philipps *et al.* (1995) reported that a significant fraction of iodine labeled IGF-I and IGF-II remained intact in the gastrointestinal lumen of suckling rats 30 min after orogastric administration. In newborn piglets, following oral administration of iodine labeled IGF-I, radioactivity can be detected in blood circulation and up to 10% of the radioactivity can bind to the anti-IGF-I antibodies. Studies in our own laboratory also showed that a small percentage of orally administered IGF-I can be found in the blood circulation in newborn piglets and the absorption is independent of gut closure (Xu and Wang 1996).

The physiological role of milk-borne IGF-I and IGF-II remains to be established. Dietary supplementation of IGF-I at a supraphysiological dose stimulates intestinal tissue growth and epithelial cell proliferation in newborn pigs (Xu *et al.* 1994; Burrin *et al.* 1996), and in newborn calves (Baumrucker *et al.* 1994). On the other hand, oral administration of IGF-I at physiological dose appears to stimulate intestinal enzyme maturation in newborn rats (Young *et al.* 1990; Ma and Xu 1997). In fetal lambs intraluminal infusion of IGF-I led to a significant histological modification in the intestine and a rise of circulating level of the peptide (Trahair *et al.* 1997). Oral administration of insulin in newborn piglets also increases intestinal brush-border enzyme activities (Shulman 1990). It is not known if such action is through binding to the insulin receptors or IGF type I receptors.

BIOACTIVE PEPTIDES DERIVED FROM MILK PROTEINS

Milk protein consists of 80% casein and 20% whey proteins. The milk casein is further divided into α_{s1}-, α_{s2}-, β- and κ-caseins. The major whey proteins are β-lactoglobulin and α-lactalbumin, consisting of about 75% of total whey proteins. A number of bioactive peptides are encoded in the primary sequences of milk proteins (Fiat and Jolle 1989; Schlimme and Meisel 1995). Some of these bioactive peptides have significant influence on gastrointestinal functions. Phosphopeptides, for example, enhance gastrointestinal absorption of calcium, and β-casomorphins inhibit gastrointestinal contraction and fluid secretion (Schlimme and Meisel 1995). Some other bioactive peptides, such as immunostimulating peptides and antihypertensive peptides (ACE inhibitors) have significant effects on general health. These bioactive peptides encoded in milk protein may be released during natural hydrolytic processes in the gastrointestinal lumen or during food processing, and may therefore have significant biological and health implications.

Opioid Peptides

Endogenous opioid peptides, such as enkephalin, endophins and dynorphin, are derived from precursor molecules proopiomelancortin, proenkephalin and prodynorphin, and all have a typical N-terminal sequence Tyr-Gly-Gly-Phe (Kitts 1994). Opioid peptides are psychoactive compounds with hormonal and neurotransmitter activities which act both in the central nervous system and in peripheral organs. Exogenous opioid peptides stimulate pancreatic insulin and gastrointestinal somatostatin release, modulate animal behavior, stimulate intestinal absorption of electrolytes and water, modulate gastrointestinal motility, stimulate food intake, induce apnea and irregular breathing and modulate sleep patterns (Fiat and Jolles 1989).

Brantl *et al.* (1979) first reported that chloroform/methanol extracts of enzymatic digest of bovine casein displayed opioid activity. The extracts were found to contain a heptapeptide, Tyr-Pro-Phe-Pro-Gly-Pro-Ile, corresponding to the residues 60-66 of β-casein and was subsequently named β-casomorphin. Similar peptides have also been found in human and buffalo β-caseins (Brantl 1984; Petrilli *et al.* 1987). Stepwise hydrolysis from the C-terminal end of the heptapeptide generates a series of β-casomorphins of hexa-, penta- and tetrapeptides with the pentapeptide having the highest biological potency (Daniel *et al.* 1990) and C-terminal end amidation of the peptides increases their opioid potency. Immunoreactive casomorphins have also been detected in fermented milk and in infant formula.

Two further opioid peptides were found in the pepsin hydrolysates of bovine α_{s1}-casein (Zioudrou *et al.* 1979) and one from human α_{s1}-casein (Kampa *et al.* 1996), the so called α-casomorphins. The two bovine α-casomorphins, Agr-Tyr-Leu-Gly-Tyr-Leu and Agr-Tyr-Leu-Gly-Tyr-Leu-Glu, correspond to residues 90-95 and 90-96 of α-casein, respectively, and the human α-casomorphin, Tyr-Val-Pro-Phe-Pro, corresponds to residues 158-162 of human α_{s1}-casein. Three opioid peptide antagonists, casoxin A, casoxin B and casoxin C, have also been found in enzymatic digests of bovine κ-casein, with casoxin C having the highest biological potency (active at 5 μM in an *in vitro* assay) (Chiba *et al.* 1989). Casoxin A is a heptapeptide, Tyr-Pro-Ser-Tyr-Gly-Leu-Asn, corresponding to fragment 35-41 of κ-casein, casoxin B is a tetra-peptide, Tyr-Pro-Tyr-Tyr, corresponding to fragment 58-61 of κ-casein and casoxin C is a decapeptide, Tyr-Ile-Pro-Ile-Gln-Tyr-Val-Leu-Ser-Arg, corresponding to fragment 25-34 of κ-casein.

Immunoreactive β-casomorphins have been detected in the small intestinal contents of adult humans following bovine milk ingestion (Svedberg *et al.* 1985). An opioid active undecapeptide, corresponding to fragment 60-70 of β-casein, has also been identified in the duodenal contents of pigs fed bovine casein (Meisel and Frister 1989). These findings strongly suggest that opioid peptides are generated during gastrointestinal digestion of milk proteins and the peptides may modulate gastrointestinal function. Furthermore, the concentration of immunoreactive casomorphins increases significantly after ingestion of bovine casein-based milk formula or canine milk, but not after soy protein formula, in 2- and 4-week-old dogs (Singh *et al.* 1989), suggesting that casein-derived casomorphins may act at distant targets via blood circulation.

There is direct evidence that casein-derived casomorphins may regulate gastrointestinal motility. Intragastric administration of casein or casein hydrolysates reduces the amplitude and the frequency of gastrointestinal contraction in dogs (Defilippi *et al.* 1995) and in cattle (Kil and Froetschel 1994) and slows the gastric emptying and gastrointestinal transition in rats (Daniel *et al.* 1990). Such effects can be suppressed by pretreatment of the animals with an opiate receptor antagonist naloxone. It has also been speculated that casein-derived casomorphins may play a role in regulating appetite via modifying pancreatic insulin secretion (Kitts 1994) and modulating immunity development in neonates by stimulating lymphocyte proliferation (Fiat and Jolles 1989). Furthermore, due to their analgesic effect and their influence on breathing, casein-derived casomorphins have been suspected of inducing post-feeding calmness and sleep in infants (Kitts 1994) and to be one of the etiological factors for sudden infant death syndrome (Ramabadran and Bansinath 1988).

Immunostimulating Peptides

It was first reported by Jolles *et al.* (1981) that extracts from trypsin hydrolyzed human milk possessed immunostimulating activity. A hexapeptide, Val-Glu-Pro-Ile-Pro-Tyr (residues 54-59 of human β-casein), was subsequently isolated from the tryptic hydrolysate of human milk (Parker *et al.* 1984). The peptide stimulated phagocytosis of sheep red blood cells by murine peritoneal macrophages in an *in vitro* assay system, and it enhanced the resistance of mice to *Klebsiella pneumoniae* infection when given intravenously. One hexapeptide Pro-Gly-Pro-Ile-Pro-Asn (residues 63-68 of bovine β-casein), and two tripeptides, Gly-Leu-Phe (residues 51-53 of human and bovine α-lactalbumin) and Leu-Leu-Tyr (residues 191-193 of bovine β-casein), have also been isolated from tryptic hydrolysates of human and bovine milk (Berthou *et al.* 1987; Gattegno *et al.* 1988; Migliore-Samoure *et al.* 1989). These peptides have similar immunostimulating activity of the human milk hexapeptide and stimulate phagocytic activity of human and murine macrophages and exert protective effects against *Klebsiella pneumoniae* infection in mice. Specific binding sites for Gly-Leu-Phe and Val-Glu-Pro-Ile-Pro-Tyr have also been found on the surface of hyman phagocytic blood cells (Jaziri *et al.* 1992).

Antihypertensive Peptides

The blood pressure is regulated in part by the renin-angiotensin system. In this system angiotensin I converting enzyme (ACE) plays an important role. ACE converts angiotensin I to a potent vasoconstrictor, angiotensin II, through the removal of two amino acids from the C-terminal of the precursor. Inhibition of ACE activity reduces angiotensin II production and lowers blood pressure in hypertensive patients and in spontaneously hypertensive animals.

Marayama and Suzuki (1982) reported that tryptic hydrolysate of casein inhibited ACE activity *in vitro*. Four ACE inhibitory peptides, dodecapeptide Phe-Phe-Val-Ala-Pro-Phe-Pro-Glu-Val-Phe-Gly-Lys, pentapeptide Phe-Phe-Val-Ala-Pro, hexapeptde Thr-Thr-Met-Pro-Leu-Trp, and heptapeptide Ala-Val-Pro-Tyr-Pro-Gln-Arg, were later isolated from the casein hydrolysate (Maruyama *et al.* 1987). These peptides correspond to the amino acid residues 23-34, 23-27, and 194-199 of bovine α_{1s}-casein and 177-183 of β-casein, respectively. Oral administration of tryptic hydrolysate of milk casein decreased blood pressure in spontaneously hypertensive rats, but it had no effect on electrocardiogram, cardiac histopathology or serum lipid concentration (Karaki *et al.* 1990).

More recently, two potent ACE inhibitory tripeptides, Val-Pro-Pro (residues 84-86 of bovine β-casein) and Ile-Pro-Pro (residues 74-76 of bovine β-casein and 108-110 of bovine κ-casein), were isolated from sour milk fermented with a starter containing *Lactobacillus helveticus* and *Saccharomyces cerevisiae* (Nakamura *et al.* 1995). Further studies showed that oral feeding of the sour milk significantly reduced the systolic blood pressure and ACE activity in aorta in spontaneously hypertensive rats (Nukamura *et al.* 1996), but it had no effect on normotensive rats. Clinical studies also showed that systolic blood pressure decreased significantly in hypertensive patients 4 weeks after daily ingestion of 95 mL of the sour milk and diastolic blood pressure decreased significantly after 8 weeks (Hata *et al.* 1996). No significant decline in blood pressure was observed in patients receiving placebo treatment of daily ingestion of 95 mL of artificially acidified milk.

CONCLUSION

From the above discussion it is apparent that milk is not only a source of nutrients but a carrier of numerous bioactive compounds. The most interesting group of bioactive compounds in milk are milk-borne bioactive peptides, including various growth factors. Most research studies indicate that milk-borne growth factors play a role in regulating postnatal gut development in suckling animals. This knowledge will facilitate our understanding on postnatal development of mammals and improve postnatal care of nursing infants and animals. Another group of bioactive compounds found in milk are the bioactive peptides derived from *in vitro* milk protein digestion. Although any physiological role of these peptides is not yet clear, they offer a great potential for developing functional foods. It may be possible in the future by a controlled hydrolysis of milk proteins to produce food products with additional health benefits to consumers.

ACKNOWLEDGMENTS

The research work at the author's laboratory was supported by the Research Grants Council of Hong Kong and the Committee on Research and Conference Grants of the University of Hong Kong. The author thanks Mr. Y.H. Yeung for his technical assistance.

REFERENCES

ADACHI, I., LIU, H. X., HORIKOSHI, I., UENO, M. and SATO, H. 1993. Possibility of lymphatic absorption of epidermal growth factor from intestine. Yakugaku Zasshi *113*, 256–263.

BALLARD, F.J., GROBOVAC, S., NICHOLAS, K.R., OWENS, P.C. and READ, L.C. 1995. Differential changes in the milk concentrations of epidermal growth factor and insulin-like growth factor-I during lactation in the tammar wallaby, *Macropus eugenii.* Gen. Comp. Endocrinol. *98*, 262–268.

BAUMRUCKER, C.R., HADSELL, D.L. and BLUM, J.W. 1994. Effects of dietary insulin-like growth factor I on growth and insulin-like growth factor receptors in neonatal calf intestine. J. Anim. Sci. *72*, 428–433.

BERSETH, C.L. 1987. Enhancement of intestinal growth in neonatal rats by epidermal growth factor in milk. Am. J. Physiol. *253,* G662–G665.

BRANTL, V. 1984. Novel opioid peptides derived from human β-casein: human β-casomorphins. Eur. J. Pharmacol. *106*, 213–214.

BRANTL, V., TESCHEMACHER, H., HENSCHEN, A. and LOTTSPEICH, F. 1979. Novel opioid peptides derived from casein (β-casomorphins). I. Isolation from bovine casein peptone. Hoppe Seylers Z. Physiol. Chem. *360*, 1211–1216.

BRITTON, J.R., GEORGE-NASCIMENTO, C. and KOLDOVSKY, O. 1988. Luminal hydrolysis of recombinant human epidermal growth factor in the rat gastrointestinal tract: segmental and developmental differences. Life Sci. *43*, 1339–1347.

BRITTON, J.R., GEORGE-NASCIMENTO, C., UDALL, J.N. and KOLDOVSKY, O. 1989. Minimal hydrolysis of epidermal growth factor by gastric fluid of premature infants. Gut *30*, 327–332.

BURRIN, D.G., WESTER, T.J., DAVIS, T.A., AMICK, S. and HEATH, J.P. 1996. Orally administered IGF-I increases intestinal mucosal growth in formula-fed neonatal pigs. Am. J. Physiol. *270*, R1085–R1091.

CARPENTER, G. 1980. Epidermal growth factor is a major growth-promoting agent in human milk. Science *210*, 198–199.

CHIBA, H., TANI, F. and YOSHIKAVA, M. 1989. Opioid antagonist peptides derived from κ-casein. J. Dairy Res. *56*, 363–366.

DANIEL, H., VOHWINKEL, M. and REHNER, G. 1990. Effect of casein and β-casomorphins on gastrointestinal motility in rats. J. Nutr. *120*, 252–257.

DEFILIPPI, C., GOMEZ, E., CHARLIN, V. and SILVA, C. 1995. Inhibition of small intestinal motility by casein: a role of β-casomorphins? Nutr. *11*, 751–754.

DONOVAN, S. M., HINTZ, R. L., WILSON, D.M. and ROSENFELD, R. G. 1990. Insulin-like growth factors I and II and their binding proteins in rat milk. Pediatr. Res. *29*, 50–55.

ERIKSSON, U., DUC, G., FROESCH, E.R. and ZAPF, J. 1993. Insulin-like growth factors (IGF) I and II and IGF binding proteins (IGFBPs) in human colostrum/transitory milk during the first week postpartum: comparison with neonatal and maternal serum. Biochem. Biophys. Res. Commun. *196*, 267–273.

FIAT, A. and JOLLES, P. 1989. Caseins of various origins and biologically active casein peptides and oligosaccharides: structure and physiological aspects. Mol. Cell. Biochem. *87*, 5–30.

HATA, Y., YAMAMOTO, M., OHNI, M., NAKAJIMA, K., NAKAMURA, Y. and TAKANO, T. 1996. A placebo-controlled study of the effect of sour milk on blood pressure in hypertensive subjects. Am. J. Clin. Nutr. *64,* 767–771.

IACOPETTA, B.J., GRIEU, F., HORISBERGER, M. and SUNAHARA, G.I. 1992. Epidermal growth factor in human and bovine milk. Acta Pediatr. *81*, 287–291.

JAEGER, L.A., LAMAR, C.H., BOTTOMS, G.D. and CLINE, T.R. 1987. Growth-stimulating substances in porcine milk. Am. J. Vet. Res. *48*, 1531–1533.

JAEGER, L.A., LAMAR, C.H., CLINE, T.R. and CARDONA, C.J. 1990. Effect of orally administered epidermal growth factor on the jejunal mucosa of weaned pigs. Am. J. Vet. Res. *51*, 471–474.

JAMES, P.S., SMITH, M.W., TIVEY, D.R. and WILSON, T.J.G. 1987. Epidermal growth factor selectively increases maltase and sucrase activities in neonatal piglet intestine. J. Physiol. *393*, 583–594.

JAZIRI, M., MIGLIORE-SAMOUR, D., CASABIANCA-PIGNEDE, M., KEDDA, K., MORGA, J.L. and JOLLES, P. 1992. Specific binding sites on human phagocytic blood cells for Gly-Leu-Phe and Val-Glu-Pro-Ile-Pro-Try immunostimulating peptides from human milk proteins. Biochim. Biophys. Acta *1160*, 251–261.

JOLLES, P., PARKER, F., FLOC'H, F., MIGLIORE, D., ALLIEL, P., ZERIAL, A. and WERNER, G.H. 1981. Immunostimulating substances from human casein. J.

Immunopharmocol. *3*, 363–369.

KAMPA, M., LOUKAS, S., HATZOGLOU, A., MARTIN, P., MARTIN, P.M. and CASTANAS, E. 1996. Identification of a novel opioid (Tyr-Val-Pro-Phe-Pro) derived from human α_{s1}-casein (α_{s1}-casomorphin and α_{s1}-casomorphin amide). Biochem. J. *319*, 903–908.

KARAKI, H., DOI, K., SUGANO, S., UCHIWA, H., SUGAI, R., MURAKAMI, U. and TAKEMOTO, S. 1990. Antihypertensive effect of tryptic hydrolysate of milk casein in spontaneously hypertensive rats. Comp. Biochem. Physiol. C *96*, 367–371.

KIL, S.J. and FROETSCHEL, M.A. 1994. Involvement of opioid peptides from casein on reticular motility and digesta passage in steers. J. Dairy Sci. *77*, 111–123.

KITTS, D.D. 1994. Bioactive substances in food: Identification and potential uses. Can. J. Physiol. Pharmacol. *72*, 423–434.

KLAGSBRUN, M. 1978. Human milk stimulates DNA synthesis and cellular proliferation in cultured fibroblasts. Proc. Natl. Acad. Sci. USA *75*, 5057–5061.

KOLDOVSKY, O. 1994. Hormonally active peptides in human milk. Acta Pediatr. Suppl. *402*, 89–93.

MA, L. and XU, R.J. 1997. Oral insulinlike growth factor-I and hydrocortisone stimulate intestinal enzyme maturation in newborn rats. Life Sci. *61*, 51–58.

MALVEN, P.V., HEAD, H.H., COLLIER, R.J. and BUONOMA, F.C. 1987. Periparturient changes in secretion and mammary uptake of insulin and in concentrations of insulin and insulin-like growth factors in milk of dairy cows. J. Dairy Sci. *70*, 2254–2265.

MARUYAMA, S., MITACHI, H., AWAYA, J., KURONO, M., TOMIZUKA, N. and SUZUKI, H. 1987. Angiotensin-I converting enzyme inhibitory activity of the C-terminal hexapeptide of α-casein. Agric. Biol. Chem. *51*, 2557–2561.

MARUYAMA, S. and SUZUKI, H. 1982. A peptide inhibitor of angiotensin I converting enzyme in the tryptic hydrolysate of casein. Agric. Biol. Chem. *46*, 1393–1394.

MEISEL, H. and FRISTER, H. 1989. Chemical characterization of bioactive peptides from *in vivo* digests of casein. J. Dairy Res. *56*, 343–349.

MUBIRU, J.N. and XU, R.J. 1997. Growth and development of the exocrine pancreas in newborn pigs: the effect of colostrum feeding. Biol. Neonate *71*, 317–326.

NAKAMURA, Y., MASUDA, O. and TAKANO, T. 1996. Decrease of tissue angiotensin I-converting enzyme activity upon feeding sour milk in spontaneously hypertensive rats. Biosci. Biotechnol. Biochem. *60*, 488–489.

NAKAMURA, Y., YAMAMOTO, N., SAKAI, K., OKUBO, A., YAMAZAKI, S. and TAKANO, T. 1995. Purification and characterization of angiotensin I converting enzyme inhibitors from sour milk. J. Dairy Sci. *78*, 777–783.

OLANREWAJU, H.A., SANZENBACHER, E.D. and SEIDEL, E.R. 1996. Insulin-like growth factor I in suckling rat gastric contents. Digest Dis. Sci. *41*, 1392–1397.

PARKER, F., MIGLIORE-SAMOUR, D., FLOC'H, F., ZERIAL, A. WERNER, G. H., JOLLES J., CASARETTO, M., ZAHN, H. and JOLLES, P. 1984. Immunostimulating hexapeptide from human casein: amino acid sequence, synthesis and biological properties. Eur. J. Biochem. *145*, 677–682.

PETRILLI, P., PUCCI, P., PELISSIER, J.P. and ADDEO, F. 1987. Digestion by pancreatic juice of a β-casomorphin-containing fragment of buffalo β-casein. Int. J.

Pept. Protein Res. *29*, 504–508.

PETSCHOW, B.W., CARTER, D.L. and HUTTON, G.D. 1993. Influence of orally administered epidermal growth factor on normal and damaged intestinal mucosa in rats. J. Pediatr. Gastroenterol. Nutr. *17*, 49–58.

PHILIPPS, A.F., RAO, R., ANDERSON, G.G., MCCRACKEN, D.M., LAKE, M. and KOLDOVSKY, O. 1995. Fate of insulin-like growth factors I and II administered orogastrically to suckling rats. Pediatr. Res. *37*, 586–592.

RAABERG, L., NEXO, E., TOLLUND, L., POULSEN, S.S., CHRISTENSIN, S.B. and CHRISTENSEN, M.S. 1990. Epidermal growth factor reactivity in rat milk. Regul. Peptide *30*, 149–157.

RAMABADRAN, K. and BANSINATH, M. 1988. Opioid peptides from milk as a possible cause of sudden infant death syndrome. Med. Hypotheses *27*, 181–187.

RAO, R.K. 1994. Luminal processing of epidermal growth factor in mouse gastrointestinal tract in vivo. Peptides *16*, 505–513.

READ, L.C., FORD, W.D.A., FILSELL, O.H., MCNEIL, J. and BALLARD, F.J. 1986. Is orally-derived epidermal growth factor beneficial following premature birth or intestinal resection? Endocr. Exp. *20*, 199–207.

READ, L.C., UPTON, F.M., FRANCIS, G.L., WALLACE, J.C., DAHLENBERG, G.W. and BALLARD, F.J. 1984. Changes in the growth-promoting activity of human milk during lactation. Pediatr. Res. *18*, 133–139.

SCHLIMME, E. and MEISEL, H. 1995. Bioactive peptides derived from milk proteins. Structural, physiological and analytical aspects. Die Nahrung *39*, 1–20.

SCHOBER, D.A., SIMMEN, F.A., HADSELL, D.L. and BAUMRUCKER, C.R. 1990. Perinatal expression of type I IGF receptors in porcine small intestine. Endocrinol. *126*, 1125–1132.

SHEN, W.H. and XU, R.J. 1996. Stability of epidermal growth factor in the gastrointestinal lumen of suckling and weaned pigs. Life Sciences *59*, 197–208.

SHULMAN, R.J. 1990. Oral insulin increases small intestinal mass and disaccharidase activity in the newborn miniature pig. Pediatr. Res. *28*, 171–175.

SINGH, M., ROSEN, C.L., CHANG, K.J. and HADDAD, G.G. 1989. Plasma β-casomorphin-7 immunoreactive peptide increases after milk intake in newborn but not in adult dogs. Pediatr. Res. *26*, 34–38.

SVEDBERG, J., DE-HAAS, J., LEIMENSTOLL, G., PAUL, F. and TESCHEMACHER, H. 1985. Demonstration of β-casomorphin immunoreactive materials in *in vitro* digests of bovine milk and in small intestine contents after bovine milk ingestion in adult humans. Peptides *6*, 825–830.

THORNBURG, W., RAO, R.K., MATRISIAN, L.M., MAGUN, B.E. and KOLDOVSKY, O. 1987. Effect of maturation on gastrointestinal absorption of epidermal growth factor in rats. Am. J. Physiol. *253*, G68–G71.

THULESEN, J., RAABERG, L., NEXO, E., MADSEN, E.L. and POULSEN, S.S. 1993. Epidermal growth factor in mammary glands and milk from rats: the influence of insulin. Diabetes Res. Clin. Pract. *21*, 11–18.

TRAHAIR, J.F., WING, S.J., QUINN, K.J. and OWENS, P.C. 1997. Regulation of gastrointestinal growth in fetal sheep by luminally administered insulin-like growth factor-I. J. Endocrinol. *152*, 29–38.

ULSHEN, M.H., LYN-COOK, L.E. and RAASCH, R. 1986. Effects of intraluminal epidermal growth factor on mucosal proliferation in the small intestine of adult rats. Gastroenterology *91*, 1134–1140.

WANG, T. and XU, R.J. 1996. Effects of colostrum feeding on intestinal development in newborn pigs. Biol. Neonate *70*, 339–348.

WESTROM, B., EKMAN, R., SVENDSEN, L., SVENDSEN, J. and KARLSSON, B.W. 1987. Levels of immunoreactive insulin, neurotensin, and bombesin in porcine colostrum and milk. J. Pediatr. Gastroenterol. Nutr. *6*, 460–465.

XU, R.J. 1996. Development of the newborn GI tract and its relation to colostrum/milk intake: A review. Reprod. Fertil. Dev. *8*, 35–48.

XU, R.J. and CRANWELL, P.D. 1990. Development of gastric acid secretion in pigs from birth to 36 days of age: The response to pentagastrin. J. Dev. Physiol. *13*, 315–326.

XU, R.J. and CRANWELL, P.D. 1991. Gastrin in fetal and neonatal pigs. Comp. Biochem. Physiol. *98B*, 615–621.

XU, R.J., MAO, Y.L. and TSO, M.Y.W. 1996. Stability of gastrin in the gastrointestinal lumen of suckling, weanling and adult pigs. Biol. Neonate *70*, 60–68.

XU, R.J., MELLOR, D.J., BIRTLES, M.J., BREIER, B.H. and GLUCKMAN, P.D. 1994. Effects of oral IGF-I or IGF-II on digestive organ growth in newborn piglets. Biol. Neonate *66*, 280–287.

XU, R.J., MELLOR, D.J., TUNGTHANATHANICH, P., BIRTLES, M.J., REYNOLDS, G.W. and SIMPSON, H.V. 1992a. Growth and morphological changes in the small and the large intestine in piglets during the first three days after birth. J. Dev. Physiol. *18*, 161–172.

XU, R.J., TUNGTHANATHANICH, P., BIRTLES, M.J., MELLOR, D.J., REYNOLDS, G.W. and SIMPSON, H.V. 1992b. Growth and morphological changes in the stomach of newborn pigs during the first three days after birth. J. Dev. Physiol. *17*, 7–14.

XU, R.J. and SHEN, W.H. 1997. Stability and absorption of milk-borne bioactive peptides in the gastrointestinal tract of neonatal pigs. In: *Digestive Physiology in Pigs,* eds J.P. Laplace, C. Fevrier and A. Barbeau, (eds.) EAAP Publication No 88. INRA, France, pp. 171–175.

XU, R.J. and WANG, T. 1996. Gastrointestinal absorption of insulinlike growth factor-I in neonatal pigs. J. Pediatr. Gastroenterol. Nutr. *23*, 430–437.

YOUNG, G.P., TARANTO, T.M., JONAS, H.A., COX, A.J., HOGG, A. and Werther, G.A. 1990. Insulin-like growth factors and the developing and mature rat small intestine: receptors and biological actions. Digestion *46 (suppl)*, 240–252.

ZIJLSTRA, R.T., ODLE, J., HALL, W.F., PETSCHOW, B.W., GELBERG, H.B. and LITOV, R.E. 1994. Effect of orally administered epidermal growth factor on intestinal recovery of neonatal pigs infected with rotavirus. J. Pediatr. Gastroenterol. Nutr. *19*, 382–390.

ZIOUDROU, C., STREATY, R.A. and KLEE, W.A. 1979. Opioid peptides derived from food proteins. The exophins. J. Biol. Chem. *10*, 2446–2449.

ATTEMPTS TO REDUCE FAT AND CHOLESTEROL IN AUSTRALIAN FOODS

F. SHERKAT[1], M. PANTELLA[1], W. HUANG[2], D. ENG[3], and J. WILSON[4]

[1]Department of Food Science, RMIT University
124 Latrobe Street, Melbourne 3001, Australia

[2]15/F 66A Broadway St. Mei Foo
Kowloon, Hong Kong

[3]Pokka Ace (M) SDN BHD; Lot 39, 41050 Klang
Selangor, Darul Ehsan, Malaysia

[4]Simplot Foods
PO Box 177, Southland Centre
Cheltenham, 3192, Melbourne

ABSTRACT

Three research activities in relation to fat and cholesterol reduction in foods are reported. These include:

(a) The reduction of cholesterol in fermented dairy foods through its assimilation by the probiotic bacteria, Lactobacillus acidophilus *and* Bifidobacteria species. *Up to 30% cholesterol assimilation was found to be possible using this approach.*

(b) The production of a fermented 'Twin Product' with a blend of cow's milk and soy milk inoculated with the lactic and probiotic cultures (soghurt). The saturated fats and the cholesterol of cow's milk are partially replaced with the polyunsaturated oil and phytosterol from soy milk. A 60:40 blend of soy:bovine milk resulted in an acceptable texture and organoleptic qualities in the resulting soghurt. Part of the cholesterol was also assimilated by the probiotic cultures during the incubation and storage.

(c) Commercial fat replacers, bulking agents and high intensity sweeteners were used in the formulation of a low-joule product similar to ice cream. The resulting product showed higher exit temperature and low initial melt down index than the standard ice cream. The taste panel (n=39) found the product acceptable but somewhat different (p=0.01%) to the standard ice cream.

INTRODUCTION

Australians may be the fattest people in the world. The average Australian is more than three kilo-grams heavier than 15 years ago. Half of Australian men and a third of all women are now classified as overweight or obese (Cadzow 1996). According to Professor Tim Welborn of the Australian Society of the Study of Obesity, "compared with all other international statistics, including USA, Holland, the UK and France, Australians were found just about the top of the league in terms of average weights".

National Heart Foundation (NHF) surveys show that in 1980s the odds of being overweight increased by 32% for women and 13% for men. The likelihood of being obese in the 90s grew by 70% for women and 24% for men. According to Dr. Garry Egger from the University of Newcastle and a member of National Health and Medical Research Council's working party on obesity "the average Australian has been putting on about a gram a day for the past 15 years". Among other problems, obesity, especially abdominal obesity, is a risk factor for late-onset diabetes, which is growing at an enormous rate and has now taken an epidemic proportion. In 1970 only 1 percent of the population was diabetic, it is now 3 percent and is predicted to be 5 percent by 2005.

Health risks begin to increase at 20 percent overweight. Overweight people are less healthy, more prone to heart disease and early death. A state of being overweight is an abnormal physiological condition, placing strain on the biological system, often leading to *diabetese mellitus*, cardiovascular illness, hypertension, respiratory disease and respiratory failure, a stroke, coronary heart disease (CHD), and some cancers. Overweight people are also vulnerable to musculo-skeletal problems, such as sleep apnoea and cartilage damage in the joints.

One reason for the weight gain in Australians is the range of food available in this country which has never been wider or more appealing. More than fuel, food is now a primary source of pleasure and interest. Food is more tempting, we are overtly hedonistic, and it is much easier to over-consume today. To the obese patient, food may represent a form of security, satisfaction or self-esteem. Last year, Australians chumped their way through 7.6 million packets of Tim Tams. We spent A$1.3 (SA = ~US75c) billion on ice cream and A$3.9 billion on soft drinks (Flanagan 1995). Add to this, all-you-can-eat deals from most fast-food chains and you end up by not remembering when last you felt hungry!

BIS Shrapnel estimates that Australian household expenditure on take away foods more than doubled in the decade to 1994, from a weekly average of A$7.50 to A$20.00. In the last five years, the number of take away food outlets throughout the country rose by 30% from 13,300 to 17,300. The popularity of chains like McDonald's and KFC has led to a rise in our fat intake.

The fact is that the total intake of energy per person has not increased in the last 15 years, but we are moving less and less each day. "Electronic wizardry" and our endless quest for speed and convenience have significantly reduced the amount of energy expended in getting through the day. A study published last year in the *International Journal of Obesity* suggests that the average person in the United Kingdom in the 1990s is burning 190 kilojoules fewer a day than did the average person in the 1970s. This trend applies similarly to the average Australian.

Twenty-five years ago, rich Australians were fatter than poorer ones. Now, the trend is reversed. At lower socio-economic areas, three in four Australians are overweight or obese. According Garry Egger, this fattening follows a pattern: "the first group to get fat is women, the second group is men, the third group is adolescents and the fourth group is children". In 1985, between one-quarter to one-third of school children were overweight. A study of 2000 Victorian school children in 1994 suggests young Australians have got even fatter in the last decade. The main reason is that their leisure time is now devoted to sedentary activities in front of the PC or TV.

It is true that some of us are biochemically destined to be stout, while others are genetically lean, but a predisposition to obesity is obviously enhanced by "lifestyle factors". Besides, this group also has the ability of quickly and efficiently converting other food components, such as carbohydrates and/or proteins into body fat. Therefore, reducing or replacing the fat in the diet or consumption of low-joule products might only solve part of the problem.

Australians are faced with a major change in attitudes in relation to their lifestyle, eating habits and obesity. Among these changes, the choice of "adequate" food plays an important role. Commercially prepared low-fat meals and low-joule processed foods will have to play their role along with healthy lifestyle and more physical activity, in slowing down and hopefully reversing the obesity pattern.

There is an increasing consumer demand for low-energy foods, with the same flavor and textural features as the normal foods. S.M.A.R.T Research (Scriven 1993) revealed that 30 percent of all Australians used low-joule foods. Twenty seven percent of users would have liked additional low-joule foods. However, thirty percent of consumers did not consume low-joule products because they were thought to be artificial. The report concluded that as health and nutrition became key factors in consumer's purchasing decisions, the consumption of low-joule products had the potential to double.

Within the Asian Context, urbanization and rapid economic growth have resulted in a move away from traditional eating patterns in many areas. As GNP increases, an increase in the consumption of animal protein, sugar and fats and oils tends to occur with a marked decline in grain consumption.

Dr. Junshi Chen from the Chinese Academy of Preventive Medicine believes that the emergence of degenerative chronic diseases in the developed world is significantly associated with the changes in their dietary patterns. In the developing world some countries remain concerned with hunger, malnutrition and communicable diseases; while in other countries (including China), there have been considerable changes in their diets towards the Western diet.

From 1978 to 1992 the consumption of meat, poultry, eggs, fish, oil and sugar have increased in China by 150, 400, 250, 100, 290 and 60%, respectively. The changes are more profound in urban areas, where the average percentage of dietary energy from fat reached 28.4% in 1992, compared with 18.6% in rural population. A study on diet and disease mortality carried out in 1983 found that the "disease of affluence" comprised of non-communicable chronic diseases was significantly positively correlated with high consumption of egg, fish, beer and sugar, and "over-nutrition" was indicated by higher plasma total cholesterol. According to Dr. Chen, the effects of significant amounts of animal foods or "over-nutrition" on population health are already beginning to appear.

A major problem associated with energy dense diets rich in animal proteins is their high level of saturated fats and cholesterol. Milk and dairy products contain saturated fat and cholesterol. Lampert (1970) estimated milk cholesterol at levels of 0.015 per cent and that of full-fat milk powder at about 0.36 per cent. About 10 percent of the cholesterol in milk fat occurs in the form of cholesterol esters. Cholesterol ($C_{27}H_{45}OH$) is the most common animal sterol, while only trace amounts are present in vegetable oils. Cholesterol serves many functions in the human body: it acts as an insulator in the brain and nervous tissue; it is a lubricant in the skin, and a precursor of a number of biologically important compounds, ie. corticosteroids, gonadal hormones and vitamin D. The implication of cholesterol in the aetiology of arteriosclerosis and CHD is well documented (Gibbons *et al.* 1982). In view of the high mortality rates associated with cardiovascular diseases and myocardial infarction, it has been suggested that intakes of cholesterol in excess of about half a gram a day must be avoided to prevent its build-up.

Several approaches to controlling weight have been implemented, including several types of faddist diets, starvation and formula diets, each with varying degrees of success. Approaches such as starvation or reduction in the portion size or the frequency of meal intake are implicated in severe health complications such as gouty arthritis, nomochronic anaemia and hypotension. The consumers want to enjoy the food without feeling guilty, and at the same time they have a psychological need to feel and look healthier, and feel and fare better socially.

The food industry was quick in responding to this need by producing low-joule products via incorporation of more water or low-joule bulking agents, synthetic and/or alternative sweeteners, fat replacers, mimetics, synthetic fats, and carbohydrate or protein based fats. For example, in the last decade, Australian dairy companies have developed a range of low-fat and no-fat products such as "Skinny", "PhysiCal" and "Rev" milks. Soft butter with blends of milk fat and vegetable oils were successfully positioned in the market place. Research has also been conducted to reduce or remove cholesterol from foods, i.e. by supercritical carbon dioxide extraction of cholesterol from egg yolk (Bringe and Cheng 1995).

EXPERIMENTAL PROCEDURE

In our studies of fat and cholesterol reduction, we have looked at the possibility of cholesterol oxidation upon heating milk and cream, and its assimilation in fermented dairy products by selected strains of probiotic bacteria. We also studied the actual reduction of cow's milk fats by blending it with soy milk, and evaluated the acceptability of zero-fat low-joule frozen desserts.

Cholesterol Metabolism by the Probiotic Bacteria

There have been a number of claims, based on studies in laboratory animals, which suggest that milk and fermented dairy products might reduce the serum cholesterol levels (Rao *et al.* 1985). Yoghurt has long been recognized as a healthy product; however, the bacteria used in yoghurt fermentation namely *Lactobacillus delbrueckii* ssp. *bulgaricus* and *Streptococus salivarius* ssp. *thermophilus*, do not have the ability to colonize the intestinal tract of humans and animals. Other bacteria possessing this attribute, such as *Lactobacillus acidophilus* and *Bifidobacteria* species mainly *B. longum* and *B. bifidum* (AB cultures or probiotic bacteria), are finding increasing use in a range of therapeutic products. In the last decade a new generation of fermented milk products containing selected intestinal bacteria have been introduced to the world market. Today, more than 70 Bifidobacteria-containing products, most of dairy origin, are produced world wide (Hughes and Hoover 1991).

Buck and Gilliland (1994) demonstrated through feeding trials on human volunteers that certain strains of *L. acidophilus* were capable of assimilating cholesterol due to their high resistance to bile and their high bile salt deconjugation abilities. Aristova *et al.* (1994) claimed that dairy products containing probiotic bacteria had a reduced cholesterol level of up to 50% depending on the type of cultures used.

It was in the light of these reports that we decided to investigate:

- the fate of total lipid and cholesterol upon the manufacturing, incubation and storage of dairy products inoculated with probiotic cultures (*L. acidophilus and B. bifidum*), and
- to determine whether the cholesterol metabolizing ability of lactic and probiotic cultures lead to detectable changes in cholesterol content.

Procedure. Sour cream with its higher cholesterol content (50 mg/100 g) was considered for the experimental work. 0.01% freeze-dried *L. acidophilus* (strain La-5) and *B. bifidum* (strain Bb-12) and 1.0% *O-mesophile* culture (strain R-704, all Chris Hansen's) was added to the standardized-pasteurized cream at 25°C, then packed in 250 mL sanitized plastic cups, sealed and incubated at 25°C overnight (18-22 h). Once the product pH reached 4.5 it was cooled to 3-4°C and stored at this temperature until the end of its shelf-life of approximately 4 weeks.

Total lipids of sour cream were extracted using the method of Folch *et al.* (1957). The fat was redissolved in 50 mL chloroform and transferred into stoppered test-tubes flushed with N_2 gas and stored at -19°C. Chromatographic techniques (thin layer and gas) were employed to identify cholesterol species, while the colorimetric method of Boehringer Mannheim (1995) was used to determine the sterols content of fat samples calculated as cholesterol.

Results. Microbiological tests indicated that AB culture numbers increased from 8×10^6 to 8.8×10^{10} cfu/g within the first 48 h, but after 6 days storage their numbers dropped to 3.3×10^9 cfu/g and continued declining towards the end of shelf-life of 4 weeks to 6.7×10^8 cfu/g.

The logarithmic phase of AB culture growth coincided with a drop of 20-30% in total cholesterol content (Table 1). This growth also resulted in a drop in total fats content by up to 8% after a storage period of 3 weeks, which is a further step towards our aim of fat and cholesterol reduction in the product.

TABLE 1.
METABOLISM OF CHOLESTEROL IN SOUR CREAM

Samples	Cholesterol (mg/100g)		Total Reduction (mg)		Drop %	
	Product	Fat	Product	Fat	Product	Fat
Raw Cream	73	373	-	-	0.0	0.0
Sour Cream (24h)	55	292	18	81	24.7	21.7
Sour Cream (1 W)	51	287	22	86	30.1	23.1

It is evident from these findings that the cholesterol assimilation mainly takes place during the incubation period, when AB and lactic cultures grow rapidly. AB cultures have strict nutritional requirements, specifically in terms of the "bifidogenic factors". No "bifidogenic factor" was added to the cream and it is possible that by adding these factors much faster growth of AB cultures, and consequently, more efficient reduction in cholesterol content may be achievable.

Cholesterol assimilation by bifidobacteria cultures is poorly understood (Hughes and Hoover 1991), although previous studies conducted on human subjects by Homma (1988) indicated the involvement of HMG-CoA reductase. There has been some indication that probiotic bacteria, themselves being deficient in cholesterol, store it in their cell membrane, which is ultimately not absorbed as readily by the intestines (Welch 1987; Gilliland 1990).

Fat Reduction Through Blending Cow's Milk and Soy Milk

Saturated fats of milk, like the cholesterol itself, play a significant role in CHD and atherosclerosis. Polyunsaturated fatty acids (ω-3, ω-6 and ω-9) are known to alleviate these nutritional problems. Blending soy milk and cow's milk results in reduced saturated fats and cholesterol content, and an increase in polyunsaturated fatty acids in the product.

Soy milk also contain phytosterols which are known to prevent cholesterol deposition in the arteries. Lactose in the cow's milk is a restricting factor in the consumption of milk and dairy products in most Asian populations; however, blending soy and cow's milk reduced the lactose content commensurate with the blend proportion.

Soy milk extracted from natural soybean flour contains oligosaccharides which enhance the growth of the AB cultures. A range of anti-oxidants and anti-cancer compounds naturally present in soybeans, such as isoflavones, genistein and phytates, also add to the health benefits of the twin product. Soy flour also contains undesirable components such as lipoxygenases and trypsin inhibitors that need to be eliminated or denatured in order to achieve a product that is fit for human consumption.

Procedure. A mild hydrothermal process was developed for soy milk extraction from Enzyme Active Full-Fat Soy Flour (EASF). This process is capable of complete elimination of the beany flavor development and up to 30% reduction in trypsin inhibitors activity (TIA) while maintaining high protein solubility index.

Soghurt was made by blending the resulting soymilk with cow's milk (at various ratios), which was then heated to 90°C for 10 min, cooled to 42 $\pm$ 1°C, inoculated with 0.01% freeze-dried ABT-Y culture (Chr. Hansen's), packed into containers and incubated at 42 $\pm$ 1°C for 3.5-4 h and chilled to 6-8°C when the right pH was achieved.

Results. The resulting soghurt contained similar protein content as the control natural yoghurt, but less fat and 60% less lactose (Fig. 1).

Biochemical changes in soghurt during incubation and storage gave a faster pH drop, from the initial 7.1 to about 4.8 within the first 2 h of incubation, and thereafter to 4.4 by the end of the incubation period of 24 h. The fact that the soghurt contained up to 60% less lactose (at blend ratio of 60:40) implies that oligosaccharides may be involved. Ishibashi and Shimamura (1993) claimed that the AB cultures are capable of producing small amounts of acetic acid, which contribute to pH drop in the soghurt.

The oligosaccharides content of the mix dropped during incubation and storage. Raffinose appears to be used in preference to stachyose (25% vs. 4.5%). The oligosaccharides metabolism continued on a steady rate up to around one week of storage, and leveled thereafter. This coincided with the growth rate of AB cultures (Fig 2).

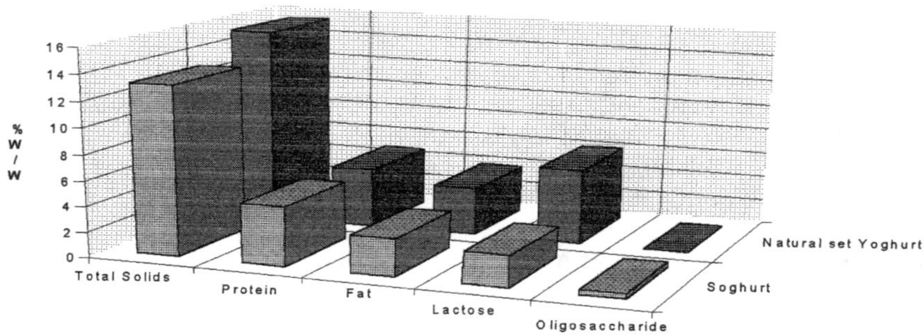

FIG. 1. COMPOSITION OF THE SOGHURT AND NATURAL SET YOGHURT

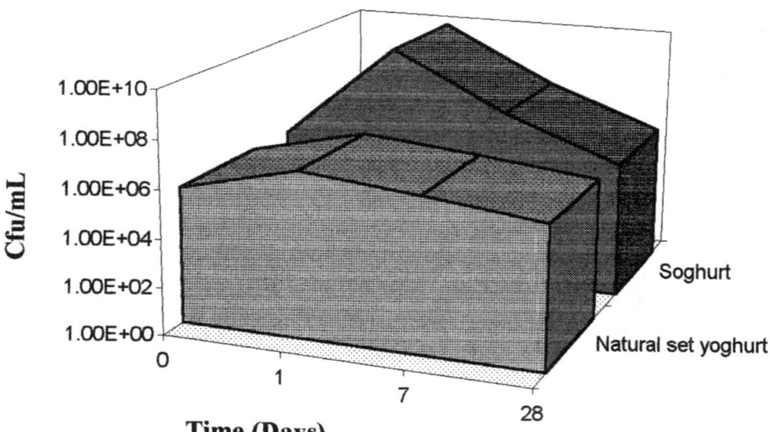

FIG. 2. GROWTH OF AB CULTURES IN SOGHURT AND NATURAL SET YOGHURT

The consistency and mouthfeel of soghurt was comparable to the control yoghurt. No beany flavor was depicted by the panelists, and the acetaldehyde levels matched that of the control yoghurt. However, slight lack of sharpness and a little "Umami" flavor was evident.

While the panelists could differentiate soghurt from yoghurt samples based on a slight lack of brightness, the acceptability level was high. This might also be due to the effect of healthy image the soghurt conveyed to panel members. The freshness of soy flour was critical to the acceptability of soghurt as the lipolysis of oils have a detrimental effect on flavor and aroma.

Trypsin inhibitors level in the soghurt dropped by 70% due to the combined effect of the hydro-thermal extraction of soy milk and the heat treatment involved in soghurt production. Literature values prove that this is an acceptable level for human consumption.

Blending soy-bovine milks achieved more than 50% reduction in the saturated fats and cholesterol level in the product. While we did not measure the amount of the residual cholesterol in the soghurt, we believe, based on the results obtained in part one of this report, that some of the cholesterol might have been metabolized by the AB cultures during their growth in soghurt.

Fat and Sugar Replacement in Frozen Desserts

Ice cream is a popular dessert and Australians are among the highest, if not the highest, consumers of ice cream and frozen desserts.

There has been attempts by the Australian food industry to produce low-fat, or reduced-energy frozen desserts, but the challenge of producing an acceptable product with zero-fat, minimum-joule by completely replacing the fat and sugar in an ice cream formulation has been an elusive goal so far. By definition, such a product can not be called ice cream, and in Australian Food Standards Codes (1994) it is referred to as "Ice Confection". An ice confection may contain less than 0.5% fat and still be classified as "zero-fat" product; however, to be classified as a low-joule product it shall not contain more than 70 kilojoules per 200 mL.

Procedure. A number of fat replacers, high intensity sweeteners, emulsifying/stabilizing agents, flavors, colors and bulking agents have been tried using a factorial experimental design and individual elimination system.

The appropriate amounts of selected fat replacer, sweetener, bulking agent, and emulsifier/stabilizer were mixed with water using the shearing action of the Damamix TR330, then heated to 60°C in a Capigani Pastocrema 32. The MSNF was added to water, mixed in the Damamix TR 330 then added to the Pastocrema.

The mixture was pasteurized at 80°C for 20 min, then homogenized at 200 psi using APV Model 15 15MR-8TBA, and returned to Pastocrema to be cooled to 4°C and aged for 4 h. At the end of this period, color and flavor was added aseptically and mixed thoroughly. The mixture was then churned in a Gelmark II to achieve an overrun of 100%. The product was dispensed from the churn, packaged and placed in a blast freezer (-40°C) to harden overnight.

Fat content, freezing point depression, hardness index, overrun and melt shock were determined using appropriate methods. Sensory evaluation was carried out according to AS 2458 (1986).

The most important attribute in selecting a suitable fat replacer was the creaminess it imparted to the product. The flavor and the absence of after-taste was the next consideration, as a bland or a 'dairy' flavor was considered most acceptable by the panelists.

The stability of high intensity sweeteners during processing and storage was also considered as some were heat sensitive and had to be added after the heat treatment stage. Other technical considerations included ease of application, hydration temperature and efficiency, the viscosity of mix and its relationship to the overrun and textural properties such as firmness of bite and iciness.

Results. At the meltdown tests, the zero-fat samples showed less meltdown up to the first 40 min, but after two h, they had 1.5-2 times more meltdown than the standard ice cream.

A combination of three bulking agents, namely polydextrose, a maltodextrin and sorbitol, gave the best result in depressing the freezing point and inhibition of ice crystal formation. No one bulking agent alone showed the ability to accomplish all the required functions.

One of the main problems encountered was the cereal flavor evident in most mixes. A reduction in the amounts of sorbitol and Litess® reduced this problem; however, it added to the cost of their bulking abilities and the total solids of the mix. The total solids could be compensated by an increase in the MSNF level, but beyond 17%, the lactose in MSNF caused a sandy texture, and generally smaller air cells resulted. The maximum usage level of Litess® was 6%, beyond which a slight bitter taste was evident. Dairy Lo® was effective in masking this cereal flavor and imparting a dairy note.

While different combinations of ingredients are possible, all with acceptable texture and mouthfeel, a typical formulation, developed and tested in our laboratory is shown in Table 2. The exit temperature of this ice convection was -1.7°C, while the standard ice cream exited at -2.5°C. This indicated the possible presence of large ice crystals resulting in a smoother product.

TABLE 2.
FORMULATION OF A LOW-JOULE ICE CONFECTION

Ingredient	%
N-Lite D®	2.00
MSNF	13.00
Maltodextrin 15 DE	6.00
Litess®	6.00
Sorbitol 50M	2.00
Pioneer®	0.80
Splenda®	0.025
Vanilla Flavour	0.50
Colour	0.005
Total Solids	29.880
Water	70.120

Sensory evaluation was conducted using an unstructured scaling method. A descriptive method was used to measure the quality of a specific sensory attribute. The taste panel (n = 39) found significant differences (p = 0.01%) between the ice confection and the standard ice cream. It is possible that a degree of bias could have affected the results. A stigma is attached to a product labelled ice confection, because it is considered to be of a lower quality. The panelists who regularly ate diet style products embraced this product more readily than those who did not.

These results indicated that there is a potential for this type of product with improved formulations. Our study found that it was feasible to produce a zero-fat, low-joule ice confection using a combination of fat replacers, high intensity sweeteners and bulking agents. However, more work needs to be done on formulation optimization to achieve better consumer appeal.

CONCLUSION AND DISCUSSION

Fat and cholesterol reduction takes different forms depending on the type of food in consideration. Application of fat replacers, while a feasible and successful approach in processed foods, may not necessarily be applicable to all kinds of foods. An important point to consider is the nutritional requirement of a minimum amount of natural fats and oils, as they act as solvents and/or carriers of a number of vitamins and other biologically significant compounds. More specifically, essential fatty acids and their long chain derivatives are an integral component of cell membranes and precursor to prostaglandins, and must be supplied by the diet. Natural fat replacers and high intensity sweeteners will be more successful with consumers who have a preconceived view of low-fat, low-joule products to be "artificial". Therefore, consumer education should accompany the development of more wholesome and tasteful products.

The opportunity for the use of probiotic cultures as a means of cholesterol reduction offers a win-win situation, as these cultures play a very important role in improving the general health of the consumer.

ACKNOWLEDGMENT

The authors acknowledge the kind support of the following companies for supplying samples of their ingredients:

A.C. Hatrick Chemicals Pty. Ltd.; Bush Boake Allen Australia; Cotter Food Services Pty. Ltd.; Essential Flavours; Germantown Australia; Givaudan-Roure; Grindsted-Bronson & Jacobs; Johnson & Johnson; National Starches; Nutrasweet Kelco Company; Pfizer Food Science Group; Quest International; Soy Products of Australia Pty. Ltd.; and Starch Australasia Ltd.

REFERENCES

ARISTOVA, V.P., ROSSIKHINA, G.A. and TUROVSKAYA, S.N. 1994. Dairy products with reduced cholesterin content. Proceedings of the 24th International Dairy Congress, 18th - 22nd September, Melbourne, Australia.

AUSTRALIAN FOOD STANDARDS CODE 1994. Australian Government Publications, Canberra, Australia.

AUSTRALIAN STANDARDS: AS 2458 - 1986 Methods of Sensory Evaluation. Australian Government publications, Canberra, Australia.

BOEHRINGER MANNHEIM GMBH-BIOCHEMICA, 1995. Methods of Biochemical Analysis and Food Analysis, Sandhofer Straze 116, 6800 Mannheim 31, Germany.

BRINGE, N.A. and CHENG, J. 1995. Low-fat, low-cholesterol egg yolk in food applications. Food Technol. *5*, 94–106.

BUCK, L.M. and GILLILAND, S.E. 1994. Comparison of freshly isolated strains of *Lactobacillus acidophilus* of human intestinal origin for ability to assimilate cholesterol during growth. J. Dairy Sci. *77*, 2925–2933.

CADZOW, J. 1996. The Big Australian, Good Weekend, The Age, May 4, 25–35.

CHEN, J. 1995. Dietary changes and disease transition in China. Australian Food-Asian Nutrition Conference, CSIRO (Human Nutrition), 21 November, Adelaide, Australia.

FLANAGAN, B. 1995. Australian Grocery Industry Marketing Guide, Melbourne.

FOLCH, J., LEES, M. and STANLEY, G.H. 1957. A simple method for the isolation and purification of total lipids from animal tissues. J. Biol. Chem. *226*, 242–250.

GIBBONS, G.F., MITROPOULOS, K.A. and MYANT, N.B. 1982. Biochemistry of Cholesterol. Elsevier, Amsterdam.

GILLILAND, S.E., NELSON, C.R. and MAXWELL, C. 1985. Assimilation of cholesterol by *Lactobacillus acidophilus*. Appl. Environ. Microbiol. *49*, 377–381.

GILLILAND, S.E. and WALDER, D.K. 1990. Factors to consider when selecting a culture of *Lactobacillus acidophilus* as a dietary adjunct to produce a hypocholesterolemic effect in humans. J. Dairy Sci. *73*, 905–911.

HOMMA, N. 1988. Bifidobacteria: a resistance factor in human beings. Bifidobacteria Microflora. *7*(1), 35.

HUGHES, D.B. and HOOVER, D.G. 1991. Bifidobacteria: Their potential for use in American dairy products. Food Technol. *45*(4), 74–83.

ISHIBASHI, N. and SHIMAMURA, S. 1993. Bifidobacteria: Research and development in Japan. Food Technol. *47*(6), 126–135.

KARATZAS, B., SHERKAT, F., TRAN, H.V. and HALMOS, A.L. 1997. Effects of probiotic culture growth on a mixture of soy-bovine milk. Presented at the 30th National Convention of AIFST and SIFST, 4–8 May, Perth, Australia.

LAMPERT, I.M. 1970. Modern Dairy Products: Composition, Food Value. Chemical Publishing Co., New York.

NOROUZ-ZADEH, J. and APPELQVIST, L. 1988. Cholesterol oxides in Swedish foods and food ingredients: Milk powder products. J. Food Sci. *53*, 74–79.

PANIANGVAIT, P., KING., A.J., JONES, A.D. and GERMAN, B.G. 1995. Cholesterol oxides in foods of animal origin, J. Food Sci. *60* (6), 1159–1174.

RAO, D.R., PULUSANI, S.R. and CHAWAN, C.B. 1985. Role of fermented milk products in milk intolerance and other clinical conditions. Adv. Nutr. Res. *7* 203–219.

SCRIVEN, F.M. 1993. Australian Consumers' Lite Survey Results, S.M.A.R.T Research, Waitara, NSW:1–3.

SHERKAT, F. and HUANG, W. 1996. Biosoghurt, A healthy product from local ingredients. 2nd International Soybean Processing and Utilisation Conference, 8–13 January, Bangkok, Thailand.

SHERKAT, F., RAZAVI, S.K. and KARATZAS, B. 1996. Protein recovery and trypsin inhibitor removal from aqueous extracts of soy flour. Presented at the Conference on Plant Proteins from European Crops, 24–27 November, Nantes, France.

WELCH, C. 1987. Nutritional and therapeutic aspects of *Lactobacillus acidophilus* in dairy products. Cultured Dairy Products J. 23–26.

PLASMA AND TISSUE LIPID DIFFERENCES AND SUSCEPTIBILITY TO OXIDATION IN HYPERTENSIVE RATS FED SATURATED AND POLYUNSATURATED DIETARY FATS

ELISA GIRARDELLI PINTO NOVAIS and DAVID D. KITTS

Department of Food Science
University of British Columbia
Vancouver, B.C. Canada V6T-1Z4

ABSTRACT

The role of dietary lipid source as well as cholesterol intake has been studied extensively; however, few studies have attempted to integrate the interactive influence of dietary fat source and cholesterol intake in subjects predisposed to hypertension. In the present study, the effect of feeding different dietary lipid sources in both non-atherogenic and atherogenic diets was studied in genetically different rat strains (Spontaneously Hypertensive (SHR) and Wistar Kyoto Normotensive (WKY)). Experimental diets consisted of 13% fat derived from butter (saturate source), soybean oil (n-6 PUFA) and menhaden oil (n-3 PUFA) and 3% from canola oil for a total of 16% total crude lipid. Cholesterol was added to the diets to final concentrations of either 0.05% (w/w) (e.g non-atherogenic diets) or 0.5% (w/w) (e.g atherogenic diets). Hypertension was confirmed at 12 weeks in the SHR. Animals fed atherogenic diets containing menhaden oil, exhibited relatively lower (P<0.001) plasma cholesterol levels compared to counterparts fed atherogenic diets containing butter or soya fat blend. Feeding rats the atherogenic diets resulted in elevated hepatic (P<0.001) cholesterol, but no change in the susceptibility of plasma LDL oxidation. All animals fed atherogenic diets increased fecal excretion of both total crude lipid and cholesterol; however, this effect was relatively greater in SHR compared to WKY counterparts. The results of this study emphasize the importance of endogenous factors (e.g. genetic) in modifying exogenous (e.g. dietary) influences on lipid metabolism and hypertension.

INTRODUCTION

Hypercholesterolemia is a well known risk factor for coronary artery disease (Barnard *et al.* 1993; Rubattu *et al.* 1993). The North American diet has traditionally contained approximately 40% of calories in the form of fat, with a relatively high saturated fatty acid content (Spencer 1995). Clinical evidence has shown that the level of dietary lipid intake influences the incidence of dyslipidemia in humans (Grundy and Denke 1990; Sanders *et al.* 1994). In animal studies, plasma and liver triacylglycerol concentrations have been found to increase when fed diets rich in saturated fatty acids (Yuan *et al.* 1997; Fernandez *et al.* 1991). Concurrent cholesterol intake is also known to modulate the fat source effect on plasma and liver lipids (Fungwe *et al.* 1994; Lin *et al.* 1995).

The importance of lipid oxidation products in the chain of events that lead to the development of atherosclerosis has been examined (Karmansky *et al.* 1996). Relatively less is known about the effect of diet on LDL-oxidation and development of hypertension. The presence of lipid oxidation products in plasma lipoproteins has been related to an increased risk for the occurrence of coronary heart disease (Steinberg *et al.* 1989). The purpose of the present study was to examine the effect of predominantly saturated vs. unsaturated fat sources, with both a high and low cholesterol concentration, on total lipid and cholesterol balance, plasma lipids and low density lipoprotein oxidation in animals with and without a predisposition to hypertension.

MATERIALS AND METHODS

Animals and Experimental Diets

Male spontaneously hypertensive rats (SHR) and Wistar Kyoto Normotensive (WKY) rats, 5 weeks old, were purchased from Charles River (Quebec), and housed in wire-mesh bottom stainless steel cages, at 23°C. Light/darkness regimen was timed in 12 h intervals, with light from 8:00 a.m. to 8:00 p.m. After two weeks adaptation, the animals were kept under a meal feeding regimen. The basal diet was prepared by mixing dry components, then incorporating fat sources to which cholesterol and cholic acid were added. Experimental diets were prepared weekly and kept refrigerated at 4°C. For detailed composition see Table 1. Deionized, distilled water was supplied ad libitum. Animals were cared for according to the principles of the Guide to the Care and Use of Experimental Animals, Vol.1, of the Canadian Council of Animal Care (Olfert *et al.* 1993).

On week 6 of the experiment the animals were placed in metabolic cages (Nalgene, Rochester, NY) for 150-300 g rats. Excreta were collected for 5 days, weighed, pooled and kept frozen until analysis. Animals were returned to their cages and continued with the previous regimen until 15 weeks of age.

Blood Pressure Measurements

Systolic blood pressure recordings were obtained from the SHR and WKY animals at 13 weeks of age, after a 1 week training period. Measurements were taken in conscious rats by an indirect tail-cuff method (Harvard Apparatus Ltd., South Natick, MA; Kitts *et al.* (1992)). Each recorded value represents the mean of three successive determinations over a period of 10-15 min.

Tissue Sample Collection and Preparation

At 15 weeks of age the animals were sacrificed under halothane (Fluothane Halothane B.P.N°3125, Ayerst Laboratories, Montreal, Que.) anaesthesia. Blood was collected by cardiac puncture into cooled heparinized tubes for plasma separation at 100 × g, 5 min, 4°C (refrigerated centrifuge, IEC CENTRA-7R, International Equipment Co., Massachusetts, USA). RBC were collected and washed twice with isotonic (0.88%) saline. Plasma aliquots were dispensed into Eppendorf tubes and frozen at -35°C until analysis. Hearts and livers were collected into chilled 50 mM Tris (Tris (hydroxymethyl) aminomethane, BioRad Laboratories, Richmond, CA), 0.1 mM EDTA (ethylenediaminetetraacetic acid; Sigma Grade, St. Louis, MO), pH 7.6 homogenizing buffer, blotted dry and frozen in a -30°C freezer until analysis.

TABLE 1.
COMPOSITION OF EXPERIMENTAL DIETS

Component	Content in % weight
Casein[1]	25.0
CaCO[2]	2.0
Ca free mineral mix[3]	3.5
Vitamin mix[4]	3.0
Choline chloride	0.2
D,L-methionine[3]	0.3
Alphacel[4]	5.0
Sucrose[4]	3.0
Canola[5]	3.0
Test fat source	13.0
Butter[7]	
Soybean Oil[8]	
Menhaden Oil[9]	
Monophosphate[6]	3.0
Corn Starch[1]	39.0
Cholesterol[1]	0.5 or 0.05
Cholic Acid[1]	0.25 or 0.025
Total	100.0

[1]ICN Biomedicals Inc., Aurora, Ohio
[2]Pacific Gardens Galore & Co., Delta, B.C.
[3]US Biochemical Corporation, Cleveland, Ohio
[4]ICN Biochemicals, Inc., Cleveland, Ohio
[5]Neptune Food Services, Richmond, B.C.
[6]Van Waters and Rogers, Abbotsford, B.C.
[7]Dairy World Foods, Burnaby, B.C.
[8]Bioforce Canada, Burnaby, B.C.
[9]Napata Haynie, Reedville, VA

Plasma Analyses

Plasma aliquots were thawed at refrigeration temperature and analyzed for total cholesterol based on the method of Siedel *et al.* (1983) for phospholipids according to Takayama *et al.* (1977) and Trinder (1969), and for triacylglycerols following the method of Trinder (1969) and Wahlefeld (1974) using biochemical assay kits (Boehringer Mannheim, Laval, Quebec).

Plasma - Lipoprotein Fraction Separation

The separation of plasma lipoprotein fractions was carried out according to the ultracentrifugation sucrose density method of Terpstra *et al.* (1981). Sudan black was added to the tubes to prestain the plasma. LDL was isolated at density fraction of $1.019 < p_{20} < 1.063$ and collected for further analysis. Samples of LDL were dialyzed against cold, degassed, N_2-saturated HEPES-NaCl buffer, pH = 7.4 overnight. The protein content of each fraction was determined by the method of Lowry *et al.* (1951) using serum albumin as a standard. Cholesterol, triacylglycerol and phospholipid analyses of the different fractions were performed as outlined above.

Lipoprotein Oxidation

Oxidation of LDL lipoprotein fraction was carried out according to the method of Comminacini *et al.* (1991). Aliquots of each fraction, corresponding to an equal amount of protein (0.5 mg/ml), were placed in a sealed test-tube containing copper (50 μM) which was used to catalyze the reaction. Reaction tubes were kept in a water bath (37°C) for up to 4 h at prefixed time intervals (0, 1 h, 2 h and 4 h). Aliquots were removed for fluorescence measurements at 430 nm, with excitation at 360 nm using a Shimadzu spectrophotofluorometer (Shimadzu, UV-visible recording spectrophotometer, UV-160, Tekscience, Oakville, On).

Liver Tissue Analysis

Liver tissue was removed from the freezer and thawed at refrigeration temperature (4°C). Lipid extraction was performed according to Folch's method (1957) with minor modifications. Total crude lipid was determined from an aliquot of the Folch's liver extract and calculated as percent weight of sample. Aliquots of the total crude lipid were also analyzed for cholesterol and triacylglycerol content as described by Siedel *et al.* (1983) and Ziegenhorn *et al.* (1975).

Fecal Lipid Extraction. Fecal material collected from balance studies was ground, while kept on ice and freeze dried (freeze-dryer Model 10-145-MRBA, Virtis Research Equipment, Gardner, NY). Samples were weighed into dried glass tubes. Freeze-dried samples were further ground using a Polytron after the addition of Folch's solution. Samples in Folch's were dispensed into Erlenmeyer flasks, which were sealed and left overnight in a shaker at 60 rpm for lipid extraction. The solution was then filtered (Whatman #1) into fat-free glass-stoppered graduated cylinders. Folch's was used to rinse flasks, which were then filtered into a separate vessel. Saline (0.9%) was added (first wash), and the solutions were mixed. The methanol-aqueous layer was suctioned off and 10 ml of 3:47:48 ($CHCl_3$:CH_3OH:dH_2O) were added (second wash), and the solutions mixed, and left overnight for phase separation. The final bottom layer volume was recorded and aliquots were recorded for further analysis. The total crude lipid content was calculated as above for liver lipid extract. Analysis of the fecal lipid extract for cholesterol was performed according to the method described above for the liver extract.

Statistical Analyses

Values are expressed as means with their standard errors. Differences between treatment means were tested by one-way analysis of variance (SPSS Inc., Chicago, IL.). Where differences existed, the sources were identified by the Student-Newman-Keuls multiple range test at $p < 0.05$ (SPSS). Interactions between treatments were identified by two-way ANOVA (MANOVA; SPSS). Correlation coefficients were determined by the method of least squares.

RESULTS

Blood Pressure

Blood pressure readings showed that SHR exhibited significantly ($p < 0.001$) higher blood pressure than WKY rats as early as 12 weeks of age. There were no other significant main treatment effects or interactions (Fig.1 A,B).

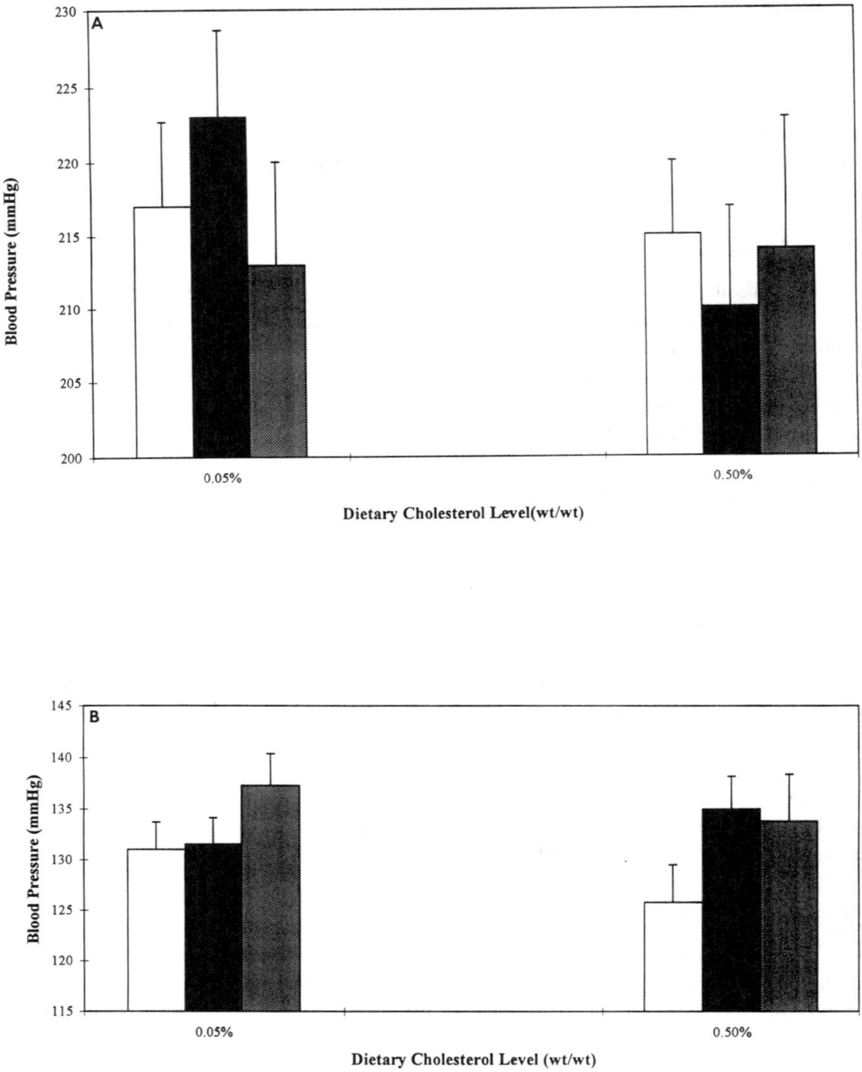

FIG. 1. BLOOD PRESSURE IN SHR (A) AND WKY (B) FED DIFFERENT DIETARY FAT SOURCES[1,2]

[1]Values indicate blood pressure (mm Hg); mean ± SEM; n = 8. [2]SHR = Spontaneously Hypertensive rat; WKY = Wistar Kyoto Normotensive rat. Fat sources identified: Butter = ▭, Soybean = ■, Menhaden = ▨. A significant ($P<0.001$) treatment effect for animal strain was observed.

Total Crude Lipid Balance

Total fecal crude lipid excreted was significantly ($p<0.001$) different between cholesterol treatments. Low cholesterol fed animals from both rat strains excreted between 0.42 g and 0.49 g total crude lipids during the balance study, compared to counterparts on a high cholesterol fed rats, which eliminated fat in feces in amounts that ranged from 0.69 g to 0.82 g fat during the same period of time for both WKY and SHR, respectively.

Lipid Digestibility

Lipid digestibility was calculated as the ratio of the difference between lipid ingested minus lipid excreted over lipid ingested. The digestibility of the dietary fat blends were significantly affected by dietary cholesterol intake ($p<0.001$) and dietary fat source ($p=0.048$). Lipid digestibility was lowered by cholesterol intake in both rat strains (Table 2).

TABLE 2.
LIPID DIGESTIBILITY OF EXPERIMENTAL DIETS[1,2] FED TO SHR AND WKY RATS

Rat Strain	SHR		WKY	
Dietary Cholesterol (% w/w)	0.05	0.5	0.05	0.5
Dietary Fat Source				
Butter	0.964 ± 0.002	0.931 ± 0.008	0.957 ± 0.004	0.934 ± 0.003
Soybean	0.955 ± 0.004	0.936 ± 0.010	0.950 ± 0.004	0.928 ± 0.007
Menhaden	0.965 ± 0.004	0.905 ± 0.030	0.947 ± 0.013	0.931 ± 0.003

Main effect:		Interactions:	
ANOVA p-value[3]:		MANOVA p-value[4]:	
S	N.S.	SxF	N.S.
C	$p<0.001$	SxC	N.S.
F	$p<0.048$	CxF	$p=0.032$

[1] Values indicate mean + SEM, n = 8, SHR = Spontaneously Hypertensive rat, WKY = Wistar Kyoto Normotensive rat

[2] Lipid digestibility = 1 - (g lipid excreted/g lipid ingested)

[3] S = strain effect, C = cholesterol level intake effect, F = dietary fat source effect, by MANOVA.

[4] Interactions: S x F = strain x fat, S x C = strain x cholesterol, C x F = cholesterol x fat

Fecal Cholesterol Output

Differences in fecal cholesterol output over the 5 day balance study were highly significant ($p<0.001$) for such treatment effects as rat strain, dietary cholesterol level and fat blend (Table 3).

TABLE 3.
FECAL CHOLESTEROL OUTPUT FROM SHR AND WKY RATS FED EXPERIMENTAL DIETS[1,2]

Rat Strain	SHR		WKY	
Dietary Cholesterol (% w/w)	0.05	0.5	0.05	0.5
Dietary Fat Source				
Butter	2.0 ± 0.1	3.4 ± 0.5	1.3 ± 0.1	2.0 ± 0.2
Soybean	2.9 ± 0.2	5.6 ± 0.5	2.7 ± 0.2	4.5 ± 0.2
Menhaden	2.5 ± 0.3	6.3 ± 0.5	1.4 ± 0.1	3.7 ± 0.3

Main effect: ANOVA p-value[3]:	Interactions: MANOVA p-value[4]:
S p<0.001	SxF p=0.032
C p<0.001	SxC p=0.05
F p<0.001	CxF p=0.004

1 Values indicate mean + SEM, n = 8, SHR = Spontaneously Hypertensive rat, WKY = Wistar Kyoto Normotensive rat

2 Fecal cholesterol concentration (mg/g dried feces/5 days)

3 S = strain effect, C = cholesterol level intake effect, F = dietary fat source effect, by MANOVA

4 Interactions: S × F = strain × fat, S × C = strain × cholesterol, C × F = cholesterol × fat, N.S. = non significant

Cholesterol Balance

Dietary fat sources also had a significant ($p \leq 0.05$) effect on cholesterol balance. SHR fed the high cholesterol menhaden diet exhibited a lower cholesterol balance than either SHR fed a high cholesterol soybean or rats fed a high cholesterol-butter diets. Among the high cholesterol fed WKY, butter fed animals exhibited a higher cholesterol balance compared to menhaden and soy lipid fed animals (Fig.2 A,B).

Liver Lipid Analysis

Total Crude Lipids. Total crude lipid content of livers varied significantly ($p<0.001$) according to the level of dietary cholesterol intake, more so than the fat

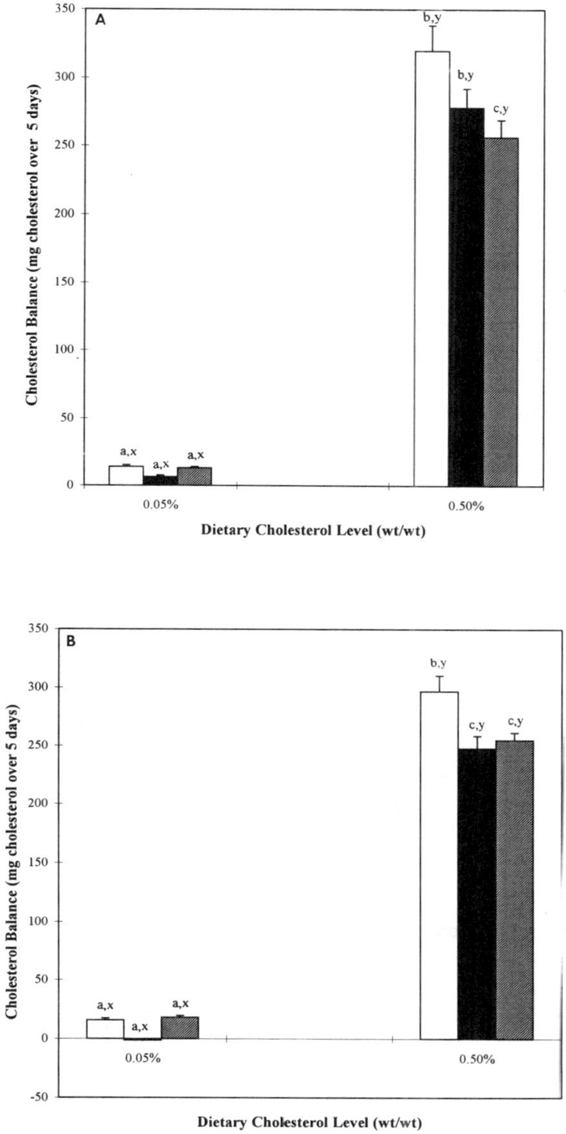

FIG. 2. CHOLESTEROL BALANCE IN SHR (A) AND WKY (B) FED DIFFERENT DIETARY FAT SOURCES[1,2]

[1]Values indicate cholesterol balance (mg): (chol. ingested (mg) - chol. excreted (mg)) over 5 days; mean ± SEM; n = 8.

[2]SHR = Spontaneously Hypertensive rat; WKY = Wistar Kyoto Normotensive rat. Fat sources identified: Butter = ▭, Soybean = ■, Menhaden = ▨.

a,b,c - denotes statistical significance for differences between dietary fat sources, $p \leq 0.05$.

x,y - denotes statistical significance for differences between dietary cholesterol levels, $p \leq 0.05$.

source fed to rats. There was no difference in liver lipid content between SHR and WKY animals. Livers from rats consuming high cholesterol diets had a total crude lipid content that was approximately three times that observed in rats fed corresponding low cholesterol diets. The intake of individual fat blends in animals fed high cholesterol diets resulted in lower ($p<0.05$) % crude lipid content in livers from menhaden fed animals, with 22.7 and 23.1% in SHR and WKY, respectively. Rats fed either butter or soy diets, in combination with high cholesterol, had a liver total crude lipid content that ranged from 27.7% in butter fed SHR to 29.8% in soybean oil fed SHR. The interaction between dietary cholesterol level and fat type was significant for liver total crude lipid ($p=0.021$).

Liver Cholesterol. Liver cholesterol concentrations corresponded to the proportions of dietary cholesterol consumed by the rats. For example, low cholesterol soybean fed SHR rats had an average of 8.19 ± 0.94 mg liver cholesterol/g tissue wet weight, while those on a high cholesterol diet had 88.18 ± 5.61 mg cholesterol/g tissue wet weight. Of the high cholesterol fed animals, the menhaden fed SHR group exhibited the lowest liver cholesterol concentration (67.88 ± 5.02 mg cholesterol/g tissue wet weight), whereas the WKY animals deposited more sterol (87.05 ± 5.76 mg cholesterol/g tissue wet weight) in the menhaden group. Both cholesterol intake ($p<0.001$) and fat type ($p=0.016$) produced significant effects on liver cholesterol concentration. The interaction between fat type and dietary cholesterol level in total liver cholesterol concentration was significant ($p=0.012$).

Liver Triacylglycerol. Liver triacylglycerol concentrations were lowest in SHR fed a high cholesterol menhaden diet (86.63 ± 2.76 mg/g liver wet weight). Rats fed menhaden diets had lower ($p\leq0.05$) triacylglycerol concentration than soybean fed counterparts. Animals fed butter diets showed no change in triacylglycerol levels with an increase in cholesterol intake. All main treatment effects were significant ($p<0.001$), as were the interactions between animal strain and fat type ($p=0.001$) and animal strain and cholesterol intake ($p<0.001$) (Fig.3 A,B).

Plasma Lipid Analysis

Total Plasma Cholesterol. Total plasma cholesterol concentration was elevated ($p=0.001$) in animals fed high cholesterol diets. This effect was especially pronounced in WKY animals fed the butter and soybean-high cholesterol diets. Comparing the values for SHR and WKY, it was noted that the differences in plasma cholesterol concentration from animals fed high and low dietary cholesterol were relatively small. For example WKY animals had higher plasma cholesterol levels than SHR counterparts, indicating a strain effect ($p < 0.001$). Menhaden oil fed animals generally had lower plasma cholesterol levels when compared to those fed other fats, but that difference reached statistical significance only for high cholesterol fed menhaden WKY. The animal strain and fat source ($p = 0.010$), and cholesterol and fat source interactions ($p = 0.001$) were also significant (Table 4).

Plasma Triacylglycerol. Plasma triacylglycerol concentrations were significantly modified by dietary cholesterol ($p<0.001$) and fat type ($p<0.001$). The interaction of dietary cholesterol and fat type on plasma triacylglycerol was also highly significant

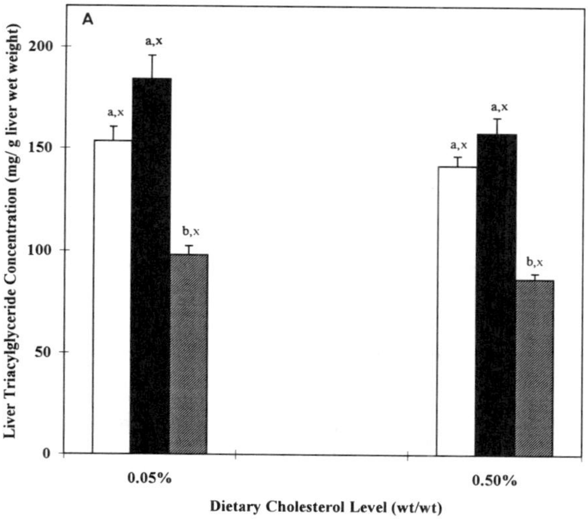

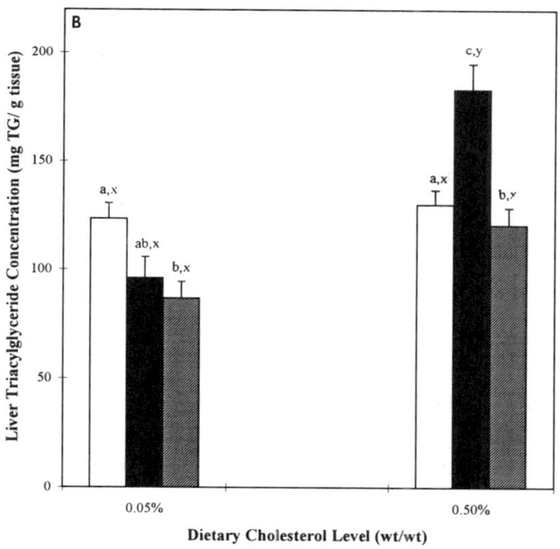

FIG. 3. LIVER TRIACYLGLYCEROL CONCENTRATION IN SHR (A) AND WKY (B) FED DIFFERENT DIETARY FAT SOURCES[1,2]

[1]Values indicate liver triacylglycerol concentration (mg/g liver weight); mean ± SEM; n = 8.

[2]SHR = Spontaneously Hypertensive rat; WKY = Wistar Kyoto Normotensive rat

Fat sources identified: Butter = ▭, Soybean = ■, Menhaden = ▨.

a,b,c - denotes statistical significance for differences between dietary fat sources, $p \leq 0.05$.

x,y - denotes statistical significance for differences between dietary cholesterol levels, $p \leq 0.05$.

($p=0.005$). Plasma triacylglycerol levels were highest in low cholesterol butter fed animals (66.60 ± 3.59 mg/dl for the SHR; 70.47 ± 7.56 mg/dl for the WKY group). The lowest triacylglycerol levels observed were in SHR fed high cholesterol, soybean (36.87 ± 1.84 mg/dl) diets.

TABLE 4.
PLASMA CHOLESTEROL CONCENTRATION IN SHR AND WKY RATS FED EXPERIMENTAL DIETS[1,2]

Rat Strain	SHR		WKY	
Dietary Cholesterol (% w/w)	0.05	0.5	0.05	0.5
Dietary Fat Source				
Butter	86.22 ± 8.88	112.85 ± 14.31	118.62 ± 4.34	246.08 ± 16.78
Soybean	102.82 ± 8.95	111.30 ± 21.30	135.67 ± 6.36	206.20 ± 12.71
Menhaden	83.75 ± 5.92	97.23 ± 6.12	121.78 ± 8.99	134.72 ± 25.84
Main effect: ANOVA p-value[3]:			Interactions: MANOVA p-value[4]:	
S $p<0.001$			SxF $p=0.010$	
C $p<0.001$			SxC $p<0.001$	
F $p<0.001$			CxF $p=0.001$	

[1] Values indicate mean + SEM, n = 8, SHR = Spontaneously Hypertensive rat, WKY = Wistar Kyoto Normotensive rat

[2] Plasma cholesterol concentration (mg/dl plasma)

[3] S = strain effect, C = cholesterol level intake effect, F = dietary fat source effect, by MANOVA.

[4] Interactions: S × F = strain × fat, S × C = strain × cholesterol, C × F = cholesterol × fat

Plasma Phospholipids. Plasma phospholipid concentrations were significantly altered by animal strain ($p<0.001$) and dietary cholesterol intake level ($p=0.005$). Phospholipid levels were higher in WKY than in SHR. Animals fed low cholesterol levels had higher plasma phospholipid concentration than counterparts fed high cholesterol diets. The interaction between rat strain and cholesterol level on plasma phospholipids was significant ($p=0.004$).

Plasma Low Density Lipoprotein Fraction Lipid Analysis

LDL-Cholesterol. LDL-cholesterol concentrations were not affected by the different treatment effects, except for the rat strain effect. WKY animals showed higher ($p<0.001$) LDL-cholesterol levels compared to their SHR counterparts. The interactions between main treatments were not significant.

LDL-Triacylglycerol. LDL-triacylglycerol did not show any significant main treatment effects or interactions (data not shown).

LDL Phospholipids. LDL-phospholipid plasma concentrations were significantly affected by both cholesterol intake level ($p<0.001$) and rat strain ($p=0.012$), but not by dietary fat type. Low cholesterol diets fed to SHR produced higher ($p = 0.05$) phospholipid values than those observed in rats fed high cholesterol diets, with the exception of SHR fed a low cholesterol butter diet. Soybean based diets resulted in the highest phospholipid concentrations in the low cholesterol treated animals. There were no significant interactions between the different main effects.

LDL Oxidation. This assay was carried out using two levels of copper sulfate. At a low level of copper sulfate, no significant differences were found for the main treatment effects. No significant interactions between the main treatment effects were detected either. The results for LDL oxidation at the higher copper sulfate concentration were analogous to those obtained at the low Cu-concentration. There were neither significant treatment effects nor significant interactions thereof with forced peroxidation of LDL (Fig. 4 A,B).

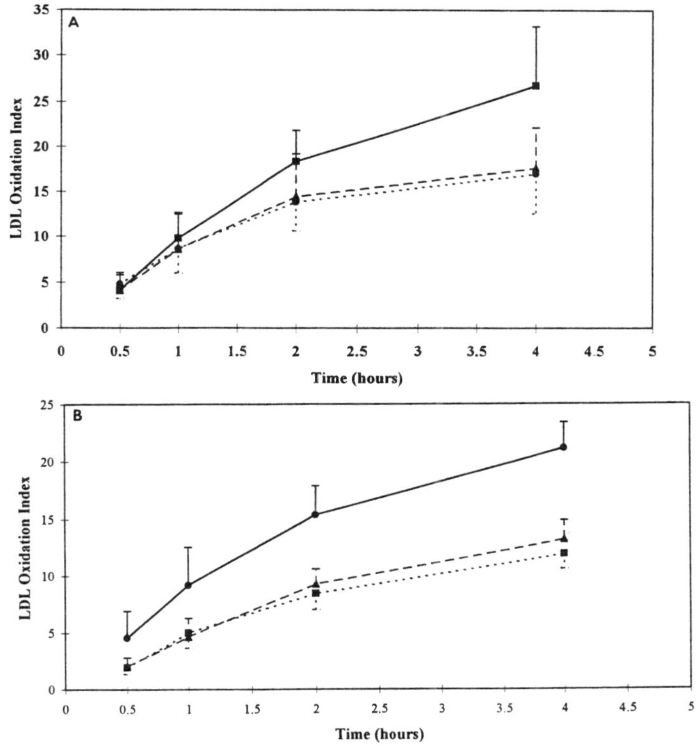

FIG 4. CU^{+2}-INDUCED LDL OXIDATION IN SHR (A) AND WKY (B) FED DIFFERENT DIETARY FAT SOURCES CONTAINING 0.5% CHOLESTEROL (W/W)[1,2]

[1]Values indicate LDL oxidation index; mean ± SEM; n = 8.

[2]SHR = Spontaneously Hypertensive rat; WKY = Wistar Kyoto Normotensive rat

Fat sources identified: Butter = ■, Soybean = ●, Menhaden = ▲

No significant treatment effect was observed.

DISCUSSION

Blood pressure in humans can be modified by consuming low fat diets in which the polyunsaturated fat content is relatively increased (Iacono *et al.* 1989). High blood pressure in SHR appears to be related to an imbalance in Na^+/K^+ transport and/or Ca metabolism (Kitts *et al.* 1992). An attempt to modify the blood pressure in rats by altering lipid source, either by varying the fat blend or the cholesterol content in the diet, was not successful.

In this experiment, high cholesterol-butter fed WKY consistently had higher total plasma cholesterol than counterparts fed menhaden oil. Since food intake and weight gain were similar among treatment groups, these parameters can be discarded as factors for differences in plasma cholesterol concentrations. Elevated plasma cholesterol in WKY was in part explained by the higher saturated fatty acid content of the butter based diet. For example, myristic acid in particular has been found to raise plasma cholesterol in gerbils (Pronczuk *et al.* 1994) and the butter blend diet contained the highest myristic acid content. The myristic acid content of soybean diets in this experiment was nearly negligible (0.3%), but it is noteworthy that the menhaden based diets also contained myristic acid (8.9%). In a study where guinea pigs were fed tallow, corn oil and olive oil at 15 g dietary fat/100 g diet, only those animals fed corn oil, with a high (C18:1) content, exhibited a lower plasma cholesterol level (Fernandez and McNamara 1993; De Schrijver *et al.* 1984). Palmitic acid enriched diets have raised plasma cholesterol in monkeys in comparison with oleic acid, only when in combination with dietary cholesterol at 0.3% (w/w) (Khosla and Hayes 1993). Other studies have not detected changes in plasma cholesterol levels when feeding fish oil, rich in n-3 fatty acids, compared to corn oil (Zampelas *et al.* 1994). Our results therefore demonstrate that the presence of n-3 PUFA from menhaden was important in possibly negating the cholesterolemic effect of myristic acid.

In SHR, changes in plasma cholesterol following an intake of different fat source blends in combination with a high cholesterol level were not as evident. These results point to a lack of responsiveness in SHR plasma cholesterol to dietary fat and or cholesterol intake. These apparent differences between the two strains also point to a genetic factor in the regulation of plasma cholesterol. The importance of this observation lies with the fact that potentially atherogenic diets may not always lead to hypercholesterolemia.

The pattern of liver cholesterol concentrations was similar for both SHR and WKY, in that liver cholesterol concentrations were consistently raised by high cholesterol intake. Lower liver cholesterol concentrations in menhaden-fed SHR were likely the result of a number of factors. In rats, cholesterol delivered to the liver via chylomicrons will up-regulate 7α-hydroxylase, and suppress HMGCoA reductase, thereby causing a decrease in cholesterol biosynthesis. The increase in dietary cholesterol intake was possibly greater than the inhibition of cholesterol synthesis in the liver of animals in this study. Preferred hepatic uptake of PUFA from chylomicrons may lead to an inhibition of hepatic cholesterol synthesis and a reduction in ACAT activity (Smit *et al.* 1994). Furthermore, n-6 PUFA, but not n-3 PUFA, have been found to stimulate the disposition of cholesterol into bile by potentiating bile-acid dependent cholesterol secretion (Smit *et al.* 1994; Berr *et al.* 1993).

Monounsaturated fatty acid rich diets in combination with a high cholesterol content have been found to raise liver triacylglycerol concentrations less than diets containing butter with high cholesterol content combination in baboons (Fox *et al.* 1987). Bouziane *et al.* (1997) observed that the ratio of PUFA/monounsaturated fatty acids determined liver triacylglycerol concentrations more so than monounsaturated fatty acids alone. Increased synthesis and decreased secretion of triacylglycerol combined to result in raised liver triacylglycerol concentrations (Lin *et al.* 1995). In the present study the dietary fat blend was found to be an important cofactor in the deposition of sterol in hepatic tissue of hypercholesterolemic rats.

Separation of plasma LDL lipoprotein fractions and subsequent lipid analysis enabled the determination of specific dietary effects on LDL lipid composition and susceptibility to oxidation. Rats are known to transport most of their cholesterol in HDL, thus the absence of statistically significant dietary fat source or cholesterol effects on LDL oxidation may likely be due to the minimal role in LDL metabolism in the rat and to the relative resistance to atherosclerosis in rats. LDL oxidation is an important component in atherosclerotic lesions and the lack of development thereof, in the presence of atherogenic factors, indicates possibly compensatory mechanisms that counterbalance dietary risk factors. Our results indicate that the predisposition of hypertension in SHR does not involve a sustained susceptibility to LDL oxidation.

CONCLUSIONS

Although lipid digestibility was relatively lower in high cholesterol fed animals in general, the total crude lipid and cholesterol excretion patterns and subsequent balances varied between WKY and SHR. Dietary fat blends modulated changes in liver crude lipid content, with high cholesterol-menhaden fed animals exhibiting a relatively lower liver total crude lipid content. Therefore, while dietary fat sources may have an impact on factors associated with coronary heart disease, such as hyperlipidemia, the concurrent dietary intake of cholesterol must be taken into account to properly assess the potential for enhanced liver lipid deposition and changes in plasma lipid levels. The hypertension tendency of SHR was not an apparent factor in the susceptibility of atherogenic induced changes in LDL oxidation.

Finally, since dietary lipid intake did not modify blood pressure in either SHR or WKY, it is concluded that high blood pressure in SHR is determined more by endogenous (e.g. genetic predisposition) then exogenous (dietary lipid intake) factors.

ACKNOWLEDGMENTS

This work was supported from a grant by the dairy farmers of Canada. The study reported was taken from the M.Sc. thesis of Elisa Girardelli P. Novais.

REFERENCES

BARNARD, R.J., FARIA, D.J., MENGES, J.E. and MARTIN, D.A. 1993. Effects of a high-fat sucrose diet on serum insulin and related atherosclerotic risk factors in rats. Atherosclerosis *100*, 229–236.

BERR, E.M., GOETZ, A., SCHREIBER, E. and BAUMGARTNER, G. 1993. Effect of dietary n-3 versus n-6 polyunsaturated fatty acids on hepatic excretion of cholesterol in the hamster. J. Lipid Res. *34*, 1275–1284.

BOUZIANE, M., BELLEVILLE, J. and PROST, J. 1997. Hepatic storage of n-3 and n-6 polyunsaturated fatty acids by very-low-density lipoproteins in growing rats fed low- or adequate-protein diets with sunflower, soybean, coconut and salmon oils. Am. J. Clin. Nutr. *65*, 750–760.

CARRELLA, M., CSILLAGHY, A., MERCATO, R. and D'ARIENZO, A. 1995. Biliary excretion of chylomicron remnant cholesterol in the rat: Responses to the expansion of their plasma pool and promoting role of stimulated bile-acid synthesis. Clin. Sci. *89*, 121–128.

DE SCHRIJVER, R., VERMEULEN, D. and DAEMS, V. 1992. Dose-response relationship between dietary (n-3) fatty acids and plasma and tissue lipids, steroid excretion and urinary malondialdehyde in rats. J. Nutr. *122*, 1979–1987.

DOUGHERTY, R.M., GALLI, C., FERRO-LUZZI, A. and IACONO, J.M. 1987, Lipid and phospholipid fatty acid composition of plasma, red blood cells, and platelets and how they are affected by dietary lipids: a study of normal subjects from Italy, Finland and the USA. Am. J. Clin. Nutr. *45*, 443–455.

FERNANDEZ, M.L. and MCNAMARA, D.J. 1991. Regulation of cholesterol and lipoprotein metabolism guinea pigs mediated by dietary fat quality and quantity. J. Nutr. *121*, 934–943.

FERNANDEZ, M.L. and MCNAMARA, D.J. 1994. Dietary fat saturation and chain length modulate Guinea pig hepatic cholesterol metabolism. J.Nutr. *124*, 331–339.

FOLCH, J., LEES, M. and STANLEY, G.H.S. 1957. A simple method for the isolation and purification of total lipid from animal tissues. J. Biol. Chem. *226*, 242–250.

FOX, J.C., MCGILL, H.C., CAREY, K.D. and GETZ, G.S. 1987. In vivo regulation of hepatic LDL receptor mRNA in the baboon. Differential effects of saturated and unsaturated fat. J. Biol. Chem. *262*, 151–163.

FUNGWE, T.V., FOX, J.E., CAGEN, L.M., WILCOX, H.G. and HEIMBERG, M. 1994. Stimulation of fatty acid biosynthesis by dietary cholesterol and of cholesterol synthesis by dietary fatty acid. J. Lip. Res. *35*, 311–318.

GRUNDY, S.M. and DENKE, M.A. 1990. Dietary influences on serum lipids and lipoproteins. J. Lip. Res. *31*, 1149–1172.

IACONO, J.M., DOUGHERTY, R.M., PUSKA, P. and PIETINEN, P. 1989. Dietary polyunsaturated fat and hypertension. Ann. Med. *21*: 251–254.

KARMANSKY, I., SHNAIDER, H., PALANT, H. and GRUENER, N. 1996. Plasma lipid oxidation and susceptibility of low-density lipoproteins to oxidation in male patients with stable coronary artery disease. Clin. Biochem. *29*, 573–579.

KHOSLA, P. and HAYES, K.C. 1993. Dietary palmitic acid raises plasma LDL cholesterol relative to oleic acid only at a high intake of cholesterol. Biochim. Biophys. Acta. *1210*, 13–22.

KITTS, D.D., YUAN, Y.V., NAGASAWA, T. and MORIYAMA, T.T. 1992. Effect of casein, casein phosphopeptides and calcium intake on ileal 45Ca disappearance and temporal systolic blood pressure in spontaneously hypertensive rats. Br. J. Nutr. 68: 765–781.

LIN, M.H., LU, S.C., HSIEH, J.-W. and HUANG, P.C. 1995. Lipoprotein responses to fish, coconut and soybean oil diets with and without cholesterol in the Syrian hamster, J. Formos. Med. Assoc. *94*, 724–731.

MILLS, D.E., MURTHY, M. and GALEY, W.R. 1995. Dietary fatty acids, membrane transport, and oxidative sensitivity in human erythrocytes. Lipids *30*, 657–663.

OLFERT, E.D., CROSS, B.M., and MCWILLIAM, A.A. (eds.) 1993. Guide to the care and use of experimental animals (VOL. 1). Canadian Council of Animal Care. Ottawa, On.

PRONCZUK, A., KHOSLA, P. and HAYES, K.C. 1994. Dietary myristic, palmitic and linoleic acids modulate cholesterolemia in gerbils. FASEB *8*, 1191–200.

RUBATTU, S., VOLPE, M., ENEA, I., RUSSO, R., ROMANO, M. and TRIMARCO, B. 1993. Influence of hypercholesterolemia on adrenal steroid metabolism and electrolyte balance in spontaneously hypertensive rats. Endocrinology *5*, 2015–2021.

RUSSELL, D.W., YAMAMOTO, T., SCHNEIDER, W.J., SLAUGHTER, C.J., BROWN, M.S. and GOLDSTEIN, J.L. 1983. cDNA cloning of the bovine low-density lipoprotein receptor: Feedback regulation of a receptor mRNA, Proc. Natl. Acad. Sci. USA *80*, 7501–7505.

SANDERS, K., JOHNSON, L., O'DEA, K. and SINCLAIR, A. 1994. The effect of dietary fat level and quality on plasma lipoprotein lipids and plasma fatty acids in normocholesterolemic subjects. Lipids *29*, 129–138.

SIEDEL, J., HAGELE, E.O., ZIEGENHORN, J. and WAHLEFELD, A.W. 1983. Reagent for the enzymatic determination of serum cholesterol with improved lipolytic efficiency. Clin. Chem. *29*, 1075–1080.

SMIT, M.A., VERKADE, H.J., HAVINGA, R., VONK, R.J., SCHERPHOF, G.L., IN'T VELT, G. and KUIPERS, F. 1994. Dietary fish oil potentiates bile acid-induced cholesterol secretion into bile in rats. J. Lipid Res. *35*, 301–310.

SPENCER, H.C. 1995. Perspectives of public health and prevention. Am. J. Med. Sci. *310* (Suppl.), S83–S85.

STEINBERG, D., PARSATHARATHY, S., CAREW, T.E. and KHOO, J.C. 1989. Beyond cholesterol. Modification of low density lipoprotein that increases athergenicity. N. Engl. J. Med. *320*, 915–924.

TAKAYAMA, M., ITOH, S., NAGASAKI, T. and TANIMIZU, I. 1977. A new enzymatic method for determination of serum choline-containing phospholipids. Clin. Chim. Acta *79*, 93–98.

TRINDER, P. 1969. Determination of glucose in blood using blood glucose oxidase with an alternative oxygen receptor. Ann. Clin. Biochem. *6*, 511–516.

YUAN, Y.V., KITTS. D.D. and GODIN, D.V. 1997. Influence of dietary cholesterol and fat source on atherosclerosis in the Japanese Quail. Brit. J. Nutr. (in press).

WAHLEFELD, A.W., MUNZ, E. and BERNT, E. 1974. An evaluation of a fully enzymatic method for creatinine determination. Zeitschr. Klin. Chem. Klin. Biochem. *12*, 259–263.

ZAMPELAS, H., PEEL, A.S., GOULD, B.J., WRIGHT, J. and WILLIAMS, C.M. 1994. Polyunsaturated fatty acids of the n-6 and n-3 series: Effects of postprandial lipid and apolipoprotein in healthy men. Eur. J. Clin. Nutr. *48*, 842–848.

ZIEGENHORN, J. 1975. Improved method for enzymatic determination of serum triglycerides. Clin. Chem. *21*, 1627–1629.

HYPOCHOLESTEROLEMIC EFFECT OF THE INSOLUBLE FRACTION OF TOFURU AS A DIETETIC SUPPLEMENT

PING-FAN RAO, RONG-ZHEN ZHANG, LONG LI, JIAN-CAI LI, HONG FU, SHU-TAO LIU, RU-MING CHEN, GONG-RUI CHEN, YU-QIANG ZHENG, BI-HONG SHI, and WEN-HONG GAO

Institute of Biotechnology, Fuzhou University
523, Gong-ye Road, Fuzhou, Fujian
P.R. China 350002

ABSTRACT

An enormous number of studies since the 1970s indicate that soy proteins can lower plasma cholesterol concentration in a variety of experimental animals as well as in humans. One of the major mechanisms proposed for soy proteins hypocholesterolemic effect is impairing of cholesterol absorption and bile acid reabsorption due to hydrophobic binding between bile acids and proteins. An indigestible fraction of soy protein hydrolyzed with microbial proteases was reported to show remarkably stronger hypocholesterolemic effect than the whole soy proteins. A correlation was proposed between hydrophobicity of peptic digests of proteins of various food sources and hypocholesterolemic effect. Protein peptic digests containing more than 25% of hydrophobic amino acids have been demonstrated to have hypocholesterolemic effect.

Tofuru, fermented Tofu, is a soy product popular in China for more than 1,000 years as a condiment and daily delicacy. Extensive fermentation of 3-4 months with Mucor *and other microorganism results in complete hydrolysis of soy proteins, and the unique flavor and texture of Tofuru. In our studies of Tofuru proteins, soy proteins were found to be completely digested into peptides with molecular weights lower than 10,000 and hydrophobic amino acid composition in the insoluble fraction of Tofuru increased to 43.6% from 35.7% in soy protein isolate. The binding of sodium deoxycholate to Tofuru was determined to be more than ten times higher than bovine serum albumin, suggesting a promising prospect of the insoluble fraction of Tofuru as a powerful hypocholesterolemic agent.*

The objective of this work was to investigate the hypocholesterolemic effect of the Tofuru insoluble fraction. Twenty-nine male weanling golden Syrian hamsters were fed rations containing 15g/100 g protein from either isolated soy protein (ISP), soy protein concentrate (SPC) or Tofuru peptides for 35 days. Serum total cholesterol concentrations were determined by HPLC. The results will be discussed.

INTRODUCTION

An enormous number of studies since the 1970s indicate that soy proteins can lower plasma cholesterol concentration in a variety of experimental animals (Potter 1995). One of the major mechanisms proposed for soy proteins hypocholesterolemic effect is impairing of cholesterol absorption and bile acid reabsorption due to hydrophobic binding between bile acids and proteins (Beynen 1980). An indigestible fraction of soy protein hydrolyzed with microbial proteases was reported to show remarkably stronger hypocholesterolemic effect than the whole soy proteins (Sugano and Koda 1993). A correlation was proposed between hydrophobicity of peptic digests of proteins of various food sources and hypocholesterolemic effect. Protein peptic digests containing more than 25% hydrophobic amino acids have been demonstrated to have hypocholesterolemic effect (Iwami *et al.* 1985).

Tofuru, fermented Tofu, is a soy product popular in China for more than 1,000 years as a condiment and daily delicacy. Extensive fermentation for 3-4 months with Mucor and other microorganism results in complete hydrolysis of soy proteins, and the unique flavor and texture of Tofuru. In our studies of Tofuru proteins, soy proteins were found to be completely digested into peptides with molecular weights lower than 10,000 and hydrophobic amino acid composition in the insoluble fraction of Tofuru increased to 43.6% from 35.7% in soy protein isolate (Chen *et al.* 1997). The binding of sodium deoxycholate to Tofuru was determined to be more than ten times higher than bovine serum albumin (Li *et al.* 1997), suggesting a promising prospect of the insoluble fraction of Tofuru as a powerful agent for binding deoxycholate.

Possible hypocholesterolemic effect of the insoluble fraction of Tofuru was investigated using animal models in this work.

EXPERIMENTAL

Preparation of Tofuru Peptides

Tofuru cubes were first smashed and mixed with three volumes of boiled water to form a slurry, which was then packed into a cloth bag and dialyzed against running water for 24 h to remove salt. The desalted slurry was then dehydrated first by pressing the bag overnight then by microwave heating to obtain dry Tofuru powder. The dried Tofuru powder was further defatted in a Soxhlet extractor using ethyl acetate (30-60°C). The completely defatted Tofuru powder for animal experiments contained 55.6% protein, as determined by Kjeldahl semi-microquantitification of nitrogen, 4.85% mineral and 10.5% water.

Animal Experiments

Forty male weanling ICR mice of 6-7 weeks were divided into four groups, and fed *ad libitum* four kinds of feed. One was commercial feed for test animals (about 30% protein); the other three groups were diets containing 20 g protein/100 g of diet protein from three different sources: casein, soy protein isolate (SPI) and Tofuru powder for 35 days. The diet containing either SPI or Tofuru powder as a protein source was further supplemented with 0.6% L-methionine or with 0.6% L-lysine and 0.2% L-threonine to avoid significant difference in mouse growth among the dietary groups caused by the lower concentration of these amino acids in soy protein. After 35 days feeding, weight gains of the different groups were recorded and mice were sacrificed by carotid amputation to collect the blood. The plasma was separated by centrifugation at 2,500 rpm for 15 min and its cholesterol and triglycerides were determined.

Determination of Serum Total Cholesterol and Triglycerides

Serum total cholesterol concentration of ICR mice was determined by the enzymatic method of Allain *et al.*(1974), and serum triglyceride concentration was determined by the method of Bucolo and David (1973).

RESULTS AND DISCUSSION

After 30 days of feeding with three different diets containing proteins from different sources, gains in weight of the four groups of mice are listed in Table 1.

As is clear from the data of Table 1, there is a great difference in weight gain between mice of group #1 which were fed with commercial feed for experimental animals and the other three groups (P<0.001). The group #1 weights almost doubled during the feeding period of 35 days, while the rest of mice fed with the prepared diets remained at basically the same weights. This great difference can be attributed to the difference in feed intakes because the mice were *ad libitum* fed. It was observed that feed intakes by mice of group #1 were remarkably more than the rest of the three groups. One more reason is that the commercial feed contains 10% higher contents of protein. No apparent difference in weight gain among the three groups of mice fed with diet containing different protein sources, indicating similar growth conditions among those three groups of mice regardless of different diets.

TABLE 1.
EFFECTS OF CASEIN, SPI, AND TOFURU POWER ON THE WEIGHT OF ICR MOUSE

	n=10			
	#1 (Control)	#2 (Casein)	#3 (SPI)	#4 (Tofuru powder)
Weight (g)[1]	28.5 ± 2.6^a	14.9 ± 0.9^b	14.0 ± 0.7^b	14.1 ± 1.1^b

n, Numbers of mice tested in each group.
[a,b] Means with different superscripts are significantly different (P < 0.001).
1, $\bar{x} \pm$ SD.

Results of serum cholesterol determination are shown in Table 2, as well as serum triglycerides concentration. Mice of group #2 fed with casein exhibited similar serum triglyceride concentration with mice fed with the commercial feed in group #1 in spite of great difference in weight gains of the two groups, while the other two groups fed with soy protein and insoluble fraction of Tofuru, respectively, displayed no difference in their serum triglycerides level, which are much lower than mice fed with casein (P<0.001). Relatively low serum triglyceride level in mice fed with soy protein, intact or degraded, can be attributed to the effect of plant proteins on hormone and on lipid metabolism (Sugano 1988).

TABLE 2.
EFFECTS OF CASEIN, SPI, AND TOFURU POWDER ON THE PLASMA CHOLESTEROL AND TRIGLYCERIDE LEVELS OF ICR MOUSE

	n=10			
	#1 (Control)	#2 (Casein)	#3 (SPI)	#4 (Tofuru power)
Cholesterol (mmol/L)[1]	2.77 ± 0.50^{a}	1.98 ± 0.44^{b}	1.07 ± 0.37^{c}	0.76 ± 0.20^{d}
Triglyceride (mmol/L)[1]	1.77 ± 0.35^{a}	1.87 ± 0.97^{a}	0.61 ± 0.17^{b}	0.46 ± 0.11^{c}

n, Numbers of mice tested in each group.

a,b,c,d Differences between means of different superscripts within the same row are significant (all of $P < 0.001$), except that between a and b for cholesterol content ($P < 0.01$) and that b and c for triglyceride content ($P < 0.05$).

1, $\bar{X} \pm SD$.

Remarkable differences in serum cholesterol concentration were observed among the three groups with similar weight gains ($P<0.001$). There is a major difference between mice fed with casein and those with soy protein, intact or degraded ($P<0.001$). This result once again confirms conclusions of numerous studies on the hypocholesterolemic effect of soy protein. Meaningful difference in serum cholesterol concentration was observed between mice fed with isolated soy protein and the insoluble fraction of Tofuru ($P<0.001$), with 1.07 mmole/L for the former and 0.76 mmole/L for the latter. In the reported studies, mice serum cholesterol level decreased from 70 mg/dl to about 52 mg/dl, a decrease by 25.6% when casein was replaced with isolated soy protein (Iwami *et al.* 1986), and from 291 mg/dl to 125 mg/dl, a decrease by 57.0% when isolated soy protein was replaced with the insoluble fraction of soy protein hydrolysate (Sugano *et al.* 1988). In our studies, serum cholesterol level was lowered by 46% when casein was replaced by isolated soy proteins, comparable to the reported data, whereas decrease of the cholesterol by Tofuru powder was only 29% in comparison with soy protein isolate, much less dramatic than the reported data.

Correlation between hypocholesterolemic effect of peptides and its *in vivo* binding ability of cholic acid was reported (Sugano 1988). The insoluble fraction of Tofuru, which was determined to exhibit the strongest binding ability to cholic acid, however, exhibited less potent hypocholesterolemic effect than the insoluble fraction of soy protein hydrolysate. This may be attributed to loss of soy phospholipid and other components with hypocholesterolemic effect from the insoluble fraction of Tofuru when soy oil was removed by ether extraction. It was reported that the hypocholesterolemic effect was reduced as the result of methanol treatment of the insoluble fraction of soy protein hydrolysate (Sugano *et al.* 1988). It is possible that a more potent hypocholesterolemic effect can be expected of the insoluble fraction of Tofuru without defatting treatment by ether extraction. Further work will be carried out to test the hypocholesterolemic effect of the untreated insoluble fraction of Tofuru.

In this preliminary work to test the health benefit of Tofuru with animal models, the insoluble fraction of Tofuru has been demonstrated to be effective in lowering serum cholesterol as a dietetic supplement. Although more work is necessary to confirm the effect and to determine conditions for the best effect, this preliminary result is encouraging. Tofuru, whose health benefit when once confirmed, can possibly become the most consumed health food after minor modification.

REFERENCE

ALLAIN, C.C., POON, L.S., CHAN, C.S.G., RICHMOND, W. and FU, P.C. 1974. Enzymatic determination of total serum cholesterol. Clin. Chem. *20(4),* 470–475.

BEYNEN, A.C. 1990. Comparison of the mechanism proposed to explain the hypocholesterolemic effect of soybean protein versus casein in experimental animals. J. Nutr. Sci. Vitaminol. *36,* S87–S93.

BUCOLO, G. and DAVID, H. 1973. Quantitative determination of serum triglycerides by the use of enzymes. Clin. Chem. *19,* 476–482.

CHEN, G.R., CHEN, R.M., LI, L. and RAO, P.F. 1997. Protein study of Tofuru. Acta Nutrimenta Sinica (Chinese) *19,* 183–187.

IWAMI, K., SAKAKIBARA, K. and IBUKI, F. 1986. Involvement of post-digestion 'hydrophobic' peptides in plasma cholesterol-lowering effect of dietary plant proteins. Agric. Biol. Chem. *50(5),* 1217–1222.

LI, L., NI, L., ZHANG, R.Z. and RAO, P.F. 1997. HPLC determination of binding of sodium deoxycholate to insoluble fraction of Tofuru. Acta Nutrimenta Sinca (Chinese), in preparation.

POTTER, S.M. 1995. Overview of proposed mechanisms for the hypocholesterolemic effect of soy. Am. Inst. Nutr. 606S–611S.

SUGANO, M. 1988. Expression of nutritional function by protein digestion: Formation of peptides regulating lipid metabolism. *In* Food Functions, Basis for Creation of Functional Foods (in Japanese). Fujimaki, M. (ed.). Gakkai Publishing Center, Tokyo, Japan.

SUGANO, M. and KOBA, K. 1993. Dietary protein and lipid metabolism: A multifunctional effect. Ann. NY Acad. Sci. *676,* 215–222.

SUGANO, M., YAMADA, Y., YOSHIDA, K., HASHIMOTO, Y., MATSUO, T. and KIMOTO, M. 1988. The hypocholesterolemic action of the undigested fraction of soybean protein in rats. Atherosclerosis *72*, 115–122.

FOOD PROTEINS AND PEPTIDES PRESENTING SPECIFIC PROTECTION TO HUMAN HEALTH (A REVIEW)

VALDEMIRO C. SGARBIERI

Centro de Química de Alimentos e Nutrição Aplicada
Instituto de Tecnologia de Alimentos
C.P. 139, Campinas, São Paulo, Brasil

ABSTRACT

Recent advances in biomedical research have helped reveal some of the complex relationships between nutrition and disease, suggesting that some food proteins and peptides may be useful in the treatment and/or prevention of a number of pathological conditions arising from malnutrition, diseases or injuries.

Among important physiological functional properties which have been attributed to food proteins are: stimulation of the immune system (milk whey proteins, casein peptides); hypotensive effect (casein peptide, zein peptide, glycinin peptide, myofibril peptide); hypocholesterolemic effect (glycinin); stimulation of hormone synthesis (trypsin inhibitor, whey protein, glycinin, lectins); tumor growth inhibition (milk whey proteins, protease inhibitors); antibacterial and antiviral effects (lactoferrin, chicken cystatin and oryzacystatin); stimulation of intestinal functions and inhibition of diarrhea (casomorphins and lactorphins); and stimulation of mineral absorption (caseinophosphopeptides). These are just a few examples of food proteins and peptides exhibiting physiological functional properties.

Proposed mechanisms and potential applications will be discussed.

INTRODUCTION

Recent advances in nutrition and biomedical research have helped reveal some of the complex relationships between nutrition and disease, suggesting that some food proteins and peptides may be useful in the treatment and/or prevention of a number of pathological conditions arising from malnutrition, diseases or injuries.

The foods or food components offering special protection to humans against disease have been named by different designations such as functional foods, nutraceuticals, pharmafoods, healthy foods and designer foods (Goldberg 1994). They form a very large and heterogeneous group of food components and ingredients including the so-called food fiber components, polyunsaturated fatty acids, isoprenoid pigments and vitamins, antioxidants, phenolic and other phytochemicals in addition to some proteins and peptides.

Japan is currently the world leader in the development of functional foods. Currently called foods for specified health use, functional foods are considered as a major new product opportunity - a new dimension of a wide range of food and drink products (Potter 1990; Arai 1993, 1996).

This review will describe the physiological functional properties of some food proteins or their peptide components. Among important physiological functional properties which have been attributed to proteins and peptides are: stimulation of the immune system, hypotensive effect, hypocholesterolemic effect, stimulation of hormone synthesis, inhibition of tumor growth, antibacterial and antiviral effects, stimulation of absorption and intestinal function (Goldberg 1994; Arai 1996).

PROTEINS AND PEPTIDES WITH STIMULATORY EFFECTS ON THE IMMUNE SYSTEM

Perhaps the class of food proteins more directly related to immunity are the immunoglobulins (IgG_1, G_2, A, and M) which occur in the blood serum and other fluids such as colostrum and milk whey. The term immunoglobulins describes a family of high molecular weight proteins sharing common physical and chemical characteristics and antigenic determinants (Butler 1969). Immunoglobulins occur in high concentration in colostrum, the first fluid secreted by the mammary glands of mammals immediately post-partum. These high molecular weight proteins are partially assimilated by the new borne and serve to transfer passive immunity to the young, protecting them against disease until their own immune defenses are activated.

When milk is fractionated by precipitation or coagulation of casein the immunoglobulins remain in the liquid whey; therefore both the colostrum and concentrated whey are rich sources of immunoglobulins (de Crignis *et al.* 1989).

The effect of various levels and different types of dietary proteins such as lactalbumin (L), casein (C), soy (S), wheat (W) and Purina stock diet was studied comparatively by using different strains of mice and measuring the specific humoral immune response to sheep red blood cells (SRBC) and horse red blood cells (HRBC). The nutritional efficiency of these diets was normal and similar. The immune response of mice fed the L diets was found to be about five times higher than that of mice fed the corresponding C diets (Bounous *et al.* 1983a, 1985, 1988a). The above-described immune effect of all tested proteins was obtained at 20 g/100 g concentration in the diet, with no further increments with 30- and 40 g protein/100 g diet.

Some of the reported results from these experiments are graphically shown in Fig. 1 and 2. The immune-enhancing effect was manifest after two weeks feeding of 20 g/100 g diet of lactalbumin and persisted for at least eight weeks of dietary treatment. Mixing lactalbumin with either casein or soy protein in a 20 g protein/100 g diet formula significantly enhanced the immune response in comparison to that of mice fed diets containing 20% soy protein or casein (Fig. 2).

Dietary cysteine is considered to be a rate-limiting substrate for the synthesis of glutathione which is necessary for lymphocyte proliferation. To the extent that cysteine can be considered a factor in promoting higher immune response and glutathione tissue levels, reported data show that cysteine administration with the whey protein mixture is far more effective than when administered as free cysteine. This suggests that the specific amino acid profile of whey protein or a cysteine-containing peptide is an important factor in determining the fate of the ingested cysteine (Bounous *et al.* 1989; Bounous and Gold 1991).

Some results (Fig. 3 and Fig. 4) also indicate that mice fed diets containing any one of the four major protein components of the whey protein mixture developed a plaque-forming cells response to sheep red blood cells significantly lower than that of mice fed

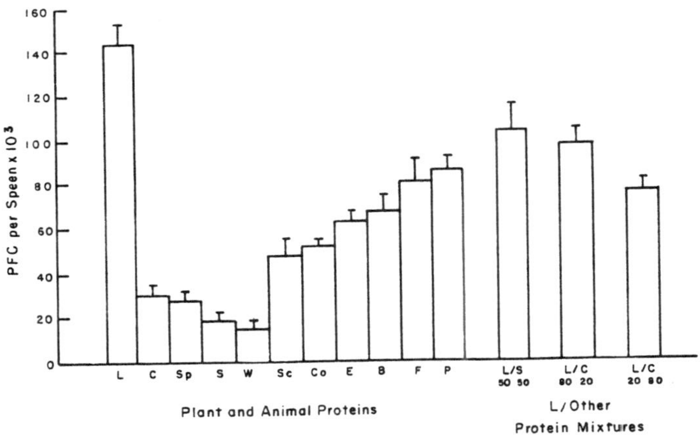

FIG. 1. PLAQUE FORMING CELLS (PFC) FOLLOWING IMMUNIZATION WITH 10^6 SHEEP RED BLOOD CELLS (SRBC)

Effect of 2 weeks dietary treatment with 20 g/100 g diet of either (L) lactalbumin, (C) Casein, (Sp) *Spirulina maxima* protein, (S) soy protein, (W) wheat protein, (Sc) Scenedesmus protein, (Co) corn protein, (E) egg albumin, (B) beef protein, (F) fish protein, (P) Purina mouse chow, or 20 g/100 g diet of a mixture containing 50:50, 80:20, and 20:80%, respectively, of L/S, L/C, and L/C (From Bounous *et al.* 1988a).

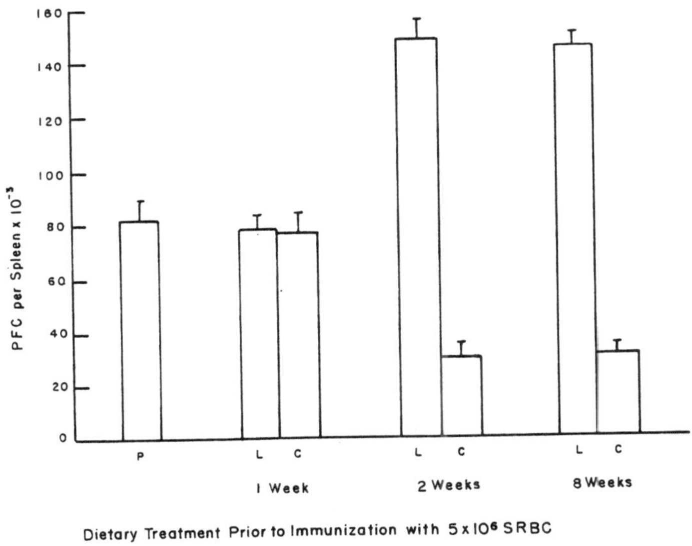

FIG. 2. PLAQUE FORMING CELLS (PFC) AFTER IMMUNIZATION WITH 10^6 SHEEP RED BLOOD CELLS (SRBC)

Effect of 1, 2 or 8 weeks of dietary treatment with 20 g/100 g diet of either lactalbumin (L) or casein (C). Each value represents the mean $\pm$ SD. LxC after 2 weeks and 8 weeks ($P \leq 0.001$). From Bounous *et al.* 1988a.

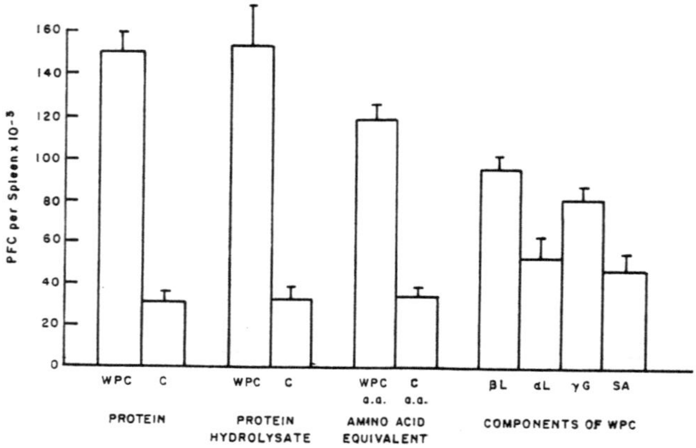

FIG. 3. PLAQUE FORMING CELLS (PFC) FOLLOWING IMMUNIZATION WITH 10^6 SHEEP RED BLOOD CELLS (SRBC)

Effect of 3 weeks of dietary treatment with 20 g/100 g diet of either whey protein concentrate (WPC), casein (C), whey protein concentrate hydrolysate, casein hydrolysate, whey protein concentrate amino acid equivalent (WPC.a.a.), casein amino acid equivalent (C.a.a.), β-lactoglobulin (βL), α-lactalbumin (αL), γ-globulin (γG), or bovine serum albumin (SA). Each value represents the mean ± SD. From Bounous *et al.* 1989.

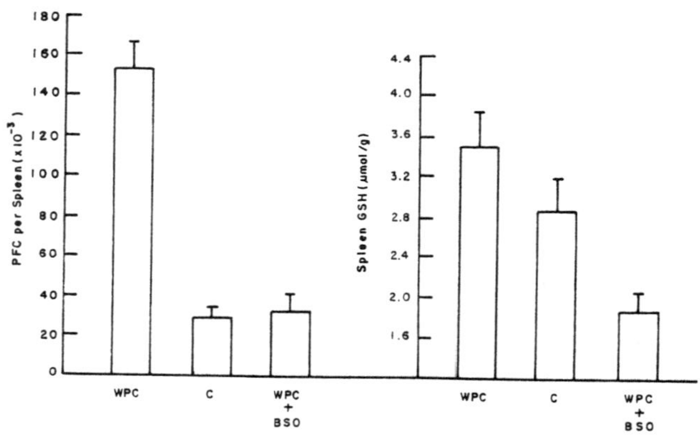

FIG. 4. LEFT: PLAQUE FORMING CELLS (PFC) FOLLOWING IMMUNIZATION WITH 10^6 SHEEP RED BLOOD CELLS (SRBC)

Effect of 3 weeks of dietary treatment with 20 g/100 g diet of either whey protein concentrate (WPC), casein (C) or whey protein concentrate plus buthionine sulfoximine (WPC + BSO). Each value represents mean ± SD: (WPC × WPC + BSO or C), $p \leq 0.005$.

RIGHT: SPLEEN GLUTATHIONE (GSH) FOLLOWING IMMUNIZATION WITH 10^6 SHEEP RED BLOOD CELLS (SRBC)

Effect of 3 weeks of dietary treatment with 20 g/100 g diet of either whey protein concentrate (WPC), whey protein concentrate plus BSO (WPC+BSO) or casein (C). Each value represents the mean ± SD (WPC × WPC+BSO, or C), $p \leq 0.005$. From Bounous *et al.* 1989.

the corresponding whey protein mixture. This led to the conclusion that the observed immunoenhancing effect of whey protein is dependent upon the overall amino acid pattern resulting from the contribution of all its protein components. Support for the importance of glutathione production in the immunoenhancing effect of milk whey protein was obtained by i.p. administration of buthionine sulfoximine (BSO) after three weeks of whey protein feeding and one day prior to immunization with sheep red blood cells (Fig. 4). The BSO treatment reduced by half the spleen glutathione level and produced a 4-5 fold drop in the immune response of whey protein diet-fed mice, thereby abolishing the difference in immune response between whey protein diet and casein diet-fed mice.

The immunoenhancing effect of whey protein concentrate is maintained when the proteins are replaced in formula diet by a pancreatic hydrolysate (oligopeptides with MW < 1000) of undenatured whey protein concentrate, as illustrated in Fig. 3 (Bounous *et al.* 1989).

The current findings indicate that the previously described biological activity of dietary whey protein is restricted to the undenatured form of the protein, and it is not related to its nutritional efficiency.

It has been demonstrated that, whereas concentrations of glutathione are dependent on the supply of cysteine, administration of cysteine is not an ideal way to increase glutathione concentration because cysteine is rapidly metabolized and furthermore, it is toxic (Estrela *et al.* 1983). On the other hand, tissue glutathione concentration may be increased by administration of γ-glutamylcysteine; glutathione increased in the kidney by about 50%, 40 to 60 min after s.c. injection in mice, returning to control values 2 h later (Anderson and Meister 1983).

According to Bounous and Gold (1991) an extensive search of all available data on amino acid sequencing of edible proteins reveals that the Glu-Cys group with disulfide link is limited to some whey proteins and to ovomucoid, a fraction of egg white which contains two of these groups.

It is interesting to note that the cysteine residues of all glutamylcysteine groups in β-lactoglobulin and serum albumin are connected by intramolecular disulfide bonds. It is also relevant to note that pancreatic trypsin does not hydrolyze the disulfide cross-linkage characteristic of the native whey proteins.

Canadian researchers hypothesized that the glutathione-promoting activity of dietary whey protein concentrate is dependent on the glutamylcysteine groups contained in serum albumin fractions, in the β-lactoglobulin and possibly in the immunoglobulin G fraction. Preservation of the disulfide bonds (which involves the cysteine) may be crucial to the release, upon digestion, of intact glutamylcysteine peptide for absorption by the intestinal mucosa.

Further benefits of dietary whey protein to human health that might be related to glutathione levels and immune-enhancing activity have been reported. Glutathione peroxidase eliminates H_2O_2 generated by mitochondrial O_2 consumption employing glutathione as a hydrogen donor to reduce H_2O_2 to H_2O (Kaplowitz *et al.* 1985).

Intracellular glutathione appears to play an important role in the defense of endothelium cells against oxidized low density lipoproteins, hence in the pathogenesis of arteriosclerosis (Kuzuya *et al.* 1989). The level of lipid peroxidation is higher in the brain of subjects affected by Alzheimer's disease than in the brain of the non-demented elderly (Chia *et al.* 1984).

Finally, a recent multicenter study has demonstrated that glutathione concentration was significantly lower in the putamen, globus pallidus, substantia nigra, and frontal cortex of Parkinsonian brains. A direct positive correlation between the severity of cellular deficit and the glutathione content could be demonstrated (Riederer *et al.* 1989).

Considering the ubiquitous distribution and multifunctional activity of glutathione and the demonstrated capacity of dietary whey protein to significantly raise glutathione levels in the tissues, several important functional properties can be suggested for whey protein concentrate and hydrolysates (Bounous *et al.* 1993; Brink 1996), as illustrated in Fig. 5.

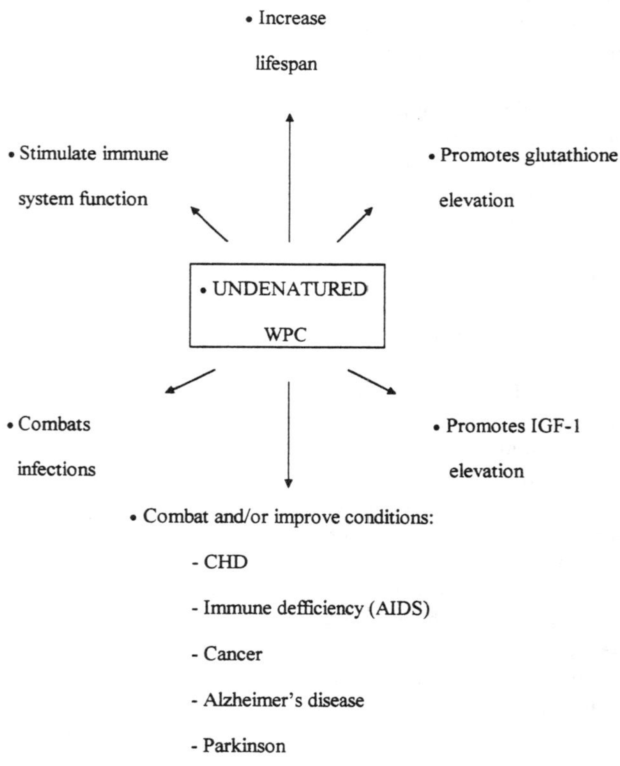

FIG. 5. PROPOSED MULTIFUNCTIONAL PROPERTIES FOR UNDENATURED WHEY PROTEINS AND THEIR PANCREATIC HYDROLYSATES

ANTIHYPERTENSIVE PEPTIDES

Japan has been the leading country for research in this area and a recent comprehensive review on the subject has been published (Ariyoshi 1993).

Angiotensin-converting enzyme (ACE) raises blood pressure by converting the inactive decaptide angiotensin I to the potent vasoconstrictor octapeptide angiotensin II, as well as inactivating the vasodilating nonapeptide bradykinin.

The blood pressure regulation mechanism by the renin-angiotensin system is illustrated in Fig. 6. Angiotensin-converting enzyme peptides have been identified and isolated from a fairly large number of food proteins (Ariyoshi 1993) including: gelatin, bovine casein, sardines, tuna, porcine glyceraldehyde-3-phosphate dehydrogenase (GAPDH), bonito, fig tree latex, α-zein, porcine plasma, soy bean, and antarctic krill muscle.

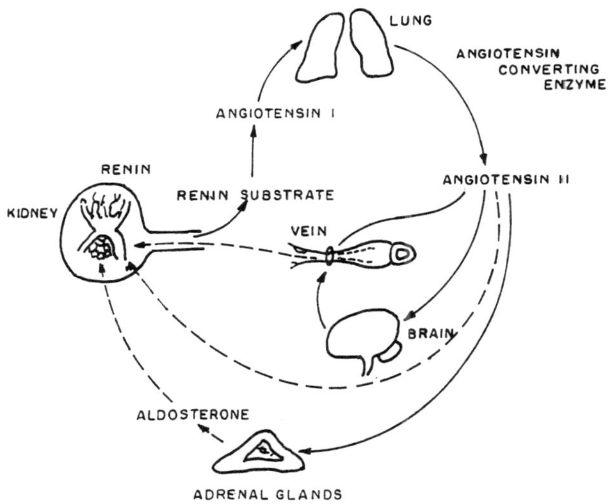

FIG. 6. SCHEMATIC DRAWING OF ORGANS AND FACTORS INVOLVED IN THE BLOOD PRESSURE CONTROL BY THE ANGIOTENSIN-CONVERTING ENZYME SYSTEM

The amino acid sequences established for various peptides are shown in Table 1. According to Table 1 some sequences obtained from bovine casein (peptide 3), from tuna fish (peptide 10), from baker's yeast GAPDH (peptides 13 and 14), from bonito (peptide 16), from fig tree latex (peptide 17), and from α-zein (peptides 19, 20, 21) showed the highest activity.

Antihypertensive activity was also observed in peptide fractions isolated from rice glutelin (Muramoto and Kawamura 1991) and rice prolamin (Saito *et al.* 1991). In all cases noted above, the bioactive peptides are not present in the food studied, but arise from proteolytic digestion of the food protein.

TABLE 1.
ACE INHIBITOR PEPTIDES FROM VARIOUS FOOD PROTEINS

	Amino Acid Sequence[c]	Source of Compound[a]	$IC_{50}(\mu M)$[b]
1.	GPAGAHYP	Gelatin	8.4
2.	FFVAPFPEVFGK	Bovine casein	77.0
3.	FFVAP	Bovine casein	6.0
4.	AVPYPQR	Bovine casein	15.0
5.	LKVGVKQY	Sardine	11.0
6.	VKAGF	Sardine	83.0
7.	KVLAGM	Sardine	30.0
8.	LKL	Sardine	188.0
9.	HQAAGW	Sardine	60.0
10.	PTHIKWGD	Tuna*	1-2
11.	PANIKWGD	Porcine GAPDH*	21.0
12.	PANKPWGSSNV	Yeast GAPDH*	18.0
13.	GHKIATFQER	Yeast GAPDH*	0.4
14.	GKKIATYQER	Yeast GAPD*	2.0
15.	IKPLNY	Bonito	43.0
16.	IKP	Bonito	1.7
17.	LYPVK	Fig tree latex	4.5
18.	LVR	Fig tree latex	14.0
19.	LRP	α-zein	0.27
20.	LSP	α-zein	1.7
21.	LQP	α-zein	1.9
22.	YRILEF	Soy bean	-
23.	LKY	Antarctic Krill	-

Adapted from Ariyoshi, 1993.
[a] Peptide obtained by enzymatic hydrolysis unless otherwise stated.
[b] IC_{50} concentration inhibiting 50% of ACE activity.
* Peptide obtained by heating the protein under acidic conditions.
[c] The single letter notation: A, alanine; C, cysteine; D, aspartic acid; E, glutamic acid; F, phenylalanine; G, glycine; H, histidine; I, isoleucine; K, lysine; L, leucine; M, methionine; N, asparagine; P, proline; Q, glutamine; R, arginine; S, serine; T, threonine; V, valine; W, tryptophan; Y, tyrosine.

The structures of peptide fragments produced by enzymatic hydrolysis of a protein depend on the specificity of the enzyme used.

An alkaline protease hydrolysate of defatted sardine meat inhibited ACE activity *in vitro* (IC_{50} = 0.18 mg/mL), and was also active *in vivo* when the hydrolysate was administered orally to spontaneously hypertensive rats at a dosage of 2 mg/kg; their blood pressure was significantly reduced. When stroke-prone spontaneously hypertensive rats were fed a diet consisting of the hydrolysate as the sole protein source, their blood pressure was significantly reduced and their lifespan were significantly prolonged, according to Ariyoshi (1993).

OPIOID, ANTI-OPIOID AND PHOSPHOPEPTIDES

Opioid peptides are defined as peptides like enkephalins that have both affinity for opiate receptors and opiate-like effects which are stereospecifically reversed by naloxone. Substances like naloxone that have both affinity for opiate receptors and anti-opiate effects are called opioid antagonists.

The opioid peptides may exert physiological effects both at the central and peripheral nervous systems. At the central nervous system, the main effects are: analgesia, catalepsy, sedation and torpor, respiratory depression, hypotension, regulation of body temperature, regulation of food intake, suppression of gastric secretion, increase and/or decrease of certain hormone levels, and regulation of sexual behavior. The peripheral effects may include suppression of intestinal motility and potentiation of melanocyte stimulating hormone (MSH) activity.

A fairly large number of opioid peptides and opioid antagonists have been isolated mainly from caseins and some from whey protein (Arai 1996; Chiba and Yoshikawa 1986). Some representative peptides isolated from caseins are shown in Tables 2, 3, and 4.

According to Drewnowski (1992), the pleasure response to palatable foods, notably those rich in sugar and fat, may be mediated through the endogenous opioid peptide systems. Preferences for sweet taste appeared to be under opioid control. Studies on rats showed that opioids most effectively reduced intakes of preferred sweet liquids such as glucose, sucrose or saccharin solutions. Studies on animals have suggested that preferences for dietary fats may also be under opioid control.

TABLE 2.
OPIOID AND OTHER PEPTIDES DERIVED FROM ALFA-S_1 CASEIN

↓43 58↓ 66↓
K D I G SP E SP T E D Q A M E D I K Q M E A Q SP I
74↓ 79↓ ↓90↓ 95↓96↓
SP SP SP Q Q I V P N SP V E Q K H... E R Y L G Y L E
↓106 119↓ ↓194
Q... K V P Q L Q I V P N SP A E E R L... K T T
↓199
M P L W

Peptide	Residues		Activity
Casomorphines	90 - 95		opioid
	90 - 96		opioid
	91 - 96		opioid
Caseinophosphopeptides	43 - 58		mineral transport
	59 - 79		mineral transport
	106 - 119		mineral transport
	66 - 74		mineral transport
Immunopeptide	149 - 199	(not shown above)	Immunostimulation

SP = serine phosphate

TABLE 3.
OPIOID AND OTHER PHYSIOLOGICALLY ACTIVE PEPTIDES FROM BETA-CASEIN

↓2 10 20 25↓
R E L E E L R V P G E I V E SP L SP SP E E S I T R I
28↓ ↓60 ↓ ↓ ↓ ↓ ↓ ↓ ↓ 70↓ ↓191 193↓
N K K... V Y P F P G P I P N S L P... F L L Y Q

Peptide	Residues	Activity
Casomorphines	60 - 63	opioid
	60 - 63[a]	opioid
	60 - 64	opioid
	60 - 65	opioid
	60 - 66	opioid
	60 - 70	opioid
Caseinophosphopeptides	1 - 28[b]	mineral transport
	1 - 25	mineral transport
	1 - 28[c]	mineral transport
Immunopeptides	63 - 68	Immunostimulation
	191 - 193	Immunostimulation

[a]Amide form; [b]casein proteolysis; [c]Isolated from intestine; SP = serine phosphate

TABLE 4.
OPIOID ANTAGONISTS AND OTHER ACTIVE PEPTIDES DERIVED FROM KAPA-CASEIN

↓25 ↓33↓34↓35 38↓ 41↓
K Y I P I Q Y V L S R Y P S Y G L N Y Y Q Q K P V
↓58 61↓
A L I N Q F L P Y P Y Y A...

Peptide	Residues		Activity
Casoxins	35 - 38[a]		Opioid antagonist
	34 - 38[a]		Opioid antagonist
	33 - 38[a]		Opioid antagonist
	25 - 34		Opioid antagonist
	35 - 41		Opioid antagonist
	58 - 61		Opioid antagonist
Glycopeptide	169 - 186	(not shown above)	Antigastric

[a] Methoxylated

Among the bioactive peptides produced by enzymatic hydrolysis, both *in vitro* and *in vivo*, the caseinophosphopeptides (CPP) are the best characterized and the most intensely studied.

Studies of Sato *et al.* (1986) and Berrocal *et al.* (1989) confirmed the function of CPP in preventing formation of insoluble calcium phosphate complexes over a range of Ca:P ratios. However, Yuan and Kitts (1991) and Yuan *et al.* (1991) failed to confirm an increase in calcium absorption with an increase in femural deposition of radiolabeled calcium, bone calcium mineralization, and bone strength in animals fed casein or soy protein diets. Therefore, the role of CPP in directly enhancing active calcium transport and absorption remain controversial (Kitts and Yuan 1992).

PROTEINS PRESENTING HYPOCHOLESTEROLEMIC EFFECT

Different dietary proteins determine different serum cholesterol levels if fed in a semi-synthetic diet to some, but not all animal species. In one species, the rabbit, this metabolic response is elicited without adding high sucrose or cholesterol supplements that have to be added to rat or pig diets in order to cause similar response (Barth and Pfeuffer 1988).

In rabbit, steady-state concentrations of serum cholesterol show a difference of more than 150 mg/dL when diets based on casein or soy protein are compared, the lower concentration caused by soy protein. The species-specificity of the hypercholesterolemic response of rabbit to casein cannot be illustrated better than by the findings of Raaij *et al.* (1981, 1982), illustrated in Fig. 7.

For atherogenesis-sensitive species like rabbit and rats a unified hypothesis has been put together (Barth and Pfeuffer 1988) which is schematized in Fig. 8 to explain the mechanism of protein-induced serum cholesterol changes. Primates and particularly normal humans seem to be resistant to cholesterol changes with dietary protein manipulation.

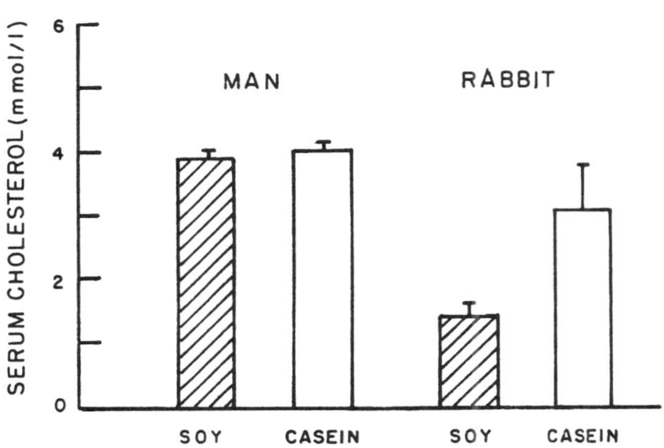

FIG. 7. DIFFERENTIAL EFFECT OF SOY PROTEIN AND CASEIN ON BLOOD SERUM CHOLESTEROL LEVEL OF NORMOCHOLESTEROLEMIC MAN AND RABBIT
From van Raaij *et al.* (1981)

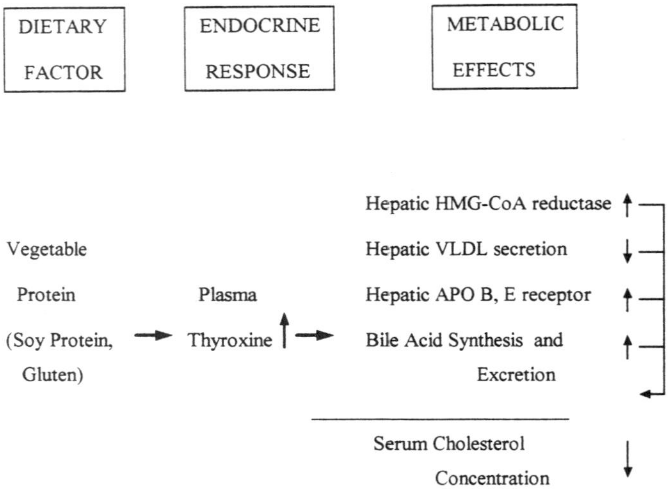

FIG. 8. PROPOSED UNIFYING CONCEPT FOR MECHANISM OF PROTEIN-INDUCED SERUM CHOLESTEROL CHANGES
Taken from Barth and Pfeuffer (1988)

Hodges *et al.* (1967) were among the first to demonstrate a clear effect of vegetable protein on lowering serum cholesterol levels in hypercholesterolemic men. Serum cholesterol decreased over 40% by the end of the study. The decrease was observed at relatively high fat intakes (45% of calories) as well as at low fat intakes (15% of calories). Other researchers have observed the cholesterol lowering potential of soy protein in hypercholesterolemic outpatients (Goldberg *et al.* 1982), hypercholesterolemic children (Widhalm 1986) and normocholesterolemic women (Carroll *et al.* 1978). In regard to hormonal responses, soy protein seems to stimulate glucagon production, thereby inhibiting both cholesterol and triacylglycerol synthesis (Sugano *et al.* 1982). Over the past 25 years, experimental data have suggested that the inclusion of soy protein in the human diet may provide cholesterol- and triacylglycerol- lowering benefits to certain individuals who are hypercholesterolemic and/or hypertriglyceridemic.

Despite numerous studies attesting to the beneficial effect of dietary soy protein in humans the topic seems to be still controversial, and the mechanism by which soy protein lowers blood lipid concentrations is uncertain.

DIETARY PROTEINS AND TUMORIGENESIS

The influence of dietary protein and specific amino acids on tumor growth has not been as extensively studied as it has for several other dietary components. Epidemiological studies suggesting that the intake of high protein foods is positively correlated with cancer are generally complicated by the simultaneous presence of excess fat. Thus, available data on the influence of protein and amino acids come primarily from laboratory investigations (Goldberg 1994).

Silverstone and Tannenbaum (1951) observed that a low protein diet (9%) suppressed the development of spontaneous hepatomas. The impact of dietary protein on chemically induced tumors reveals that tumor formation and growth are depressed when protein quality or quantity is limited. The explanation for inhibition was that changes in drug metabolizing enzymes should account for the observed inhibitory effect of inadequate protein or amino acid intake on tumor induction (Singletary and Milner 1987; Yang *et al.* 1992).

Using an *in vitro* assay, José and Good (1973a, b) observed that protein or amino acid deprivation in mice dramatically depressed antibody production while increasing or permitting maintenance of a vigorous cell-mediated immunity against tumor cells.

Data reported by Canadian researchers (Bounous *et al.* 1981) emphasized the tumor-enhancing effect of excessive amino acids in the diet rather than the inhibitory effect of dietary restriction of amino acids. Different dietary levels of amino acids could influence different parameters of cell-mediated immunity.

Bounous *et al.* (1983b) reported on the growth of tumors in mice fed two different dietary proteins, namely casein and lactalbumin hydrolysates, and also correlated immunological findings with those found in non-tumor-bearing mice fed the same diets (Bounous and Kongshavn 1982). Diets containing 12% (w/w) and 28% of casein or lactalbumin hydrolysate on the growth of implanted mammary adenocarcinoma H2712 in C3H mice strain and fibrosarcoma 1038 in DBA-2J mice strain were compared. The results obtained indicated that amino acid intake above the minimum requirement for normal growth of non-tumor-bearing mice (28% casein and lactalbumin diets) enhances the growth of implanted fibrosarcoma and mammary carcinoma (Bounous *et al.* 1983b), while not stimulating body growth above normal in comparable mice without tumors.

The above mentioned authors concluded that the dietary nitrogen intake that exceeds the minimum requirement stimulate the growth of implanted tumors. This effect is not related to protein nutritional quality and appears to be dependent on a direct enhancement of tumor growth.

The influence of two formula diets containing 20 g/100 g diet of either whey protein concentrate or casein or Purina mouse chow on the humoral immune responsiveness and dimethylhydrazine (DMH) induced colon carcinogenesis in A/J mice was reported (Bounous *et al.* 1988b). After 24 weeks of DMH treatment (15 mg DMH/kg body weight) the incidence of tumors in the whey protein-fed mice was substantially lower (Fig. 9) than that in mice fed either the casein or Purina diet. Similarly, the tumor area was less in the whey protein group in comparison to either the casein or Purina groups, with some difference between casein and Purina groups. Body weight gain was similar in all dietary groups.

It is well known that the incidence and size of tumors are influenced by the immune system. In advanced phase of the disease in which plaque-forming cell measurements were made, the humoral immune response was greatly reduced in all dietary groups. It is, hence, conceivable that, particularly in the early phase of tumor development, the protein related difference in immune reactivity among the dietary groups may have influenced the observed difference in tumor development and whey protein diet appears to significantly inhibit the incidence and growth of chemically induced colon cancer in mice.

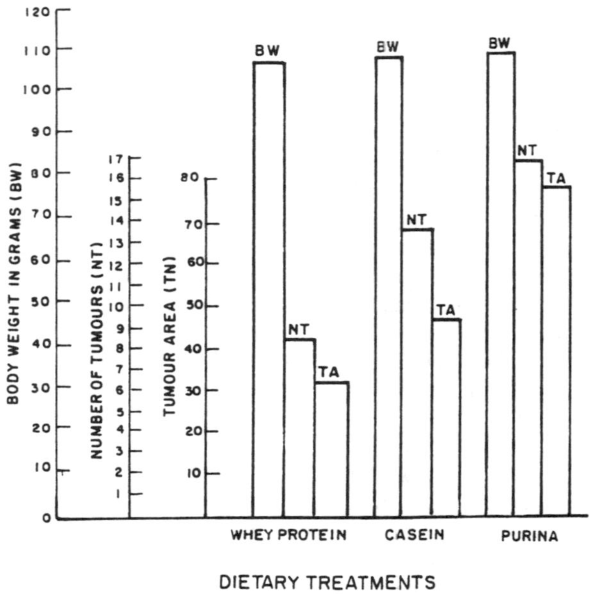

FIG. 9. EFFECT OF DIETARY PROTEIN REGIMEN ON BODY GROWTH AND TUMOR DEVELOPMENT IN 1,2-DIMETHYLHYDRAZINE TREATED A/J MICE (MEAN OF 10 MICE PER GROUP)

NT: Whey protein × casein ($p \leq 0.01$); whey protein × Purina ($p \leq 0.02$).

TA: whey protein × Purina ($p \leq 0.001$); whey protein × casein ($p \leq 0.02$).

Adapted from Bounous *et al.* (1988b).

Several pathological conditions associated with carcinogenesis are related to changes in proteases responsible for tumor promotion and neoplastic transformation. The inhibition of such activities explains the effectiveness of protease inhibitors in the prevention of some type of cancers (Garcia-Carreño 1996). For comprehensive reviews of this topic see De Clerk and Imren (1994), Das and Mukhopadhyay (1994) and Steinmetz and Potter (1991).

Several serine proteinase inhibitors from soybean and potato suppressed oral carcinogenesis in hamsters that was induced by 7,12-dimethylbenz(a)anthracene (Kennedy *et al.* 1993). Details about the mechanisms of action of the preventive effects of proteinase inhibitors on cancer remain to be elucidated. The authors postulated a mechanism to explain how plant proteinase inhibitors affect enzymes produced by neoplastic cells, reducing damage to the extracellular matrix caused by the tumor proteinases, and thus limiting tissue invasion.

Japanese researchers (Kawamura and Ishikawa 1993) extracted and isolated from the fruit body of matsutake mushroom a high molecular weight protein (MW 210 kD) with a selective cytotoxicity against virus transformed cells. The purified protein showed antitumor activity not only against mouse cell lines but also human tumor cell lines. In a preliminary experiment, the protein had strong cytotoxic activity against human cell lines and was also very effective against a primary culture from a uterine cancer from which a malignant type of HPV-18 virus was separated. The data presented by the Japanese researchers suggested that this antitumorigenic protein may be useful as an antitumor drug.

Cystatin is a general term denoting a superfamily of proteins which specifically inhibit enzymes belonging to the cysteine class of proteinases. In the field of medical sciences, a variety of animal cystatins have long been extensively investigated for their structure, function and physiological significance. Some cystatins occur in various tissues of animal and human bodies, probably acting as biodefense substances against microbial and viral infections. Oryzacystatin was found in rice by Abe *et al.* (1987) and was the first well defined cystatin of plant origin (Abe *et al.* 1991).

Some human viruses require cysteine proteinases for processing their polyproteins during their proliferation in infected cells. This suggests that the application of a cystatin could show an antiviral effect as it enters the cells. Potent inhibitory effects of two species of oryzacystatin on the replication of poliovirus in infected Vero Cells has been observed (Kondo *et al.* 1992).

REFERENCES

ABE, K., EMORI, Y., KONDO, H., SUZUKI, K. and ARAI, S. 1987. Molecular cloning of a cysteine proteinase inhibitor of rice (oryzacystatin). J. Biol. Chem. *262*:16793–16797.

ABE, K., KONDO, H., WATANABE, H., EMORI, Y. and ARAI, S. 1991. Oryzacystatins as the first well defined cystatins of plant origin and their target proteinases in rice seeds. Biomed. Biochim. Acta *50*:637–641.

ANDERSON, M.E. and MEISTER, A. 1983. Transport and direct utilization of γ-glutamylcysteine for glutathione synthesis. Proc. Natl. Acad. Sci. *80*, 807–811.

ARAI, S. 1993. Physiological functions of foods. Proceedings Sixth Internat. Congress Engin. Food, 23–27 May, Makuari Messe, Chiba, Japan.

ARAI, S. 1996. Studies on functional foods in Japan - State of the art (Review). Biosci. Biotech. Biochem. 60, 9–15.

ARIYOSHI, Y. 1993. Angiotensin-converting enzyme inhibitors derived from food proteins. Trends Food Sci. Technol. *4*, 139–144.

BARTH, C.A. and PFEUFFER, M. 1988. Dietary protein and atherogenesis. Klin. Wochenschr. *66*, 135–143.

BERROCAL, R., CHANTON, S., JUILLERAT, M.A., PAVILLARD, B., SHERZ, J.C. and JOST, R. 1989. Tryptic phosphopetides from whole casein. II. Physiochemical properties related to the solubilization of calcium. J. Dairy Res. *56*, 335–341.

BOUNOUS, G. and GOLD, P. 1991. The biological activity of undenatured dietary whey proteins: role of glutathione. Clin. Invest. Med. *14*, 296–309.

BOUNOUS, G. and KONGSHAVN, P.A.L. 1982. Influence of dietary proteins on the immune-system of mice. J. Nutr. *112*, 1747–1755.

BOUNOUS, G., SADARANGANI, C., PANG, K.C. and KONGSHAVN, P.A.L. 1981. Effect of dietary amino acids on tumor growth and cell-mediated immune responses. Clin. Invest. Med. *4*, 109–115.

BOUNOUS, G., LÉTOURNEAU, L. and KONGSHAVN, P.A.L. 1983a. Influence of dietary protein type on the immune system of mice. J. Nutr. *113*, 1415–1421.

BOUNOUS, G., LÉTOURNEAU, L. and KONGSHAVN, P.A.L. 1983b. The effect of concentration and type of dietary protein hydrolysates on tumor growth in mice. Clin. Invest. Med. *6*, 197–201.

BOUNOUS, G., SHEOUDA, N.; KONGSHAVN, P.A.L. and OSMOND, D.G. 1985. Mechanism of altered β-cell response induced by changes in dietary protein type in mice. J. Nutr. *115*, 1409–1417.

BOUNOUS, G., KONGSHAVN, P.A.L. and GOLD, P. 1988a. The immunoenhancing property of dietary whey protein concentrate. Clin. Invest. Med. *11*, 271–278.

BOUNOUS, G., PAPENBURG, R., KONGSHAVN, P.A.L., GOLD, P. and FLEIZER, D. 1988b. Dietary whey protein inhibits the development of dimethylhydrazine induced malignancy. Clin. Invest. Med. *11*, 213–217.

BOUNOUS, G., BATIST, G. and GOLD, P. 1989. Immunoenhancing property of dietary whey protein in mice: role of glutathione. Clin. Invest. Med. *12*, 154–161.

BOUNOUS, G., BARUCHEL, S., FALUTZ, J. and GOLD, P. 1993. Whey proteins as a food supplement in HIV-seropositive individuals. Clin. Invest. Med. *16*, 204–209.

BRINK, W. 1996. The life extension protein that fights disease and extends lifespan. Life Extension Report, January, pp. 21–28.

BUTLER, J.E. 1969. Bovine immunoglobulins: a review. J. Dairy Sci. *52*, 1985–1909.

CHIA, L.S., TOMPSON, J.E. and MOSCORELLO, M.A. 1984. X-Ray diffraction evidence for myelin disorder in brain from humans with Alzheimer's disease. Can. Biochem. Biophys. Acta Ser. Biomembr. *775*, 308–312.

CHIBA, H. and YOSHIKAWA, M. 1986. Biologically functional peptides from food proteins: new opioid peptides from milk proteins. *In* Protein Tailoring for Food and Medical Uses. R.E. Feeney and J.R. Whitaker (eds.), Marcel Dekker Inc., New York, pp. 123–153.

CARROLL, K.K., GIOVANNETTI, P.M., HUFF, M.W., MOASE, O., ROBERTS, D.C.K. and WALFE, B.M. 1978. Hypercholesterolemic effect of substituting soy bean protein for animal protein in the diet of healthy young women. Am. J. Clin. Nutr. *31*, 1312–1321.

DAS, S. and MUKHOPADHYAY, P. 1994. Protease inhibitor in chemoprevention of cancer. Acta Oncol. *33*, 859–865.

DE CLERK, Y. and IMREN, S. 1994. Protease inhibitors: role of potential therapeutic use in human cancer. Eur. J. Cancer *30A*, 2170–2180.

DE CRIGNIS, G.L., MANK, H.H., ELBERTZHAGEN, H. and KLOSTERMEYER, H. 1989. Colostrum as a source of antibodies. *In* Milk Proteins: Nutritional, Clinical, Functional and Technological Aspects. C.A. Barth and E. Schilimme (eds.), Springer-Verlag, New York, pp. 165–167.

DREWNOWSKI, A. 1992. Food preferences and the opioid peptide system. Trends Food Sci. Technol. *3*, 97–99.

ESTRELA, J.M., SAEZ, G.T., SUCH, L. and VINA, J. 1983. The effect of cysteine and N-acetylcysteine on rat liver glutathione (GSH). Biochem. Pharmacol. *32*, 3483–3485.

GARCIA-CARREÑO, F.L. 1996. Proteinase inhibitors. Trends Food Sci. Technol. *7*, 197–204.

GOLDBERG, A.P., LIM, A., KOLAR, J.B., GRUNDHAUSER, J.J., STEINKE, F.H. and SCHONFELD, G. 1982. Soybean protein independently lowers plasma cholesterol levels in primary hypercholesterolemia. Atherosclerosis *43*, 355–368.

GOLDBERG, I. (ed.). 1994. Functional Foods. Chapman & Hall Inc., New York, 571p.

HODGES, R.E., KREHL, W.A., STONE, D.B. and LOPEZ, A. 1967. Dietary carbohydrates and low cholesterol diets: effects on serum lipids of man. Am. J. Clin. Nutr. *20*, 198–208.

JOSÉ, D.G. and GOOD, R.A. 1973a. Quantitative effects of nutritional protein and calories deficiency upon immune responses to tumors in mice. Cancer Res. *33*, 807–812.

JOSÉ, D.G. and GOOD, R.A. 1973b. Quantitative effects of nutritional essential amino acid deficiency upon immune responses to tumors in mice. J. Exp. Med. *137*, 1–9.

KAPLOWITZ, N., AW, T.Y. and OOKTENS, M. 1985. The regulation of hepatic glutathione. Ann. Rev. Pharmacol. Toxicol. *25*, 715–744.

KAWAMURA, Y. and ISHIKAWA, M. 1993. Antimurogenic and immunoactive protein and peptide factors in food stuffs (I) - an antitumorigenic protein from *Tricholoma matsutake*. *In* Food and Cancer Prevention: Chemical and Biological Aspects. K.W. Waldron, I.T. Johnson, and G.W. Fenwick (eds.), Royal Society of Chemistry, pp. 327–330.

KENNEDY, A., BILLINGS, P., MAKI, A. and NEWBERNE, P. 1993. Effect of various preparations of dietary protease inhibitors on oral carcinogenesis in hamster induced by DMBA. Nutr. Cancer *19*, 191–200.

KITTS, D.D. and YUAN, Y.V. 1992. Caseinophosphopeptides and calcium bioavailability. Trends Food Sci. Technol. *2*, 31–35.

KONDO, H., IJIRI, S., ABE, K., MAEDA, H. and ARAI, S. 1992. Inhibitory effect of oryzacystatins and a truncation mutant on the replication of poliovirus in infected cells. FEBS Lett. *299*, 48–50.

KUZUYA, M., NAITO, M., FUNAKI, C., HAYASHI, T., ASAI, K. and KUZUYA, F. 1989. Protective role of intracellular glutathione against oxidized low-density lipoprotein in cultured endothelial cells. Biochem. Biophys. Res. Commun. *163*, 1466–1472.

MURAMOTO, M. and KAWAMURA, Y. 1991. Properties of rice proteins and angiotensin-converting enzyme-inhibiting peptides from proteins. Shokuhin Kogyo *34*, 18–26.

POTTER, D. 1990. Functional foods - a major opportunity for the dairy industry? Dairy Ind. Int. *55*, 32–33.

van RAAIJ, J.M.A., KATAN, M.B., HAUTVAST, J.G.A.J. and HERMUS, R.J.J. 1981. Effects of casein versus soy protein diets on serum cholesterol and lipoproteins in young healthy volunteers. Am. J. Clin. Nutr. *34*, 1261–1271.

van RAAIJ, J.M.A., KATAN, M.B., WEST, C.E. and HAUTVAST, J.A.G.J. 1982. Influence of diets containing casein, soy isolate and soy concentrate on serum cholesterol and lipoproteins in middle-aged volunteers. Am. J. Clin. Nutr. *35*, 925–934.

RIEDERER, P., SOFIC, E., RAUSCH, W.D., SCHMIDT, B., REYNOLDS, G.P., JELLINGER, K. and YOUDIM, M.B.H. 1989. Transition metals, ferritin, glutathione, and ascorbic acid in Parkinsonian brains. J. Neurochem. *52*, 215–220.

SAITO, Y., KAWATO, S., ABE, Y. and IMAYASU, S. 1991. Oral angiotensin-converting enzyme inhibitors for hypertension control. Japanese Patent 4,279,529.

SATO, R., NOGUCHI, T. and NAITO, H. 1986. Casein phosphopeptide (CPP) enhances calcium absorption from the ligated segment of rat small intestine. J. Nutr. Sci. Vitaminol. *32*, 67–76.

SINGLETARY, K.W. and MILNER, J.A. 1987. Influence of prior dietary protein intake on metabolism, DNA binding and adduct formation of 7,12-dimethyl-benz(a)anthracene in isolated rat mammary epithelial cells. J. Nutr. *117*, 587–592.

SILVERSTONE, H. and TANNENBAUM, A. 1951. Proportion of dietary protein and the formation of spontaneous hepatomas in the mouse. Cancer Res. *11*, 442–446.

STEINMETZ, K. and POTTER, D. 1991. Vegetables, fruit and cancer. Cancer Causes Control *2*, 427–442.

SUGANO, M., ISHIWAKI, N., NAGATA, Y. and IMAIZUMI, K. 1982. Effects of arginine and lysine addition to casein and soybean protein on serum lipids, apolipoproteins, insulin and glucagon in rats. Brit. J. Nutr. *48*, 211–221.

WIDHALM, K. 1986. Effects of diets on serum cholesterol lipids and lipoproteins in hypercholesterolemic children. *In* Nutritional Effects of Cholesterol Metabolism. A.C. Beyen (ed.), Transmondial Voorhuzen, pp. 133–140.

YANG, C.S., BRADY, J.F. and HONG, J-Y. 1992. Dietary effect on cytochrome P_{450} xenobiotic metabolism, and toxicity. FASEB J. *6*, 737–744.

YUAN, Y.V. and KITTS, D.D. 1991. Confirmation of calcium absorption and femoral utilization in spontaneously hypertensive rats fed casein phosphopeptide diets. Nutr. Res. *11*, 1257–1272.

YUAN, Y.V., KITTS, D.D., NAGASAWA, T. and NAKAI, S. 1991. Paracellular calcium absorption, femur mineralization, and biomechanics in rats fed selected dietary proteins. Food Chem. *39*, 125–137.

AN EFFICIENT PRODUCTION OF DFA III AND ITS POTENTIAL UTILITY AS A PHYSIOLOGICALLY FUNCTIONAL FOOD

FUSAO TOMITA, ATSUSHI YOKOTA, TAKANORI KASAI[1], HIROSHI HARA[1] and KOUJI SAYAMA[2]

Laboratory of Applied Microbiology
Faculty of Agriculture
Hokkaido University

[1]Laboratory of Foods and Nutrition
Faculty of Agriculture
Hokkaido University

[2]Research Laboratories
Nitten Co., Ltd.
Hokkaido Japan

ABSTRACT

In the course of our screening program for the oligosaccharides production from inulin, it was found that Arthrobacter sp. H65-7 produces α-D-fructofuranose-β-D-fructofuranose 2',1:2,3'-dianhydride(DFA III) efficiently. The responsible enzyme was purified and identified as inulase II whose gene was subsequently cloned and expressed in Escherichia coli *at much higher levels than in the original bacterium. Thus it became possible to provide a large amount of DFA III for evaluating its efficacy as a physiologically functional food.*

DFA III has a half sweetness of sucrose. It was not digested in rat and human digestive systems and did not stimulate the growth of lactic acid bacteria including Bifidobacteria. *It stimulated the growth of a certain type (lecithinase-negative) of* Clostridium sp. *in rat. In rat, it stimulated the uptake of calcium much higher than known stimulants such as fructo-oligosaccharides and raffinose, although DFA III was not digested at all in this system.*

INTRODUCTION

Inulin is one of most abundant natural carbohydrates and is extracted easily from such plants as Jerusalem artichoke and chicory. However, its use is rather limited, since it is not digested in the human digestive systems. Inulin is a linear β-2,1-linked fructan terminated with sucrose residues. In order to utilize inulin for the production of useful compounds, high fructose syrup is produced in some amounts, but competition with other conventional products such as inverted sugar is high. Thus we initiated studies to produce other useful sugars such as oligosaccharides, from the view of current development of oligosaccharides as a physiologically functional foods.

Several enzymes such as 2,1-β-D-fructan fructoanhydrolase (EC 3.2.1.7; inulinase) and inulin fructotransferase (depolymerizing) (EC 2.4.1.93; inulase II) have been shown to degrade inulin to give fructose and/or oligosaccharides (Nakumara *et al.* 1978; Negro

1978; Xiao 1988). However, their amounts or activities are not good enough to use them for the production of oligosaccharides. And thus the use of oligosaccharides has not been well developed.

Thus we have initiated to search for inulin degrading enzymes of microbial origin, in order to produce value-added oligosaccharides from inulin. We found a useful bacteria to produce a novel type of inulin fructotransferase (depolymerizing) (EC 2.4.1.93) which converts inulin efficiently into α-D-fructofuranose-β-D-fructofuranose 2',1:2,3'-dianhydride (DFA III) (Yokota *et al.* 1991). In order to obtain a large amount of DFA III, we also attempted the cloning of the gene for inulase II, expression of the gene in *E. coli* (Sukurai *et al.* 1997). Furthermore we found unique physiological functions of DFA III in rat (Nagura *et al.* 1996; Suzuki *et al.* 1997).

RESULTS AND DISCUSSION

Isolation of Inulin from Chicory (Inoue *et al.* 1996; Sakurai and Tomita 1997)

Among inulin producing plants, chicory (*Chicorium intybus* L.) is the most suitable one as a source of inulin from its high content of inulin and higher degree of polymerization (more than 30 fructose units). It is also an important crop that could replace sugar beet in Hokkaido, for recent trends in decline of sucrose consumption will result in decrease in its cultivation and these trends will demolish sugar industry including agriculture in such areas as Hokkaido. Chicory is one of the most suitable crops in cool areas, since it can tolerate cool temperature, disease, and desiccation and it can be cultivated without much trouble in these areas.

Furthermore, its yields per ha are as high as 45 t, which is much higher than those of corn or sugar beet. Inulin can be extracted easily as shown in Fig. 1 and Table 1. After seven cycles of extractions with hot water, liming, carbonation and several cycles of crystallization, pure inulin can be obtained in the yield of 46% as shown in Table 1. All the instruments used here were those for sucrose extraction from sugar beet.

Screening of Inulin-degrading Enzymes from Microbes (Yokota *et al.* 1991b)

As stated in Introduction, it is very important to have a very active enzyme for the production of oligosaccharides from inulin. We have searched for oligosaccharide-producing microorganisms from soil samples. Inulase II producers were selected from inulin-assimilating microbes. Soil microbes were subjected to the screening of their inulin decomposing activity by selecting them to grow on a medium containing inulin as a sole carbon source. The screening medium consisted of 10 g inulin, 1.4 g ammonium sulfate, 2 g KH_2PO_4, 0.3 g $CaCl_2$, 0.3 g urea, 0.3 g $MgSO_4 \cdot 7H_2O$, 5 mg $FeSO_4 \cdot 7H_2O$, 1.6 mg $MnSO_4 \cdot H_2O$, 1.4 mg $ZnSO_4 \cdot 7H_2O$, 2 mg $CoCl_2$, 1 g polypeptone, 2 g Tween 80, and 20 g agar per liter of deionized water (pH 5.2). Microbes showing a clear zone around their colonies were selected as plausible candidates for having inulin decomposing ability.

These isolates were grown in the production medium containing 10 g inulin, 2 g $NaNO_3$, 0.5 g $MgSO_4 \cdot 7H_2O$, 0.5 g KCl, 0.5 g KH_2PO_4, 0.01 g $FeSO_4 \cdot 7H_2O$, 0.2 g yeast extract and NaOH to adjust the pH to 7.0 per liter of deionized water and the culture supernatants were tested for their inulin decomposing activity. Among 84 microbes, one strain, the strain H65-7 was selected for further study.

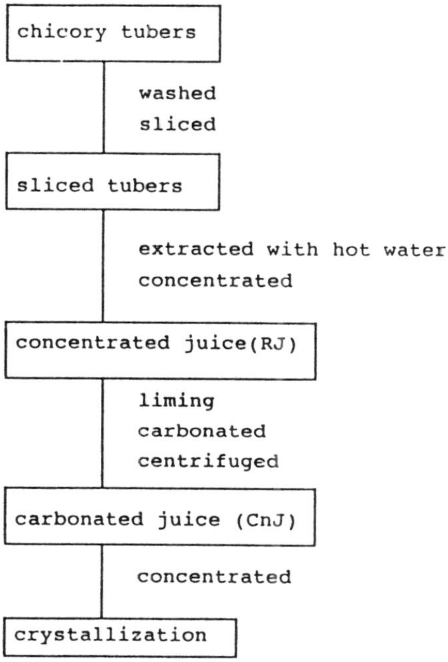

FIG. 1. PURIFICATION PROCEDURE OF INULIN FROM CHICORY

TABLE 1.
MATERIAL BALANCE IN PURIFICATION PROCESSES OF INULIN

	Weight (kg)	Inulin (g/100 g)	Total Inulin (kg)	Recovery Yield (%)
Sliced Chicory	1792	18.62	334	100
Water	2707			
Pulp	2199	6.92	152	46
RJ (twice)	2300	6.34	146	
Conc. RJ	1560	11.26	76	53
CnJ (7 times)	1470	10.40	153	46

Isolation and Identification of Reaction Products (Yokota *et al.* 1991b; Tomita *et al.* 1992)

The reaction mixture, consisting of 550 ml of culture supernatant and the same volume of 0.1 M citric acid-NaOH buffer (pH 5.5) containing 10% inulin, was incubated at 60°C for 2 h. The reaction was stopped by heating for 5 min in boiling water, and was concentrated under reduced pressure. This concentrate was subjected to silica gel chromatography. Purified material had the molecular weight of 324, and $[a]^{20}$ +134.9° (c 1.0,H_2O, authentic (Jackson and McDonald 1931), +135.64°). It was analyzed by ^{13}C-NMR spectra as shown in Table 2 and was identified as DFA III.

TABLE 2.
^{13}C-NMR CHEMICAL SHIFTS OF DFA III

Assignment	Chemical shift of ^{13}C resonance of			
Carbon atom number	α-D-Fructofuranose		β-D-Fructofuranose	
2	106.3	(106.6)	104.1	(103.8)
3	83.9	(83.6)	84.6	(84.4)
4	78.1	(77.9)	75.0	(74.8)
5	82.9	(82.6)	81.8	(81.4)
1	66.2	(65.8)	61.7	(61.4)
6	63.3	(63.2)	63.8	(63.5)

δ in ppm at 125 MHz with tetramethylsilane as an external standard in D_2O.
Data in parenthesis are from published data (Uchiyama 1982).

Classification of the Strain H65-7 (Yokota *et al.* 1991b)

The strain H65-7 is a Gram positive, non-sporeforming bacterium, which has rod-coccus growth cycle. It has lysine as a diamino acid in the cell wall and MK-9(H2) as a menaquinone. It has the peptidoglycan type of either Lys-Ala-Thr-Ala or Lys-Thr-Ala_2. The cell wall contains rhamnose and galactose. Thus the strain H65-7 was identified as *Arthrobacter sp.* H65-7.

Characteristics of the Enzyme (Yokota *et al.* 1991a)

The enzyme was purified as shown in Table 3. The purified enzyme showed a single band on PAGE and molecular weight of the enzyme was estimated to be 100,000 consisting of two identical subunits. The isoelectric point of the enzyme was estimated to be pH 4.7. The optimum pH and temperature for the enzyme activity were found to be 5.5 and 60°C. The enzyme could not react with sucrose, 1-kestose, nystose, 1-fructofuranosyl-nystose, raffinose, melibiose, melezitose, stachyose, and lean. The enzyme activity was not affected by 1 mM of Ca^{2+}, Co^{2+}, Mg^{2+}, Mn^{2+}, Zn^{2+}, Pb^{2+}, Cu^{2+}, Hg^{2+}, Ba^{2+}, Fe^{2+}, and Ni^{2+}. These characteristics are different from those of other inulases and our enzyme seems to be the best to produce DFA III, for this enzyme can degrade inulin completely in a short reaction time as shown in Table 4.

N-terminal and Inner Amino Acid Sequence of Inulase II (Sakurai *et al.* 1997).

Inulase II was purified from culture supernatant of Arthrobacter sp. H65-7 in the medium shown above except yeast extract was 0.5 g per liter. The purified enzyme (10 nmol) was digested overnight with lysyl endopeptidase at 30 °C in 0.1 M Tris-Cl buffer (pH 8.5) containing 8.0 M urea and 100 mM dithiothreitol. The digested peptide fragments were separated on a reverse-phase HPLC. The amino acid sequences of these peptide fragments and N-terminal sequence of intact enzyme were analyzed with a gas-phase protein sequencer. N-Terminal region sequence was determined to be ADSTEETNRYDVTSWKIKGRPEVT) and one of internal regions to be DNVDTSGWLELQPG.

TABLE 3.
PURIFICATION STEPS OF INULASE II FROM *ARTHROBACTER SP.* H65-7

Purification step	Protein (mg)	Total activity (units)	Specific activity (units/mg)	Yield (%)
Culture supernatant	132.8	10074	75.9	100
$(NH_4)_2SO_4$(60%)	26.6	5432	204	54
DEAE-Toyopearl 650M	2.16	1305	604	13

Purification started from 714 ml of the crude enzyme (culture supernatant)

TABLE 4.
PRODUCTION OF DFA III BY CRUDE INULASE II

Inulin (mg/ml)	DFA III Production (mg/ml)	Yield(%)*
50	46.5	93.0
100	84.8	84.8
150	127.7	85.1
200	167.4	83.7
250	206.2	82.5

*Weight % based on the initial inulin.

Cloning and Nucleotide Sequence of Inulase II, Inulin Fructotransferase, (*ift*) gene (Sakurai *et al.* 1997)

According to the above amino acid sequences, probes were prepared as follows. Probe 1 (5'-TAC GAC GT(G/C) AC(G/C) TC(G/C) TGG AAG AT-3') corresponds to N-terminal region amino acid sequence and probe 2 (5'-GT(G/C) GAC AC(G/C) TC(G/C) GG(G/C) TGG CT(G/C) GA-3') corresponds to the internal region sequence shown above.

The genomic library of *Arthrobacter sp.* H65-7 was screened by colony hybridization with probes 1 and 2. Colonies hybridized with both probes were selected and examined for the presence of ift gene according to conventional procedures.

As shown in Fig. 2, the deduced primary structure of inulase II had a homology with inulin fructotransferase (DFA I-producing) from *Arthrobacter globiformis* S14-3.

However, almost no homology was observed between inulase II and exo-inulinase, and inulin-hydrolyzing enzyme from *Kluyveromyces marxianus*.

```
H    1  MMDPSRRRLLGAGAVATLTGALALGAAAPAQAADSTEETNRYDVTSWKIKGRPEVTAQID
                                                 ****.*   . ..... .*
S    1                                      MANTVYDVTTW---SGATISPYVD

H   61  IGAVINDIIADVKKRQTTADARPGAVITIPPGDYDLRTQVVVDVSYLTIAGFGHGFFSRS
        ******.****.* .**...******* ****.*** *.******.* * * ****.* .
S   22  IGAVINQIIADIKANQTSQAARPGAVIYIPPGHYDLLTRVVVDVSFLQIKGSGHGFLSEA

H  121  IKDNVDTSGWLELQPGGSHIRVLTPSTAPQAFLVRRAGSP----RLSGVVFRDFCLDGVE
        *.*. .*..*.* ***.*****  ......****.*.*.*    **... *..******
S   82  IRDESSTGSWVETQPGASHIRVKNTDGNREAFLVSRSGDPNVVGRLNSIEFKGFCLDGV-

H  177  FPPDGNSYRNG--RTGIEVASDNDSFHITGMGFVYLEHALIVRGADALRVHDNMIAECGN
          .*...*. *  ..**.*.*******..**********.**.****  ...*.*****.
S  141  --TDSKPYSPGNSKIGISVQSDNDSFHVEGMGFVYLEHAIIVKGADAPNITNNFIAECGS

H  235  CVELTGAGQATIVSNNLMGAGPEGATLLAENHEGLLITGNNLFPRGRSLVELTGCNRCSV
        *.*****.*.. ..**..  .. * .. *** ** *****.*. .. . ..*..*** *.
S  199  CIELTGASQVAKITNNFLISAWAGYSIYAENAEGPLITGNSLL-WAAN-ITLSDCNRVSI

H  295  TSNRFQGFFPGIMRLINNCKENLITGNHFRRGMEGFPPFLGTSNGLDDLYGVVHIAGDNN
        .**.. . **... *..**.****..*****      .  ***. .***.*.***.*.**
S  257  SSNKLLSNFPSMVALLGNCSENLIAANHFRR-----VSGDGTSTRFDDLFGLVHIEGNNN

H  355  FFANNLIAYDVSPDRIVPPNAQPTMILVAGGDSNVVATNHVVSNVETQHVVLDASTVRSK
          ..*.....*....* *..* **.*** .**** .***..****..  ****.**. ..
S  312  TVTGNMFSFNVPASSISPSGATPTIILVKSGDSNYLATNNIVSNVSAM-VVLDGSTTATR

H  415  VLDSGPASKVTSYSADTAIRPTP
        .. *. .*....*... .. ***
S  371  IIYSAKNSQLNAYTTSYTLVPTP
```

FIG. 2. COMPARISON BETWEEN THE DEDUCED AMINO ACID SEQUENCE OF INULASE II FROM *ARTHROBACTER SP.* H65-7(H) AND THAT OF INULIN FRUCTOTRANSFERASE (DFA I-PRODUCING) FROM *A. GLOBIFORMIS* S14-3(S)
(Haraguchi *et al* 1995).
Asterisks indicate identical residues. Functionally similar residues are shown by dots. Gaps are introduced to improve alignment.

Effective Expression of ift Gene in Escherichia coli (Sakurai *et al.* 1997)

Ift gene hooked on pUC18 (pIFT-A) was transformed to *E. coli* and the transformant was checked for its expression of inulase II. The transformant expressed it effectively and the expression is under the control of IPTG and no expression was observed in the opposite direction. Thus it was concluded that a functional promoter sequence for ift gene could not be detected in the *E. coli* background in the genomic fragment of *Arthrobacter sp.* H65-7.

Improvement of expression was attempted to increase the productivity of DFA III. Upstream region of ift gene was eliminated as shown in Fig. 3 to construct pIFT-B. As shown in Fig. 3, the activity in the cell-free extract increased 72-fold higher than that of *E. coli* carrying pIFT-A. The enzyme produced by this transformant was the same as that obtained from *Arthrobacter sp.* H65-7 and an effective method to prepare DFA III has now been established.

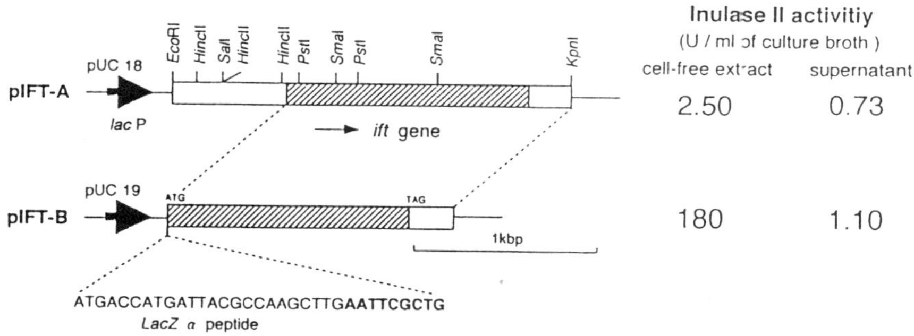

FIG. 3. INULASE II ACTIVITIES OF *E. COLI* TRANSFORMANTS
The lac promoter of pUC18 and pUC19 is shown by large arrows. The hatched box shows ORF of ift gene. The small arrow in pIFT-A indicates the direction of transcription. The bold letters in pIFT-B indicate the sequence from cloned DNA fragment.

Effects of DFA III to Microbial Flora in Rat Cecum (Nagura *et al.* 1996)

DFA III has about 52% sweetness of sucrose, low hygroscopic property, and high stability to acid and heat. Furthermore, it is not digested by intestinal enzymes of rat, nor absorbed by inverted intestinal sac. Thus DFA III is expected to be a non-digestible oligosaccharide. When rats were fed with diets containing 2% DFA III or 5% raffinose, lowering of pH and increase of organic acids and contents were observed in cecum; thus it is clear that DFA III was digested in cecum. As shown in Fig. 4, *Bifidobacteria* increased when raffinose was given, while lecithinase-negative *Clostridia* increased when DFA III was given. However, there was no difference in the composition of organic acids in both cases.

Effects of DFA III on Absorption of Ca^{2+} in Bowel of Rats (Suzuki *et al.* 1997)

In order to examine effects of DFA III on mineral absorption in rats, rats were given a sucrose diet (30 g/kg diet) for one week and then test diets containing fructo-oligosaccharides, raffinose, or DFA III for 2 weeks. Amounts of Ca^{2+} in diets were 3 g/kg diet and chromium oxide (0.5 g/kg diet) was added as a marker of non-absorbable mineral. As shown in Fig. 5, calcium absorption in small and large intestines was enhanced greatly in the presence of DFA III. As shown in Fig. 6, apparent increases in calcium solubility occurred in the cecum and colon with DFA III and other oligosaccharides. Amounts of calcium absorbed were proportionally elevated to the amounts of DFA III *in vitro* experiments using everted sac of jejunum and ileum.

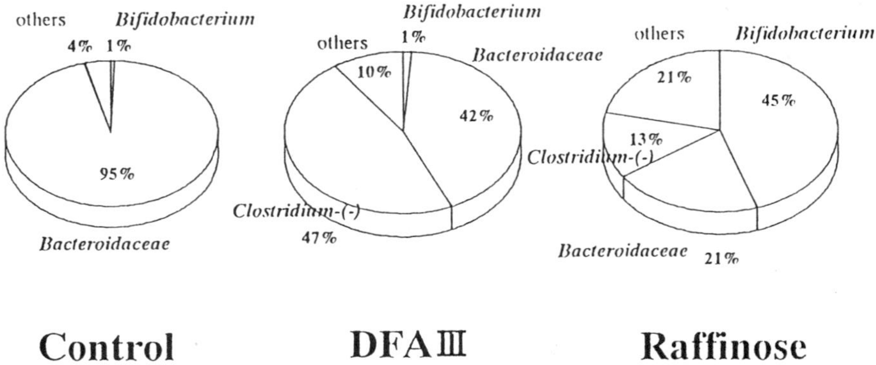

FIG. 4. EFFECTS OF VARIOUS OLIGOSACCHARIDES TO MICROFLORA IN RATS

SD rats (5 weeks old, male) were fed with a basic diet (casein 230 g, corn starch 614 g, cellulose 50 g, corn oil 50 g, mineral mixture 40 g, vitamin mixture 10 g, DL-methionine 3 g, choline-HCl 2 g per kg diet for 1 week and then fed with diets replacing corn starch with 20 g DFA III or 50 g raffinose for 4 weeks. Cecal contents were taken out and were subjected to study of microflora according to Mitsuoka (Mituoka 1984).

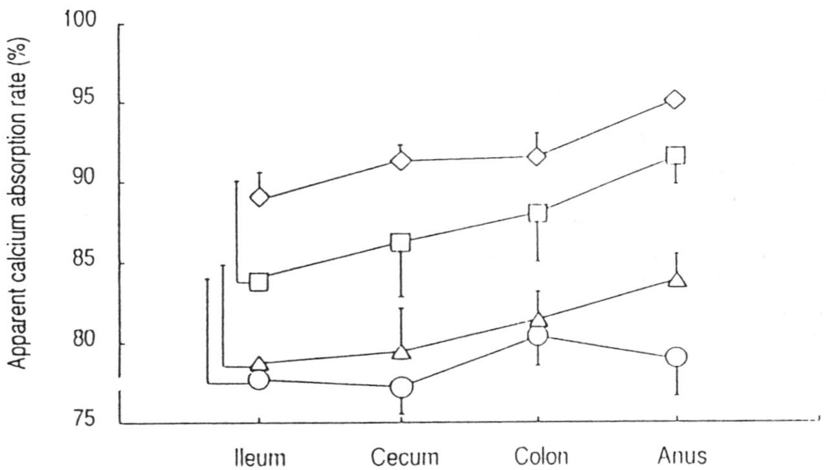

FIG. 5. CALCIUM ABSORPTION WAS INCREASED IN THE SMALL AND LARGE INTESTINE IN RATS FED WITH DFA III

○, Control; Δ, Fructooligosaccharides; □, Raffinose; ◇, DFA III. n=6 ($p<0.05$).

SD rats (5 weeks old, male) were fed with a basic diet consisting of 250 g casein, 50 g corn oil, 29 g mineral mixture, 11 g vitamin mixture, 3 g calcium, 50 g cellulose, and sucrose to make up 1 kg for one week and then were fed with test diets containing DFA III, fructooligosaccharide, or raffinose (0-30 g/ kg diet) in place of sucrose for 2 weeks. Chromium oxide (0.5 g/kg diet) was added as a non-absorbable marker to measure apparent absorption of Ca^{+2}. Apparent calcium absorption rate (%) were determined by Cr^{2+}.

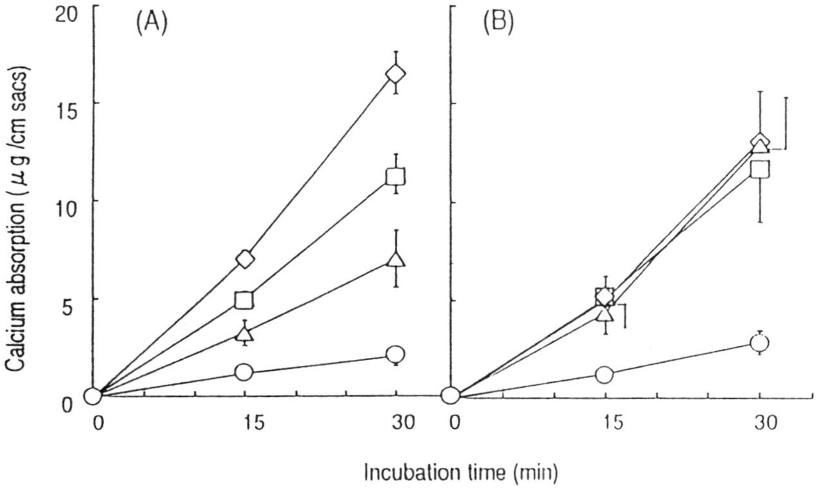

FIG. 6. EFFECTS OF DFA III CONCENTRATION ON CALCIUM ABSORPTION IN THE EVERTED JEJUNAL(A) AND ILEAL SEGMENTS (B)
○, mM; Δ, mM; □, 100 mM; ◇, 200 mM. n=6 ($p<0.05$)

As shown above, it was clearly demonstrated that DFA III stimulated calcium absorption both in the small and large intestines. Elevated absorption in the large intestine was observed as consequence of fermentation of DFA III by intestinal microbes, while DFA III stimulated absorption of calcium in the small intestine in the simultaneous presence of calcium.

REFERENCES

HARAGUCHI, K., SEKI, K., KISHIMOTO, M., NAGATA, T., KASUMI, T., KAINUMA, K. and KOBAYASHI, S. 1995. Purification and properties of inulin fructotransferase (DFA I-producing) from *Arthrobacter globiformis* S14-3.Biosci. Biotech. Biochem. *59*, 1809–1812.

INOUE, M., KIKUCHI, H., YOKOTA, A., TOMITA, F. and SAYAMA, K. 1996. Large scale preparation of DFAIII from inulin. Presented at the Annual Meeting of Hokkaido Branch of Japan Society for Biotechnology, Bioscience, and Agrochemistry, July 26–27, Abashiri City.

JACKSON, R.F. and MCDONALD, E. 1931. Two new crystalline difructose anhydrides from hydrolyzed inulin. Bur. Stand. J. Res. *6*, 709–715.

MITUOKA, T. 1984. A Color Atlas of Anaerobic Bacteria. Sobunsha, Tokyo.

NAGURA, T., NAKAMURA, N., KISHIDA, T., YOKOTA, A., TOMITA, F. and SAYAMA, K. 1996. Characteristics of DFA III – its effects on intestinal microflora of human and rat. Presented at the Annual Meeting of Hokkaido Branch of Japan Society for Bioscience, Biotechnology, and Agrochemistry, July 26-27, Abashiri City.

NAKAMURA, T., HOASHI, S. and NAKATSU, S. 1978. Culture conditions for inulase production by *Aspergillus*. Nippon Nougeikagaku Kaishi (Japan) *52*, 105–110.

NEGRO, H. 1978. Inulase from *Kluyveromyces fragilis*. J. Ferment. Technol. *56*, 102–107.

SAKURAI, H. and TOMITA, F. 1997. A new perspective on inulin as a carbohydrate resource. Bioscience and Industry (Japan), *55*, 25–29.

SAKURAI, H., YOKOTA, A. and TOMITA, F. 1997. Molecular cloning of an inulin fructotransferase (depolymerizing) gene from *Arthrobacter sp*. H65–7 and its expression in *Escherichia coli*. Biosci. Biotech. Biochem. *61*, 87–92.

SUZUKI, T., HARA, H., KASAI, T. and TOMITA, F. 1997. Enhanced uptake of calcium by DFA III in rat. Presented at the Annual Meeting of Japan Society for Bioscience, Biotechnology, and Agrochemistry, March 30–April 4, Tokyo.

TOMITA, F., YOKOTA, A. and ENOMOTO, K. 1992. Microbial production of difructose anhydride from inulin. Microbial Utilization of Renewable Resources *7*, 483–488.

UCHIYAMA, T. 1982. Anomeric configurations of di-D-fructose anhydride, produced by inulin D-fructotransferase. Carbohydr. Res. *101*, 138–140.

XIAO, R., TANIDA, M. and TAKAO, S. 1988. Inulinase from *Chrysosporium pannorum*. J. Ferment. Technol. *66*, 553–558.

YOKOTA, A., ENOMOTO, K. and TOMITA, F. 1991a. Purification and properties of an inulin fructotransferase (depolymerizing) from *Arthrobacter sp*. H65-7. J. Ferment. Bioeng. *72*, 262–265.

YOKOTA, A., HIRAYAMA, S., ENOMOTO, K., MIURA, Y., TAKAO, S. and TOMITA, F. 1991b. Production of inulin fructotransferase (depolymerizing) by *Arthrobacter sp*. H65–7 and preparation of DFA III from inulin by the enzyme. J. Ferment. Bioeng. *72*, 258–261.

HPLC DETERMINATION OF ANGIOTENSIN-CONVERTING ENZYME ACTIVITY ON TOYOPEARL HW-40S COLUMN

GONG-RUI CHEN, SHU-TAO LIU, BI-HONG SHI, RONG-ZHEN ZHANG, JIAN-CAI LI, RU-MING CHEN, LONG LI, WEN-HONG GAO, TIAN-BAO CHEN, YU-QIANG ZHENG and PING-FAN RAO

Institute of Biotechnology
Fuzhou University
523, Gong-Ye Road
Fuzhou, Fujian, 350002, P.R. China

ABSTRACT

Angiotensin-converting enzyme (EC 3.4.15.1; ACE), is a membrane-bound dipeptidyl carboxypeptidase that mediates the cleavage of the C-terminal dipeptide His-Leu of the decapeptide angiotensin, generating the most powerful endogenous vaso-constricting angiotensin.

Some ACE inhibitors, such as Captopril, have been used as anti-hypertensive drugs. Moreover in recent years, large quantities of ACE inhibitors have been identified and isolated from peptides derived from food material such as casein, soy protein, fish protein and so on. Functional food with hypotensive effect has been developed on the basis of these works.

Typical procedures for screening hypotensive peptides of food origins are separation of products of peptic and tryptic digestion of proteins followed by inhibitory activity determination of each fraction. A method developed by Cushman has been the most widely used, in which ACE activity is determined by the amount of hippuric acid generated as a product of enzymatic reaction of ACE with tripeptide of hippuryl-L-histidyl-L-leucine. Hippuric acid is determined spectrophotometrically at 228 nm after its isolation from the reaction system by ethylacetate extraction, which not only requires a large quantity of reagent but also results in large error.

An improved method based on Cushman's method is proposed in this paper. In this method, an enzymatic reaction system is based on Cushman's method, while isolation and determination of hippuric acid is performed by medium performance gel chromatography on a Toyopearl HW-40S column. Due to the size exclusion nature of the column with somewhat hydrophobic properties, complete separation of four existing fractions in the reaction system is obtained within a small fraction of the time necessary in Cushman's method, with ideal reproducibility.

INTRODUCTION

Angiotensin-converting enzyme (EC 3.4.15.1; ACE) is a membrane-bound dipeptidyl carboxypeptidase that mediates the cleavage of the C-terminal dipeptide His-Leu of the decapeptide angiotensin I, generating the more powerful endogenous vaso-constricting angiotensin II (Ballerman *et al.* 1991).

Some ACE inhibitors, such as Captopril, have been used as anti-hypertensive drugs. Moreover, in recent years large quantities of ACE inhibitors have been identified and isolated from peptides derived from food material which include: casein, soy protein and fish protein, and functional food with hypotensive effect has been developed on the basis of this research (Matsuda *et al.* 1983; Suzuki *et al.* 1983; Natarajan *et al.* 1984; Lantz *et al.* 1991; Matsumura *et al.* 1992; Saito *et al.* 1992; Suetsuna 1992; Tsuzuki *et al.* 1992; Yoshikawa *et al.* 1992; Kinoshita *et al.* 1993; Yamamoto *et al.* 1994; Teranaka *et al.* 1995).

The typical procedure for screening hypotensive peptides of food origin consists of separation of the products of peptic and tryptic digestion of proteins followed by ACE activity determination of each fraction. The most widely-used method to determine ACE activity has been proposed by Cushman *et al.* (1971), in which ACE activity is determined spectrophotometrically at 228 nm by the amount of hippuric acid generated in a fixed time as a product of enzymatic reaction of ACE with the tripeptide hippuryl-L-histidyl-L-leucine and after it is isolated from the reaction system by ethyl acetate extraction. The procedure has been useful but it not only requires a relatively large quantity of sample and reagents but also results in considerable error due to complicated procedures such as extraction. Efforts have been made to improve the accuracy and convenience by employing high performance liquid chromatography by which isolation and quantification of hippuric acid can be attained in a single step (Hugo *et al.* 1982; Meng *et al.* 1995; Nagamatsu *et al.* 1978). All the reported methods use reverse phase chromatography, which inevitably involves organic solvents such as acetonitrile and methyl alcohol of HPLC grade.

Toyopearl HW-40S is a medium performance gel chromatographic media with some degree of reverse phase media properties especially at a relatively high salt concentration (Rao *et al.* 1997). The combination of gel chromatography and reverse phase chromatography under certain conditions has produced satisfactory separation of 18 amino acids and some small peptides on a Toyopearl HW-40S column (Zhang 1996; Rao *et al.* 1997). The purpose of this paper is to report a simpler method to determine ACE activity using HPLC on a Toyopearl HW-40S column.

EXPERIMENTAL

ACE Assay

The ACE assay was based on the method proposed by Saito *et al.* (1992), which was modified from the method of Cushman *et al.* (1971). Angiotensin-converting enzyme (ACE) from rabbit lung with a marked activity of 2.5 units/mg protein, hippuryl-L-histidyl-L-leucine (HHL) and hippuric acid were purchased from Sigma Chemical Co. Other reagents was all analytical grade. To begin the assay, 30 μL of ACE solution was added to 60 μL deionized water, and incubated at 37°C for 3 min in a water incubator (Model 501, Shanghai, China). In case of ACE inhibitory activity determination, a 60 μL inhibitor sample solution was used instead of deionized water, while a corresponding buffer solution was used in the blank assay. Three hundred (300) μL of the substrate solution was added to the mixture and then incubated at 37°C for 30 min. The enzymatic reaction was terminated by the addition of 500 μL of 1 M HCl. Then, 10 μL of the thoroughly mixed reaction solution was applied to an HPLC system for further separation and quantification of hippuric acid. The substrate solution of 5.82 mM HHL and ACE solution of 100 mU/ml marked activity, were used as a test solution in this method. Here boric acid-borax buffer solution, pH 8.3, (Gerald 1989) with 0.5 M NaCl were used to dissolve substrate and enzyme.

High Performance Gel Chromatography (HPLC)

The column matrix for HPLC was Toyopearl HW-40S purchased from Tosoh Co., Japan. It was packaged into a stainless steel column (7.5 ID × 160 mm), and connected to a CCPD 8000 HPLC system (Tosoh Co., Japan). The effluent was monitored by a UV 8000 detector (Tosoh Co., Japan) at 228 nm measured by a recorder (BD112, Kipp & Zonen, Holland). Sample loop volume was 10 μL. The eluant was borate buffer, pH 8.3, containing 300 mM NaCl (Gerald 1989) at a flow rate of 0.500 mL/min. The chromatography was conducted at room temperature. The other conditions are shown in the legend for each related figure.

Calibration of Hippuric Acid Concentration

Hippuric acid (10.5 mg) was dissolved in 10 ml of the same borate buffer to prepare 0.117 mM stock solution, and then this solution was diluted 2, 4, 8, 16-fold with the same buffer to make five standard solutions with concentrations of: 0, 0.1172, 0.0586, 0.0293, 0.0146 and 0.0073 mM. Each of these standard and control solutions was applied to the HPLC system. The peak height of hippuric acid (H, mm), was measured from the chromatogram. A calibration curve was established as the regression of hippuric acid concentration (C, mM) vs. peak height (H, mm).

Calculation of ACE Activity

Since a unit of ACE activity (AU) is defined as the amount catalyzing the formation of 1 μ mole of hippuric acid from HHL in 1 min at 37°C under the given conditions, the ACE activity of each sample applied to the chromatogram could be easily calculated by the quantification of hippuric acid.

Determination of K_m for ACE

To determine the reliability of this method, K_m of the standard ACE was determined and compared with the reported data. ACE activity assay was carried out at various substrate concentrations such as: 0, 0.150, 0.300, 0.600, 1.200, 2.25 and 4.50 mM by adding 0, 10, 20, 40, 80, 150 and 300 μL of the substrate solution. The difference between the added volume of the substrate solution and the standard 300 μL was made up by the same borate buffer. The velocities of the ACE catalyzed reaction were calculated from the amounts of hippuric acid generated at different substrate solutions but within the same enzymatic reaction time. K_m and V_{max} of ACE were obtained according to the method of Lineweaver-Burk.

Statistics

A software package of Statistica V4.5 for WINDOWS was used for the major data processing throughout this work.

RESULTS AND DISCUSSION

Separation of ACE Assay Reaction Mixture

A typical chromatogram of ACE reaction mixture separated by a Toyopearl HW-40S column is shown in Fig. 1. Identified by comparison with the retention time of the standard samples, all the major components of the ACE activity assay reaction including: ACE, HHL, hippuric acid and histidyl leucine, were satisfactorily separated, as is clearly shown in the chromatogram. The void volume time (T_0) is also marked on Fig. 1.

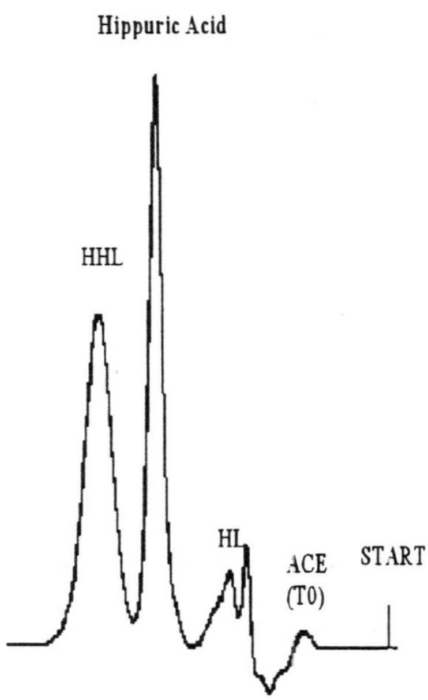

FIG. 1. A TYPICAL CHROMATOGRAM OF ACE REACTION MIXTURE ON TOYOPEARL HW-40S COLUMN

Chromatographic conditions were described in the Experiment Section. ACE, histidyl-leucine (HL), hippuric acid and HHL were separated from each other, with retention time of 5.00, 11.00, 15.00 and 18.50 min, respectively. Void volume time (T_0) and total volume time (T_t) were 5.00 and 14.10 min, respectively.

Angiotensin-converting enzyme was eluted at the void volume, since the upper limit of globin molecular weight for separation by Toyopearl HW-40S is 10 KDa, while the molecular weight of ACE is 146 KDa (Meng *et al.* 1996), much higher than the limit. The remaining components, which differ from each other only by one amino acid and can thus be theoretically expected to be eluted in the same fraction at the total volume, were completely separated. Increasing NaCl concentration in the elution buffer effectively improved the separation, with 300 mM NaCl as the optimum for achieving the best separation. Furthermore, histidyl leucine was eluted first, followed by hippuric acid and then hippuryl histidyl leucine. It is apparent that the separation of these three components is based on the reverse phase chromatographic properties rather than gel filtration properties of this matrix. The same matrix has been reported to be used to separate amino acids based on similar principles (Rao *et al.* 1997). In this case, a combination of both gel filtration properties and reverse phase chromatographic properties of the matrix has successfully made the simultaneous separation of proteins from peptides and peptide and amino acid separation possible.

A remarkable advantage of the procedure proposed in this study involving separating ACE assay mixture on a Toyopearl HW-40S column is that no organic solvents are required, which not only means lower operation cost and easier availability of the required reagents, but also means that the simplest HPLC apparatus can be used in the analysis since no solvent gradient is used. Consequently, this method may find much wider applications in ACE assay.

Since the amount of the sample required for each HPLC analysis is only 10 μL, only a tiny fraction of the sample required by traditional extraction and spectrophotometric methods, a total volume of 890 μL of the enzymatic reaction mixture can be used for up to 85-89 batches of HPLC analysis. It is therefore apparent that samples, enzyme and the substrate required can be proportionally and drastically reduced by using this procedure.

Calibration of Hippuric Acid Amount and Calculation of ACE Activity

Since hippuric acid is completely separated as is shown in Fig. 1, its peak height on the chromatogram can be easily used to calibrate its concentration. Calibration curve of hippuric acid concentration with its peak height is shown in Fig. 2. Peak heights of all 5 hippuric acid solution samples with different concentrations fell exactly on the same line when plotted against their concentration, indicating a strict correlation between the hippuric acid concentration and peak height on the chromatogram. The correlation between hippuric acid concentration (C, mmole) and its peak height (H, mm), as illustrated in Fig. 2, can be expressed by the following equation:

$$C = 0.6314*H \tag{1}$$

From a chromatogram, the peak height of hippuric acid (H, mm), was easily measured and its concentration was determined by Eq. 1. In addition, the ACE activity (AU), was calculated according to the following equation:

$$A = (890\ \mu l)*C/30\ \text{min} = 1.873*10\hat{\ }(-5)*H \tag{2}$$

Here 890 μl and 30 min represent the total ACE reaction solution volume and reaction time, respectively.

Determination of K_m of ACE

Using this new method and Eqs. (1) and (2), hippuric acid generated from cleavage of HHL by ACE at various HHL concentrations was determined and plotted against each

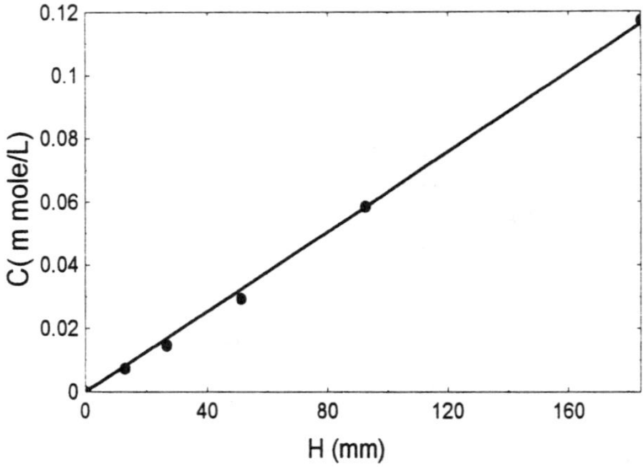

FIG. 2. CURVE OF CORRELATION BETWEEN HIPPURIC ACID CONCENTRATION (C, mmoles/L) AND ITS PEAK HEIGHT (H, mm)
It was concluded that C has a linear relationship with H, with relative coefficient K=0.6314 [(mmole/L)/mm]

substrate concentration, as shown in Fig 3. The Michaelis curve shown in Fig. 3 indicates precision of this proposed new method. The Michaelis equation for ACE derived from rabbit lung was expressed as the following:

$$V = 5.000*S/(0.615+S) \quad (3)$$

From Eq. (3), K_m and V_{max} were found to be 0.615 mM and 5.000 nmoles/min respectively. Compared with the reported values of Cushman *et al.* (1971) and Friedland *et al.* (1983), which were 2.6 mM and 1.2 mM, respectively, K_m obtained with our method is lower. The difference might be attributed to the different buffer systems for the enzyme assay with borate buffer in our method and phosphate in the reported works. In addition, from the V_{max} value of 5.000 nmole/min, we can infer that the test enzyme solution had a ACE activity of 150 mU/mL, higher than the marked activity value of 100 mU/ml. This may also be attributed to the different buffer system and ionic strength, as well as the method of extraction in the reported work, since inevitably some hippuric acid remains un-extracted. Hence, a higher V_{max} and lower K_m were observed by our method.

SUMMARY

Satisfactory separation of ACE activity assay reaction system and precise quantification of its products can be achieved by HPLC on a Toyopearl HW-40S column under chromatographic conditions, exploiting both the gel filtration property and hydrophobic property of this matrix, as is well demonstrated in the example of K_m determination. The procedures can be used to make fast and precise determination of ACE activity with small amount of samples, without using organic solvent and using the simplest of HPLC apparatus.

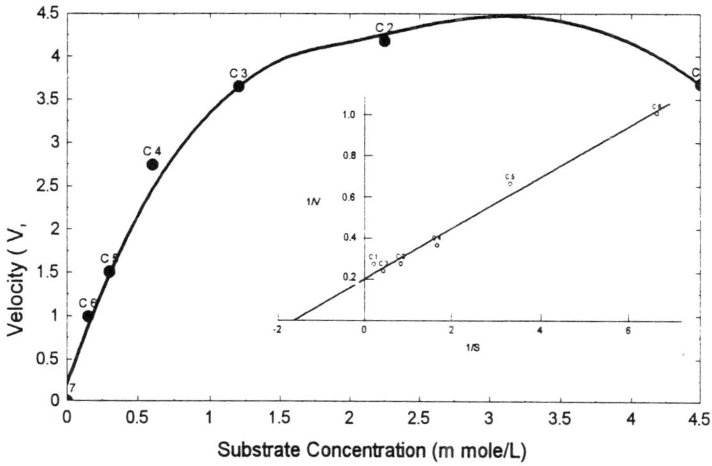

FIG. 3. EFFECT OF SUBSTRATE CONCENTRATION ON THE ACTIVITY OF ACE OF RABBIT LUNG

Activity measured as the rate of hydrolysis of HHL, using the test ACE assay system described in the text. The insert shows a Lineweaver-Burk plot of the same data.

REFERENCES

BALLERMAN, B.J., ZEIDEL, M.L., GUNNING, M.E. and BRENNER, B.M. 1991. Vasoactive peptides and the kidney. *In* The Kidney, 4th Edn. BRENNER, B.M. and RECTOR, F.C. (eds.). pp. 510–583. Saunders, Philadelphia.

CUSHMAN, D.W. and CHEUNG, H.S. 1971. Spectrophotometric assay and properties of the angiotensin converting enzyme of rabbit lung. Biochem. Pharmol. *20*, 1637–1648.

FRIEDLAND, J. and SILVERSTEIN, E. 1983. Properties of soluble and particulate angiotensin-converting enzymes of rabbit lung, induced macrophage and serum. Int. J. Biochem. *15* (11), 1337–1343.

GERALD, D.F. 1989. Practical Handbook of Biochemistry and Molecular Biology, CRC Press, Inc., Florida, USA.

HUGO, M.N., SIMON, L.S., MARC, E.V.S., ROBERT, M.V. and KAREL, J.V.A. 1982. Improved micromethod for assay of serum angiotensin converting enzyme. Clin. Chem. *28* (6), 1352–1355.

KINOSHITA, E., YAMAKOSHI, J. and KIKUCHI, M. 1993. Purification and identification of an angiotensin I-converting enzyme inhibitor from soy sauce. Biosci. Biotechnol. Biochem. *57*, 1107–1110.

LANTZ, I., GLAMSTA, E.L., TALBACK, L. and NYBERG, F. 1991. Hemorphins derived from hemoglobin have an inhibitory action on angiotensin converting enzyme activity. FEBS Lett. *287*, 39–41.

MATSUDA, H., NAGAOKA, T., MORITA, H., OSAJIMA, K. and OSUJIAM, Y. 1983. Angiotensin I converting enzyme inhibitory peptides generated from sardine muscle by protease for food industry. Nippon Shokuhin Kogyo Gakkaishi *39* (8), 678–683.

MATSUMURA, N. and SHIMAZU, T. 1992. Angiotensin I Converting Enzyme Inhibitory Peptides and Their Manufacture. Jpn. Kokai Tokkyo Koho JP 04, 149, 196.

MENG, Q.C., BALCELLS, E., DELL'ITALIA, L., DURAND, J. and OPARIL, S. 1995. Sensitive method for quantitation of angiotensin-converting enzyme (ACE) activity in tissue. Biochem. Pharmacol. *50*, 1445–1450.

MENG, Q.C. and SUZANNE, O. 1996. Purification and assay methods for angiotensin-converting enzyme. J. Chromatog. A. *743*, 105–122.

NAGAMATSU, A., SOEDA, S. and INOKUCHI, J.I. 1978. Rapid estimation of angiotensin I-converting enzyme activity by high-speed liquid chromatography, Yakugaku Zasshi (Japanese) *98*, 1296–1299.

NATARAJAN, S., GORDON, E.M., SABO, E.F., GODFREY, J.D., WELLER, H. N., PLUSCEC, J., ROM, M.B. and CUSHMAN, D.W. 1984. Ketomethyldipeptides I. A new class of angiotensin converting enzyme inhibitors. Biochem. Biophys. Res. Commun. *124*, 141–147.

RAO, P.F., LIU, S.T., ZHANG, R.Z., CHEN, G.R., ZHENG, Y.Q. and SHI, B.H. 1997. Deviation of size-exclusion chromatographic behavior of tryptophan on TOYOPEARL HW-40S column, Chinese J. Chromatog. *3*, 193–196.

SAITO, Y., NAKAMURA, K., KAWATO, A. and IMAYASU, S. 1992. Angiotensin I converting enzyme inhibitor in sake and its by-products. Nippon Nogeikagaku Kaishi *66* (7), 1081–1087.

SUETSUNA, K. 1992. Novel Peptides, Jpn. Kokai Tokkyo Koho JP 04, 120, 093.

SUZUKI, T., ISHIKAWA, N. and MEGURO, H. 1983. Angiotensin I-converting enzyme inhibiting activity in foods. Nippon Nogeikagaku Kaishi *57* (11), 1143–1146.

TERANAKA, T., EZAWA, M., MATSUYAMA, J., EBINE, H. and KIYOSAWA, I. 1995. Inhibitory effects of extracts from rice-koji miso, barley-koji miso, and soybean-koji miso on the activity of angiotensin converting enzyme. Nippon Nogeikagaku Kaishi *69* (9), 1163–1169.

TSUZUKI, W., KIKUCHI, Y. and SHINOKARA, M. 1992. Fluorometric assay of angiotensin I-converting enzyme inhibitory activity of vinegars. Nippon Shokuhin Kogyo Gakkaishi *39* (2), 188–192.

YAMAMOTO, N., AKINO, A. and TAKANO, T. 1994. Anti-hypertensive effect of the peptides derived from casein by an extracellular proteinase from *Lactobacillus helveticus*. J. Dairy Sci. *77* (4), 917–922.

YOSHIKAWA, M., SASAKI, M. and CHIBA, H. 1992. Bioactive Peptides and Their Salt, Jpn. Kokai Tokkyo Koho JP 04, 154, 798.

ZHANG, R.Z., LIU, S.T., CHEN, R.M., LI, J.C., LI, L. and RAO, P.F. 1996. Isolation and identification of substances with angiotensin converting enzyme inhibitory activity in Fujian rice wine. J. Fuzhou University (Natural Science) *24* (6), 114–118.

A STUDY OF PROTEINS IN PIDAN (CHINESE EGGS)

RONG-ZHEN ZHANG, SHU-TAO LIU, LONG LI, RU-MING CHEN,
BI-HONG SHI, WEN-HONG GAO, GONG-RUI CHEN,
YU-QIANG ZHENG and PING-FAN RAO

Institute of Biotechnology
Fuzhou University
Fuzhou, Fujian, 350002, P.R. China

ABSTRACT

Egg proteins in pidan, a traditional Chinese processed duck egg product, were investigated by SDS-PAGE and amino acid analysis. It was shown that almost all the proteins in both egg white and yolk of duck egg were hydrolyzed by alkali into small peptides, with only a small portion of free amino acids. Contents of four amino acids were found to decrease as the result of degradation by alkaline hydrolysis processing. Up to 80% of cystine or cysteine in duck egg was destroyed, resulting in the characteristic flavor and texture of pidan.

INTRODUCTION

Pidan, a traditional processed egg product in China, is prepared by incubating fresh duck eggs with a slurry consisting of lime, soda, salt, tea and water. It is very much favored by Chinese for its unique flavor and texture.

Because of strong alkaline substances used in processing, the physical and chemical properties of egg proteins have been completely changed. Egg white becomes gellified with dark color, while egg yolk turns a dark color as well as having a strong thiol smell. Needless to say, it is extremely important to investigate these changes in terms of nutritional evaluation of pidan or product quality control in manufacturing practice.

The most plausible tentative theory for pidan processing attributes and unique characteristics is a result of alkaline hydrolysis by sodium hydroxide, which is a product of reaction between lime and soda. Proteins in egg white and yolk are in part hydrolyzed by sodium hydroxide to amino acids, and thiol amino acids are further degraded into ammonia and sulfur constituting the unique smell and flavor of pidan. This is a reduction based on well known biochemical principles, and experimental confirmation is necessary to complete a convincing theory for pidan processing.

In this work, pidan proteins were studied by sodium dodecyl sulfate-polyacrylamide gel electrophoresis (SDS-PAGE), amino acid analysis and protein quantification in comparison with proteins in fresh duck egg.

EXPERIMENTAL

Pretreatment of Samples

Egg White and Yolk of Pidan. Pidan was purchased from Taizhou Egg Processing Factory (Zhejiang, China) as a commercial product. After removing the egg shell, egg white and egg yolk were carefully separated and grounded. Ground egg white and egg yolk were then homogenized with an FG-101A electric grinder (Shanghai, China). Homogenized pidan egg white and yolk were used as egg white sample and yolk sample throughout this work.

Fresh Egg White and Yolk of Duck Egg. Fresh duck eggs were purchased from the grocery store. Egg white and yolk were carefully separated and homogenized to make the samples for further investigation.

Protein Quantification by Semi-Micro-Kjeldahl Method

Protein quantification was carried out with all four egg samples on a modified Kjeldahl apparatus according to the method by Huang (1989).

SDS-PAGE

SDS-PAGE was conducted according to the method of Laemmli (1970) on a Bio-Rad Mini-PROTEIN II electrophoretic apparatus (CA, USA). Constant voltage of 100 V was applied in this work, and the gel was stained with Coomassie Brilliant-Blue G-250 purchased from Sino-American Biotechnology Company (Luo-yang, China). The stacking gel and separation gel were 4% and 15%, respectively. Electrophoretic samples of fresh duck egg white and yolk were prepared from homogenized duck egg white and yolk samples. Appropriate amounts of the samples were first heated in test tubes with 0.1% SDS, 1,4-dithiotheitol (DTT) and distilled water at 100°C for 3 min. The mixture was then centrifuged at 4,000 rpm for 5 min to remove the precipitate. The sample for electrophoretic analysis was prepared by adding an appropriate amount of Phenol Blue and glyceride to the supernatant. Pidan egg white and yolk samples were prepared much the same way except that the prepared pidan samples were first subjected to overnight dialysis before being dissolved in 0.1% SDS solution.

Amino Acid Analysis

After hydrolysis with 6 N HCl at 110°C and removal of HCl, amino acid analysis was conducted on the homogenized pidan egg white and yolk, as well as the homogenized fresh duck egg white and yolk with a Shimazu 835-50 Amino Acid Analyzer (Tokyo, Japan).

RESULTS AND DISCUSSION

Protein Quantification

The results of semi-micro-Kjeldahl protein quantification of pidan egg white and yolk as well as fresh duck egg white and yolk are 19.0, 14.3, 12.1 and 18.0%, respectively. Protein concentration in egg white increased as a result of pidan processing while that in the yolk decreased. This result is in good accord with the previously reported study (Gao 1991). It can be attributed to the movement of egg white water into both egg yolk and outside slurry due to diffusion, resulting in decrease of water content in the egg white and increase in the egg yolk.

SDS-PAGE

SDS-PAGE patterns of the four samples are shown in Fig. 1 and 2. Four protein molecular weight markers were included in both figures. They were lysozyme (LYS), carbonic anhydrase (CA), chicken egg white ovalbumin (OVA) and bovine serum albumin (BSA), corresponding to molecular weights of 14.3, 29.0, 45.0 and 68.0 KDa.

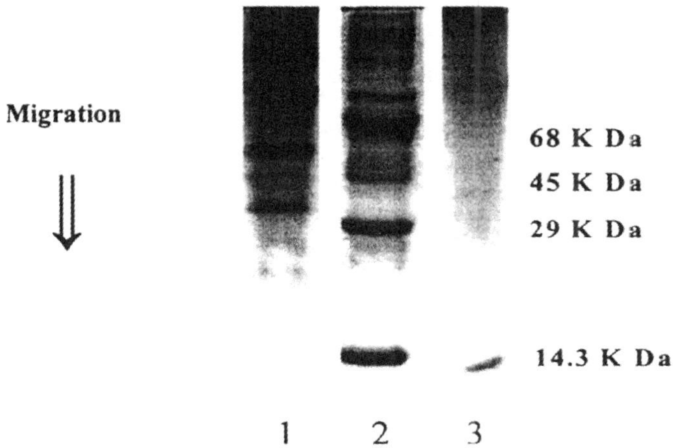

FIG. 1. ELECTROPHORETIC PATTERN OF PIDAN AND FRESH DUCK EGG YOLK
Electrophoresis condition was described in the Experimental Section. 1, 2, and 3 were pidan yolk, standard proteins and fresh yolk, respectively.
Migration direction was from top to bottom.

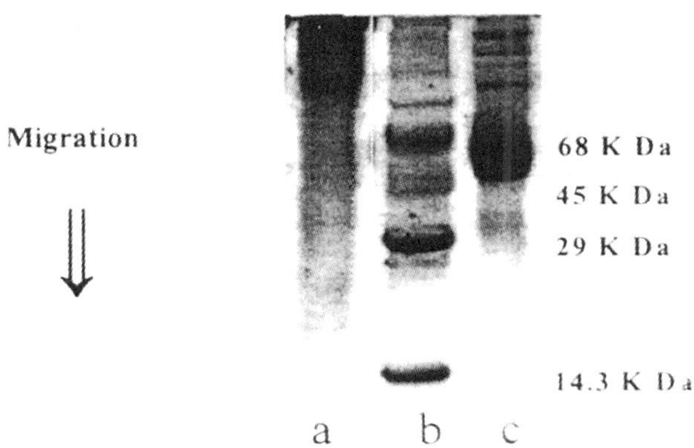

FIG. 2. ELECTROPHORETIC PATTERN OF PIDAN AND FRESH DUCK EGG WHITE
Electrophoresis condition was described in the Experimental Section. a, b, c were fresh egg white, standard proteins and pidan white, respectively.
Migration direction was from top to bottom.

Molecular weight of each protein band was determined from a standard plot of logarithm of molecular weight against their migration rate for the standard proteins. Listed in Table 1 are molecular weights of the protein bands present in the fresh duck egg yolk.

TABLE 1.
PROTEIN BANDS OF DUCK EGG YOLK

Location	Quantity of Protein Bands	Molecular Weight (KDa)
Above BSA	10	122.7, 120.6, 106.5, 99.9, 95.7, 92.1, 87.7, 76.6, 73.1
Between BSA and OVA	3	66.2, 63.7, 52.1
Between OVA and LYS	3	44.7, 42.1, 34.8

The only protein bands left in pidan egg yolk were the one above the BSA band and the one below the LYS band, corresponding to 76.6 KDa and 10.0 KDa (Fig. 1). The latter band apparently represents a product of degradation of a larger protein, since no corresponding band was observed in the electrophoretic pattern of the fresh duck egg yolk. As to the 76.6 kDa band, there seems to be a corresponding band in the electrophoretic patterns of the fresh duck egg white. If these two bands really represent the same protein, it could be a protein with amazingly strong resistance to alkaline degradation.

Listed in Table 2 are the molecular weights of protein bands present in fresh duck egg white sample. Basically, no protein bands are discernable with the pidan egg white sample.

TABLE 2.
PROTEIN BANDS OF DUCK EGG WHITE

location	Quantity of Protein Bands	Molecular Weight (KDa)
Above BSA	5	138.0, 125.9, 120.8, 112.0, 105.7
Between BSA and OVA	1	55.0
Between OVA and LYS	1	34.7

It can be concluded based on Fig. 1 and 2 that most duck egg proteins have been degraded into peptides of small molecular weights as a result of pidan processing.

Amino Acid Analysis

The results of amino acid content determination of pidan egg white and yolk are listed together with the fresh duck egg white and yolk in Table 3.

TABLE 3.
AMINO ACID ANALYSIS RESULTS OF EGG WHITE AND YOLK IN FRESH DUCK EGG AND PIDAN

Amino Acid	Sample							
	Fresh duck Egg				Pidan			
	Egg White		Egg Yolk		Egg White		Egg Yolk	
	Content W/V (g/100 ml)	Percentage (%)	Content W/W (g/100 g)	Percentage (%)	Content W/W (g/100 g)	Percentage (%)	Content W/W (g/100 g)	Percentage (%)
Asparagine	1.2616	9.57	1.4267	9.50	1.5485	10.10	1.1059	11.02
Threonine	0.8158	6.19	0.8340	5.56	0.9392	6.10	0.6389	5.85
Serine	1.0306	7.82	1.1712	7.81	1.1376	7.40	0.7288	6.67
Glutamic Acid	1.9479	14.78	2.4061	16.00	2.4931	16.28	1.6075	14.72
Proline	0.2169	1.65	0.2736	1.80	0.2862	1.87	0.2312	2.12
Glycine	0.4847	3.68	0.4840	3.20	0.5941	3.88	0.3784	3.46
Alanine	0.5964	4.53	0.7599	5.07	0.7469	4.88	0.5789	5.30
Cystine	0.3344	2.54	0.2264	1.51	0.0751	0.49	0.0562	0.51
Valine	0.7868	5.97	0.7907	5.27	0.9758	6.37	0.6447	5.90
Methionine	0.7707	5.85	0.4207	2.80	0.9470	6.19	0.3863	3.54
Isoleucine	0.7028	5.33	0.7911	5.27	0.8979	5.86	0.6508	5.96
Leucine	1.1049	8.39	1.3143	8.76	1.3195	8.60	1.0193	9.30
Tyrosine	0.5284	4.01	0.6175	4.10	0.6455	4.20	0.4661	4.27
Phenylalanine	0.6825	5.18	0.4618	3.08	0.7751	5.06	0.3662	3.35
Lysine	0.7078	5.37	0.9631	6.40	0.6649	4.34	0.5999	5.49
Tryptophan				ND[1]				
Histidine	0.3019	2.29	0.4733	3.16	0.3871	2.53	0.3392	3.11
Arginine	0.9019	6.85	1.5867	10.60	0.8773	5.73	1.1259	10.31
Total	13.176[2]	100	15.001	100	15.311	100	10.924	100

[1] Tryptophan was destroyed in the course of sample acid hydrolysis, so no data are shown on tryptophan

[2] Density of fresh duck egg white was determined to be 1.05 g/ml, so content (w/w) in fresh duck egg white was set as 13.176 g/100 g

Most amino acids exhibit the same content variation in egg white and egg yolk in comparison with those in the fresh egg except for glutamic acid, threonine, phenylalanine and histidine, and the content change was more radical in egg white than in egg yolk. Contents of more than 10 amino acids were found to have increased in pidan egg white and yolk from the fresh egg white and yolk. Increase of glycine and alanine may be attributed to alkaline degradation of serine and cystine (Walsh *et al.* 1979). Among amino acids exhibiting content decrease, two were basic amino acids: lysine and arginine, and the cystine content decreased to 1/5 and 1/3 in egg white and egg yolk, respectively. Mechanism of alkaline degradation of cystine and cysteine has been elucidated (Walsh *et al.* 1979) and sulfur and lanthionine are identified among the products. Apparently, the sulfur and the reaction products of sulfur with metallic ions present are the major chemicals attributing the special smell, color and patterns of the gel to pidan.

The total amino acid content obtained from amino acid analysis represents the total protein content, which is listed in Table 4 in comparison with the data obtained by semi-micro Kjeldahl quantification. As is clear from Table 4, while there is no remarkable difference in protein content values determined by the two methods, the value obtained by Kjeldahl quantification for pidan egg is much greater than the value obtained by amino acid analysis, indicating that duck egg proteins have not only been degraded to peptides and amino acids but also into other nitrogen-containing substances.

TABLE 4.
COMPARISON OF TOTAL PROTEIN CONTENT OBTAINED BY AMINO ACID ANALYSIS WITH THE DATA OBTAINED BY SEMI–MICRO KJELDAHL QUANTIFICATION

	fresh white	pidan white	fresh yolk	pidan yolk
Kjeldahl quantification	12.1%	19.0%	18.0%	14.3%
amino acid analysis	12.5%	15.3%	15.0%	10.9%

One concern arises for the food nutritive value of pidan, which has undergone radical processing such as alkaline hydrolysis. Racemization of amino acids by alkaline hydrolysis of protein causes half of the total generated amino acids to be unusable by humans, while some amino acids are destroyed by alkaline hydrolysis. Fortunately, as shown in Table 3, only a few amino acids decreased by 5-80%, and SDS-PAGE data suggest that the greatest portion of protein was hydrolyzed into peptides, and only a small portion to free amino acids. Although pidan processing somewhat affects the duck egg original nutritional value, it is not serious. On the other hand, complete cleavage of duck proteins in pidan egg not only generate the unique flavor, but also can possibly improve its digestion and lower the risk of duck egg as a source of food allergies.

SUMMARY

Preliminary investigation on proteins of pidan shows that almost all the proteins in both egg white and yolk of duck egg were hydrolyzed into small peptides, with a small portion further hydrolyzed into free amino acids. Among four amino acids whose contents decreased by alkaline hydrolysis during pidan processing, cystine/cysteine were the most destroyed, resulting in the characteristic flavor and texture of pidan.

REFERENCES

GAO, Z. 1991. Egg Product Technology. Commercial Publication Co., Beijing, China, pp. 134–163.

HUANG, W.S. 1989. Foodstuff Identification and Analysis (Chinese). Light Industry Publication Company, Beijing, China, pp. 51–53.

LAEMMLI, U.K. 1970. Cleavage of structural protein during the assembly of the head of bacteriophage T_4. Nature *227*, 680.

WALSH, R.G., NASHEF, A.S. and FEENEY, R.E. 1979. Intramolecular cross-linking of proteins by formation of lysinoalanine or lanthionine. Modification of disulfides in ovomucoids. Int. J. Pept. Prot. Res. *14*, 290–295.

HPLC DETERMINATION OF CHOLIC ACID BINDING TO PROTEIN ON TSK G3000SW COLUMN

YU-QIANG ZHENG, LONG LI, LI NI, JIAN-CAI LI, RONG-ZHEN ZHANG, SHU-TAO LIU, RU-MING CHEN, BI-HONG SHI, WEN-HONG GAO, GONG-RUI CHEN and PING-FAN RAO

Institute of Biotechnology, Fuzhou University
523 Gong-Ye Road, Fuzhou, Fujian, 350002
P.R. China

ABSTRACT

One of the proposed mechanisms for hypocholesterolemic effect of soy protein is the enhancement of bile acids excretion due to their binding to soy proteins. Removal of bile acids by the binding lowers cholesterol level directly by interrupting enterohepatic circulation in which bile acids are converted into cholesterol, and results in shift of hepatic cholesterol metabolism to provide cholesterol for enhanced bile acid synthesis. This consequently leads to increased removal of cholesterol from the blood. Evidence shows a correlation between binding capacity of proteins to bile acids and the hypocholesterolemic effect.

The current method to determine bile salts binding to proteins is equilibrium dialysis with combination of bile salts quantification by scintillation counter. It is not only tedious and time-consuming but also with poor reproducibility. The method is even more complicated by the employment of isotopes for bile acid quantification.

Described in this paper is a simple method of determining sodium deoxycholate binding to proteins using high performance liquid chromatography. The method can be applied to determine sodium deoxycholate binding to both water-soluble and water-insoluble protein and peptides. Binding equilibrium is attained in the process of the gel chromatography on a TSK 300SW column, and sodium deoxycholate is quantified by a differential refractometer. A typical run of this method can be completed in 2 h with a reproducibility of ± 1.0%.

INTRODUCTION

One of the proposed mechanisms for hypocholesterolemic effect of soy protein is the enhancement of bile acids excretion due to their binding to soy proteins (Potter 1995). Removal of bile acids by the binding lowers cholesterol level directly by interrupting enterohepatic circulation in which bile acids are converted into cholesterol, and results in shift of hepatic cholesterol metabolism to provide cholesterol for enhanced bile acid synthesis; this consequently leads to increased removal of cholesterol from the blood. Evidence shows a correlation between binding capacity of proteins to bile acids and the hypocholesterolemic effect (Markino *et al.* 1988).

The current method to determine bile salts binding to proteins is equilibrium dialysis with combination of bile salts quantitation by scintillation counter (Iwami *et al.* 1986).

It is not only tedious and time-consuming but also has poor reproducibility. The method is even further complicated by the employment of isotopes for bile acid quantitation.

Gel chromatography is very useful in studying the interaction between large molecules such as proteins and small molecules such as surfactants. High performance gel chromatography (HPGC) is used to determine the binding of sodium dodecyl sulfate to proteins, in which binding equilibrium and quantitation of binding can be attained in the same chromatographic run (Rao and Takagi 1988). Compared with the traditional dialysis binding equilibrium, binding determination by HPGC is not only much more efficient but also precise and reliable.

Based on similar principles, a simple method to determine the binding of deoxycholate proteins is developed in this work in order to provide a more convenient and efficient tool to study sodium deoxycholate (SDC) binding to proteins and peptides.

EXPERIMENTAL

This new method consists of two major steps: 1. calibration of a precisely known SDC concentration with the SDC peak area on a chromatogram of HPGC obtained by a differential refractometer; 2. equilibration of SDC binding to the protein against the elution buffer quantitation of SDC by high performance gel chromatography. In this work SDC binding to bovine serum albumin in 0.01 M sodium phosphate buffer, pH 7.0, with various SDC concentrations was determined.

Sodium phosphate buffer (0.01 M), pH 7.0, was prepared and used throughout the whole work as a starting buffer for other solutions. The elution buffer for HPLC was prepared by adding precisely weighed SDC to the above phosphate buffer according to the equilibrium SDC concentration required, which was 0.3-3 mM.

Standard SDC solution was prepared by adding precisely weighed SDC to the elution buffer to create a 3 mM SDC solution.

Samples for SDC calibration were prepared by diluting the standard SDC solution with the elution buffer to make 0.1-3 mM SDC in the elution buffer.

Samples for binding determination were prepared by adding about 0.2 g BSA into 3 ml of the standard SDC solution, and incubating at 37°C for 1 h. BSA concentration was determined by a Lambda Bio10 UV-VIS Spectrophotometer (Perkin-Elmer, U.S.A.) assuming an absorbance of a 1% solution at 280 nm with 1 cm optical length to be 6.78.

Both standard SDC solution and BSA sample were subject to high performance gel chromatography on a 0.75 × 15 cm TSK3000SW (Tosoh, Japan) column using a CCPD 8000 HPLC pump (Tosoh, Japan) connected with a RI8000 differential refractometer (Toshoh, Japan). SDC binding to BSA was determined by the SDC peak height difference on the chromatograms of the standard SDC solution and BSA solution.

HPGC was conducted at 37°C at a flow rate of 1.0 ml/min; the sample loop used was 10 μl. Other conditions are shown in the legend of the related figures.

Sodium deoxycholate of biochemical reagent grade was purchased from Shanghai Biotech Co. (Shanghai, China), bovine serum albumin was a product of Shanghai Dongfeng Biotech Co. (Shanghai, China). All the other chemical reagents used were analytical purity grade.

RESULTS AND DISCUSSION

Typical chromatograms of a standard SDC solution and SDC-BSA binding sample are shown in Fig. 1. SDC was eluted as a sharp peak at the total liquid volume of the column as is shown in Fig. 1A. In Fig. 1B, widely separated bovine serum albumin and SDC peaks are both sharp and the baseline is stable, suggesting completeness of a rapid binding equilibrium in the course of chromatographic run within 10 min. The SDC peak is remarkably lower than that in Fig. 1A because of SDC binding to BSA. As is clear from Fig. 2, SDC peak height correlated linearly and strictly to SDC concentration. The strict linearity and the passage through the origin of the plot indicate that the gel media have no affinity to SDC and the feasibility of calibration of SDC peak against its concentration with a single standard SDC solution sample.

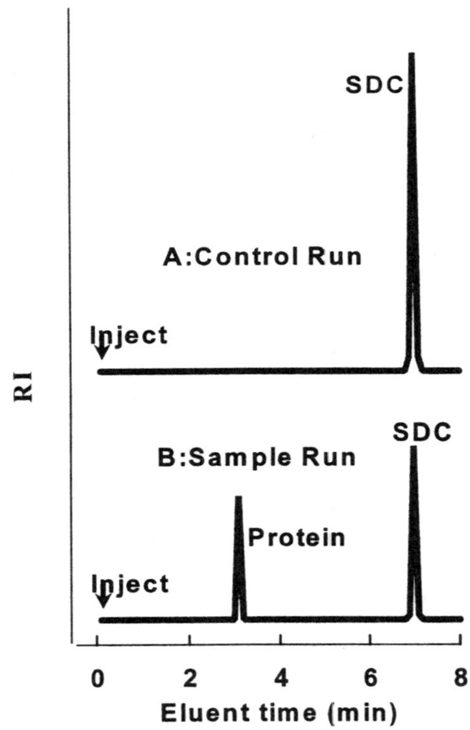

FIG. 1. CHROMATOGRAPHIC PATTERN OF BSA AND SDC
Experimental conditions: column: 0.75 × 15 cm TSK-G3000SW; mobile phase: 0.01 M sodium phosphate buffer, pH 7.0, with various SDC concentrations; flow rate: 1.0 ml/min; temperature: 37°C; sample loop: 10 μl; monitor: RI8000 differential refractometer.

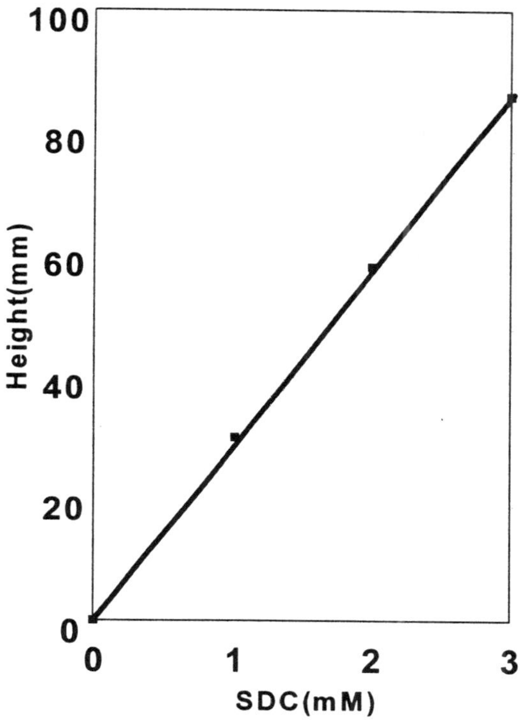

FIG. 2. PLOT OF THE PEAK HEIGHT OF THE SDC PEAK DETECTED WITH RI DETECTOR AGAINST THE CONCENTRATION OF SDC

Comparing Fig. 1A with Fig. 1B, it is clear that when BSA was added into the standard SDC solution, the SDC peak on the chromatogram of Fig. 1B was remarkably reduced due to SDC binding to BSA. Apparently, the difference of the SDC peak height in the two chromatograms represents the amount of SDC bound to BSA. The amount of SDC bound to BSA, D (SDC/g protein) can be easily calculated according to the following equation:

$$D = (H_0\text{-}H)\ C_0/(H_0C) \qquad (1)$$

where H_0 is the height of the SDC peak in the standard SDC run, H is the height in the sample run, C_0 is the SDC concentration of the standard SDC solution, and the C is BSA concentration in the sample run.

In spite of the great difference in mechanism of binding of SDS with BSA from that of SDC with BSA, binding equilibrium can all be attained rapidly by gel chromatography in both cases. This new method, therefore, is an extension or development of the HPLC determination of SDS binding to BSA (Rao and Takagi 1988).

With an excellent reproducibility of chromatogram on TSK G3000SW column a typical SDC binding determination which consists of a standard SDC solution run and an SDC-BSA binding sample run can be completed with ease within 20 min. In comparison with the reported methods of SDC binding determination such as equilibrium dialysis, scintillation, selective electrode and ultracentrifuge, this is not only convenient, but the accuracy has also been greatly improved.

As an application example of this method, a SDC binding isotherm with BSA was determined, as shown in Fig. 3. As the equilibrium SDC concentration increases, the binding of SDC with BSA increases accordingly, which is basically consistent with a SDC binding isotherm obtained by gel chromatography on a Sephadex G-150 column to achieve binding equilibrium in combination with quantitation by isotope scintillation (Markino *et al.* 1973).

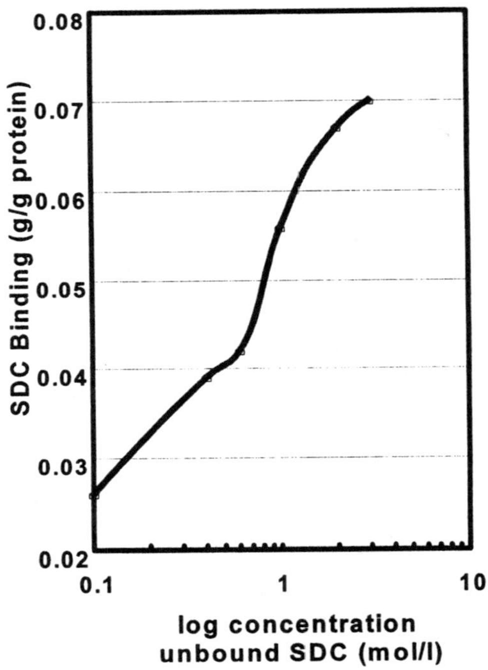

FIG. 3. BINDING OF SDC TO BSA AT 37°C

REFERENCES

IWAMI, K., SAKAKIBARA, K. and IBUKI, F. 1986. Involvement of post-digestion hydrophobic peptides in plasma cholesterol-lowering effect of dietary plant proteins. Agric. Biol. Chem. *50*(5), 1217–1222.

MARKINO, S., NAKASHIMA, H., MINAMI, K., MORIYAMA, R. and TAKAO, S. 1988. Bile acid-binding protein from soybean seed: Isolation, partial characterization and insulin-stimulating activity. Agric. Biol. Chem *52* (3), 801–809.

MARKINO, S., REYNOLDS, J.A. and TANFORD, C. 1973. The binding of deoxycholate and Triton X-100 to proteins. J. Biol. Chem. *248* (14), 4926–4932.

POTTER, S.M. 1995. Soy and cholesterol reduction: Hypothesized mechanisms: Overview of proposed mechanisms for the hypocholesterolemic effect of soy. J. Nutr. *125*, 606S–611S.

RAO, P.F. and TAKAGI, T. 1988. Differential refractometric determination of binding of sodium dodecyl sulfate to protein using high-performance gel chromatography. Anal. Biochem. *174*, 251–256.

IMPROVED METHODS FOR THE SEPARATION AND PURIFICATION OF IMMUNOGLOBULIN FROM EGG YOLK BY FILTRATION AND ONE STEP ANION-EXCHANGE CHROMATOGRAPHY

JIAN-CAI LI, TIAN-BAO CHEN, RONG-ZHEN ZHANG, RU-MING CHEN, LONG LI and PING-FAN RAO

Institute of Biotechnology, Fuzhou University
523 Gong-ye Road, 350002, Fuzhou, Fujian
P.R. China 350002

ABSTRACT

Reported in this paper is an improved method for isolation of antibodies by filtration and anion-exchange chromatography from egg yolk. Egg yolk was diluted 7 times with distilled water without pH adjustment and then frozen at -10°C. The frozen diluted egg yolk was then thawed at 15°C. Celite was added to the diluted egg yolk prior to filtration to facilitate the process. The diluted yolk solution was then filtered through cellulose acetate filters with pore size of 0.22 um at 15°C. An industrially feasible filtration velocity was achieved with the system, hundreds of times faster than reported data. A clear water-soluble fraction (WSF) contained approximately 15-18% by weight of antibodies compared to the weight of total proteins obtained. The WSF was then adjusted to contain 75 mM sodium phosphate buffer, pH 6.8, and applied to a DEAE-Toyopearl 650M column. The electrophoretically pure IgY was obtained in the eluate eluted with 150 mM sodium phosphate buffer, pH 6.8. It is a method most likely to be developed into a commercial scale process to produce IgY suitable for industrial applications in terms of cost and scale.

INTRODUCTION

The use of egg yolks as a source of antibodies provides a convenient and cost effective alternative to preparing polyclonal antibodies from mammals such as rabbits and goats. Advantages of egg yolk immunoglobulin (IgY) compared to mammalian IgG include greater specificity to mammalian antigens, lower cost and convenience of egg collection, and application for use in serological tests affected by rheumatoid factors. Some of the suggested potential uses of IgY in immunotherapy include fortification of infant formula (Shimizu *et al.* 1988), prevention of dental caries (Otake *et al.* 1991), protection of neonatal piglets against fatal enteric colibacillosis (Yokohama *et al.* 1992) and treatment of fish diseases (Hatta 1992), especially under conditions where use of antibiotics and other drugs may present a problem.

Although egg yolk has been recognized before as a convenient and inexpensive source of antibodies, IgY has not found widespread use as one might expect. This can apparently be attributed mostly to difficulties in IgY isolation from the yolk, especially separation of the water-soluble fraction (WSF) containing IgY from water-insoluble components (lipids and lipoproteins). It is an urgent task to establish a more efficient method of IgY isolation in terms of cost and scale before any meaningful industrial applications of IgY can be realized.

Several methods have been described for fractionation of WSF from water-insoluble components in egg yolk. Most of these methods used water dilution, followed by centrifugation or filtration, to achieve separation of WSF. Prior to centrifugation, there was usually a need to carry out precipitation of lipoproteins with polyethylene glycol (PEG) (Polson *et al.* 1985), sodium dextran sulfate (DS) (Jensenius *et al.* 1981), polysaccharide (Hatta *et al.* 1990; Shah and Singh 1992), or ethanol (Horikoshi *et al.* 1993). However, most of the published methods inevitably involve long ultracentrifugation time, repeated precipitation, and thus are difficult to scale-up. Moreover, they can not remove lipoproteins effectively. Direct filtration of the diluted yolk was not possible due to clogging of filtration media with mucous lipoproteins (Akita and Nakai 1992). In the simplest method of the reported ones for WSF separation, WSF is obtained by diafiltration of the freeze-thaw treated diluted egg yolk solution (Kim and Nakai 1996). Replacing processes such as centrifugation, polyelectrolyte precipitation or organic solvent precipitation, complete removal of lipids and lipoproteins is achieved with this direct filtration. Simple enough though, the method suffers from a fatal problem of excessive slowness of filtration, practically eliminating its prospects as a candidate for industrial scale process.

To isolate IgY from WSF, many kinds of chromatography have been used including DEAE-anion exchange chromatography (McCannel and Nakai 1990; Akita and Nakai 1992), gel-filtration (Hassl and Aspock 1988; Akita and Nakai 1992), and cation-exchange chromatography (Fichtali *et al.* 1992). Ultrafiltration (UF) was employed to fractionate WSF obtained by centrifugation and filtration of diluted yolk (Akita and Nakai 1992). Successful isolation of IgY, however, inevitably involves a combination of more than one chromatographic technique.

The objective of this work was to develop a simple system for WSF separation and IgY isolation, with a prospect of eventual development into an industrial scale process.

MATERIALS AND METHODS

Eggs were obtained from the local market and stored at 4-6°C. IgY used as a reference standard in electrophoresis was isolated according to the method of Horikoshi *et al.* (1993). All other chemicals were of analytical grade.

Egg yolk was separated from egg white and rolled on paper towels to remove adhering albumin. After removing its membrane, yolk was diluted with distilled water and adequately stirred at room temperature, the diluted yolk was frozen at various temperatures for a period of time, then thawed. Prior to filtration, celite was added to the diluted egg yolk to enhance the filtering speed. The diluted yolk was then filtered through cellulose acetate filters with pore size of 0.22 μm at 15°C. The protein content of delipidated WSF was measured by the method of Lowry *et al.* (1951); the total triglyceride content of WSF was determined according to the method of Bucolo and David (1973).

Anion-exchange chromatography was carried out on a DEAE-Toyopearl 650M (Tosho, Japan). Prior to isolation by chromatography, the WSF was adjusted to pH of 6.8 and a final molarity of 0.075 M sodium phosphate, then directly applied to the column equilibrated with 0.075 M sodium phosphate buffer, pH 6.8. The adsorbed proteins were eluted at 1.0 mL/min with 0.15 M sodium phosphate buffer, pH 6.8. The elution profile was monitored at 280 nm. The eluted peak was collected, then applied to SDS-PAGE for purity analysis.

Sodium dodecyl sulfate-polyacrylamide gel electrophoresis (SDS-PAGE) was carried out according to Laemmli (1970), on a separating gel of 10% acrylamide and 4% stacking gel using a Bio-Rad MINI-PROTEIN II Cell. Proteins were stained with 0.04% Coomassie brilliant blue G-250 in 40% ethanol and 10% acetic acid.

Recovery of separated immunoglobulin was calculated by comparing IgY content in the filtrated WSF and the eluted fraction by anion-exchange chromatography.

RESULTS AND DISCUSSION

Separation of Water Soluble Fraction from Yolk by Filtration

A colorless and transparent water soluble fraction (WSF) of egg yolk was obtained by filtration of the freeze-thaw treated diluted yolk solution. The lipid content of the WSF obtained was determined to be less than 1.2%, indicating satisfactory removal of lipid, while its protein concentration was determined to be 0.5%, equivalent to 80% recovery of the water-soluble proteins in egg yolk. Excellent WSF could be obtained by this method without addition of any chemical reagents but with the greatest operation convenience in comparison with other reported methods.

What is more important with this new method of WSF separation is that filtration velocity was very fast. With a filtration area of 10 cm^2, typical filtration time for 25 ml of 7-times diluted egg yolk solution was less than a min, only a tiny fraction of the filtration time required by the reported method of Kim and Nakai (1996), in which 50 ml of 10-times diluted yolk was diafiltrated through No. 52 filter paper with 200 ml of buffer at 1 ml/min. While it would be very difficult for the latter method to develop into an industrial application, possibility of preparation of WSF by filtration (our method) is very good with our new results.

The greatest difference between these two ways of filtration is that one is direct filtration and the other filtration with filter aid. Effect of celite addition to the suspension before filtration is shown in Fig. 1. Addition of filter aid is the most common practice to improve the filtration efficiency. Nevertheless, such a single practice has made an incredible difference to the outcome in at least three ways: 1. as stated above, filtration velocity has been increased by hundreds of times with a suspension pretreated very much the same way but with higher concentration; further investigation into the filtration properties should show even greater difference in the velocities since no dramatic decrease of filtration velocity was observed with increasing filtrate volume in this system; 2. requirements for the sample conditions are much lower, for example, thawing temperature of the diluted yolk can be much higher, to 15°C vs. 4-6°C at a wider pH range of pH 4-7 and lower dilution folds; 3. a layer of porous filter cake consisting of yolk granules and celite effectively prevents the mucous lipid materials in yolk from directly contacting with the membrane and blocking the pores of cellulose acetate membrane filters; this prevents the membrane from easy fouling. All these differences can be attributed to a great extent to the great difference between the filter cake consisting of solely yolk granules and of celite and the granules. The cake structure is impossible to be maintained with soft granules which are impervious to changes in the solution conditions, but addition of celite helps construct a solid, a chemically and physically stable framework for the cake.

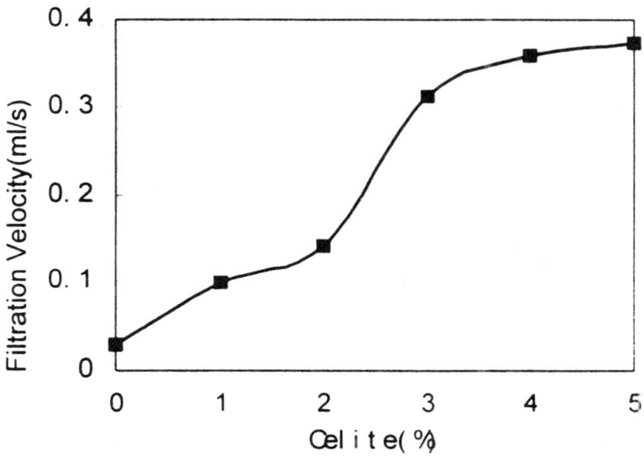

FIG. 1. EFFECT OF ADDITION OF CELITE ON THE FILTRATION SPEED

SDS-PAGE patterns of the obtained WSF are shown in Fig. 2 (lane 2). Antibodies are apparently one of the four major proteins detected in WSF. No evidence is available at present but further investigation is very likely to show that adsorption of some minor lipoprotein might help clear the protein patterns of WSF.

Based on our preliminary results, it can be concluded that filtration of the diluted yolk in the presence of the filter aid can be a very promising candidate for an industrial scale process to prepare WSF from egg yolk.

Isolation of IgY from WSF by DEAE-Toyopearl Anion-Exchange Chromatography

Only four protein bands were detected in the SDS-PAGE patterns, as is shown in Fig. 2 (lane 2). The proteins in the WSF include α-, β-, and γ-livetins with molecular weights of 80, 45, and 150 kD (Martin *et al.* 1957; Martin and Cook 1958) with a little almost indiscernible amount of low-density lipoproteins.

Shown in Fig. 3 is the anion-exchange chromatogram of the WSF on DEAE-Toyopearl 650M column. As is clear from the chromatogram, most proteins were not adsorbed to the column at 75 mM sodium phosphate buffer, pH 6.8. Only one peak was obtained from the column when the adsorbed protein was eluted with 0.15 M sodium phosphate buffer, pH 6.8. SDS-PAGE patterns of the fraction obtained are shown in Fig. 2 (lane 4), displaying a single IgY band, indicating that IgY was successfully isolated from the water-soluble fraction by a one-step anion-exchange chromatography to electrophoretic purity.

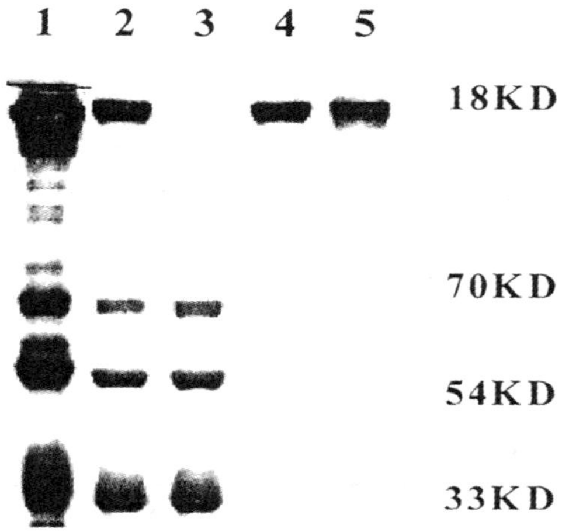

FIG. 2. SDS-PAGE PATTERNS OF IGY DURING THE SEPARATION PROCEDURE
Lane 1, egg yolk; Lane 2, WSF; Lane 3, fraction unbound to DEAE-Toyopearl 650M; Lane 4, fraction bound to DEAE-Toyopearl 650M; Lane 5, standard IgY

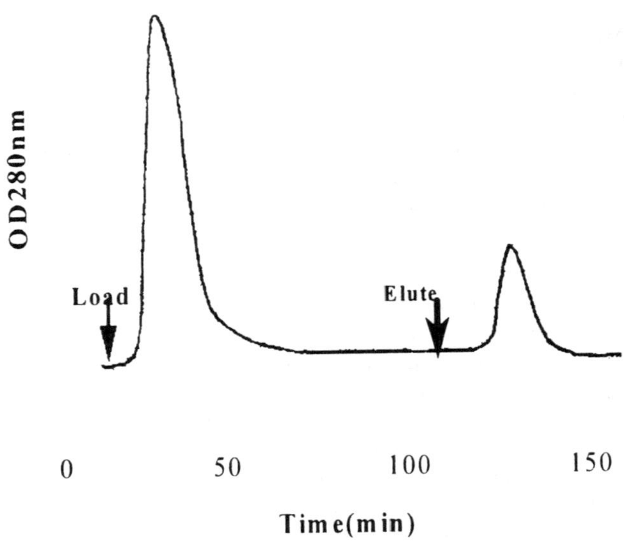

FIG. 3. DEAE ANION EXCHANGE CHROMATOGRAM OF WSF
Experimental Condition: column: DEAE-Toyopearl 650M (1.6 × 10 cm); starting buffer: 0.075 M phosphate buffer, pH 6.8; Eluting buffer: 0.15 M phosphate buffer, pH 6.8; flow rate: 1.0 ml/min; monitor wavelength: 280 nm

Although the WSF contains relatively few proteins, isolation of IgY from the WSF was performed only by a combination of several purification techniques in the previously reported studies. Prior to chromatography, the WSF is usually subjected to some other purification processes including salt precipitation, alcohol precipitation, utrafiltration, and so on. One-step isolation of IgY as demonstrated here has greatly simplified the procedure, and this process can easily be scaled-up since the medium performance anion-exchanger, DEAE-Toyopearl 650M is designed for commercial scale processes.

SDS-PAGE patterns of samples at the various stages of purification are shown in Fig. 2. The yield of IgY by one-step ion-exchange chromatography on DEAE-Toyopearl 650M column is estimated to be about 90-95%.

SUMMARY

A water soluble fraction (WSF) was efficiently separated from chicken egg yolk by filtration of freeze-thaw treated dilute yolk without adding any chemicals at a velocity possibly good enough for industrial scale production. IgY was isolated from the WSF with 90-95% recovery by a one-step anion exchange chromatography on a DEAE-Toyopearl 650M column. Combination of these two methods will possibly provide a complete solution to industrial scale preparation of low-cost IgY, which is the premise to industrial scale application of IgY.

REFERENCES

AKITA, E.M. and NAKAI, S. 1992. Immunoglobulins from egg yolk: Isolation and purification. J. Food Sci. *57,* 629–634.

BUCOLO, G. and DAVID, H. 1973. Quantitative determination of serum triglycerides by the use of enzymes. Clin. Chem. *19,* 476–482.

FICHTALI, J., CHARTER, E.A., LO, K.V. and NAKAI, S. 1992. Separation of egg yolk immunoglobulins using an automated liquid chromatography system. Biotechnol. Bioengin. *40,* 1388–1394.

HASSL, A. and ASPOCK, H. 1988. Purification of egg yolk immunoglobulins. A two step procedure using hydrophobic interaction chromatography and gel filtration. J. Immunol. Meth. *110,* 225–228.

HATTA, H., KIM, M. and YAMAMOTO, T. 1990. A novel isolation method for hen egg yolk antibody, "IgY". Agric. Biol. Chem. *54,* 2531–2535.

HATTA, H. 1992. Prevention of fish disease using egg yolk antibody (IgY). Presented at International Symposium on Non-Conventional Egg Uses and Newly Emerging Processing Technologies. Banff, Alberta, Canada. *April 23.*

HORIKOSHI, T., HIRAOKA, J., SAITO, M. and HAMADA, S. 1993. IgY antibody from hen egg yolks: Purification by ethanol fractionation. J. Food Sci. *58(4),* 739–742.

JENSEIUS, J.C., ANDERSEN, I., HAU, J., CROVE, M. and KOCH, C. 1981. Eggs: Conveniently packaged antibodies. Methods for purification of yolk IgG. J. Immunol. Methods *46,* 63–68.

KIM, H. and NAKAI, S. 1996. Immunoglobulin separation from egg yolk: A serial filtration system. J. Food Sci. *61,* 510–523.

LEAMMLI, U.K. 1970. Cleavage of structural protein during the assembly of the head of bacteriophage T4. Nature *227,* 680–685.

LOWRY, O.H., ROSEBROUGH, N., FARR, A. and RANDALL, J. 1951. Protein measurement with the Folin phenol reagent. J. Biol. Chem. *193,* 265–275.

MARTIN, W.G., VANDEGAER, J.E. and COOK, W.H. 1957. Fractionation of livetin and the molecular weights of the α- and β-components. Can. J. Biochem. Physiol. *35,* 241–250.

MARTIN, W.G. and COOK, W.H. 1958. Preparation and molecular weight of γ-livetin from egg yolk. Can. J. Biochem. Physiol. *36,* 153–160.

McCANNEL, A.A. and NAKAI, S. 1990. Separation of egg yolk immunoglobulins into subpopulations using DEAE-ion exchange chromatography. Can. Inst. Food Sci. Technol. J. *23,* 42–46.

OTAKE, S., NISHIHARA, Y., MAKIMURA, M., HATTA, H., KIM, M., YAMAMOTO, T. and HIRASAWS, M. 1991. Protection of rats against dental caries by passive immunization with hen-yolk antibody (IgY). J. Dent. Res. *70,* 162–166.

POLSON, A., COETZER, T., KRUGAR, J., von MALTZAHN, E. and VAN DER MERWE, K.J. 1985. Improvements in the isolation of IgY from the yolk of eggs laid by immunized hen. Immunol. Invest. *14,* 323–327.

SHAH, B.B. and SINGH, R.K. 1992. Separation of egg yolk proteins and lipids with carboxymethyl cellulose. J. Food Process. Preserv. *16,* 257–288.

SHIMIZU, M., FITZSIMMONS, R.C. and NAKAI, S. 1988. Anti-*E. coli* immunoglobulin Y isolated from egg yolk of immunized chickens as a potential food ingredient. J. Food Sci. *53(5),* 1360–1366.

YOKOHAMA, H., PERALTA, R.C., DIAZ, R., SENDO, S., IKEMORI, Y. and KODAMA, Y. 1992. Passive protective effect of chicken egg immunoglobulins against experimental enterotoxigenic *Escherichia coli* infection in neonatal piglets. Infect. Immun. *60,* 998–1007.

ISOLATION AND CHARACTERIZATION OF A PROTEASE FROM CHINESE FISH SAUCE MATERIAL, *ENGRAULIS JAPONICUS*

CHUN-JIAN HUANG, SHAO-YUN WANG, HONG FU, JIAN-CAI LI, SHU-TAO LIU, RONG-ZHEN ZHANG, RU-MING CHEN, LONG LI, PING-FAN RAO

Institute of Biotechnology, Fuzhou University
523 Gong-ye Road, Fuzhou, Fujian
350002 P.R. China

ABSTRACT

Activity of an alkaline protease was detected from the muscle of a Chinese fish sauce material, Engraulis Japonicus. *Soluble proteins and enzymes of the ground fish muscle were extracted with 0.5% KCl, and fractionated by DEAE-ion-exchange chromatography and gel chromatography to obtain electrophoretically pure protease with a molecular weight of 39,000 as estimated by SDS-PAGE, and an isoelectric point (pI) of pI 5.6. The optimum temperature and pH of protease activity were 60°C and pH 8.0, respectively.*

INTRODUCTION

Fish sauce has been one of major condiments in China for more than 2,500 years, especially in the coastal areas. The manufacturing procedure remains basically the same all these years among most Chinese fish sauce manufacturers. It is natural fermentation, in which fresh fish is suspended in a high concentration brine and kept outdoors for 2-3 years before the extraction can be collected as fish sauce. Efforts have been made by a few manufacturers to accelerate the process by keeping fish autolysis in an incubator rather than a simple container in the outdoors. The processing period has been remarkably shortened to about 1 month. One of the major improved practices is the usage of *Engraulis Japonicus* extract. *E. Japonicus,* one of the most commonly used sea fish for fish sauce, is incubated at 50-60°C for hours and the extract is added to the incubator as starter. This practice has been in use for more than 2 decades but its mechanism has never been elucidated.

On the other hand, a large volume of studies on protease in fish muscle has been reported. Protease isolated from fish has found its applications as rennet substitutes and fish sauce processing (Haard *et al.* 1990; Wasson 1992).

As the first step to modernize traditional Chinese fish sauce production, a protease in *E. Japonicus* muscle was investigated in this work.

EXPERIMENTAL

Extraction of Soluble Protease from Muscle of *Engraulis Japonicus*

Fifty (50) grams of fresh *E. Japonicus* muscle was ground and crude proteins were extracted with different solutions and different volume proportions, by stirring for 4 min with an electric stirrer. After standing 60 min, the mixture was centrifuged at 10,000 × g for 30 min. The supernatant was collected, and protease activity was determined. The supernatant with the highest protease activity was used as the crude protease extract sample for further separation on ion-exchange chromatography.

Protease Activity Determination. This was determined by the method of Lowry *et al.* (1951).

Anion-Exchange Chromatography. Chromatography was carried out on a DEAE-Toyopearl 650M (Tosho, Japan) column. The column (1.6 × 10 cm) was equilibrated with the starting buffer of 0.02 M sodium phosphate buffer, pH 6.8. The crude protein extract was adjusted to contain the same buffer concentration as the starting buffer of the column and applied to the column followed by washing with 3 column volumes of the starting buffer. Adsorbed proteins were eluted at 1.0 mL/min with a linear gradient of NaCl from 200 mL starting buffer and 200 mL starting buffer containing 1.0 M NaCl. The elution profile was monitored at 280 nm with a UV-monitor (Zhejiang, China) and collected in 3 ml fractions by a DSJ fraction collector. Protease activity of each fraction was determined and analyzed by SDS-PAGE.

Gel Chromatography

The fractions with high protease activity from ion-exchange chromatography were pooled and concentrated with polyethylene glycol and further fractionated by gel chromatography using a Sephacryl S200 (Phamacia LKB, Uppsala, Sweden) as media. One mL of the concentrated sample was applied to the column (1.5 × 60 cm) equilibrated with the same buffer. The eluate was monitored at 280 nm and collected.

SDS-PAGE

Sodium dodecyl sulfate-polyacrylamide gel electrophoresis (SDS-PAGE) was carried out according to Laemmli (1970), on a separating gel and a stacking gel containing 12.5% and 4% acrylamide, respectively. A constant voltage of 100 V was applied. Protein were stained with 0.04% Coomassie brilliant blue G-250 (Sigma, St, Louis, MO) in 40% ethanol and 10% acetic acid.

RESULTS AND DISCUSSION

Extraction of Protease from *Engraulis Japonicus* Muscle

Effects of different extraction solution on the yield of proteolytic activity is shown in Table 1. The highest yield of enzymatic activity was obtained at a relatively low salt concentration (0.5% KCl), a typical property of alkaline protease with maximum solubilization in 0.5% KCl (Bonete *et al.* 1984). About 1970 units activity were recovered from 1 gram of fresh *E. Japonicus* muscle.

Fractionation of Crude Protease Extract on DEAE Ion-Exchange Chromatography

Most proteins were not adsorbed when the crude protease sample was loaded onto a DEAE-Toyopearl 650M column. Figure 1 shows the elution pattern of the adsorbed proteins from the DEAE-Toyopearl 650M column with a linear salt gradient, as well as the protease activity of each fraction. The adsorbed proteins were fractionated into two peaks. Protease activity was detected only in the first peak (P1).

TABLE 1.
EFFECTS OF DIFFERENT EXTRACTION MEDIA ON ISOLATION OF EJ PROTEASE

Extracted solution	Protein content (mg/mL)	Specific activity (units/mg)[1]	Activity yield (units/g)[2]
0.5% KCl	6.13	402	1971
0.2 M KCl	7.50	260	1560
0.05 M phosphate buffer (pH7.2)	8.44	142	959
0.05 M phosphate buffer + 0.5% KCl (pH7.2)	8.41	223	1500
0.05 M phosphate buffer + 0.2M KCl (pH7.2)	9.00	194	1390
0.05 M Tris-HCl (pH7.2)	5.70	266	1213
0.05 M Tris-HCl + 0.5% KCl(pH7.2)	8.10	197	1277
0.05 M Tris-HCl + 0.2 M KCl(pH7.2)	8.60	148	1018

[1] EJ Protease activity was measured as nanomoles of tyrosine liberated per hour.
[2] Activity yield per gram of fresh *Engraulis Japonicus* muscle.

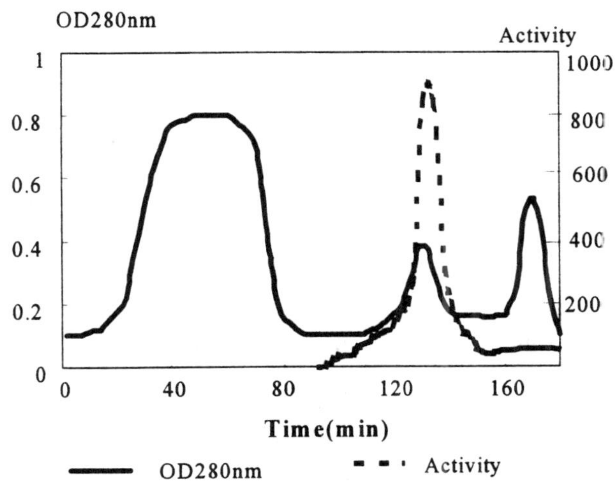

FIG. 1. DEAE ION-EXCHANGE CHROMATOGRAM OF THE EXTRACTED SUPERNATANT
Conditions: column, DEAE-Toyopearl 650M column (1.6 × 10 cm); Eluent, a linear gradient of NaCl from starting buffer (0.02 M sodium phosphate buffer, pH 6.8) and starting buffer containing 1.0 M NaCl; flow rate, 0.1 mL/min; detector, UV-280 nm.

Purification of Protease by Gel Chromatography

Fractions of the P1 in Fig. 1 were pooled and concentrated with polyethylene glycol. The gel chromatographic pattern of the concentrated P1 sample on an Sephacryl S200 column is shown in Fig. 2, and the protease activity of each collected fraction is shown in the same figure. As is clear from Fig. 2, P1 was fractionated into three peaks, and the third peak exhibited the highest protease activity.

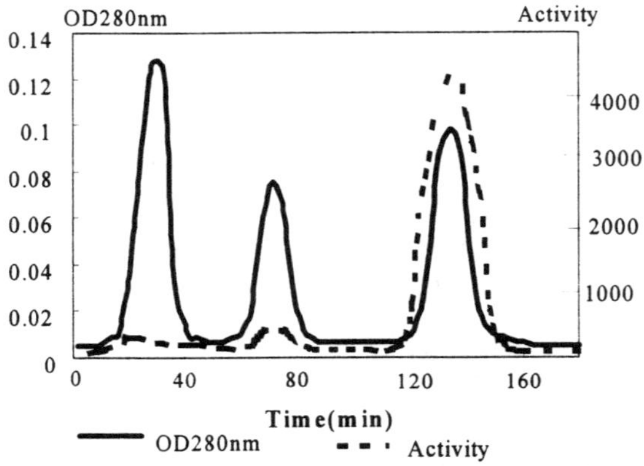

FIG. 2. SEPHACRYL S200 GEL CHROMATOGRAM OF THE SAMPLE CONTAINING EJM-PROTEASE OBTAINED FROM DEAE ION-EXCHANGE CHROMATOGRAPHY
Conditions: column, Sephacryl S200 column (1.5 × 60 cm); eluent, 0.02 M phosphate buffer, pH 6.8; flow rate, 0.1 mL/min; detector, UV-280 nm.

SDS-PAGE electrophoretic patterns of each fraction with the highest protease activity obtained in every separation step are shown in Fig. 3. As shown in Fig. 3, most soluble proteins extracted from fresh *E. Japonicus* muscle were not adsorbed to the DEAE-Toyopearl 650M column. The electrophoretic patterns for the third peak obtained by gel chromatography of P1 gave a single band, corresponding to a molecular weight of 39 K, indicating the *E. Japonicus* protease obtained was of high purity.

The Optimum pH and Temperature of *E. Japonicus* Protease

The optimum pH and temperature of the protease obtained are shown in Fig. 4 and 5 to be pH 8.0 and 60°C, respectively.

Effect of heat treatment on the remaining activity of the purified protease is shown in Table 2. The data indicate good heat stability in comparison with the commercially available enzyme AS1.398 from *Bacillus subtilis* (Jiangsu, China).

Listed in Table 3 are properties of the Protease in comparison with some of the reported proteases from different fishes, including cathepsin B (Sherekar 1988), cathepsin D (Doke *et al.* 1980), and serine proteinase (Kimoto 1983). The optimum temperature is higher for the Protease than those from other fishes.

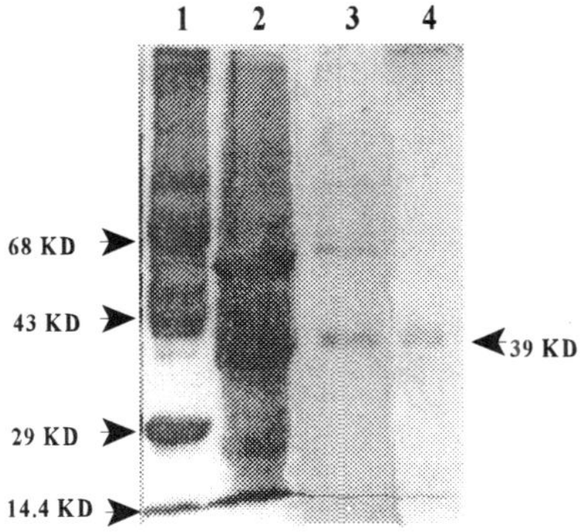

FIG. 3. THE SDS-PAGE PATTERN OF SAMPLES OF EVERY PURIFICATION STEP

Lane 1. Standard molecular mass markers: bovine serum albumin (68 KDa); ovalbumin (43KDa); carbonic anhydrase (29KDa); lysozyme (14.4 KDa);

Lane 2. The supernatant extracted by 0.5% KCl;

Lane 3. The first peak obtained by ion-exchange chromatography;

Lane 4. The third peak separated by gel chromatography.

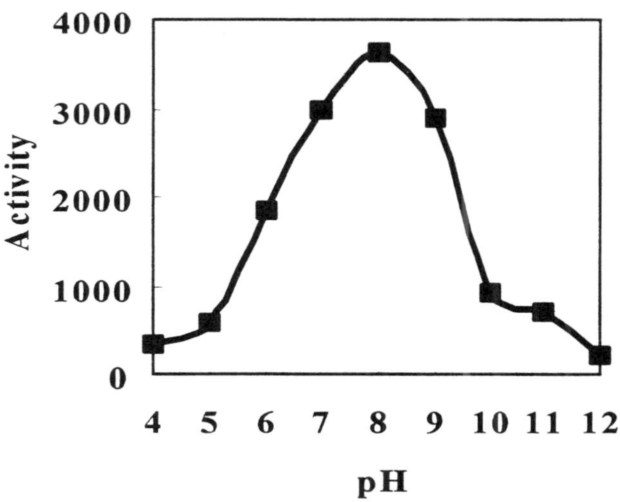

FIG. 4. EFFECT OF pH ON THE PROTEASE ACTIVITY

In our studies, the protease obtained from *E. Japonicus* muscle hydrolyzed casein efficiently, and hemoglobin and bovine serum albumin to some extent (results not shown).

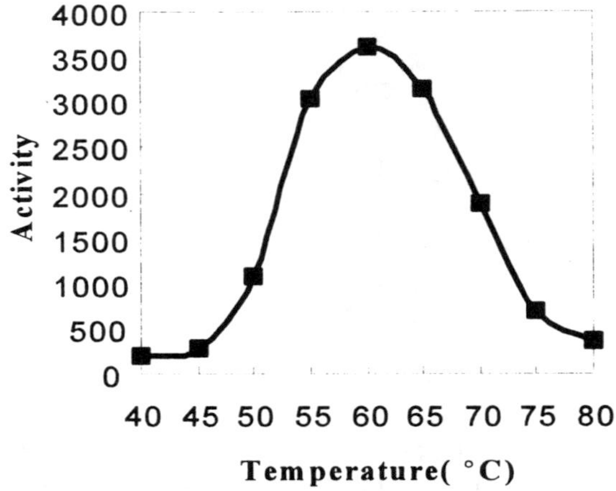

FIG. 5. EFFECT OF TEMPERATURE ON THE ENZYMES ACTIVITY

TABLE 2.
EFFECTS OF HEAT TREATMENT ON THE ENZYME ACTIVITY

	Remaining activity (%)					
	Incubation 5 min		Incubation 10 min		Incubation 30 min	
Temperature (°C)	EJ Protease	AS1.398	EJ Protease	AS1.398	EJ Protease	AS1.398
40	100	100	100	100	100	95
50	100	90	98	80	92	49
60	100	45	95	7	90	4
70	60	5	55	0	41	0
80	45	1	36	0	27	0

TABLE 3.
THE COMPARISON OF CHARACTERISTICS OF EJM-PROTEASE AND OTHER PROTEASES

Sample	EJ Protease	Cathepsin B	Cathepsin D	Serine Proteinase
Recovery (%)	12.8	8.7	13.8	5.4
Purification ratio (fold)	46.8	42.77	113.5	80.4
Molecular weight	39,000	23,500	38,000	30,000
pI (isoelectric point)	5.6	Non data	Non data	2.6
Substrate	Casein	Z-arg-arg-NNap	Non data	TAME[1]
Optimum temperature (°C)	60	42	50	55
Optimum pH	8.0	6.0	5.0	5.0

1, Tosyl-arginine-methylester

It seems that the protease isolated in this work, with a relatively high heat stability and optimum temperature, is one of the major factors contributing to remarkable reduction of production time for Chinese fish sauce from 2-3 year to about 1 month when *E. Japonicus* extract is added.

REFERENCES

BONETE, M.J., MANJION, A., LLORCA, F. and IBORRA, J.L. 1984. Acid proteinase activity in fish I. Comparative study of extraction of cathepsins B and D from *Mujul auratus*. Comp. Biochem. Physiol. *78B,* 203–209.

DOKE, S.N., NINJOOR, V. and NADKARNI, G.B. 1980. Characterization of cathepsin D from the skeletal muscle of fresh water fish, *Tilapia mossambica*. Agric. Biol. Chem. *44,* 1521–1527.

HAARD, N.F. 1990. Enzymes from food myosystems. J. Muscle Foods. *1,* 293–338.

KIMOTO, K., KUSAMA, S. and MURAKAMA, K. 1983. Purification and characterization of serine proteinases from *Euphausia superba*. Agric. Biol. Chem. *47 (3),* 529–534.

LAEMMLI, U.K. 1970. Cleavage of structural protein during the assembly of the head of bacteriophage T4. Nature *227,* 680–685.

LOWRY, O.H., ROSEBROUGH, N., FARR, A. and RANDALL, J. 1951. Protein measurement with the Folin phenol reagent. J. Biol. Chem. *193,* 265–275.

SHEREKAR, S.V., GORE, M.S. and NINJOOR, V. 1988. Purification and characterization of cathepsin B from the skeletal muscle of fresh water fish, *Tilapia mossambica*. J. Food Sci. *53 (4),* 1018–1023.

WASSON, D.H. 1992. Fish muscle protease and heat-induced myofibrillar degradation: A review. J. Aquatic Food Product Technol. *1* (2), 23–41.

ANTI-INFLAMMATORY ACTIVITY OF ANTELOPE HORN KERATIN AND ITS TRYPTIC HYDROLYSATE

LONG LI, WEN WANG, BI-HONG SHI, JIAN-CAI LI, RONG-ZHEN ZHANG, SHU-TAO LIU, RU-MING CHEN, WEN-HONG GAO, GONG-RUI CHEN, YU-QIANG ZHENG and PING-FAN RAO

Institute of Biotechnology, Fuzhou University
523 Gong-Ye Road, Fuzhou, Fujian, 350002
P.R. China

ABSTRACT

In this research, the biosynthesis of metabolites of arachidonic acid by rabbit-washed platelets was investigated. Major products of metabolism were 12-hydroxy-5,8,10-heptadecatrienoic acid (HHT) and 12-hydroxy-6,8,11,14-eicosatetraenoic acid (12-HETE). Inflammation was the result. Since antelope horn is used to cure inflammation in China, the effects of hydrolyates of antelope horn keratin on the formation were investigated. The results show that all products were decreased by the addition of hydrolyates of the keratin.

INTRODUCTION

In China, keratin prepared from animal horns, shells and scales have not only been used as a food protein source but also as an important medicine for more than two thousand years. Antelope horn, ram horn, turtle shell and pangolin scales are the most important anti-inflammatory agents in traditional Chinese medicine for both oral intake and external applications.

Inflammation is characterized by pain, redness, swelling, heat, and eventual loss of function of the affected area. All these conditions are caused in part by lipid-derived mediators such as the eicosanoids, which are 20-carbon oxygenation products derived from arachidonic acid and are generated, in part, by the action of three major classes of intracellular enzymes: cyclo-oxygenases, lipoxygenases and epoxygenases. The prostaglandins (PGs) and leukotrienes (LT), formed by the actions of cyclo-oxygenase and lipoxygenase on arachidonic acid, have been found to play an important role in inflammation (Sigal and Ron 1994). Substances inhibiting these two enzyme activities can be used as anti-inflammatory agents. A biochemical model for screening these substances is a platelet system with arachidonic acid as the substrate. Anti-inflammatory properties can be determined by how much the production of prostaglandins (PGs) and leukotrienes from arachidonic acid are inhibited by the intracellular enzyme system within platelets.

Antelope horn contains calcium phosphate, insoluble organic salts and keratin which is the main component. Its sulfate content is only 1.2%, making it the keratin with the least sulfate.

Antelope horn is used as a major ingredient in several powerful prepared Chinese medicines used to fight inflammation. Acid and alkaline hydrolysates have also been shown to be effective as anti-inflammatory agents and are used in many commercially available medicines that are administered intravenously (Ding 1977; Xue *et al.* 1995; Yao *et al.* 1995).

While keratin is an object of interest in biochemistry primarily because of its structure, it is of interest to determine its anti-inflammatory activity using the above-mentioned platelet model, since its biological activity has already been clearly suggested by Chinese medicine, but it has not been investigated by modern Western science. Antelope horn is used mostly in medicines administered orally, and acid hydrolysis and alkaline hydrolysis are reported to enhance its anti-inflammatory activity. It is also of interest to investigate how enzymatic digestion, rather than non specific hydrolysis, influences antelope horn anti-inflammatory activity.

MATERIAL AND METHODS

Preparation of Samples for Anti-inflammatory Activity Test

Antelope horn purchased from a local drug store was shredded and ground into powder as fine as possible. The antelope horn powder (100 mg) was then boiled with 25 ml of 0.50 mM phosphate buffer (pH 7.0) in a loosely capped test tube for 60 min to obtain a water-soluble extract of antelope horn. Insoluble powder was removed and the supernatant of the antelope horn water-extraction was used for the activity test.

The extract was subjected to tryptic digestion by adding 10 mg of trypsin and incubated at 37°C for 5 h. Trypsin, with a specific activity of 10400 U/mg, was a product of Sigma Chemical Company (St. Louis, MO, USA). The hydrolysate was used as antelope horn digest sample.

Both extracted sample and digested sample of antelope horn were used in the anti-inflammatory test and peptide mapping by capillary liquid chromatography.

Peptide mapping was performed with an ABI 173 capillary liquid chromatograph (CA, USA). Experimental conditions are listed in the legend for the related figures.

Preparation of Suspensions of Washed Platelet

Rabbit blood was collected by marginal ear venipuncture. The blood was collected into plastic containers containing 0.2% EDTA. Platelet-rich plasma (PRP) was obtained from the top layer after the blood was centrifuged at room temperature for 10 min at 200 g. The PRP was re-centrifuged at 4°C for 15 min at 2,000g. The precipitated platelets were washed twice with 20 mM Tris-HCl buffer, pH 7.5, containing 1 mM EDTA and 5 mM glucose. The precipitated platelets were then suspended in 20 mM Tris-HCl buffer, pH 7.5, containing 5 mM glucose (Yue *et al.* 1989). The platelet content in this suspension was determined in a modified Neubauer Cell Counter.

Determination of Anti-Inflammatory Activity

Platelets (0.5 ml) were incubated at 37°C for 20 min with the extracted sample, the digested sample and with physiological saline (blank). Then 5 μl of arachidonic acid (sodium salt, 10 mg/6 ml), purchased from Sigma Chemical Company (St. Louis, MO, USA) was added to the mixture and incubated for another 5 min. A series of platelet-enzymatic reactions were terminated by adjusting the system to pH 3.5 with formic acid. The products were extracted twice by ethyl acetate (0.5 ml), the ethyl acetate was collected and evaporated to dryness under a stream of nitrogen gas and the residue was dissolved in methanol (25 μl). The obtained solution was subjected to reverse-phase chromatography for separation and quantification of the products of platelet- enzymatic reactions.

Reverse-phase chromatography was carried out with a Shimazu LC-4 HPLC equipment on a C18 Zorbas column (0.46 × 25 cm, DuPont) using water/methanol/acetic acid (24:76:0.01) as eluant. The flow rate was 0.8 ml/min. The eluate was monitored at 235 nm which was set to detect 12-hydroxy-5,8,10-heptadecatrienoic acid (HHT) and 12-hydroxy-6,8,11,14-eicosatetraenoic acid (12-HETE).

Anti-inflammatory activity was determined by comparing HHT and 12-HETE contents from the chromatograms.

RESULTS AND DISCUSSION

Factors Influencing Products of Platelet System

Influence of Addition of Arachidonic Acid. Chromatograms of platelet system products with and without addition of arachidonic acid are shown in Fig. 1(2#) and Fig. (1#), respectively. It is clear that there is a large difference in the content of substances eluted at 10 and 19 min. They were identified as HHT and 12-HETE, respectively. When the exogenous arachidonic acid was added into the platelet system, the amount of major metabolites increased remarkably. The production of HHT and 12-HETE with addition of arachidonic acid were 22- and 27-fold larger than those without addition of arachidonic acid, as is shown in Table 1. The amount of metabolite of endogenous arachidonic acid was small enough to be ignored in comparison with biosynthesis of exogenous arachidonic acid.

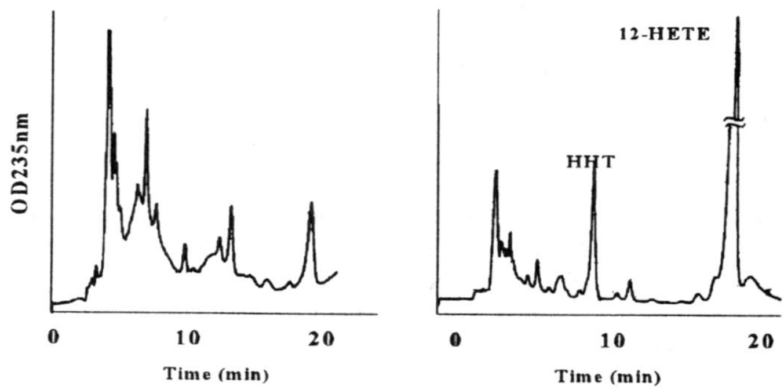

1#   2#

FIG. 1. EFFECT OF ARACHIDONIC ACID ON THE METABOLISM
1#; incubation in the absence of arachidonic acid
2#; incubation in the presence of arachidonic acid
Experimental Conditions: column: Zorbax ODS, 0.46 × 25 cm (Du Pont Instruments); Mobile phase: 76% methanol: 24% H_2O: 0.01% acetic acid; flow rate: 0.8 ml/min, pressure: 110 atm; chart speed: 5 mm/min, 30°C; Range: 1#: 0.01 AUFS; 2#: 0.04 AUFS; monitor wavelength: UV 235 nm

TABLE 1.
EFFECT OF ADDITION OF ARACHIDONIC ACID ON INFLAMMATION

	1#	2#	3#
	0.5 ml suspension of washed rabbit platelet		
	/	5 μl AA-Na	5 μl AA-Na
platelet amount (10^9/L)	513	513	119
metabolite (HHT)[a]	22	488	52
12-(HETE)[a]	68	1808	61

[a]height of HHT or 12-HETE in the chromatograms (mm)

Effect of Platelet Amount. Effect of platelet amount on the formation of HHT and 12-HETE is also shown in Table 1. As is clear from the table, platelet amount played a vital role in determining the formation of HHT and 12-HETE. Under the same conditions, more HHT and 12-HETE formed with more platelets, implying the importance of platelet amount to the final results. Platelet amount was controlled to be 500×10^9/L throughout this work.

Anti-inflammatory Effect of Water-extraction and Hydrolysate of Antelope Horn Keratin

Figure 2 shows results of product analysis of the platelet-arachidonic acid system with three samples: physiological saline, water-extraction and hydrolysate. The overall chromatographic patterns are similar to Fig. 1 except for larger differences in peak heights of HHT and 12-HETE. In comparison with the chromatograms of physiological saline, HHT and 12-HETE peaks are remarkably lower than those with water-extraction and hydrolysate. The result implies that both the extract and tryptic hydrolysate of antelope horn keratin inhibited the metabolism. In other words, they exhibited anti-inflammatory activity. This is the first biochemical evidence of anti-inflammatory activity of antelope horn, affirming a scientific foundation for the traditional utilization of antelope horn by Chinese to cure inflammation.

Apparently, the difference of the HHT and 12-HETE peak height in the two chromatograms represents difference in inhibition rate. The inhibition effect can be easily expressed by the following equation:

$$\delta = (H_0 - H_S)/H_0 \times 100\% \qquad (1)$$

where H_0 is the height of the HHT or 12-HETE peak in the control run, which is physiological saline; H_S is the height for the sample run.

As is shown in Table 2, much more powerful activity was detected in the hydrolysate of the extract than the original extract, indicating possibility of existence of peptides with strong anti-inflammatory activity as products of tryptic digestion of the keratin.

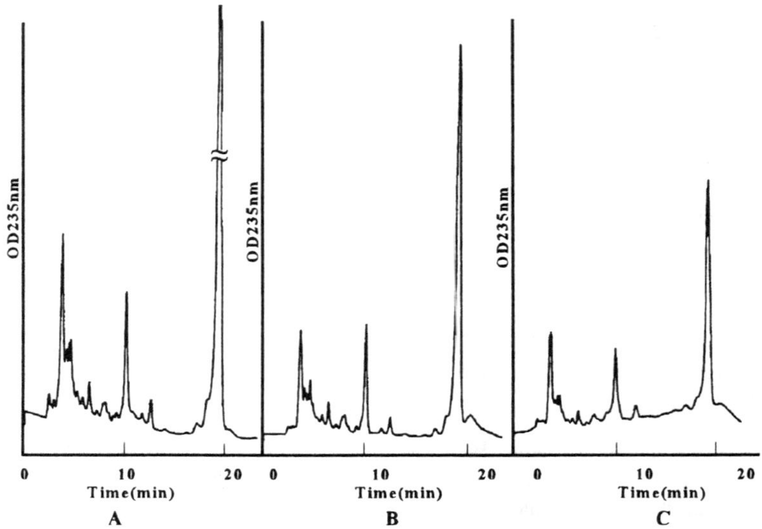

FIG. 2. ANTI-INFLAMMATORY EFFECT OF EXTRACT AND HYDROLYSATE OF ANTELOPE HORN KERATIN

A: physiological saline; B: water-extraction; C: hydrolysate

Experimental Conditions: same as listed in Fig. 1. Range: 0.04 AUFS

TABLE 2.
ANTI-INFLAMMATORY EFFECT OF HYDROLYSATE OF ANTELOPE HORN KERATIN

A (control run)	B (sample run)	C (sample run)
	0.5 ml suspension of washed rabbit platelet	
50 μl physiological saline	50 μl extract	50 μl hydrolysate (5 hr)
	5 μl AA-Na	
	Inhibition (%)	
/	14.8 (a)	47.5 (b)
/	19.9 (a)	53.7 (b)

(a) inhibition of HHT; (b) inhibition of 12-HETE

Analysis of the Extract and the Hydrolysate of Antelope Horn Keratin

Figure 3 is a chromatographic pattern of the hydrolysate of antelope horn keratin. Because of interference of trypsin autolysis products, it is rather difficult to decide the degree of hydrolysis, and the amount of hydrolytic products. A peak at 22 min, however, constantly increased with keratin hydrolysis. The peaks at 34 min, 36 min and 45 min also increased. It seems likely that these peptides may be the candidates for anti-inflammatory peptides.

Anti-inflammatory activity was confirmed by a platelet-arachidonic acid system with water-extract and tryptic hydrolysate of antelope horn keratin in this work. In order to revitalize the traditional remedy of antelope horn, much more work is necessary such as isolation and characterization of tryptic products, elucidation of the factors determining the activity of antelope horn keratin and so on, which is under way at the present.

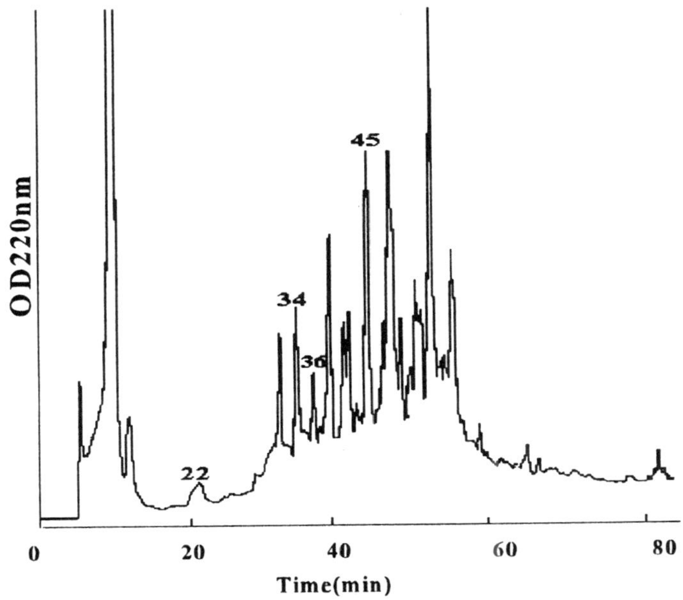

FIG. 3. CHROMATOGRAPHIC PATTERNS OF EXTRACT AND HYDROLYSATE OF ANTELOPE HORN KERATIN

Experimental Conditions: column: C18, 5 μ, 0.05 × 15cm (ABI cLc system); mobile phase: A: water (0.1% TFA); B: acetonitrile (0.085% TFA); 5% ~ 80% B (0 ~ 75 min); 80% ~ 5%B (75 ~ 80 min) flow rate: 5 μl/min; pressure: 760 psi; chart speed: 1 mm/min; 30 °C; range: 0.5 AUFS

REFERENCES

REN, D. 1977. Preparation of antelope injection by hydrolysation. Zhongcaoyaotongxun (Chinese), *17*(1), 17–19.

SIEGEL, M.I., MCCONNELL, R.T. and CUATRECASAS, P. 1979. Aspirin-like drugs interfere with arachidonate metabolism by inhibition of the 12-hydroperoxy-5,8,10,14-eicosatetraenoic acid peroxidase activity of the lipoxygenase pathway. Proc. Natl. Acad. Sci. USA *76*, 3774–3778.

SIGAL, L.H. and RON, Y. 1994. Immunology and Inflammation: Basic Mechanisms and Clinical Consequences. McGraw-Hill, Inc. p. 272.

XUE, S.Y., WANG, M.W., CHEN, S.W. and CHEN, J.M. 1995. Pharmaceutical study of antelope tonic. Zhongchenyao (Chinese), *17*(8), 34–35.

YAO, Y.J., LI, Y., LIU, Y.L., LI, X.Z. and WANG, Y.J. 1995. Pharmaceutical study of antelope antidote pill. Zhhongchenyao (Chinese), *17*(4), 31–33.

YUE, T.L., CHEN, X.S. and LI, J. 1989. Effect of Anisodamine on the metabolism of arachidonic acid by rat platelets. Acta Pharm. Sinica (Chinese), *24*(9), 647–652.

CHEMICAL COMPOSITION OF BOVINE COLOSTRUM

GRUO BEN HENG

Shang Hai Dairy Training and Research Center
101 Peng Lian Road
Shanghai, China 200072

ABSTRACT

Chemical compositions of bovine colostrum were studied very carefully in the paper, which included changing levels of gross composition, proteins, fatty acids and minerals as lactation time lengthened. Fats, total proteins, whey proteins, ash and total solids were higher than those in milk and they decreased as lactation time increased. Lactose was lower than that in milk and increased as lactation time increased. Whey proteins of colostrum such as immunoglobulin G, β-lactoglobulin, bovine serum albumin, lactoferrin and lactoperoxidase were obviously higher than those in milk. They decreased as lactation time increased. There were high levels of unsaturated fatty acids in colostrum when it was compared with bovine milk. Na, Cl, Fe, Zn, Cr and Mg in colostrum were higher than those in milk. They fell as lactation time increased. I, K, P, Mn and Cu increased as lactation time increased. Co, As and Pb were not detected by the ICP method.

INTRODUCTION

Bovine colostrum is very different from milk in chemical composition (French 1988; Ishikawa 1992). All compositions change as the lactation time increases. Carroll (1961) studied whey proteins, Cl^- and pH of bovine colostrum. Some specialists researched the properties, structures and physiological functions of whey proteins in colostrum such as immunoglobulins, lactoferrin, lactoperoxidase, lysozyme, α-lactalbumin and β-lactoglobulin (Bezkorovaing 1977; Schanbaccber and Smith 1975; Yoshida 1988). Some trace composition of proteins, enzymes, minerals and vitamins were found in bovine colostrum by use of affinity and gel chromatography in recent years, which included insulin-like growth factor, epidermal growth factor, transforming growth factor and fibroblast growth factor (Ozawa *et al.* 1991; Yoshida 1988).

Although chemical composition of bovine colostrum has been analyzed very carefully, the following problems have not been resolved very well: (1) changing levels of whey proteins in colostrum were reported during lactation period (3 h-72 h). Other compositions except for whey proteins were not measured, which included changes of fatty acids, lactose and mineral elements; and (2) chemical compositions of bovine colostrum were related to breeds, rearing conditions (climate and temperature, etc.), age and seasons. Bovine colostrum data in other countries would not necessarily represent our own country (China).

Now, because there are not any biologically active substances in infant foods, some nutritional and physiological problems such as malnutrition and disease are produced for infants who eat the foods. Therefore, it is very valuable to study and develop a new type of infant food, which is very close to the gross and trace components of human milk. Studies on the chemical components of bovine colostrum are very important and worthwhile because it is one of the best materials which can be used to produce the new infant food. Chemical composition of bovine colostrum was researched very systematically and carefully in this paper. The data will be helpful to produce a new type of infant food.

MATERIALS AND METHODS

Materials

Bovine colostrum was collected in our university after 3, 12, 36, 48, 60 and 72 h of calf-birth. Three cow samples in the same collecting time were mixed from the sample.

Anti-bovine IgG was bought from ChangChun Biological Institute. Other reagents were bought from Harbin Chemical Co. shops.

Methods

Proteins, fats and carbohydrates were measured by an infrared milk composition analyzer. IgG content was determined by a single immunodiffusion technique. Whey proteins were measured by electrophoresis and a density scanner (Andrews 1981; Tokuyama and Tokuyama 1993). Fatty acids were determined by gas chromatography. Minerals were determined by coupled plasma atomic emission spectrometer.

Instruments

The instruments used were:

(1) Milko-scan 104 Infra Analyzer (Denmark);

(2) electrophoresis apparatus (Beijing Liou Yi factory), measuring conditions: current 8 mA. voltage 60-80 V, electrophoresis time 5-6 h;

(3) density scanner, dual-wavelength scanner cs-390 (Shimadzu), applied wavelength, wavelength 1 was 370 and wavelength 2 was 600;

(4) GC-9A gas chromatographic analyzer, working conditions were as follows: column length 160 $\pm$ 3 mm (12% DEGS/Chromsorb WAW DMCS was filled in it), column temperature 195°C, sample temperature 250°C, carrier gas, N_2 (35 ml/min), N_2 pressure 0.5 kg/cm^2, H_2 35 ml/min, air pressure 0.5 kg/cm^2 and air rate 500 ml/min, paper rate 2.5 mm/min and sample amount 1 μl.

(5) P.E. 6500 coupled plasma atomic emission spectrometer. R_f forward power 1.1 kW, plasma gas flow: 20 L/min, auxiliary gas flow: zero, carrier gas flow: 0.45 L/min, observation height: 14 min above the load coil, sample flow: 1.1 ml/min, wavelengths: Co = 238.892 nm, Cr = 205.552 nm, Fe = 238.204 nm, Pb = 220.353 nm, Cu = 324.754 nm, Zn = 213.856 nm, Cd = 214.438 nm, Al = 309.271 nm, As = 228.812 nm, Mn = 257.610 nm, Mg = 279.553 nm, Ca = 393.366 nm, P = 253.565 nm.

RESULTS AND DISCUSSION

Gross Components of Bovine Colostrum

Gross compositions of bovine colostrum are arranged in Table 1.

Total solids, fats, proteins and ash in colostrum were much higher than those in milk. They decreased as lactation time increased. In particular, whey proteins have the biggest change in composition; whey protein in colostrum at 3 h is six times that at 72 h and its content at 72 h is three times higher than that in milk. At a lactation time of 72 h, all compositions except for proteins were very close to the contents in milk. Lactose increased as lactation time lengthened and was very close to its content in milk after 72 h of calf-birth.

TABLE 1.
GROSS COMPOSITIONS IN BOVINE COLOSTRUM

Calf-birth time (h)	3	12	24	36	48	60	72	bovine[a] milk
fats (%)	6.80	6.10	5.42	5.12	4.83	3.60	3.72	3.50
Total protein (%)	9.42	9.24	9.16	5.28	4.18	5.68	4.68	3.20
whey proteins (%)	8.50	8.41	7.46	4.24	3.00	4.25	1.60	0.47
casein (%)	0.92	0.83	1.70	1.04	1.18	1.43	3.18	2.73
lactose (%)	2.38	2.93	3.02	4.00	3.72	5.11	4.27	4.60
ash	1.02	0.93	0.86	0.82	0.78	0.81	0.74	0.70
total solids (%)	19.62	19.20	18.42	15.22	13.51	15.20	13.41	12.00

[a]Jinshilin 1987. Dairy Industry Handbook, China

Whey Proteins in Bovine Colostrum

All whey proteins in colostrum are shown in Table 2.

TABLE 2.
COMPOSITIONS OF WHEY PROTEINS IN BOVINE COLOSTRUM (mg/ml)

	Lactation time (h)							
Calf-birth	3	12	24	36	48	60	72	milk[(3)]
IgG	45.00	61.50	40.00	15.00	13.60	15.80	6.00	0.50
IgA	7.08	9.55	6.98	3.17	0.56	0.56	0.12	0.09
α-La	5.97	8.4	8.56	6.42	8.12	8.12	2.36	2.0
β-Lg	40.50	39.88	26.54	18.47	19.42	19.42	6.18	4.0
BSA	5.07	5.21	1.97	1.20	1.15	1.15	0.44	0.273
Lf	3.06	4.28	1.77	—[(1)]	0.94	0.94	—[(1)]	0.02~0.35
Lp	3.46	4.29	2.45	1.00	—[(2)]	—[(2)]	—[(2)]	0.03

Notes (1) (2) not detected; (3) Jinshilin. 1987. Dairy Industry Handbook, China.

Whey proteins in bovine colostrum have some regular changes during 3 to 72 h lactation (Fig. 1). Whey proteins in our research include α-lactalbumin (α-La), β-lactoglobulin (β-lg), bovine serum albumin (BSA), lactoferrin (Lf) and lactoperoxidase (Lp). α-La in colostrum was a little higher than that in milk. The highest value of α-La in colostrum was four times of that in milk. α-La fell as lactation time increased. β-Lg at 3 h was ten times of that in milk and at 72 h it was very near that in milk. BSA decreased regularly during 3 to 72 h lactation. BSA of colostrum at 72 h was one eleventh of that at 3 h and was a little higher than that in milk.

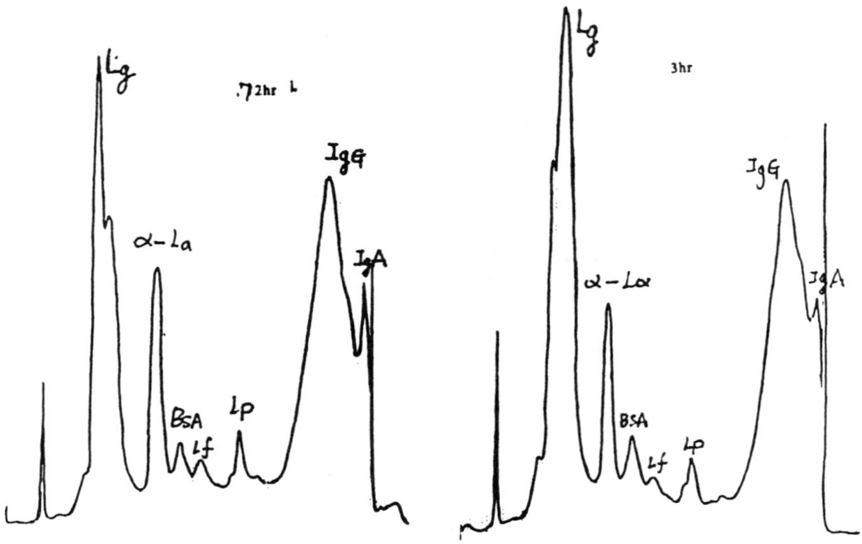

FIG. 1. COMPOSITION OF PROTEINS IN BOVINE COLOSTRUM AT 72 AND 3 H AFTER CALF-BIRTH

Lf was very high in colostrum and at 3 h it was 9-153 times of that in milk. It was much higher than that in milk after 72 h of calf-birth. Lf fell regularly as lactation period changed from 3 to 72 h.

Lp is a very important enzyme in milk. Lp in colostrum had a very high content and at 3 h it was one hundred times that in milk. It decreased very rapidly during 3 to 72 h lactation. We could not measure Lp contents by electrophoresis after 48 h of calf-birth.

Chemical Compositions of Fatty Acids in Colostrum

Chromatographic data are for standard and tested samples. Eight fatty acids could be separated very well (Table 3). Therefore, the method was appropriate and effective to measure fatty acids in dairy products.

TABLE 3.
FATTY ACIDS IN BOVINE COLOSTRUM (g/100 g fat)

Sample	Lactation time (h) 3	12	24	36	48	60	72	bovine[1] milk (ranges)	human[1] milk
Lauric acid	2.69	2.49	1.81	2.43	1.93	2.64	1.23	2.96(2.40-4.50)	3.1
Myristic acid	9.88	10.06	7.85	8.06	7.24	7.79	7.79	11.2(8.39-14.60)	5.1
Palmitic acid	27.95	27.09	23.50	21.27	19.78	20.03	20.03	27.8(22.05-30.20)	20.2
Stearic acid	8.28	8.19	10.05	10.44	12.83	14.97	14.97	12.1(10.50-15.20)	6.0
Oleic acid	33.49	33.52	37.63	37.90	37.69	32.06	32.06	30.3(18.7-30.40)	46.4
Linoleic acid	4.49	4.46	4.15	4.12	3.84	3.51	3.51	2.22(1.23-2.50)	13.0
Linolenic acid	0.95	0.97	1.17	1.42	1.33	1.86	1.86	1.03(0.90-2.61)	1.40
Total fatty acids	87.84	87.00	86.63	85.64	84.76	84.63	84.63	87.61	95.2
Unsaturated fatty acids	38.93	38.95	42.95	43.44	42.86	37.43	37.43	33.55	60.8

[1]Jensen 1973; Paul and Southgate 1978

Fatty Acids in Colostrum. Composition of fatty acids in colostrum are shown in Table 3.

Fatty acids in human and bovine milk were reported very carefully (Tokuyama and Tokuyama 1993; Yoshida 1988). When composition of fatty acids were compared in bovine milk, human milk and bovine colostrum, some conclusions were found. They are: (1) lauric acid, myristic acid and palmitic acid in colostrum are lower than that in bovine milk. They decreased as lactation time lengthened. Lauric acid in colostrum was lower than that in human milk, but myristic acid and palmitic acid were higher than that in human milk. Stearic acid in colostrum was lower than in bovine milk and it increased as lactation time increased. There were higher total unsaturated fatty acids in colostrum when bovine milk and colostrum were compared. Linoleic acid decreased and linolenic acid increased as lactation time increased; (2) Total fatty acids in colostrum were lower than in bovine and human milk and fell as lactation time increased. The unsaturated fatty acids in colostrum were higher than that in bovine milk and lower than that in human milk.

Minerals in Bovine Colostrum

.Contents of minerals in bovine colostrum are arranged in Table 4.

There were great differences for minerals of bovine milk and colostrum; some of them were higher at 3 h than those in milk such as Na, Cl, Fe, Zn, Cr and Mg. They fell as lactation time increased. Na, Cl and Mg in colostrum were close to those in bovine milk after 72 h of calf-birth. Fe, Zn and Cr in 72 h colostrum were four, four and eight times those in bovine milk, respectively. Some minerals increased as lactation time increased which included I, K, P, Mn and Cu. K, Cu and I in 3 h colostrum were lower than those in milk and in 72 h colostrum were close to those in milk. P in the beginning lactation period was close to milk and Mn was higher than in milk during 3 to 72 h lactation time. Co, As and Pb were not detected by the ICP method.

TABLE 4.
MINERALS IN BOVINE COLOSTRUM

Elements	Lactation time (h)							bovine
	3	12	24	36	48	60	72	milk(4)
Na (mg)	1447.4	1083.62	976.35	874.36	746.83	706.49	548.46	350-900
K (mg)	608.40	724.49	810.25	862.94	958.45	1011.24	1028.43	1100-1700
Cl (mg)	2708.65	1806.95	1558.45	1554.90	1526.50	1498.10	1246.05	900-1100
Ca (mg)	1150.01	1116.35	1402.53	1016.09	1193.02	1443.38	1080.12	1100-1130
Mg (mg)	140.23	101.59	85.82	74.74	70.00	69.20	65.17	90-140
P (mg)	933.54	944.99	1023.76	1033.11	1248.00	1329.11	962.31	900-1000
Al (mg)	112.75	10.95	10.00	10.75	14.41	15.25	12.49	—
Fe (μg)	3575.64	3025.57	2896.82	2219.77	2416.23	2354.81	1929.93	300-600
Zn (μg)	18929.91	8717.28	7854.54	7397.83	7586.39	8160.29	12905.71	2000-6000
Cu (μg)	172.57	132.73	123.32	150.25	318.68	407.74	307.82	100-600
Mn (μg)	83.34	65.78	79.19	65.51	92.51	99.42	101.03	20-50
I (μg)	132.50	148.76	150.24	190.86	208.74	245.37	256.64	260
Cr (μg)	141.51	129.20	106.90	107.38	88.96	81.54	80.16	8-13
Co (μg)	-	-	-	-	-	-	-	0.5 - 1.3
As (μg)	-	-	-	-	-	-	-	-
Pb (μg)	-	-	-	-	-	-	-	-

"-" Not detected (Fox 1982)

CONCLUSIONS

The following conclusions can be reached from the results.

1. Bovine colostrum is different from bovine milk. Fats, total protein, whey proteins, ash and total solids in colostrum are higher than those in milk and they decrease as lactation time increases. Lactose in 3 h colostrum is lower than that in milk and it increases as lactation time increases.
2. Some whey proteins in colostrum such as IgG, β-Lg, BSA, lf and lp are higher than those in milk. They decrease as lactation time increases.
3. Unsaturated fatty acids including oleic acid, linoleic acid and linolenic acid in colostrum are higher than those in milk. Oleic acid and linoleic acid decrease and linolenic acid increases as lactation time increases. Saturated fatty acids (lauric acid, myristic acid and palmitic acid) in 3 h colostrum are lower than those in milk and increase as lactation time increases. Stearic acid is low and increases as lactation time increases.
4. Some elements such as Na, Cl, Fe, Zn, Cr and Mg fall as lactation time increases. Na, Cl and Mg in 72 h colostrum are very close to those in milk, but Fe, Zn and Cr are still higher in colostrum. I, K, P, Mn and Cu increase as lactation time increases. Moreover, K, Cu and I in 3 h colostrum are lower than those in milk and Mn is higher than that in milk during 3 - 72 h lactation time.

REFERENCES

ANDREWS, A. 1981. Electrophoresis. Clarendon Press, Oxford.

BEZKOROVAING, A. 1977. Human milk and colostrum proteins: a review. J. Dairy Sci. *60*, 1023–1037.

CARROLL, E.J, MURPHY, F.A. and AALUND, O. 1965. Changes in whey proteins, between drying and colostrum formation. J. Dairy Sci. *48*(9), 1246–1249.

FOX, P.F., ed. 1982. Developments in Dairy Chemistry - 1. Proteins. Applied Science Publishers, London.

FRENCH, M.A.H. 1988. Immunoglobulins in Health and Disease. MTP Press, Ltd., London.

HUANG, M. 1991. Measuring fatty acids of milk powder by gas chromatography. China Dairy Ind. (Chinese) *18* (3), 109–112.

ISHIKAWA, H. 1992. Changes in the chemical composition of colostrum from Japanese black cows. Anim. Sci. Techn. (Jpn) *63*(11), 1153–1156.

JENSEN, R.G. 1973. Chemical composition of human and bovine milk. J. Am. Oil Chem. Soc. *50*, 186–195.

OZAWA, A., HODATE, K. MIYAMOTO, S., OHTANI, F., TSUSHIMA, T. and JOHKE, T. 1991. Plasma profiles of insulin-like growth factor-1 for 24 hours and after injection of bovine growth hormone in dairy heifers. Anim. Sci. Techn. (Jpn) *62*(11), 933–938.

SCHANBACCBER, F.L. and SMITH, K.L. 1975. formation and role of unusual whey proteins and enzyme relation to mammary function. J. Dairy Sci. *58*, 1048–1062.

TOKUYAMA, Y. and TOKUYAMA, H. 1993. Purification and identification of TGF-β2-related growth factor from bovine colostrum. J. Dairy Res. *60*, 99–109.

YOSHIDA, S. 1988. Isolation of some minor milk proteins, distributed in acid whey, from approximately 100,000 to 250,000 daltons of particle size. J. Dairy Sci. *71* 1–9.

DEVELOPMENT OF A WATER-SOLUBLE CARBOXYMETHYL-β-(1→3)-GLUCAN DERIVED FROM *SACCHAROMYCES CEREVISIAE*

XIAO LIN DING and MIAO WANG

School of Food Science and Technology
Wuxi University of Light Industry
Wuxi, China

ABSTRACT

The report describes a method for the solubilization of micro-particulate β-(1→3)-glucan. Insoluble glucan is suspended in sodium hydroxide and partially carboxymethylated at 65°C. The resulting water-soluble product is called CMG. The solubility is up to 98%. The substituted degree is about 0.2-0.3. Molecular weight and intrinsic viscosity were determined by gel permeation chromatography and viscometer. ^{13}C-NMR spectroscopy confirmed the β-(1→3) interchain linkage. In solution CMG self-associates partly in a triple helix. The ability to prepare an immunologically active, water-soluble β-(1→3)-glucan preparation will greatly enhance the utility of this class of compounds.

INTRODUCTION

Glucan is a β-(1→3)-linked polyglucose immune stimulant that is isolated from the inner cell wall of *Saccharamyces cerevisiae*. Glucan exerts a beneficial effect on a variety of experimental disease states of bacterial, viral, fungal and parastitic origin (Williams *et al.* 1992). Glucan has also been shown to ameliorate immunosuppression and modify the course of experimental neoplastic disease (Di Luzio *et al.* 1985). These observations have stimulated research into the potential biomedical or functional food factor applications of polymeric β-1,3-D-glucan.

A major obstacle to the utilization of β-1,3-D-glucan is its relative lack of solubility in aqueous media. Specifically, β-1,3-D-glucan is an insoluble microparticulate (1-2 μm) upon initial isolation from *Saccharamyces cerevisiae*. Although topical or intralesional administration of insoluble microparticulate β-1,3-D-glucan induces no toxicity, it is limited in its application to medicine and food. The feasibility of preparing water-soluble β-1,3-D-glucans with immunological activity from insoluble yeast glucan has been demonstrated (Williams *et al.* 1991).

This report describes 1) a method for the solubilization of yeast derived β-1,3-D-glucan that results in a water soluble carboxymethylated glucan (CMG); 2) preliminary data on the physicochemical characteristics of CMG; 3) preliminary animal test data on the immunological activity of CMG.

EXPERIMENTAL PROCEDURES

Preparation of Water-insoluble, Microparticulate Glucan from Yeast Autolyzed Residues

Particulate glucan was isolated from autolyzed residues of *S. cerevisiae* by a modification of the method of Manners *et al.* 1973a,b).

Preparation of Carboxymethylated Glucan

Soluble CM-glucan was prepared as outlined in Fig. 1.

---

10 g of water-insoluble particulate glucan + 20 ml of aqueous NaOH (200g/L) and 18 ml of ethanol

↓ mixed for 30 min at 50°C

added 8 g sodium salt of monochloracetic acid in 20 ml of 95% ethanol

↓ stirred at 65°C for 6 h

excess of NaOH was neutralized with concentrated hydrochloric acid

↓

centrifuged and discarded supernatant

↓

washed with 80% ethanol three times

↓

dried at 37°C by air

↓

The yield of the sodium salt of carboxymethylated glucan(CMG-Na) derivative, with a substitution degree (DS) of 0.2-0.3.

FIG. 1. FLOW CHART DESCRIBING THE PREPARATION OF CMG-NA FROM INSOLUBLE B-GLUCAN

Determination of Molecular Weight and Instrinsic Viscosity of CMG

Molecular weight of CMG-Na was determined by gel permeation chromatography (GPC). GPC was performed in a glass column (120 × 1 mm i.d.) packed with Sepharose CL-2B, using 0.1 M NaCl as the mobile phase. The elution rate was 0.1 ml/min, the concentration of the applied sample was 3 mg/ml in the mobile phase and injected sample volume was 1 ml. The concentration of the polymer in the effluent (2 ml fractions) was determined by the phenol-sulfuric acid method (Zhang 1987). A set of dextrans was used as molecular weight standard. The characteristic sample elution volume, V_e, was that corresponding to the maximum of its chromatographic curve.

Viscosity measurements were performed with a capillary viscometer. Intrinsic viscosity values ($[\eta]$), in milliliters per gram, were determined from at least four concentrations, and evaluated using the equation:

$$\eta sp/c = [\eta] + k_H[\eta]^2 c$$

Where η_{sp} is specific viscosity, k_H is Huggins' constant and C is concentration.

^{13}C-NMR Spectroscopy of CMG

To investigate the type of interchain linkage and elucidate the polymer backbone microparticulate glucan and CMG-Na were dissolved in DMSO-d_6 and D_2O, respectively and analyzed by ^{13}C-NMR spectroscopy. Analyses were performed on a FX-9OQNMR spectrometer (JEOL Inc., Japan).

Helix-Coil Transition Analysis of CMG

The conformational structure of CMG-Na in aqueous solution was established by helix-coil transition analysis according to a modification of the Ogawa and Hatano procedure (Williams 1992; Ogawa and Hatano 1978). Briefly, Congo Red was dissolved in 1.0 mM NaOH to a final concentration of 88 μM. CMG-Na was dissolved in 1.0 mM NaOH. Laminarin was employed as a β-(1-3)-linked triple-helical control. Dextran (40 kDa) was employed as a random-coil control. CMG-Na or polysaccharide standards (250 μl) were added to 10 mM microcuvettes containing 750 μl of either Congo Red-NaOH or water-NaOH. Absorbance (λ_{max}) was determined using an W-240 spectrophotometer (Shimadu Inc., Japan). Polysaccharides existing in an ordered conformation form a complex with Congo Red in dilute aqueous NaOH solution. To assess the order-disorder transition, the λ_{max} for solutions of Congo Red-CMG-Na or Congo Red-polysaccharide standards were determined at NaOH concentrations ranging from 0.001-1.0 M.

Preliminary Animal Test of Immunological Activity

ICR mice (18-20 g) were obtain from Shanghai Laboratory Animal Company. Phagocytic activity of the peritoneal cavity of mice was assayed by a method described in the literature (Xu *et al.* 1996).

RESULTS AND DISCUSSION

The Solubility of CMG

Herein we describe a method for the solubilization of β-D-glucan from *S. cerevisiae*. The resulting water-soluble preparation (CMG) is a biological response modifier (BRMs). Solubilization was achieved by partially carboxymethylating the β-D-glucan polymer with monochloroacetic acid in an alkaline medium. The heterogeneous etherification of the particulate β-D-glucan yielded the sodium salt of the carboxymethylated β-D-glucan. Based on determination of substituted degree (DS), DS of the soluble β-D-glucan was about 0.2-0.3. Table 1 shows the solubility of CMGs with different DS's. The solubility of CMG depends not only on DS, but also the distribution of substituted groups as well on the backbone. In fact, it is difficult to control the DS of soluble glucan exactly, so we can use the solubility as an indicator in the preparation of soluble glucan.

TABLE 1.
THE SOLUBILITY OF CMGS

NO.	DS	Solubility(%)
CMG1	0.276	96.20
CMG2	0.265	86.40
CMG3	0.210	83.48
CMG4	0.193	76.53
CMG5	0.188	43.33
CMG6	0.170	30.83

Physicochemical Characteristics of CMG

The molecular weight averages and intrinsic viscosity of CMG-Na (DS=0.276) are presented in Table 2. Two polymer peaks were resolved. Peak 1, which represents 41.4% of the total polymer weight, has a weight average M_w of 4.23×10^5. Peak 2, which comprises 10.2% of the polymers, has a weight average M_w of 3.73×10^4. The average intrinsic viscosity was 4.48 dL/g (solution in 0.1M NaCl).

TABLE 2.
MOLECULAR WEIGHT AVERAGES AND INTRINSIC VISCOSITY
(in 0.1 M NaCl)

Parameter	peak1		peak2
M_w (weight-average mol. wt.)	4.23×10^5		3.73×10^4
M_n (number-average mol. wt.)	3.82×10^5		3.64×10^4
$d=M_W/M_n$ (polydispersity)	1.1073		1.0247
$[\eta]$ (intrinsic viscosity) (dL/g)		4.48	
% of total polymers	41.4		10.2

The Structure of CMG

To confirm the type of interchain linkage associated with CMG, samples were analyzed by ^{13}C-NMR spectroscopy in D_20 or DMSO-d_6. This allows elucidation of the polymer backbone and can also be employed to evaluate the type of side-chain branching, if any, along the backbone. The ^{13}C-NMR spectrum of water insoluble, microparticulate β-D-glucan isolated from *Saccharomyces cerevesiae* and water-soluble CMG prepared from the insoluble material are presented in Fig. 2. Laminarin in DMSO-d_6 served as the β-(1→3)-linked triple-helical control. Comparison of the insoluble, microparticulate glucan and CMG peak shows excellent correspondence with laminarin. In addition, the ^{13}C-NMR spectrum of laminarin reported earlier agreed well with the present laminarin spectrum. ^{13}C-NMR chemical shifts in ppm for insoluble glucan, CMG and laminarin are presented in Table 3. Comparison of the chemical shift of insoluble glucan and CMG with laminarin confirms the β-(1→3) assignment. These data also indicate that the solubilization procedure does not substantially alter the basic molecule.

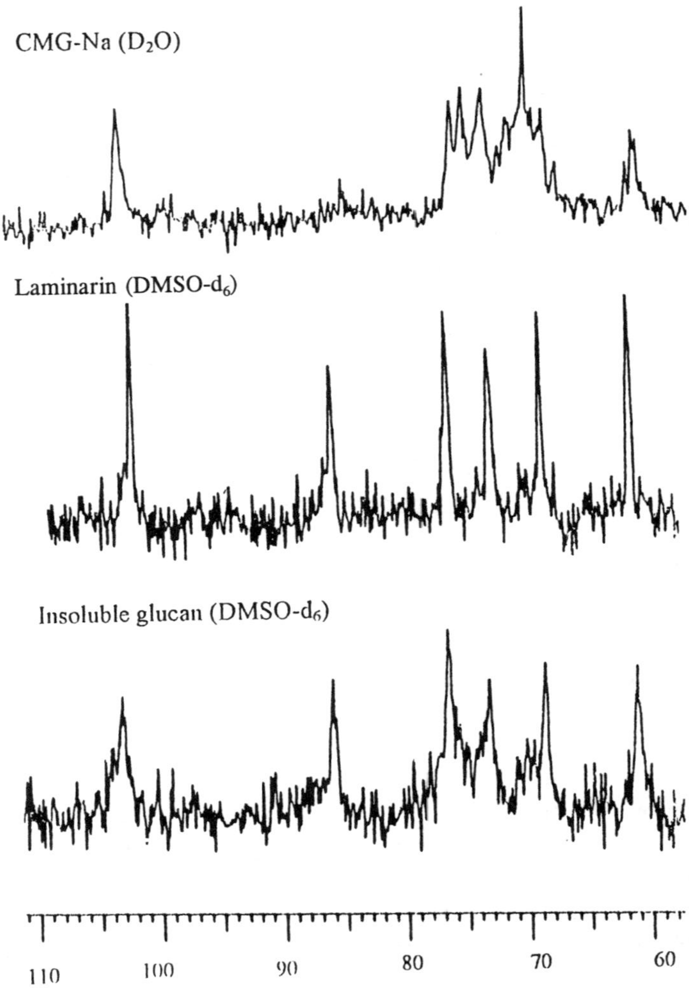

FIG. 2. THE ^{13}C-NMR SPECTRUM OF WATER-INSOLUBLE YEAST, LAMINARIN AND CMG-Na

TABLE 3.
^{13}C-NMR CHEMICAL SHIFTS OF WATER INSOLUBLE GLUCAN, LAMINARIN IN DMSO-d_6 AND CMG-Na IN D_2O

C-atom	laminarin-DMSO-d_6	Insoluble glucan-DMSO-d_6	CMG-Na-D2O
C-1	101.1	103.2	103.3
C-2	71.8	73.6	73.5
C-3	85.1	86.2	86.8
C-4	67.5	68.9	69.0
C-5	76.1	76.8	76.5
C-6	60.7	61.4	61.5

Helix-Coil Transition Analysis of CMG

Previous reports indicate that the immunological and antitumor activity of certain β-(1→3)-D-glucan BRMs is related to the higher structure of the polymer. Maeda *et al.* (1988) reported that the denaturation of lentinan, a triple-helical β-linked glucan BRM, decreases antitumor activity. Renaturation of the polymer restored antitumor activity. These data suggest that the higher structure, specifically the solution conformation, may be critically important with regard to induction of immunobiological activity. The solution conformation of CMG was determined by the technique of Ogawa and Hatano (1978). CMG may exhibit some triple-helical conformation as denoted by a slight shift in the absorption maxima in 0.2 M NaOH (Fig. 3). Laminarin, which served as the triple-helical control, exhibited a shift in absorption maximum between 0.1 and 0.2 M NaOH. Examination of a 40 kDa dextran, which served as the random coil control, revealed no shift in absorption maximum. Congo Red in NaOH served as the negative control. The possibility exists that shifts in absorption maximum observed for CMG may be attributable to chain ionization effects. However, laminarin, a β-(1-3)- linked water soluble, triple-helical polyglucose that has no group substitution showed a shift in

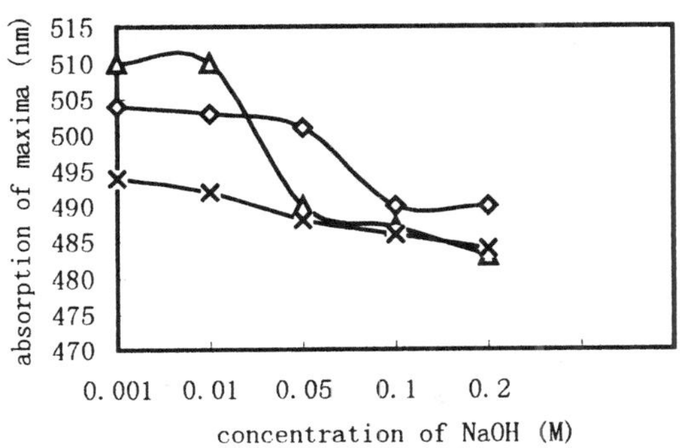

FIG. 3. ANALYSIS OF HELIX-COIL TRANSITION OF CMG-Na IN THE PRESENCE OF CONGO RED AND VARYING CONCENTRATIONS OF NaOH
Δ, Laminarin; ◇, CMG-Na; ×, Dextran 40 kDa

absorption maximum similar to that observed with CMG. In addition, previous work showed a branched, water-soluble β-(1-3)-linked polyglucose derived from *Sclerotium glucanicum* has no charged groups. The shift in absorption maximum observed with *S. glucanium*-derived glucan is similar to that observed with CMG. These observations tend to argue against chain ionization effects in CMG polymers being solely responsible for the observed shifts in absorption maximum.

The Immunological Activity of CMG

Numerous studies have shown that β-(1-3)-D-glucan belongs to a class of biological response modifiers (BRMs). Glucan from the inner cell wall of *Saccharomyces cerevisiae* is an immune stimulant. In order to prove the immunological activity of CMG, studies were conducted to determine whether CMG would stimulate macrophage-enhancing phagocytic activity. The oral administration of CMG (40-160 mg/kg) was done for 12 consecutive days. A positive control for macrophage activity is laminarin. A negative control is saline, carboxymethylated cellulose (CMC) and carboxymethylated starch (CMS). Tables 4 and 5 show the effect of orally administration of CMG on the phagocytic activity of peritheal macrophage. Marked enhancement of phagocytic activity was observed. The highest enhancing effect was observed in mice given 160 mg/kg. The effect seemed to be dose-dependent in the range from 40-160 mg/kg. The reason for the results may be related to the ratio of helices to coils in CMG. The effect of CMG on macrophage is similar to laminarin. Both have a similar backbone structure of β-(1-3)-linked glucan. CMG is a kind of β-3-(1-4)-linkage polyglucose. CMS is a kind of α-(1-4)-linkage polyglucose. Their structures are different from that of CMG and laminarin, so it is a very important backbone-linked type.

TABLE 4.
THE EFFECT OF ORALLY ADMINISTRATION CMG-Na ON THE IMMUNOLOGIC ACTIVITY OF MICE

No.		kind administration	of dose (mg/kg)	phagocytic activity (%)	phagocytic index
1	blank	saline		57.31±9.20	1.42±0.95
2	group of low dose	CMG	40	66.02±9.55*	2.75±1.09**
3	group of middle dose	CMG	80	72.43±9.55**	3.77±1.09**
4	group of high dose	CMG	160	82.02±6.63***	6.32±1.63***
5	positive control	Lentinan	80	72.35±7.03**	4.28±1.35**
6	negative control	CMS	80	64.85±5.52	4.14±0.98
7	negative control	CMC	80	67.74±3.03	3.49±1.00

***P<0.001, **P<0.01, *P<0.05
CMC: carboxymethyl-cellulose, CMG: carboxymethyl-glucan, CMS: carboxymethyl-starch.

TABLE 5.
THE EFFECT OF ORALLY ADMINISTRATION CMG-Na ON THE IMMUNOLOGIC ACTIVITY OF MICE

No.		kind administration	of dose (mg/kg)	spleen index (wt./mice wt.)	Thymus index (wt./mice wt.)
1	blank	saline		6.31±1.62	8.17±0.97
2	group of low dose	CMG	40	8.50±2.52	8.82±1.08
3	group of middle dose	CMG	80	8.38±2.95	8.19±0.94
4	group of high dose	CMG	160	9.17±2.24	8.68±1.23
5	positive control	Lentinan	80	8.75±1.47	8.29±1.63
6	negative control	CMS	80	6.37±0.87	9.23±0.89
7	negative control	CMC	80	7.76±1.41	8.94±0.80

***$P<0.001$. **$P<0.01$. *$P<0.05$
CMC: carboxymethyl-cellulose, CMG: carboxymethyl-glucan, CMS: carboxymethyl-starch.

REFERENCES

DI LUZIO, N.R. 1985. Update on the immunomodulating activities of glucan. Springer Semin. Immunopathol. *8*, 387–400.

MAEDA, Y.Y., WATANABE, S.T., CHIHARA, C. and ROKUTANDA, M. 1988. Denaturation and renaturation of a beta-1,6:1,3-glucan, lentinan, associated with expression of T-cell-mediated response. Cancer Res. *48*, 671–675.

MANNERS, D.J., MASSON, A.J. and PATTERSON, J.C. 1973a. The structure of a beta-(1→3)-D-glucan from yeast cell walls. Biochem. J. *135*, 19–30.

MANNERS, D.J., MASSON, A.J., PATTERSON, J.C., BJORNDAL, H. and LINDBERG, B. 1973b. The structure of a beta-(1→3)-D-glucan from yeast cell walls. Biochem. J. *135*, 31–36.

OGAWA, K. and HATANO, M. 1978. Circular dichroism of the complex of a (1→3)-beta-D-glucan with Congo Red. Carbohydr. Res. *67*, 527–535.

WILLIAMS, D.L., McNAMEE, R.B., JONES, E.L., PRETUS, H.A., ENSLEY, H.E., BROWDER, I.W. and DI LUZIO, N.R. 1991. A method for the solubilization of a (1→3)-beta-D-glucan isolated from *Saccharomyces cerevisiae*. Carbohydrate Res. *219*, 203–213.

WILLIAMS, D.L., PRETUS, H.A., McNAMEE, R.B., JONES, E.L., ENSLEY, H.E., BROWDER, I.W. and DI LUZIO, N.R. 1992. Development physiocochemical characterization and preclinical efficacy evaluation of a water-soluble glucan sulfate derived from *Saccharomyces cerevisiae*. Carbohydr. Res. *235*, 247–257.

XU, S.Y. *et al.* 1996. The methods of evaluation and test on functional foods. People's Hygiene Press. Beijing, China.

ZHANG, W.J. 1987. The application of biochemistry in complex polysaccharides. Shanghai Science and Technology Press. Shanghai, China.

THE HEMAGGLUTINATING AND CYTOTOXIC ACTIVITIES OF EXTRACTS FROM MEXICAN LEGUMES ON HUMAN TUMOR CELLS

NURIA ROCHA, LUIS A. SALAZAR-OLIVO, FIKRAT ABDULLAEV and ELVIRA GONZALEZ de MEJIA

Department of Food Research and Postgraduate Studies
Autonomous University of Queretaro, Mexico
Cerro de las Campanas, Queretaro, Qro 76010, Mexico

ABSTRACT

The present study compared the hemagglutinating activities and cytotoxic effect of extracts from different Mexican legumes on tumor cell proliferation, colony formation and DNA synthesis. Considerable variation was observed in protein content and hemagglutinating activity between extracts from different plants, but no correlation was found between these parameters. Crude extracts from Mexican legumes possess cytotoxic activity against human tumor HeLa cells as evaluated by inhibition of cell proliferation, colony formation and DNA synthesis.

INTRODUCTION

A major problem in the use of synthetic chemopreventing agents in different disease treatments is the potential toxicity of these drugs to normal cells. Recent interest has focused on curative properties of various extracts and naturally occurring compounds from food plants which have biological activity (Yu *et al.* 1993; Abdullaev and Gonzalez de Mejia 1997).

It is well known that legumes, among other plant foods, are very important sources for the diet in developing countries. In Mexico, legumes such as beans, are widely consumed and represent very good sources of proteins, vitamins, minerals and other nutrients despite the fact that beans also contain a significant amount of toxic and antinutrient factors such as lectins. However, diets based on raw legume seed meals are not well utilized by humans or animals mainly because of the presence of antinutrients and in some cases can be toxic. In kidney bean (*Phaseolus vulgaris*) seed lectin (phytohemagglutinin; PHA) was identified as the main antinutrient compound (Sharon and Lis 1989; Pusztai 1991).

The cytotoxic effect of different plant lectins, including lectins from legumes, on growth of normal and malignant cells has been reported (Shoham *et al.* 1970; Lin *et al.* 1970; Robinson and Mekori 1971; Ryder *et al.* 1992; Pryme *et al.* 1994; Mody *et al.* 1995). Recently, our laboratory has demonstrated that extracts of Mexican bean (*P. vulgaris*) or lectin purified from red kidney bean (*P. vulgaris*) seeds alone and in combination with synthetic selenium compounds has inhibitory effect on colony formation of cultured human cervical epitheloid carcinoma (HeLa) cells (Abdullaev and Gonzalez de Mejia 1995/1996). It is interesting to note that, by using [^{3}H]-thymidine and [^{3}H]-uridine uptake as a criterion of cell growth and proliferation, several studies have demonstrated the effect of plant lectins on nucleic acid synthesis (Yu *et al.* 1993; Ryder *et al.* 1992, 1994; Kim *et al.* 1993; Kiss *et al.* 1997).

As part of a research program directed towards the isolation and characterization of bioactive compounds from Mexican plants used in traditional food, this paper describes the cytotoxic screening of crude extracts obtained from Mexican legumes on cultured human tumor cells.

MATERIALS AND METHODS

Seeds and Extracts

Tepary bean (*P. acutifiolius*) seeds were purchased from a public market in Sonora (Mexico) and common bean (*P. vulgaris*) seeds were purchased from a public market in Queretaro (Mexico). Seeds of mezquite trees (*Prosopis juliflora*) were collected in the garden of University of Queretaro (Mexico). We used also a commercial lectin from red kidney bean (*P. vulgaris*; PHA-E; Sigma, Chemical Co., St. Louis, USA). Dry bean seeds were ground into flour in a Wiley mill. Flour was extracted overnight at 4°C with phosphate buffer, pH 7.4 (10 ml/g flour), and then centrifuged at 4500 rpm for 20 min to give the crude extract. Protein content was determined using bovine serum albumin as standard (Bradford 1976). The crude extract was stored at -20°C before use.

Hemagglutinating Activity

Hemagglutinating activity was determined as described by Jaffe (1980), employing a 2% rabbit erythrocyte suspension prepared from fresh blood. HeLa cells, a generous gift from Dr. Alejandro Garcia-Carranca (University National Autonomous of Mexico, Mexico D.F.), were grown in Dulbecco's Modified Eagle's Medium (DMEM, GIBCO) with 10% calf serum (Hyclone), insulin (5 μg/ml) (Sigma, Chemical Co., St. Louis, USA) and antibiotics. Incubation was carried out at 37°C in a humidified atmosphere of 5% CO_2 and 95% air.

Cell Proliferation Assay

For cell proliferation assays, cells were transferred into 35 mm dishes at a density of 1.5×10^5 per dish in 3 ml of DMEM with serum. After 48 h incubation at 37°C in a humidified atmosphere of 5% CO_2 and 95% air, each dish was washed with 3 ml of phosphate buffer saline (PBS) and then 3 ml of serum-free DMEM containing 0.05 mg/ml of extract were added to each dish and incubation was continued for 6 h. Then the medium was changed by DMEM supplemented with serum and incubation was continued another 48 h. At the end of the culture period, the cells were trypsinized and the cell suspension was counted with a Coulter Counter.

Colony Formation Assay

To examine the effect of crude extracts of lectins from Mexican legumes on tumor cell colony formation, HeLa cells were transferred into 100 mm dishes at 2×10^4 cells per dish with 10 ml of medium. After three days, the above indicated crude extracts were added to the culture at the concentrations indicated in the individual experiments and incubation was continued for 2 h. Then the cells were treated as described previously (Abdullaev and Frenkel 1992). At least four replicates were carried out for each culture.

[^{3}H]-Thymidine Incorporation

Nucleic acid synthesis was monitored by incorporation of a radioactive precursor ^{3}H-thymidine for DNA (final concentration 3 μCi/ml) into acid-insoluble materials, i.e. DNA, as described previously (Abdullaev and Frenkel 1992). All determinations were carried out in duplicate.

Statistical Analysis

We used regression analysis module STATGRAPHICS V 5.0 for the linear regression analyses.

RESULTS

The protein content and hemagglutinating activity of extracts from Mexican legumes are shown in Table 1. In these assays cultivated tepary bean extract had the highest hemagglutinating activity against rabbit erythrocytes in comparison with the other tested extracts. It was also shown that the extracts had significant differences in content of total protein. No correlation was found between protein content and hemagglutinating activity in the tested extracts.

TABLE 1.
PROTEIN CONTENT AND HEMAGGLUTINATING ACTIVITY OF EXTRACTS FROM MEXICAN LEGUMES

Legumes	Protein (mg/ml extract)	Lectin (U/mg protein)[1]
Tepary Cultivated	9.24 ± 2.48	10,240 ± 1,827
Tepary Wild Type	15.24 ± 2.73	4,266 ± 1,206
Common Bean	8.10 ± 2.31	2,133 ± 603
Mezquite	2.80 ± 0.19	1,706 ± 600

[1]U, titer of agglutination is defined as a double serial dilution.

Table 2 presents results on the effect of the legume extracts on *in vitro* proliferation of HeLa cells. In these experiments we chose a concentration of 0.05 mg protein/ml because experimental results with commercial PHA lectin demonstrated about 50% inhibition of cell proliferation at this concentration. A comparison of the effects of the different legume extracts on growth of human tumor cells demonstrated that extracts from mezquite seeds have a significant (49%) inhibitory effect on tumor cell proliferation. Extracts from common bean also showed ability to inhibit tumor cell proliferation but extracts from tepary beans at this concentration had very little inhibitory effect. These results indicate that mezquite seeds have cytotoxic activity which is comparable with the activity of purified lectin. Our preliminary results with partially purified lectins from mezquite indicated an inhibition of cell proliferation higher than 90% (data not shown) with a concentration of 0.05 mg protein/ml.

TABLE 2.
CYTOTOXIC EFFECT OF EXTRACTS FROM MEXICAN LEGUMES ON CELL PROLIFERATION

Legumes (0.05 mg protein/ml)	Number of cells $\times$ 10^5 after treatment	Inhibition (%)
Control	7.05 $\pm$ 0.63	0
Tepary Cultivated	6.32 $\pm$ 0.24	10.35
Tepary Wild Type	6.88 $\pm$ 0.35	2.41
Common Bean	5.60 $\pm$ 0.39	20.56
Mezquite	3.60 $\pm$ 0.18	48.93
Lectin PHA	3.70 $\pm$ 0.18	48.51

The effects of crude extracts of the three legumes on HeLa cells plating efficiency are presented in Fig. 1. In these experiments HeLa cells were incubated with three concentrations of extracts for 2 h, trypsinized, diluted (200 cells/dish) and seeded on plates to determine the number of cells which could produce colonies. Results (Fig. 1) showed that under these conditions there was a dose-dependent inhibition of colony formation by all four extracts. Extract from mezquite seeds showed higher significant inhibitory effect in comparison with other tested extracts.

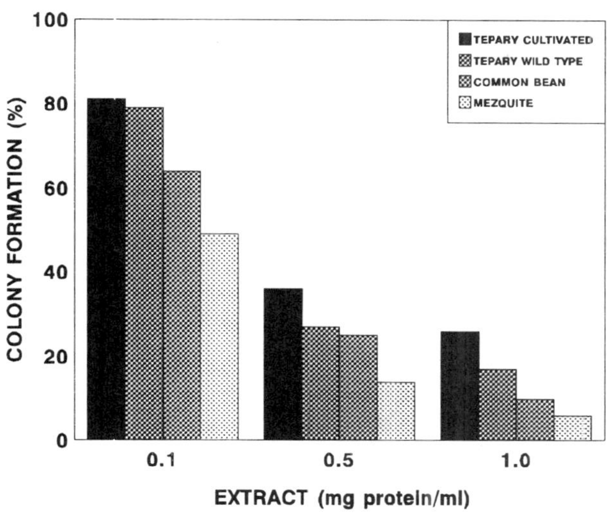

FIG. 1. EFFECT OF CRUDE EXTRACT FROM MEXICAN LEGUMES ON TUMOR CELL COLONY FORMATION

Cells were exposed to indicated concentrations of extracts for 2 h, after which they were trypsinized and counted. The number of cells which formed colonies were determined as described in Materials and Methods. The results are presented as a percentage of the number of colonies formed by untreated cells (100% = 102 colonies/dish)

The effect of legume extracts on DNA synthesis in Hela cells is shown in Fig. 2. Treatment of these cells with different concentrations of extracts from Mexican legumes resulted in a dose-dependent decrease in DNA synthesis. All concentrations of mezquite seed extracts showed significant inhibitory effect in comparison with the other plant extracts.

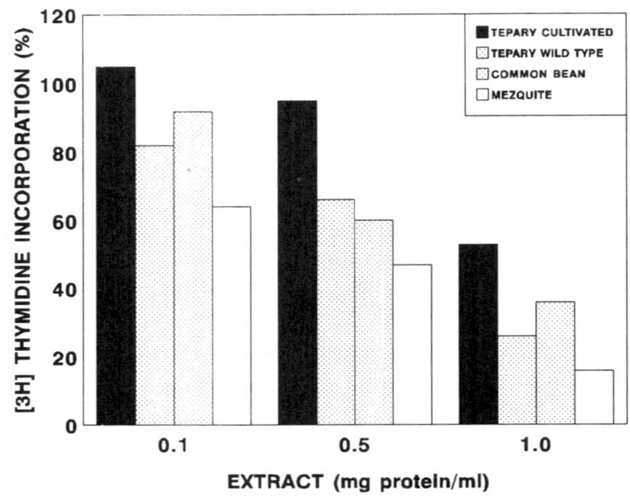

FIG. 2. EFFECT OF EXTRACTS FROM MEXICAN LEGUMES ON DNA SYNTHESIS
Cells were exposed to indicated concentrations of extracts for 2 h, after which ^{3}H-thymidine was added and incubation continued for 30 min. The radioactivity incorporated into DNA was then determined as described in Materials and Methods. The results are presented as a percentage of incorporation into untreated cells. (100% = 135,500 c.p.m.)

The results in Table 3 involved 12 points at least and the results in Table 4 involved 3 points at least, so in all cases we used simple regression analysis. Table 3 shows significant correlation between colony formation and DNA synthesis ($r = 0.8929$ and $r^2 = 0.7974$). As a function of legume type (Table 4), the correlation analysis shows that common bean had the higher correlation in relation to the other extracts between DNA synthesis and colony formation ($r = 0.9857$ and $r^2 = 0.9717$). Mezquite beans had a significant correlation ($r = 0.8704$ and $r^2 = 0.7577$). Tepary beans had a significant correlation (cultivated and wild type), but showed lower correlations in this experiment than did extracts from mezquite.

TABLE 3.
CORRELATION AMONG HEMAGGLUTINATION, CELL PROLIFERATION, COLONY INHIBITION AND DNA SYNTHESIS

	c.p./Hem	c.f./Hem	c.p./c.f.	c.p./DNA syn	c.f./DNA syn
r	0.7013	0.3195	0.3275	0.3770	0.8929
r^2	0.4919	0.1021	0.1073	0.1422	0.7974

c.p., cell proliferation; Hem, hemagglutinating activity; c.f., colony formation; DNA syn., DNA synthesis.

TABLE 4.
CORRELATION AMONG DIFFERENT EXTRACTS WITH DNA SYNTHESIS, COLONY INHIBITION AND DNA SYNTHESIS

Extract		DNA syn/c.f.
Tepary (cult)	r	0.7690
	r^2	0.5914
Tepary (Wild)	r	0.8165
	r^2	0.6668
Common bean	r	0.9857
	r^2	0.9717
Mezquite	r	0.8704
	r^2	0.7577

c.f., colony formation; DNA syn, DNA synthesis.

DISCUSSION

Of the results presented above, three findings in particular deserve attention. First, the data show no correlation among protein content, hemagglutining activity and cytotoxic activity of extracts from the Mexican legumes. Second, extracts from different Mexican plants had a differential inhibitory effect on cell proliferation, colony formation and DNA synthesis, although in all cases inhibition was dose-dependent. Third, extracts of mezquite seeds had significant effects on cell proliferation, colony formation and DNA synthesis in comparison with the other tested extracts. The relatively higher cytotoxic activity of extract from mesquite seeds indicates that selection of Mexican legumes for research by reference to their use in cancer prevention may be useful for identification of new anticancer agents.

Further experiments are in progress to isolate and characterize the lectins of these plants and to determine their mechanism(s) of action.

REFERENCES

ABDULLAEV, F.I. and FRENKEL, G.D. 1992. Effect of saffron on cell colony formation and cellular nucleic acid and protein synthesis. BioFactors *3*(3), 201–204.

ABDULLAEV, F.I. and GONZALEZ DE MEJIA, E. 1995/1996. Inhibition of colony formation of Hela cells by naturally occurring and synthetic agents. BioFactors *5*(3), 133–138.

ABDULLAEV, F.I. and GONZALEZ de MEJIA, E. 1997. Antitumor activity of natural agents: Lectins and saffron. Arch. Latinoamericanos Nut. *47*(3), 23–29.

BRADFORD, M.M. 1976. A rapid and sensitive method for the quantitation of microgram quantities of protein utilizing the principle of protein dye binding. Anal. Biochem. *72*, 248–254.

JAFFE, W. 1980. Hemagglutinins (lectins). *In* Toxic Constituents in Plant Foodstuff. Chap. 3, Liener I.E., ed. pp. 73–102. Acad. Press. New York, NY.

KIM, M., RAO, M.V., TWEARDY, D.L., PRAKASH, M., GALILI, U. and GORELIK, E. 1993. Lectin-induced apoptosis of tumour cells. Glycobiol. *3*, 447–453.

KISS, R., CAMBY, I., DUCKWORTH, C., DECKER, R., SALMON, I., PASTEELS, J.L., DANGUY, A. and YEATON, P. 1997. *In vitro* influence of *Phaseolus vulgaris, Griffonia licifolia*, Concanavalin A, wheat germ and peanut agglutinins on HCT-15, LoVo and SW 837 human colorectal cancer cell growth. Gut *40*(2), 253–261.

LIN J.K., TSERNG, K.Y., CHEN, C.C., LIN, L.T. and TUNG, T.C. 1970. Abrin and ricin. Anti-tumor substances. Nature *227*, 292–293.

MODY, R.M., JOSHI, S. and CHANEY, W. 1995. Use of lectins as diagnostic and therapeutic tools for cancer. J. Pharmacol. Toxicol. Methods *33*(1), 1–10.

PUSZTAI, A. 1991. Plant Lectins. Cambridge University Press, Cambridge.

PRYME, I.F., PUSZTAI, A.J. and BARDOCZ, S. 1994. A diet containing the lectin phytohaemagglutinin (PHA) slowed down the proliferation of Krebs II cell tumors in mice. Cancer Lett. *76*, 133-137.

ROBINSON, E. and MEKORI, T. 1971. Studies on the effect of phytohemagglutinin on ascites tumor in mice. Isr. J. Med. Sci. *7*, 83–89.

RYDER, S.D., SMITH, J.A. and RHODES, J.M. 1992. Peanut lectin: a mitogen for normal human colonic epithelium and human HT29 colorectal cancer cells. J. Natl. Cancer Inst. *84*, 1410–1416.

RYDER, S.D, SMITH, J.A., PARKER, N. and RHODES, J.M. 1994. Proliferative responses of HT29 and Caco2 human colorectal cancer cells to a panel of lectins. Gastroenterology *106*(1), 85–93.

SHARON, N. and LIS, H. 1989. Lectins. Chapman and Hall, London.

SHOHAM, J., INBAR, M. and SACHS, L. 1970. Differential toxicity on normal and transformed cell *in vitro* and inhibition of tumour development *in vivo* by Concanavalin A. Nature *227*, 1244–1246.

YU, L., FERNING, D.C., SMITH, J.A., MILTON, J.D. and RHODES, J.M. 1993. Reversible inhibition of proliferation of epithelial cell lines by *Agaricus bisporus* (edible mushroom) lectin. Cancer Res. *53*, 4627–4632.

PRELIMINARY ANALYSIS OF CRYSTALLIZATION CONDITIONS OF GAMMA CONGLUTIN OF LUPIN

ALMA L. MARTÍNEZ-AYALA[1], ALEXANDER McPHERSON[2], OCTAVIO PAREDES-LÓPEZ[3] and GLORIA S. DÁVILA-ORTÍZ[1]

[1]Departamento de Biotecnología, Centro de Desarrollo de Productos Bióticos
del Instituto Politécnico Nacional
Apartado Postal 24
62730 Yautepec, Mor., Mexico

[2]University of California, Riverside
Department of Biochemistry
Riverside, CA 92521

[3]Departamento de Biotecnología y Bioquímica
Centro de Investigación y de Estudios Avanzados del Instituto Politécnico Nacional
Apartado Postal 629
36500 Irapuato, Gto., Mexico

ABSTRACT

The lupin γ conglutin is one of the most important storage proteins in the seeds of lupin and the good essential amino acid composition makes it an attractive target for genetic and protein engineering. We have purified the protein from Lupinus campestris *to a high level of homogeneity. The protein, under reducing conditions migrates on SDS-PAGE as two bands 17 and 30 kDa and under nonreducing conditions as one band of 42-47 kDa. There is one inter-subunit disulfide bond. Ten amino acid residues were determined from the end of the N-terminal amino acid of the minor subunit, along with an oligosaccharide chain; the oligosaccharide chain gives resistance to hydrolysis by trypsin. A broad range of crystallization conditions were investigated, using the method of vapor diffusion with a variety of precipitant agents and over a wide pH range. Microcrystals of the protein were obtained under different conditions. The best crystals were obtained from 2.0 M ammonium sulfate in 0.02 M MOPS buffer at pH 6.4. The crystals grew at room temperature in one week's time but at present we have not achieved a size sufficient for a detailed structural analysis by X-ray diffraction. We are continuing efforts to improve the quality of these crystals so that a crystallographic analysis may be done.*

INTRODUCTION

Lupin is a legume with one of the highest seed protein contents. As in other legumes, most of the lupin seed proteins are globulins (Gueguen and Cerletti 1994). Globulins of *Lupinus albus* have been characterized, on the basis of both their amino acid composition and their molecular weights, and have been grouped in the following categories: vicilin-like (7S) protein, legumin-like (11S) protein, γ-conglutin and other globulins (Duranti *et al.* 1981).

γ-Conglutin differs from the other globulins in its amino acid composition, with less acidic amino acids and more lysine, threonine, tryptophan and valine. This composition confers a very good methionine essential amino acid (MEAA) value to γ-conglutin compared with those of other globulins. For example, MEAA is 99.53 in *L. albus* (Duranti and Cerletti 1979; Duranti *et al.* 1981).

γ-Conglutin is conserved in white lupin cotyledons after 15 days of germination (Esnault *et al.* 1996). Therefore, this protein is not used to supply amino acids during germination. So γ-conglutin must not be considered as a storage protein.

Current knowledge on lupin protein is mostly the result of research with European *Lupinus*, with only a few biochemical studies of the American species. Here, we describe some molecular characteristics and the preliminary results of the crystallization of the γ-conglutin of *Lupinus campestris*, a wild lupin grown in Mexico.

MATERIALS AND METHODS

Preparation of the Protein

Seeds of *Lupinus campestris* grown in Morelos, Mexico were dehulled and ground to flour. The flour was defatted with hexane. γ-Conglutin was obtained by the method of Blagrove and Gillespie (1975).

Protein Determination

All protein concentrations were determined by the method of Bradford (1976) with bovine serum albumin as the standard.

Gel Electrophoresis

SDS-PAGE was carried out according to the method of Shagger and von Jagow (1987) using 13% polyacrylamide gels in the presence of 1% SDS, with or without β-mercaptoethanol. Standard proteins used were lysozyme (14.4 KDa), Kunitz soybean trypsin inhibitor (20.1 KDa), carbonic anhydrase (31 KDa), ovalbumin (45 KDa), bovine serum albumin (66 KDa) and phosphorylase b (97.4 KDa).

Digestion of γ-Conglutin Using Trypsin

The native γ-conglutin was incubated at 37°C with bovine trypsin (Sigma) over a period of 30 min to 24 h. The reaction mixture had a γ-conglutin to protease ratio of 100:1 in a volume of 100 μl. The proteolysis was stopped by mixing the digestion solution with sample buffer containing 10% SDS and immediately boiling for 1 min. The products of the digestion were subjected to SDS-PAGE.

N-Terminal Amino Acid Sequence

Sequencing was carried out according to the manufacturer's recommendations using an Applied Biosystems gas-phase sequencer model 475A.

Crystallization of the γ-Conglutin

Preliminary crystallization conditions were determined using the crystal screen crystallization kit (Hamton Research). γ-Conglutin (aliquots of 17 mg/ml) was crystallized by vapor diffusion in sitting drop plates at room temperature.

RESULTS AND DISCUSSION

γ-Conglutin was resolved into its constituent subunits by SDS-PAGE. Its electrophoretic patterns without and with reducing agent (Fig. 1) consisted of one band (40-42 KDa) and two bands (27-30 kDa and 15-17 kDa) respectively; these results indicated that there is one inter chain disulfide bond. The results reported here suggest that the γ-conglutin of *Lupinus campestris* has common features to the γ-conglutin of other species (Esnault *et al.* 1996; Duranti *et al.* 1981). In all the species studied, the protein is composed of two disulfide bonded polypeptides, one close to 30 KDa and the second to 17 kDa molecular weights.

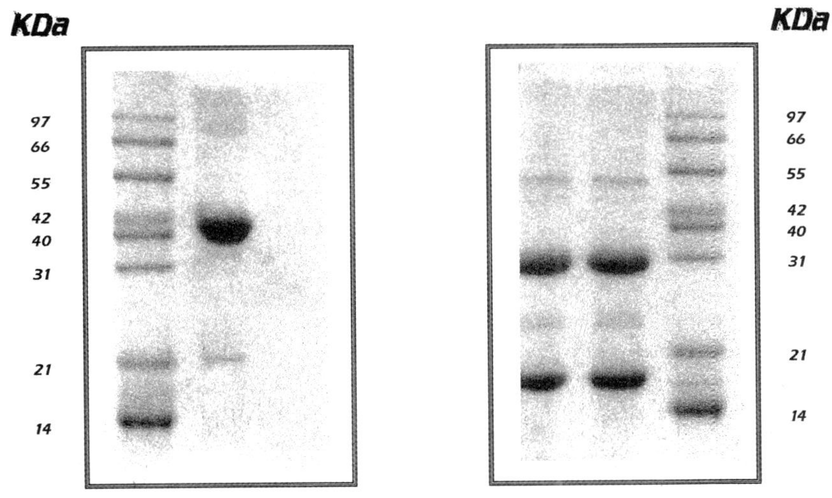

10% SDS-PAGE-ME 10% SDS-PAGE+ME

FIG. 1. SDS-PAGE OF NON REDUCED (LEFT) AND REDUCED (RIGHT) γ *LUPINUS CAMPESTRIS*

When the γ-conglutin was incubated with trypsin at different time periods, the electrophoretic profile (Fig. 2) did not show evidence for protein hydrolysis (no peptides formed). It is suggested that the resistance of the protein to trypsin hydrolysis could be associated with the presence of a carbohydrate chain.

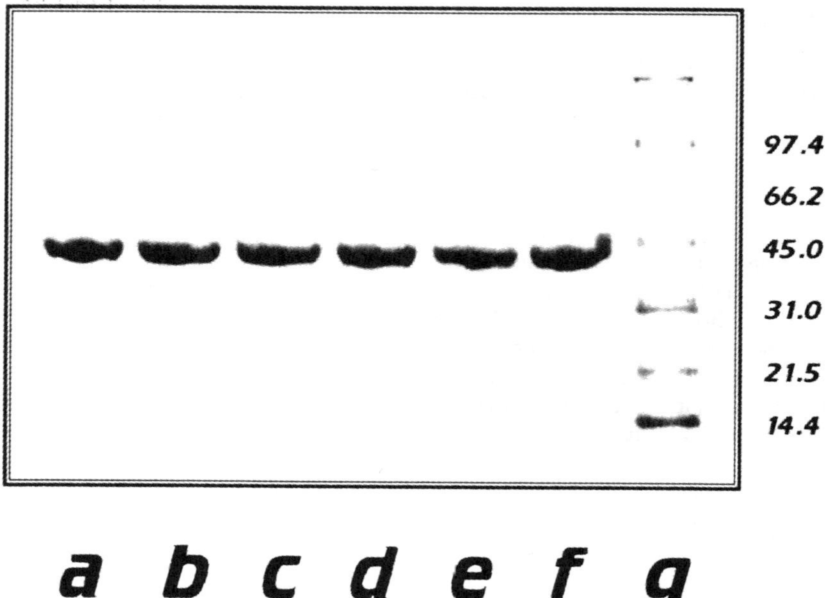

FIG. 2. SDS-PAGE OF TIME COURSE γ-CONGLUTIN DIGESTION BY TRYPSIN
Lanes: g, standard proteins; a, γ-conglutin; b, γ-conglutin and trypsin at 37°C, 0 min; c, γ-conglutin and trypsin at 37°C, 30 min; d, γ-conglutin and trypsin at 37°C, 60 min; e, γ-conglutin and trypsin at 37°C, 120 min; f, γ-conglutin and trypsin at 37°C, 24 h.

The N-terminal amino acid sequence of the smaller polypeptide was determined (Fig. 3). The sequence of 10 amino acids was identical to the N-terminal sequence of the smaller chain of *L. angustifolius* (Kolivas and Gayler 1993; Elleman 1977).

The properties observed here are similar to those reported for γ-conglutin of *Lupinus albus* (Duranti *et al.* 1995).

S T V Y H E F L E I

FIG. 3. N-TERMINAL SEQUENCE OF THE SMALLER POLYPEPTIDE IN *LUPINUS CAMPESTRIS* γ-CONGLUTIN

The crystallization studies of γ-conglutin were carried out using the procedures described by McPherson (1990), using a variety of salts, polyethylene glycols, and other precipitants over a wide range of pH. In addition, the effects of metal ions and a spectrum of detergents on crystallization were investigated. The best precipitant agent was 2.0 M ammonium sulfate in 0.02 M MOPS buffer at pH 6.4 (Fig.4). However, the crystals obtained grew like clusters, so it is still necessary to obtain monocrystals large enough for preliminary X-ray diffraction analysis.

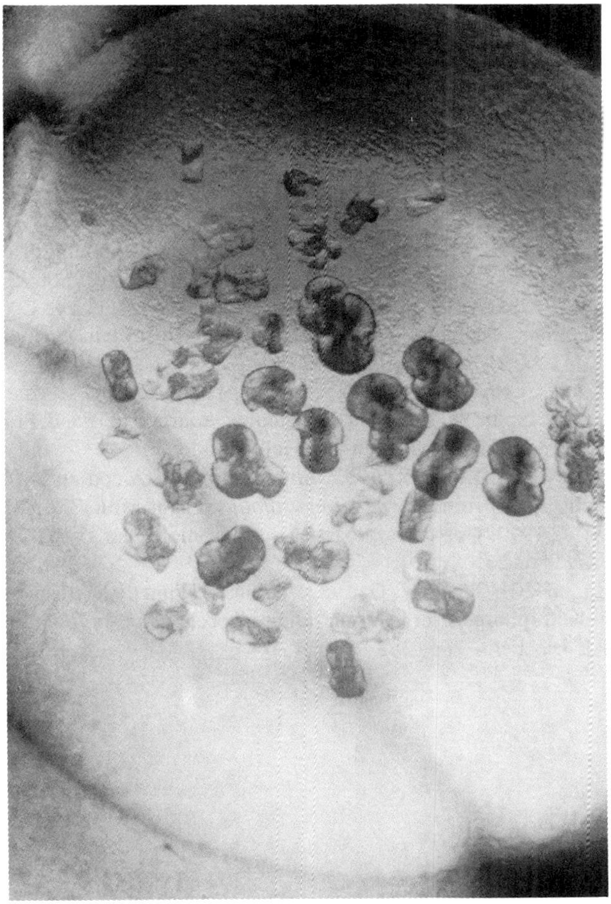

FIG. 4. γ-CONGLUTIN CRYSTALS

ACKNOWLEDGMENT

We acknowledge financial support from Consejo Nacional de Ciencia y Tecnología (CONACYT) Mexico and the Instituto Politécnico Nacional, Mexico.

REFERENCES

BLAGROVE, R.J. and GILLESPIE, J.M. 1975. Isolation, purification and characterization of the seed globulins of *Lupinus angustifolius*. Aust. J. Plant. Physiol. *2*, 13–27.

BRADFORD, M.M. 1976. A rapid sensitive method for quantitation of microgram quantities of protein utilizing the principle of protein-dye binding. Anal. Biochem. *72*, 248–254.

DURANTI, M. and CERLETTI, P. 1979. Amino acid composition of seed proteins of *Lupinus albus*. J. Agric. Food Chem. *27*, 977–978.

DURANTI, M., GIUS, C., SESSA, F. and VECCHIO, G. 1995. The saccharide chain of lupin seed conglutin γ is not responsible for the protection of the native protin from degradation by trypsin, but facilitates the refolding of the acid-treated protein to the resistant conformation. Eur. J. Biochem. *230*, 886–891.

DURANTI, M., RESTANI, P., PONIATOWSKA, M. and CERLETTI, P. 1981. The seed globulins of *Lupinus albus*. Phytochemistry *20*, 2071–2095.

ELLEMAN, T.C. 1977. Amino acid sequence of the smaller subunit of conglutin γ, a storage globulin of *Lupinus angustifolius*. Aust. J. Biol. Sci. *30*, 33–45.

ESNAULT, M.A., CITHAREL, J., THOMAS, D., GUEGAN, P. and CAVALIER, A. 1996. Behaviour of conglutin γ, a major lupin seed protein during germination. Plant Physiol. Biochem. *34*, 101–109.

GUEGUEN, J. and CERLETTI, P. 1994. Proteins of some legume seeds: soybean, pea, faba bean and lupin. *In* New and Developing Sources of Food Proteins (B.J.F. Hudson, ed.) 145–196. Chapman and Hall, London.

KOLIVAS, S. and GAYLER, K.R. 1993. Structure of cDNA coding for conglutin γ, a sulphur-rich protein from *Lupinus angustifolius*. Plant Mol. Biol. *21*, 397–401.

MCPHERSON, A. 1990. Current approaches to macromolecular crystallization. Eur. J. Biochem. *189*, 1–23.

SHAGGER, H. and VON JAGOW, G. 1987. Tricine-sodium dodecyl sulfate-poliacrylamide gel electrophoresis for the separation of proteins in the range from 1 to 100 kDa. Anal. Biochem. *166*, 368–379.

ENZYMATIC CONVERSION OF CELLULOSIC MATERIALS IN A CONTINUOUS STIRRED TANK REACTOR WITH AN ULTRAFILTRATION MEMBRANE

HANSHU DING, ELENA VLASENKO, CHARLES SHOEMAKER and SHARON SHOEMAKER

Department of Food Science and Technology
University of California, Davis, CA 95616

California Institute of Food and Agricultural Research
Davis, CA 95616

ABSTRACT

A continuous stirred tank reactor equipped with an ultrafiltration membrane was used for enzymatic hydrolysis of two cellulosic materials, Solka Floc™ cellulose and acid-pretreated mixed urban waste. An enzyme preparation, consisting of two commercially available cellulases, Spezyme CP® and Novozym 188®, was used for hydrolysis. Low molecular-weight hydrolysis products were continuously removed from the reactor through the membrane, thereby relieving end-product inhibition. The polymeric substrate and enzymes were retained in the reactor. Additional substrate was introduced into the reactor as the reaction proceeded to a more liquid state. The reaction parameters were compared for the continuous stirred tank reactor and the batch shake flask reactor using both types of cellulosic substrates.

Conversion of Solka Floc™ cellulose after enzymatic hydrolysis with two additions of substrate in the membrane reactor was 1.5 times higher when compared to the shake flask, whereas conversion of the acid-pretreated material was not improved in the membrane reactor. When pure cellulose was used as a substrate in the membrane reactor, the cellulases were active upon subsequent additions of fresh substrate. However, with subsequent additions of lignocellulose, substrate conversion rapidly decreased. This is likely due to accumulation of the insoluble lignin residue in the reaction mixture and the irreversible adsorption of cellulases onto lignin residue. The amount of enzyme required to produce 1 gram of glucose was approximately 3 times lower in the membrane reactor compared to the shake flask with pure cellulose as a substrate, and 1.3-1.4 times lower for lignocellulosic material.

The final glucose concentration in the hydrolyzate from the membrane reactor was low compared to the shake flask. Use of the second, reverse osmosis (RO) membrane, in-line with the UF membrane in a continuous mode, will be examined in order to obviate the dilution problem and concentrate the glucose solution for the subsequent microbial fermentation.

INTRODUCTION

Cellulose-containing waste materials, such as agricultural residues, waste wood, and municipal solid wastes, pose a serious problem in California for their disposal.

Biotechnology-based approaches for the conversion of cellulosic wastes to ethanol and other chemicals are being studied by different research groups (Ingram and Doran 1995; Duff and Murray 1996; Olsson and Hagerdal 1996). The key step in the cellulose-to-ethanol bioconversion process is enzymatic hydrolysis of cellulose (Klyosov 1990; Beguin and Aubert 1994). Significant progress has been achieved in this area in recent years. However, commercial large-scale processes utilizing cellulases for enzymatic hydrolysis of cellulosic wastes do not yet exist. The main reasons for this are the relatively high cost of enzymes and inhibition of cellulases by hydrolysis products (cellobiose and glucose), which results in incomplete depolymerization of cellulose to glucose.

End-product inhibition can be eliminated by continuous removal of soluble hydrolysis products from the reaction mixture. This approach was realized in a continuous stirred tank reactor (CSTR) equipped with an ultrafiltration (UF) membrane (Ghose and Kostick 1970; Henley *et al.* 1980; Ohlson *et al.* 1984; Lee and Kim 1993). High molecular-weight cellulase (enzyme) and insoluble cellulosic material (substrate) were retained within the membrane reactor, whereas low molecular-weight soluble products of hydrolysis passed through the membrane. As a result, the efficiency of cellulose conversion to soluble sugars was significantly increased (Henley *et al.* 1980; Ohlson *et al.* 1984).

Ohlson *et al.* (1984) used an UF-membrane reactor to recover enzymes during the process. Eliminating end-product inhibition drove the reaction further toward complete hydrolysis and allowed the addition of fresh portions of cellulosic materials to the reactor. The enzymes in the reactor hydrolyzed the fresh substrate and thus were reused. However, a serious disadvantage of the membrane reactor was the continuous dilution of the product, glucose. It was pointed out that substantial expense would be required to concentrate the glucose solution for the subsequent microbial fermentation (Ohlson *et al.* 1984).

We suggest that the dilution problem can be obviated by using a second, reverse osmosis (RO) membrane, in-line with the UF membrane in a continuous mode. The overall research objective is to design and evaluate a bimembrane system, accommodating both UF- and RO-membranes, for enzymatic hydrolysis of cellulose-containing materials. This article reports the results of the first part of our study, in which the UF-membrane reactor was set up and tested using two substrates, Solka Floc™ cellulose and acid-pretreated mixed urban waste.

MATERIALS AND METHODS

Substrates

Two materials were used in hydrolysis experiments: Solka Floc™ cellulose (grade 300-FCC) obtained from The Creative Food Ingredient Co., and acid-pretreated mixed urban waste provided by the U.S. DOE National Renewable Energy Laboratory (NREL). The waste material was prepared at NREL by blending five different feedstocks, fir (35% of dry weight), almond tree pruning (20%), wheat straw (20%), office waste paper (12.5%), and newsprint (12.5%), and then pretreated using dilute sulfuric acid. Compositional analysis, carried out at NREL, showed that dilute-acid pretreatment solubilized essentially all hemicellulose, giving material which contained 54.5% of glucan and 1% of non-glucose polysaccharides (xylan, galactan, arabinan, and mannan).

Content of dry solids in Solka Floc™ cellulose and in the acid-pretreated material was determined gravimetrically, after drying of samples at 105°C for 24 h, and was found to be 96.0% and 23.6%, respectively.

Enzymes

Spezyme CP® cellulase was provided by Genencor International (USA) and Novozym 188® cellobiase was obtained from Novo Nordisk (USA). The activities of enzymes toward filter paper and cellobiose are presented in Table 1. Filter-paper activity was measured according to the standard procedure recommended by the Commission on Biotechnology, IUPAC (Ghose 1987) and expressed in Filter Paper Units (FPU).

TABLE 1.
ACTIVITIES OF COMMERCIAL CELLULASES

Cellulase preparation	Filter paper activity, FPU/mL	Cellobiase activity, CBU/mL
Spezyme CP®	90.7	20.8
Novozym 188®	1.4	528

Cellobiase activity was determined as the initial rate of hydrolysis of 2 mM cellobiose to glucose at pH 5.0, 50°C, and expressed in Cellobiase Units (CBU). Glucose released during hydrolysis of cellobiose was determined by the glucose oxidase-peroxidase method using 2,2′-azino-di-(3-ethylbenzthiazoline)-6-sulfonate (ABTS) as a chromogen (Bergmeyer and Bernt 1974). One CBU corresponded to 1 μmol of β-1,4-glycosidic bonds of substrate hydrolyzed in one min during the initial stage of hydrolysis.

Enzymatic Hydrolysis in Shake Flasks

Solka Floc™ cellulose and acid-pretreated waste material were hydrolyzed with commercial enzymes in 100-mL glass flasks on a shaker (200 rpm) at pH 5.0 and 50°C. After 10 mM sodium-acetate buffer (pH 5.0) was added to a weighed amount of substrate and the pH adjusted to 5.0, the reaction was started by adding an enzyme solution to a final volume of 50 mL.

The concentration of substrate, which was expressed as the amount of dry solids per volume of the reaction mixture, varied from 10 g/L to 100 g/L. In order to promote complete conversion of cellobiose to glucose, Novozym 188® cellobiase was added to Spezyme CP® cellulase in all hydrolysis experiments. The combined enzyme preparation was formulated so as to provide a 1:1 ratio between CBU contributed by Novozym 188® and FPU contributed by Spezyme CP®. Filter paper activity in different experiments varied from 0.5 to 20 FPU per mL of the reaction mixture. Enzyme loading varied from 10 to 200 FPU per g of dry solids.

To follow the course of hydrolysis, 0.8 mL aliquots of the reaction mixture were taken at different times. The liquid phase (hydrolyzate) was separated from the solid residue by centrifugation (14,000 rpm, 3 min) and analyzed for glucose after the enzymatic reaction was stopped by an addition of one volume of the alkaline solution (512 mM Na_2CO_3, 288 mM $NaHCO_3$, pH 9.9) to four volumes of hydrolyzate. The concentration of glucose was determined using a YSI Model 2700 SELECT Biochemistry Analyzer. The degree of conversion was expressed as a percentage of dry solids hydrolyzed to glucose (biomass conversion) or as a percentage of cellulose hydrolyzed to glucose (cellulose conversion).

Enzymatic Hydrolysis in the UF-Membrane Reactor

A schematic diagram of the overall system for enzymatic hydrolysis of cellulosic materials in the reactor utilizing an ultrafiltration membrane is shown in Fig. 1.

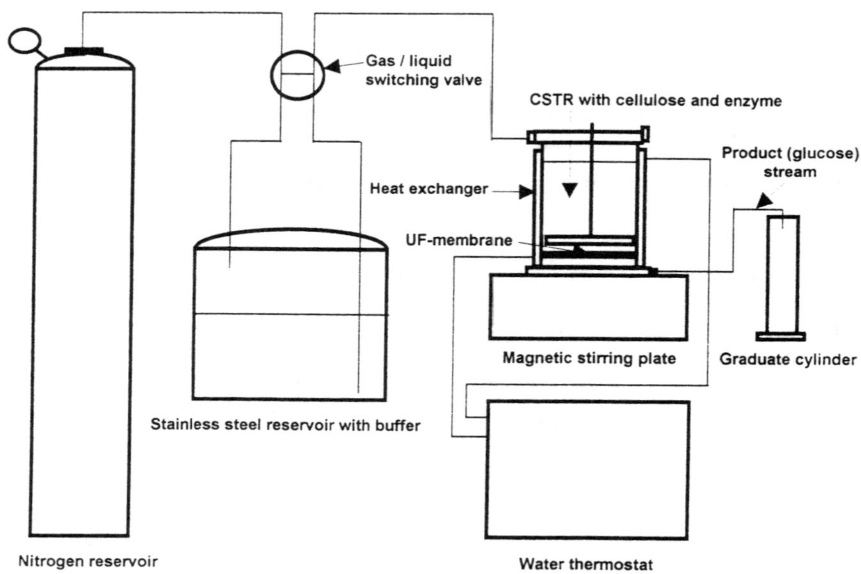

FIG. 1. EXPERIMENTAL DESIGN OF A UF-MEMBRANE REACTOR FOR HYDROLYSIS OF CELLULOSIC MATERIALS

Enzymatic hydrolysis was carried out in an Amicon ultrafiltration stirred cell (Model 8400, maximum volume 400 ml) at pH 5.0 and 50°C. Solid cellulosic substrate and cellulase enzymes were confined to the reactor by an UF membrane at the bottom of the cell. In all experiments Amicon polysulfone membrane PM10 with a 10,000 molecular-weight cutoff (MWCO) was utilized.

The stirred cell was pressurized using nitrogen. Under constant pressure, soluble products of hydrolysis were continuously removed through the UF membrane and replaced with 10 mM sodium-acetate buffer (pH 5.0) from a 4 L stainless steel reservoir

(Amicon, Model RS4). Instant switching between gas and liquid lines was performed using Amicon CDS10 valve with sliding control.

The heat exchanger shown in Fig. 1 was formed from a plastic tubing coiled around the reactor. Hot water from a water thermostat was circulating in the tubing so that the temperature in the reactor was kept at 50°C. The hydrolysis mixture was stirred using a magnetic stirring plate.

The initial concentration of Solka Floc™ cellulose and acid-pretreated material in the membrane reactor was 100 g/L and 50 g/L, respectively. Combined enzyme preparation of Spezyme CP® (1 FPU/mL) and Novozym 188® (1 CBU/mL) was used for hydrolysis. The total volume of the slurry was 200 mL for Solka Floc™ cellulose and 240 ml for the acid-pretreated material; the volume was kept constant during reaction.

The pressure in the system was kept constant at 2.5 psi for Solka Floc™ cellulose and at 20 psi for the acid-pretreated material. Dilution rate D, at which the glucose solution was continuously removed, was expressed as reciprocal h (h^{-1}) = permeate flow (mL/h) / reaction volume (mL). Due to eventual membrane fouling, the dilution rate gradually decreased with time. Average dilution rate in the course of hydrolysis was equal to 0.2 h^{-1} for Solka Floc™ cellulose and 0.1 h^{-1} for the acid-pretreated material.

Fractions of the permeate were collected into graduated cylinders and the volume measured. Glucose concentration in each fraction was determined using a YSI Model 2700 SELECT Biochemistry Analyzer. The cumulative glucose production was then calculated and compared with the quantity of dry material (or cellulose) originally loaded into the reactor to estimate the degree of biomass (or cellulose) conversion.

After completion of the first stage of hydrolysis, fresh substrate was added to the reaction mixture to restore the initial concentration of dry solids and hydrolyzed with cellulases remaining in the reaction mixture (second stage of hydrolysis).

RESULTS AND DISCUSSION

Enzymatic Hydrolysis of Cellulosic Materials in Shake Flasks

To examine the potential for hydrolysis of Solka Floc™ cellulose and acid-pretreated waste material in the batch reactor, the samples were hydrolyzed with a combined enzyme preparation in shake flasks. In this study the enzyme-to-substrate ratio was evaluated from 10 FPU to 200 FPU per gram of dry solids (Tables 2 and 3).

When the enzyme activity in the reaction mixture was kept constant at 1 FPU/mL, the use of a higher concentration of Solka Floc™ gave hydrolyzates with a higher glucose concentration, but resulted in a lower degree of cellulose conversion (Table 2). Increase in the enzyme loading up to 50 FPU/g at constant concentration of Solka Floc™ (50 g/L or 100 g/L) provided conditions for a higher degree of cellulose conversion. However, further increase in the enzyme loading (up to 100 FPU/g or even 200 FPU/g) did not improve the hydrolysis significantly (Table 2).

For the acid-pretreated material (tested at about 100 g/L) the use of the enzyme loadings at greater than 50 FPU/g was not feasible as well, since it did not bring about a proportional increase in the degree of biomass conversion (Table 3). The washing of the acid-pretreated material with water did not significantly improve hydrolysis compared to the unwashed substrate (Table 3).

TABLE 2.
HYDROLYSIS OF SOLKA FLOC™ CELLULOSE WITH COMBINED ENZYME PREPARATION OF SPEZYME CP® AND NOVOZYM 188®
AT DIFFERENT ENZYME LOADINGS
pH 5.0, 50°C, stirring in 100-ml flasks on a shaker, reaction time 96 h

Substrate, g dry solids/L	Enzyme, FPU/mL	Enzyme loading, FPU/g dry solids	Increase in glucose, g/L	Cellulose conversion, %
10.0	1.0	100.0	10.2	92.0
20.0	1.0	50.2	19.9	89.4
50.0	1.0	20.1	39.8	71.5
93.2	0.9	10.0	51.3	49.5
50.0	0.5	10.0	33.1	59.5
50.0	1.0	20.1	39.8	71.5
50.0	2.5	50.1	49.8	89.6
50.0	5.0	100.3	51.1	92.0
50.0	10.0	200.5	52.2	94.0
93.2	0.9	10.0	51.3	49.5
100.0	2.0	20.0	69.0	62.1
100.0	5.0	50.1	81.8	73.6
100.0	10.0	100.3	82.1	73.9
100.0	20.1	200.5	83.3	75.0

TABLE 3.
HYDROLYSIS OF ACID-PRETREATED URBAN WASTE WITH COMBINED ENZYME PREPARATION OF SPEZYME CP® AND NOVOZYM 188®
AT DIFFERENT ENZYME LOADINGS
pH 5.0, 50°C, stirring in 100-ml flasks on a shaker, reaction time 96 h

Substrate, g dry solids/L	Enzyme, FPU/mL	Enzyme loading, FPU/g dry solids	Increase in glucose, g/L	Biomass conversion, %
Unwashed material				
98.4	1.0	10.1	27.7	25.3
98.2	2.0	20.1	36.2	33.2
98.2	4.9	50.3	41.9	38.4
98.2	9.9	100.7	45.3	41.5
98.2	19.8	201.4	47.5	43.5
Washed material				
101.4	1.0	10.0	33.4	29.6
101.5	2.0	20.0	36.2	32.1
101.5	5.1	50.1	46.4	41.2
101.5	10.2	100.1	49.0	43.4
101.5	20.3	200.2	51.6	45.8

The enzyme digestibility of the acid-pretreated material was determined at the conditions, that were favorable for hydrolysis, i.e. at low substrate concentration (10 g/L) and at high enzyme loading (100 FPU/g dry solids). Based on the compositional analysis of the acid-pretreated substrate performed at NREL (see "Materials and Methods" section), we estimated that up to 85% of cellulose in unwashed material and 87% of cellulose in washed material was converted to glucose (compared to 92%-conversion of Solka Floc™ cellulose at the similar conditions, Table 2).

Enzymatic Hydrolysis of Cellulosic Materials in the UF-membrane Reactor

There are several factors that may limit the degree of enzymatic conversion of cellulose to soluble sugars. These factors include end-product inhibition (Holtzapple *et al.* 1990; Ramos *et al.* 1993), different kinds of enzyme inactivation (Reese 1980; Gusakov *et al.* 1992), non-specific adsorption of cellulolytic enzymes onto lignin (Chernoglazov *et al.* 1988; Ooshima *et al.* 1990), and the decrease in the reactivity of cellulosic material during the course of hydrolysis (Lee and Fan, 1983; Sinitsyn *et al.* 1991).

To reduce end-product inhibition, soluble hydrolysis products should be continuously removed from the reaction mixture. The UF-membrane reactor utilizing a membrane with MWCO of 10,000 Da was assembled (Fig. 1) and tested using Solka Floc™ cellulose or acid-pretreated urban waste. The membrane kept the larger components (cellulose, enzymes) in the reactor (retentate) while allowing low molecular-weight molecules (sugars) to pass through the membrane (permeate).

Figure 2 shows that conversion of Solka Floc™ cellulose achieved in the membrane reactor was significantly higher compared to results achieved in shake flask; using the membrane reactor, 80% of the cellulose was hydrolyzed to glucose during the first stage hydrolysis, and additional 68% during the second stage hydrolysis, whereas using shake flask only 50% of cellulose was converted to glucose.

The second addition of Solka Floc™ was made when hydrolysis of the initial substrate was nearly complete and the reaction mixture was liquefied. Since the same enzyme was used for two additions of substrate, the enzyme-to-substrate ratio in the membrane reactor was kept to a minimum (5.0 FPU/g) and was almost 2 times lower compared to the shake flask (9.7 FPU/g, Table 4). The amount of enzyme required to produce 1 g of glucose in the membrane reactor was about 3 times lower than in the shake flask (6.0 FPU/g and 17.6 FPU/g, respectively, Table 4).

Optimization of the process in the membrane reactor could reduce enzyme consumption even more and, therefore, minimize enzyme cost. Among the parameters to be optimized are substrate concentration, enzyme-to-substrate ratio, dilution rate, intensity of stirring, and frequency of adding of fresh substrate during semi-continuous hydrolysis of cellulose.

Our data indicate that end-product inhibition was the major factor limiting hydrolysis of Solka Floc™ cellulose in the batch reactor. Contribution of other factors, such as enzyme inactivation or decrease in the substrate reactivity was probably not significant. The high stability of commercial cellulases under operational conditions was demonstrated by the fact that the amount of glucose produced in the membrane reactor during the second stage hydrolysis was only slightly lower compared to the amount of glucose obtained in the first stage hydrolysis (Table 4).

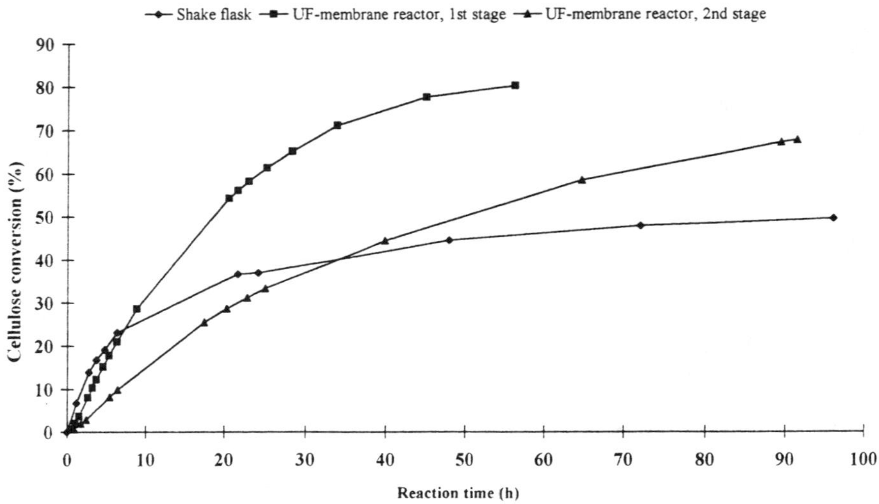

FIG. 2. HYDROLYSIS OF SOLKA FLOC™ CELLULOSE (100 g/L) WITH COMBINED ENZYME PREPARATION OF SPEZYME CP® (1 FPU/mL) AND NOVOZYM 188® (1 CBU/mL) IN THE SHAKE FLASK AND IN THE UF-MEMBRANE REACTOR, pH 5.0, 50°C, STIRRING

TABLE 4.
HYDROLYSIS OF SOLKA FLOC™ CELLULOSE WITH COMBINED ENZYME PREPARATION OF SPEZYME CP® AND NOVOZYM 188® IN THE SHAKE FLASK AND IN THE UF-MEMBRANE REACTOR (TWO SUBSEQUENT ADDITIONS OF SUBSTRATE)

Parameter	Shake flask (96 h)	UF-membrane reactor		
		1st stage hydrolysis (56 h)	2nd stage hydrolysis (91 h)	Total
Before hydrolysis				
Reaction volume, mL	200	200	220	200
Substrate, g dry solids/L	93.2	100.0	92.3	199.1
Substrate, g dry solids	18.6	20.0	20.3	39.8
Enzyme, FPU/mL	0.9	1.0	0.9	1.0
Enzyme, FPU	180	200	200	200
Enzyme, FPU/g dry solids	9.7	10.0	9.9	5.0
After hydrolysis				
Volume, mL	200	2868	3119	5986
Glucose, g/L	51.3	6.2	4.9	5.5
Glucose, g	10.3	17.8	15.2	33.1
Cellulose conversion, %	49.5	80.3	67.6	74.8
FPU/g Glc	17.6	11.2	13.1	6.0

The high reactivity of the insoluble residue of cellulose obtained after the first stage hydrolysis was demonstrated in the following experiment. Two 10-mL portions of the reaction mixture obtained after the first stage hydrolysis (containing the solid residue and cellulases) were transferred to two 25-mL flasks on a shaker and incubated at 50°C. No enzyme was added to the first flask, whereas fresh enzyme preparation consisting of Spezyme CP® (1 FPU/mL) and Novozym 188® (1 CBU/mL) was added into the second flask. After 70 h of incubation, 60% of the insoluble residue was converted to glucose in the first flask, indicating that the residue was readily digested by the cellulases remaining in the reaction mixture after the first stage hydrolysis. About the same level of conversion (65%) was observed in the second flask, containing additional fresh enzyme. This indicates that at the end of the first stage hydrolysis, the reaction was not limited by the amount of available cellulase.

The experiments in the membrane reactor were also carried out using the acid-pretreated urban waste. In contrast to the experiments using Solka Floc™ cellulose, where the suspension was that of an evenly dispersed white powder, urban wood waste gave a suspension of larger woody particles which prevented effective stirring of the hydrolysis mixture at high substrate concentrations. To obtain effective stirring in the membrane reactor, the highest concentration of the acid-pretreated material was 50 g/L.

Another problem which was experienced with the acid-pretreated material, and not with Solka Floc™ cellulose, was rapid membrane fouling. As a result, the UF pressure was increased in the experiment with urban waste, and this further increased the risk of the premature membrane damage with the rough edges of the woody substrate.

The data showed (Fig. 3) that the use of the membrane reactor compared to the shake flask did not provide such a significant increase in hydrolysis efficiency with acid-pretreated material, as it was observed in case of Solka Floc™ cellulose. Conversion of the cellulose fraction to glucose was 76.0% in the shake flask and only slightly higher (80.2%) after the first stage of hydrolysis in the membrane reactor. Hydrolysis in the second stage using the membrane reactor was much less effective than in the first stage, with only 35.7% of cellulose converted to glucose. However, the enzyme-to-substrate ratio and the enzyme consumption per gram of glucose in the membrane reactor was 1.3-1.4 times lower compared to the shake flask (Table 5).

It appeared that effective hydrolysis of the acid-pretreated urban waste in the membrane reactor was compromised by the high lignin content in this material (37.9%, according to NREL). It is known (Chernoglazov *et al.* 1988; Ooshima *et al.* 1990) that cellulases adsorb tightly and irreversibly and are inactivated by the phenolic lignin component of wood. Model experiments on recovery of cellulases have shown that, when substrates of low lignin content (4%) were used, the enzyme can be recovered by readsorption onto the fresh substrate and used in 4-5 cycles of hydrolysis without loss of activity (Lee *et al.* 1995). When lignocellulose with 32% lignin content was used, only 71 and 43% of the original activity were recovered in the second and third hydrolysis cycles, respectively (Lee *et al.* 1995).

A serious disadvantage of the membrane reactor was that the final glucose concentration in permeate was much lower than in shake flask (Tables 4 and 5). This problem could be obviated by the use of the second membrane working in a reverse osmosis (RO) mode, which would allow the in-line concentration of glucose to the levels needed for subsequent microbial fermentation. We are testing a SEPA CF membrane filtration unit from Osmonics Inc. which accommodates flat RO membranes. The results on the use of the bimembrane system for enzymatic hydrolysis of cellulose and acid-pretreated urban waste will be reported subsequently.

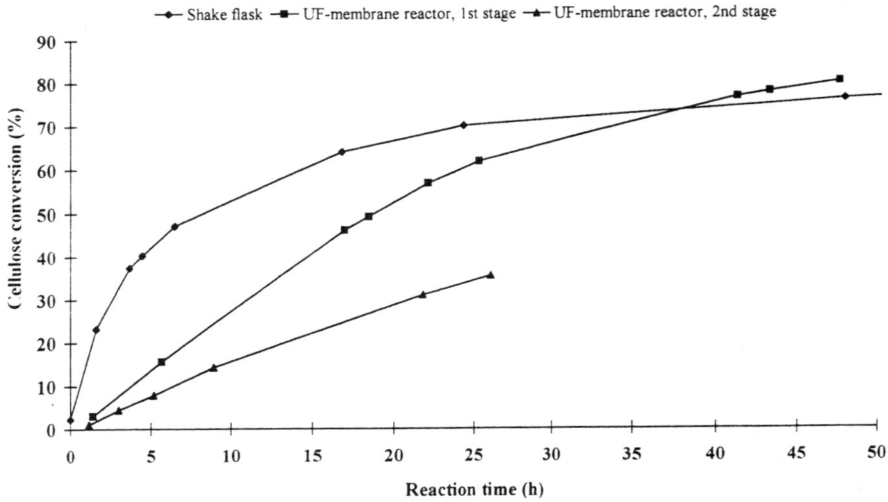

FIG. 3. HYDROLYSIS OF ACID-PRETREATED URBAN WASTE (50 g/L) WITH COMBINED ENZYME PREPARATION OF SPEZYME CP® (1 FPU/mL) AND NOVOZYM 188® (1 CBU/mL) IN THE SHAKE FLASK AND IN THE UF-MEMBRANE REACTOR, pH 5.0, 50°C, STIRRING

CONCLUSIONS

A continuous stirred tank reactor utilizing an ultrafiltration membrane with a 10,000 molecular weight cut-off was assembled and evaluated for enzymatic hydrolysis of pure cellulose (Solka Floc) and lignocellulosic material (acid-pretreated urban waste). An enzyme preparation consisting of two commercial cellulases, Spezyme CP® and Novozym 188®, was used for hydrolysis. Insoluble cellulosic substrate and enzymes were retained within the membrane reactor, whereas low molecular-weight hydrolysis products (mainly glucose) passed through the membrane.

Continuous removal of glucose from the membrane reactor allowed the reduction of end-product inhibition of cellulases and provided 1.5 times higher conversion of Solka Floc™ cellulose compared to results in the shake flask. Conversion of the acid-pretreated urban waste, however, was not improved by the use of the membrane reactor.

When pure cellulose was used in the membrane reactor, the cellulases efficiently hydrolyzed a subsequent addition of substrate. However, when lignocellulosic material was used in a substrate-feeding mode, the degree of substrate conversion rapidly decreased and the efficient use of enzyme was not achieved. The amount of enzyme required to produce 1 g of glucose was approximately 3 times lower in the membrane reactor compared to the shake flask for Solka Floc™ cellulose, and 1.3-1.4 times lower in case of the acid-pretreated material.

TABLE 5.
HYDROLYSIS OF ACID-PRETREATED URBAN WASTE WITH COMBINED ENZYME PREPARATION OF SPEZYME CP® AND NOVOZYM 188® IN THE SHAKE FLASK AND IN THE UF-MEMBRANE REACTOR
(two subsequent additions of substrate)

Parameter	Shake flask (48 h)	UF-membrane reactor		
		1st stage hydrolysis (48 h)	2nd stage hydrolysis (26 h)	Total
Before hydrolysis				
Reaction volume, mL	200	240	260	260
Substrate, g dry solids/L	50.0	50.0	51.1	66.4
Substrate, g dry solids	10.0	12.0	13.3	17.2
Enzyme, FPU/mL	1.0	1.0	0.9	0.9
Enzyme, FPU	200	240	240	240
Enzyme, FPU/g dry solids	20.0	20.0	18.1	14.0
After hydrolysis				
Volume, mL	200	1130	722	1852
Glucose, g/L	23.0	5.2	2.3	4.0
Glucose, g	4.6	5.8	1.6	7.4
Biomass conversion, %	41.4	43.7	11.1	38.9
FPU/g Glc	43.5	41.2	146.3	32.3

When pure cellulose was used in the membrane reactor, the cellulases efficiently hydrolyzed a subsequent addition of substrate. However, when lignocellulosic material was used in a substrate-feeding mode, the degree of substrate conversion rapidly decreased and the efficient use of enzyme was not achieved. The amount of enzyme required to produce 1 g of glucose was approximately 3 times lower in the membrane reactor compared to the shake flask for Solka Floc™ cellulose, and 1.3-1.4 times lower in case of the acid-pretreated material.

Since the product stream from the membrane reactor gave a low glucose concentration, the technical possibilities of using another membrane process, reverse osmosis, are being considered for concentrating the glucose solution for subsequent microbial fermentation.

REFERENCES

BEGUIN, P. and AUBERT, J.-P. 1994. The biological degradation of cellulose. FEMS Microbiol. Rev. *13*, 25–58.

BERGMEYER, H.U. and BERNT, E. 1974. Determination with glucose oxidase and peroxidase. In *Methods of Enzymatic Analysis,* ed. H. U. Bergmeyer & K. Gawehn. Weinheim: Verlag Chemie. Academic Press, New York, 2nd Edn. *3*, 1205–1215.

CHERNOGLAZOV, V.M., ERMOLOVA, O.V. and KLYOSOV, A.A. 1988. Adsorption of high-purity endo-1,4-beta-glucanases from *Trichoderma reesei* on components of lignocellulosic materials: cellulose, lignin and xylan. Enzyme Microb. Technol. *10*, 503–507.

DUFF, S.J.B. and MURRAY, W.D. 1996. Bioconversion of forest products industry waste cellulosics to fuel ethanol: A review. *Bioresource Technol.* 55, 1–33.

GHOSE, T.K. 1987. Measurement of cellulase activities. (Recommendations of Commission on Biotechnology, IUPAC). Pure and Appl. Chem. *59*, 257–268.

GHOSE, T.K. and KOSTICK, J.A. 1970. A model for continuous enzymatic saccharification of cellulose with simultaneous removal of glucose syrup. Biotechnol. Bioeng. *12*, 921–946.

GUSAKOV, A.V., SINITSYN, A.P., MANENKOVA, J.A. and PROTAS, O. V. 1992. Enzymatic saccharification of industrial and agricultural lignocellulosic wastes. Main features of the process. Appl. Biochem. Biotechnol. *34/35*, 625–637.

HENLEY, R.G., YANG, R.Y.K. and GREENFIELD, P.F. 1980. Enzymatic saccharification of cellulose in membrane reactors. Enzyme Microb. Technol. *2*, 206–208.

HOLTZAPPLE, M., COGNATA, M., SHU, Y. and HENDRICKSON, C. 1990. Inhibition of *Trichoderma reesei* cellulase by sugars and solvents. Biotechnol. Bioeng. *36*, 275–287.

INGRAM, L.O. and DORAN, J.B. 1995. Conversion of cellulosic materials to ethanol. FEMS Microbiol. Rev. *16*, 235–241.

KLYOSOV, A.A. 1990. Trends in biochemistry and enzymology of cellulose degradation. Biochemistry *29*, 10577–10585.

LEE, Y-H. and FAN, L.T. 1983. Kinetic studies of enzymatic hydrolysis of insoluble cellulose: II. Analysis of extended hydrolysis times. Biotechnol. Bioeng. *25*, 939–966.

LEE, S.-G. and KIM, H.-S. 1993. Optimal operating policy of the ultrafiltration membrane bioreactor for enzymatic hydrolysis of cellulose. Biotechnol. Bioeng. *42*, 737–746.

LEE, D., YU, A.H.S. and SADDLER, J.N. 1995. Evaluation of cellulase recycling strategies for the hydrolysis of lignocellulosic substrates. Biotechnol. Bioeng. *45*, 328–336.

OHLSON, I., TRAGARDH, G. and HAHN-HAGERDAL, B. 1984. Enzymatic hydrolysis of sodium-hydroxide-pretreated sallow in an ultrafiltration membrane reactor. Biotechnol. Bioeng. *26*, 647–653.

OLSSON, L. and HAHN-HAGERDAL, B. 1996. Fermentation of lignocellulosic hydrolysates for ethanol production. Enzyme Microb. Technol. *18*, 312–331.

OOSHIMA, H., BURNS, D.S. and CONVERSE, A.O. 1990. Adsorption of cellulase from *Trichoderma reesei* on cellulose and lignacious residue in wood pretreated by dilute sulfuric acid with explosive decompression. Biotechnol. Bioeng. *36*, 446–452.

RAMOS, L.P., BREUIL, J.N. and SADDLER, J.N. 1993. The use of enzyme recycling and the influence of sugar accumulation on cellulose hydrolysis by *Trichoderma cellulases*. Enzyme Microb. Technol. *15*, 91–125.

REESE, E.T. 1980. Inactivation of cellulase by shaking and its prevention by surfactants. J. Appl. Biochem. *2*, 36–39.

SINITSYN, A.P., GUSAKOV, A.V. and VLASENKO, E.Y. 1991. Effect of structural and physico-chemical features of cellulosic substrates on the efficiency of enzymatic hydrolysis. Appl. Biochem. Biotechnol. *30*, 43–59.

UTILIZATION OF CA AND ZN IN METAL PROTEINATE, METAL AMINO ACID COMPLEXES AND INORGANIC SALTS FOR RATS

XIAOMING ZHANG, XINGHUA YUAN and KECHANG ZHANG

Wuxi University of Light Industry
Wuxi 214036, Jiangsu, China

ABSTRACT

Seventy two Sprague-Dawley rats (half male, average BW 90 g) were used to evaluate the utilization of Ca and Zn in metal proteinate, metal amino acid complexes and $CaCO_3$, and $ZnSO_4 \cdot 7H_2O$. The rats were randomly assigned to one of six treatments. Dietary treatments were: (1) a basal diet (138 mg/kg of Ca and 12 mg/kg of Zn); (2) basal + 2000 mg/kg of Ca and 20 mg/kg of Zn from amino acid complexes; (3) basal + 4000 mg/kg of Ca and 40 mg/kg of Zn from amino acid complexes; (4) basal + 2000 mg/kg of Ca and 20 mg/kg of Zn from metal proteinates; (5) basal + 4000 mg/kg of Ca and 40 mg/kg of Zn from metal proteinates; (6) basal + 4000 mg/kg of Ca from reagent grade $CaCO_3$ and 40 mg/kg of Zn from reagent grade $ZnSO_4 \cdot 7H_2O$. The experiments were conducted for two months. Average body weight tended to be similar among treatments. The Ca utilization of Ca proteinate and Ca amino acid complexes were both higher than inorganic salts based on the thigh-bone density and thigh bone and serum Ca concentrations. Thigh-bone density was higher ($p<0.01$) for rats fed Ca proteinate than for rats fed $CaCO_3$. Ca proteinate increased ($p<0.05$) thigh-bone density more than Ca amino acid complexes. The rats fed metal proteinate had a higher serum Zn content ($p<0.01$) than the rats fed amino acid complexes or inorganic salts. There were no differences in serum and tissue Zn contents between the rats fed amino acid complexes and the rats fed inorganic salts. Zn proteinate increased ($p<0.01$) brain Zn content more than Zn amino acid complexes. The utilization of metal proteinates was higher than inorganic salts ($p<0.01$), suggesting that metal proteinates are absorbed via another mechanism that differs from that of inorganic salts, and the antagonistic relationships between minerals are overcome. The metal amino acid complexes had equal or greater bioavailability than inorganic salts.

INTRODUCTION

Interest in using organic mineral complexes as mineral sources for animals has increased because of the reported potential of higher bioavailability than from inorganic mineral sources. Theories suggested that the mineral centered inside the five or six membered chelate could more easily cross the brush border of the intestine and the entire chelate could be absorbed as small peptides (Fouad 1974). Most would agree that a chelate remains intact and avoids ionization in the stomach/rumen and is affected only minimally by phosphates, phytates and other reactions common to inorganic minerals (Sherman 1990). Spears (1989) reported that when a deficient diet was fed, apparent absorption of Zn, ZnMet or ZnO forms was similar, but Zn retention increased with ZnMet, suggesting a different metabolism following absorption. However, other studies indicated that organic Zn complexes were no more effective than $ZnSO_4$ (Hills *et al.* 1987, Schell *et al.* 1996).

Very little information is available comparing the utilization of Ca complexes with that of $CaCO_3$. Also limited research has addressed specific antagonistic relationships between minerals in organic salts or in some cases, metal proteinate forms. The objectives of the present study were to determine whether metal proteinate or metal amino acid complexes can improve the Ca and Zn utilization compared with $CaCO_3$ and $ZnSO_4$ and to evaluate Zn utilization as affected by excess calcium from different sources.

MATERIALS AND METHODS

Seventy two Sprague-Dawley rats (half male) with an average initial BW of 90 g were randomly assigned to one of six treatments. Dietary treatments were: (1) a basal diet (138 mg/kg of Ca and 12 mg/kg of Zn); (2) basal + 2000 mg/kg of Ca and 20 mg/kg of Zn from amino acid complexes; (3) basal + 4000 mg/kg of Ca and 40 mg/kg of Zn from amino acid complexes; (4) basal + 2000 mg/kg of Ca and 20 mg/kg of Zn from metal proteinates; (5) basal + 4000 mg/kg of Ca and 40 mg/kg of Zn from metal proteinates; (6) basal + 4000 mg/kg of Ca from reagent grade $CaCO_3$ and 40 mg/kg of Zn from reagent grade $ZnSO_4 \cdot 7H_2O$. The metal amino acid complexes were prepared by reacting a mixture of lysine and glycine with selected minerals. The metal proteinates were derived from the reactants of yeast hydrolysates and special minerals; most of the peptides used as ligands had molecular weights of 210 to 650 daltons.

The rats were individually housed in stainless steel wire-bottomed cages, with free-choice distilled water available. To adapt to the environment and diet, the rats were fed the basal diet for 30 d before the experiment. The experimental period was 60 d. Rats were killed at the end of each experiment. The thigh bone was excised and the thigh bone density analyzed by a density instrument. Liver, brain, thigh bone and serum were obtained for further mineral analyses. Ca and Zn in tissues and serum were determined by atomic absorption spectrophotometry.

All data were analyzed using SAS (SAS 1990). Differences among the mineral forms were determined using the least significant difference (LSD) test (SAS 1990).

RESULTS AND DISCUSSION

Thigh Bone Density and Tissue Calcium Concentration

Performance, thighbone density and tissue Ca concentrations of rats fed diets with Ca from three sources were measured. There were no differences in body weight among the treatment groups (Table 1). Rats fed Ca amino acid complexes had higher ($p < 0.01$, Table 1) thigh-bone density than rats fed $CaCO_3$. The rats fed Ca proteinate had higher ($p<0.01$, Table 1) thigh-bone density than rats fed $CaCO_3$. Ca proteinate increased thigh-bone density more than Ca amino acid complexes ($p<0.05$, Table 1).

Overall, thigh bone and serum Ca concentrations were increased by supplementation with organic Ca complexes, but the increase was not significant ($p>0.05$). The significant differences ($p<0.05$ or $p<0.01$, Table 1) of thigh-bone density among the

TABLE 1.
PERFORMANCE, THIGH-BONE DENSITY AND TISSUE CA CONCENTRATIONS OF RATS FED DIETS WITH CA FROM THREE SOURCES

	Treatment					
	1	2	3	4	5	6
		2000 mg Ca/kg			4000 mg Ca/kg	
Item	Control	CaAA[a]	CaP[a]	CaAA	CaP	$CaCO_3$
Body weight (g)	251.4 ± 56.1	232.9 ± 36.4	256.0 ± 33.4	261.8 ± 34.4	243.4 ±40.8	264.9 ±42.5
Thigh-bone density (g/cm^2)	1.63 ± 0.12	1.82 ± 0.08[c]	1.88 ± 0.09[c]	1.80 ± 0.07[c]	1.90 ± 0.10[c]	1.74 ± 0.10[b]
Thigh-bone Ca(mg/g)	36.9 ± 15.1	44.3 ± 11.7	47.9 ± 8.9[b]	51.2 ± 10.2[b]	51.5 ± 5.5[c]	49.8 ±14.9
Serum Ca(mg/g)	8.3 ± 2.8	12.1 ± 4.7[b]	12.0 ± 3.4[b]	13.2 ± 4.2[c]	12.7 ± 4.7[b]	11.9 ± 4.0[b]

[a]CaAA = Ca amino acid complex; CaP = Ca proteinate
[b]Compared with the control group, $p<0.05$.
[c]Compared with the control group, $p<0.01$.

treatment groups suggested that thigh-bone density was a sensitive indicator of Ca status and utilization of Ca by rats.

Serum and Tissue Zinc Concentration

Serum and tissue Zn concentration of rats fed diets with Zn from three different sources are shown in Table 2. There were no differences in serum Zn content among the rats fed Zn amino acid complexes and $ZnSO_4$. Zn proteinate increased ($p<0.01$, Table 2) serum Zn concentration more than Zn amino acid complexes or $ZnSO_4$. It is worth noting that rats fed 20 mg/kg of Zn from Zn proteinate had higher ($p<0.01$, Table 2) serum Zn concentration than rats fed 40 mg/kg of Zn from amino acid complexes or $ZnSO_4$. There were no significant differences in thigh bone and brain Zn content among the rats fed Zn proteinate and $ZnSO_4$, whereas 20 mg/kg of Zn from Zn proteinate increased thigh bone and brain Zn content more than 40 mg/kg of Zn from $ZnSO_4$ (Table 2). Rats fed Zn proteinate had higher ($p<0.01$, Table 2) brain Zn concentration than rats fed Zn amino acid complexes. However there were no differences in liver Zn content among the treatment groups (Table 2).

The significant differences ($P<0.01$, Table 2) of serum Zn content among the treatment groups suggested that serum Zn content was a sensitive indicator of Zn status and utilization of Zn for rats. Blood plasm serves as the immediate source of stored Zn. Overall, the results from these experiments indicated that the utilization of Ca and Zn in metal proteinate and amino acid complexes were higher than that of inorganic salts, whereas metal proteinate increased bioavailability of minerals more than amino acid complexes (Tables 1 and 2). The metal proteinate used in the present studies is a mixture of small peptide- and amino acid-metal complexes. Most of the ligands used in the metal proteinate are di- and tripeptides. Small peptides (mostly di- and tripeptides) are absorbed from the small intestine more rapidly than are free amino acids. There are different transport systems for amino acids and peptides. So the metal proteinate could be absorbed by several pathways, which could have more benefit to animals than the single peptide or amino acid complexes.

Ashmead *et al.* (1985) concluded that minerals may be transported through the intestinal mucosa both as free metal ions and in the form of intact complexes. The metal ions will be absorbed by active transport. The intestinal absorption mechanism of divalent metal ions is very similar; metal ions compete with one another for transport carrier. There are significant antagonist effects among these ionic minerals (Baker and Wedekind 1988). In this experiment, the utilization of Zn from $ZnSO_4$ or Zn amino acid complexes might be affected by excess Ca, whereas Ca and Zn from the metal proteinate could be absorbed in a peptide-like form through the secondary intestinal pathway and the antagonist effect was overcome by the ligands in complexes. As expected the serum Zn content was significantly increased ($p<0.01$, Table 2) by metal proteinates.

The utilization of Zn in amino acid complexes is lower than that in metal proteinate, indicating that both Ca and Zn amino acid complexes are not too stable. The antagonistic effect on Zn from excess Ca still existed.

IMPLICATIONS

The utilization of Ca and Zn from metal proteinate is higher than that of amino acid-metal complexes or inorganic salts. Metal proteinate had higher serum Zn content

TABLE 2.
SERUM AND TISSUE ZN CONCENTRATION OF RATS FED DIETS WITH ZN FROM THREE DIFFERENT SOURCES

	Treatment					
	1	2	3	4	5	6
		20 mg Zn/kg			40 mg Zn/kg	
Item	Control	ZnAA[a]	ZnP[a]	ZnAA	ZnP	$ZnSO_4$
Serum Zn (ug/100ml)	76.7 ± 31.2	143.0 ± 26.1	213.2 ± 53.9[c]	151.9 ± 44.2[c]	222.3 ± 42.9[c]	157.9 ± 40.3[c]
Thigh-bone Zn (ug/g)	166.0 ± 50.6	152.8 ± 63.6	203.5 ± 44.8	199.5 ± 57.6	212.1 ± 41.9[b]	202.8 ± 72.3
Brain Zn(ug/g)	16.3 ± 2.2	15.6 ± 1.2	18.8 ± 1.2[c]	16.1 ± 1.4	19.1 ± 2.6[b]	17.4 ± 4.0
Liver Zn (ug/g)	25.9 ± 15.8	31.8 ± 17.0	27.2 ± 8.6	25.2 ± 7.6	30.8 ± 9.2	32.5 ± 6.8

[a]ZnAA= Zn amino acid complex; ZnP = Zn proteinate
[b]Compared with the control group, $p<0.05$.
[c]Compared with the control group, $p<0.01$.

than the two other sources, suggesting different absorption mechanisms for metal proteinate that overcome the antagonistic relationships between minerals. Ca amino acid complexes increased utilization of Ca compared with $CaCO_3$. Supplementation with metal amino acid complexes did not increase serum Zn content. This response indicates that Ca and Zn amino acid complexes are not stable in the digestive system.

Furthermore, thigh-bone density and serum Zn concentration may be used as sensitive indicators of utilization of Ca and Zn for rats.

REFERENCES

ASHMEAD, H.D., GRAFF, D.J. and ASHMEAD, H.H. 1985. Intestinal Absorption of Metal Ions and Chelates. Charles C. Thomas, Publisher, Springfield, IL.

BAHER, D.H. and WEDEHIND, K.J. 1988. Manganese utilization in chicks as affected by excess calcium and phosphorus ingestion. Proc. Maryland Nutr. Conf. P. 29.

FOUND, M.T. 1974. Chelation and chelated minerals. J. Appl. Nutr. *26*, 6.

HILL, D.A., PEO, E.R. and LEWIS, A.J. 1987. Influence of picolinic acid on the uptake of zinc amino acid complexes by the everted rat gut. J. Anim. Sci. *65*, 173–178.

SCHELL, T.C and KORNEGAY, E.J. 1996. Zinc concentration in tissues and performance of zinc from ZnO, Zn-Methionine, Zn-Lysine, or $ZnSO_4$ J. Anim. Sci. *74*, 1584–1593.

SHERMAN, B.R. and ROWLAND, R.D. 1990. Mineral chelates. Piggyback Nutrients Feed Management *41*, 5.

SPEARS, J.W. 1989. Zinc methionine for ruminants: Relative bioavailability of zinc in lambs and effects on growth and performance of growing heifers. J Anim. Sci. *67*, 825.

WEBB, K.E. JR. 1990. Intestinal Absorption of Protein Hydrolysis Products: A Review. SAS 1990. SAS/STAT® User's Guide (Release 6.04 Ed) SAS Inst. Inc. Cary, NC.

VIRUSES AND PARASITES IN THE U.S. FOOD AND WATER SUPPLY

DEAN O. CLIVER

W.H.O. Collaborating Center on Food Virology
School of Veterinary Medicine
University of California
Davis, CA 95616-8743

ABSTRACT

Viruses and protozoan parasites are recognized as important causes of foodborne and waterborne disease in the U.S. Hepatitis A was the fourth leading cause of outbreak-associated foodborne disease in the most recent compilation by the U.S. Centers for Disease Control and Prevention, and gastroenteritis due to Norwalk-like viruses ranked number nine. Foodborne viruses come from human feces. Vehicles in outbreaks are most often bivalve mollusks that have accumulated the virus from contaminated water during their filter feeding; however, any food handled by an infected person can become contaminated. The source of hepatitis A virus contamination in a recent outbreak, in which the vehicle was frozen strawberries, remains unknown.

The principal protozoa transmitted via food and water in the U.S. are Cryptosporidium parvam *and* Giardia lamblia. *These may be of human or animal fecal origin.* G. lamblia *was the leading cause of recorded waterborne disease in the U.S. until 1993, when an outbreak of waterborne cryptosporidiosis in Milwaukee, Wisconsin, caused 403,000 illnesses. Both of these agents are occasionally transmitted via food. In 1996, a widespread outbreak of illness due to* Cyclospora cayetanensis *occurred in the U.S. and Canada in which the vehicle was found to have been fresh raspberries from Guatemala. This agent is usually seen only as imported cases in North America.*

Viruses are much smaller, and the protozoa larger, than foodborne and waterborne bacteria. These viruses and protozoa share the properties of being unable to multiply outside the host's body and being very difficult to detect in food or water. Bacterial indicators of contamination, such as the coliform group or even Escherichia coli, *are very poorly correlated with the presence of viruses or protozoa in food or water. Therefore, prevention is based on very careful control of human and animal waste and on close application of the principles of food hygiene.*

INTRODUCTION

Viruses and protozoan parasites are recognized as important causes of foodborne and waterborne disease in the U.S., even though diagnostic difficulties lead to under-reporting of the incidence of viral and protozoal illnesses (Council for Agricultural Science and Technology 1994). The agents will be discussed from the standpoints of their epidemiology, transmission, and impact on public health.

VIRUSES

Hepatitis A was the fourth leading cause of outbreak-associated foodborne disease in the most recent compilation by the U.S. Centers for Disease Control and Prevention, and gastroenteritis due to Norwalk-like viruses ranked number nine (Bean *et al.* 1996). Hepatitis E virus, which is often transmitted via water (and perhaps food) in Asia, Africa, and South America, evidently occurs only as imported cases in North America. Foodborne viruses come from human feces. This is true because the viruses transmitted to humans via food and water infect only humans and are shed only in feces (an uncommon but significant exception is the shedding of Norwalk-like viruses in vomitus) (Cliver 1997).

Hepatitis A virus infects perorally and colonizes the liver (Cromeans *et al.* 1994). Although infection does not kill the host cells in the liver, in time the body's immune system notes the invasion and sends cytotoxic T-cells to destroy the infected cells. The incubation period for illness ranges from 15 to 50 days, with a median of 28 days. During the last half of the incubation period, virus produced in the liver drains via the common bile duct into the intestine and is shed with feces; shedding typically ends as soon as the illness does. The majority of transmission apparently occurs via contact, although the food and water vehicles are important. Natural infection probably affords lifelong immunity; active immunization with vaccine is said to protect for at least 10 years, whereas passive immunization with pooled immune serum globulin protects for 6 months or less.

Vehicles in outbreaks are most often bivalve mollusks that have accumulated the virus from sewage-contaminated water during their filter feeding; however, any food handled by an infected person can become contaminated. Sandwiches, salads, and other foods served cold or uncooked are most often contaminated by handling. Prevention is based on careful hand washing and on avoiding contact of hands with food. The source of hepatitis A virus contamination in a recent outbreak, in which the vehicle was frozen strawberries, remains unknown (Centers for Disease Control and Prevention 1997a).

The Norwalk-like viruses (sometimes called small round structured viruses; Appleton 1994) are frequent causes of foodborne and perhaps waterborne gastroenteritis (vomiting and diarrhea). Onset times are typically 24 to 48 h after exposure, and the duration of illness is usually also about 24 to 48 h. Virus is shed in vomitus and diarrheal stool, and in normal stool for as long as a week after onset of illness. Food vehicles are essentially the same as for hepatitis A; transmission via water appears less common. Infection with one of these viruses evidently does not confer long-term immunity, even to the same virus type. As a result, there has been little incentive to develop vaccines against these agents. Antibody response to infection does occur, however, and can be used in diagnosis. Laboratory diagnosis is evidently not often attempted, with the result that reports of foodborne and waterborne outbreaks seem to have declined in the U.S., even though there is no reason to believe that the incidence has decreased.

Other than the agents already discussed, only the astroviruses (Appleton 1994) and rotaviruses (Sattar *et al.* 1994) are known to be transmitted via food and water in the U.S. Both cause gastroenteritis in humans, but are seldom reported to cause common-source outbreaks of illness. The rotaviruses are an important cause of infant death in developing countries.

PROTOZOA

The principal protozoa transmitted via food and water in the U.S. are *Cryptosporidium parvum* and *Giardia lamblia*. These may be of human or animal fecal origin.

G. lamblia (alias *duodenalis* or *intestinalis*) was the leading cause of recorded waterborne disease in the U.S. until 1993 (Fayer 1994). It has caused several outbreaks in communities whose water supplies derive from surface sources and rely on chemical (usually chlorine) disinfection without previous filtration. Proper filtration removes the transmission form (cysts) from water. It can cause a prolonged diarrhea in the absence of proper diagnosis and treatment. It is also a risk to people camping out and drinking untreated water from surface sources, and to children in day care centers.

In 1993, an outbreak of waterborne cryptosporidiosis in Milwaukee, Wisconsin, caused 403,000 diarrheal illnesses (Mackenzie *et al.* 1994). Several outbreaks associated with community water supplies had been recorded earlier or have occurred since. The transmission form (oocyst) is so small as to be very difficult to remove from surface water by filtration and is very little affected by chlorine at levels ordinarily used with drinking water. *C. parvum*, too, can be transmitted to campers and in day care centers. Because there is no recognized treatment for cryptosporidiosis, infected persons recover on the basis of their own immune responses. Infection with *Cryptosporidium* is typically lifelong in AIDS patients and is said to have caused approximately 100 deaths among human immunodeficiency virus-infected persons in the aftermath of the Milwaukee outbreak.

Both of these agents are occasionally transmitted via food. At least two outbreaks of cryptosporidiosis have been recorded in which the vehicle was apple juice or cider. Humans are not the only reservoir of these protozoa: several species of domestic and feral mammals may also be hosts, so nonhuman sources of contamination are a serious possibility. Indeed, the source of the oocysts in Lake Michigan that led to contamination of the Milwaukee water supply has never been established.

In 1996, a widespread outbreak of illness due to *Cyclospora cayetanensis* occurred in the U.S. and Canada, in which the vehicle was found to have been fresh raspberries from Guatemala (Centers for Disease Control and Prevention 1996). Vehicles in more recent outbreaks of cyclosporiasis in the U.S. have been raspberries from Guatemala (again in the spring of 1997), and a salad mixture of baby lettuce, and basil (Centers for Disease Control and Prevention 1997b). This agent had usually been seen only in imported cases in North America until 1996. It is not known to infect nonhuman species; and its transmission form (oocyst) has the special property of needing days to weeks, under favorable conditions, to sporulate and become infectious to another human. Therefore, direct person-to-person transmission is relatively unlikely.

PREVENTION

Viruses are much smaller, and the protozoa larger, than foodborne and waterborne bacteria. These viruses and protozoa share the properties of being unable to multiply outside the host's body and being very difficult to detect in food or water. Bacterial indicators of contamination, such as the coliform group or even *Escherichia coli*, are very poorly correlated with the presence of viruses or protozoa in food or water.

The foodborne viruses are fairly heat resistant — especially the hepatitis A virus, which also withstands drying. They are acid-resistant and are preserved by refrigeration and freezing. *Giardia* cysts and *Cryptosporidium* oocysts are supposedly killed by freezing, though the public is told not to chill drinks with ice made from water that may be contaminated with *Cryptosporidium*. The cysts and oocysts are apparently killed by heat treatments equivalent to milk pasteurization; but when a public water supply is found to be contaminated, boiling the water is recommended until the situation can be alleviated. Ultraviolet light and chemical disinfectants other than chlorine are being explored for disinfection of protozoan-contaminated food and water. Ionizing radiation is apparently effective against cysts and oocysts, which present relatively large targets, but are less effective against viruses, which present small targets and thus require large and costly doses to be inactivated.

For the reasons discussed, prevention is based on very careful control of human and animal waste and on close application of the principles of food hygiene. The "danger zone," of food storage temperatures to be avoided for fear of bacterial growth, is irrelevant. Beginning in 1997, the U.S. Environmental Protection Agency is requiring public water systems that serve at least 100,000 people to test their raw water supplies for viruses and for *C. parvum* and for *G. lamblia*. Advanced technologies are being considered for prevention of transmission via water, but a good deal of prevention of transmission via food is still based on careful washing of food workers' hands.

REFERENCES

APPLETON, H. 1994. Norwalk virus and the small round viruses causing foodborne gastroenteritis. *In* Foodborne Disease Handbook: Vol. 2. Diseases Caused by Viruses, Parasites, and Fungi. Y.H. Hui, J.R. Gorham, K.D. Murrell, and D.O. Cliver (eds.). Marcel Dekker, New York.

BEAN, N.H., GOULDING, J.S., LAO, C. and ANGULO, F.J. 1996. Surveillance for foodborne-disease outbreaks--United States, 1988-1992. CDC Surveillance Summaries, Morbid. Mortal. Weekly Rep. *45 (SS-5)*, 1–66.

CENTERS FOR DISEASE CONTROL AND PREVENTION. 1996. Update: Outbreaks of *Cyclospora cayetanensis* infection — United States and Canada, 1996. Morbid. Mortal. Weekly Rep. *45*, 611–612.

CENTERS FOR DISEASE CONTROL AND PREVENTION. 1997a. Hepatitis A associated with consumption of frozen strawberries — Michigan, March, 1997. Morbid. Mortal. Weekly Rep. *46*, 288, 295.

CENTERS FOR DISEASE CONTROL AND PREVENTION. 1997b. Outbreak of cyclosporiasis — Northern Virginia-Washington, D.C.-Baltimore, Maryland metropolitan area, 1997. Morbid. Mortal. Weekly Rep. *46*, 689–691.

CLIVER, D.O. 1997. Foodborne viruses. *In* Food Microbiology: Fundamentals and Frontiers, M.P. Doyle, L.R. Beuchat, and T.J. Montville (eds.). American Society for Microbiology, Washington, D.C.

COUNCIL FOR AGRICULTURAL SCIENCE AND TECHNOLOGY. 1994. Foodborne Pathogens: Risks and Consequences. Task Force Report No. 122, September 1994. Council for Agricultural Science and Technology, Ames, IA.

CROMEANS, T., NAINAN, O.V., FIELDS, H.A., FAVOROV, M.O. and MARGOLIS, H.S. 1994. Hepatitis A and E viruses. *In* Foodborne Disease Handbook: Vol. 2. Diseases Caused by Viruses, Parasites, and Fungi, Y.H. Hui, J.R. Gorham, K.D. Murrell and D.O. Cliver (eds.). Marcel Dekker, New York.

FAYER, R. 1994. Foodborne and waterborne zoonotic protozoa. *In* Foodborne Disease Handbook: Vol. 2. Diseases Caused by Viruses, Parasites, and Fungi. Y.H. Hui, J.R. Gorham, K.D. Murrell and D.O. Cliver (eds.). Marcel Dekker, New York.

MACKENZIE, W.R., HOXIE, N.J., PROCTOR, M.E., GRADUS, M.S., BLAIR, K.A., PETERSON, D.E., KAZMIERCZAK, J.J., ADDISS, D.G., FOX, K.R., ROSE, J.B. and DAVIS, J.P. 1994. A massive outbreak in Milwaukee of *Cryptosporidium* infection transmitted through the public water supply. New Eng. J. Med. *331*, 161–167.

SATTAR, S.A., SPRINGTHORPE, V.S. and ANSARI, S.A. 1994. Rotavirus. *In* Foodborne Disease Handbook: Vol. 2. Diseases Caused by Viruses, Parasites, and Fungi, Y.H. Hui. J.R. Gorham, K.D. Murrell, and D.O. Cliver (eds.). Marcel Dekker, New York.

DEVELOPMENT AND USE OF MOLECULAR DIAGNOSTIC TECHNIQUES FOR THE DETECTION AND SUBTYPING OF FOOD PATHOGENS

HAU-YANG TSEN

Department of Food Science
National Chung-Hsing University
Taichung, Taiwan, ROC

ABSTRACT

Conventional methods for the detection of certain food pathogens such as Salmonella, enterotoxigenic Staphylococcus aureus *and pathogenic* Escherichia coli *in food samples are time consuming and laborious, thus rapid methods for detection of these food pathogens are important. In the past years, we have developed DNA probes and polymerase chain reaction (PCR) primers and used them for the inspection of food samples. Furthermore, for some food pathogens, such as type A enterotoxigenic* S. aureus, *we have also investigated their antibiograms and genomic finger-prints, such as pulsed field gel electrophoretic (PFGE) patterns of chromosomal DNA so that the subtypes and the most disseminated strains for these bacterial strains may be elucidated. The data so established may also be useful for tracing the contamination origin of pathogenic bacteria once an outbreak occurs. Results obtained from our studies indicate that novel DNA probes and PCR primers obtained from molecular cloning technique or from 16S rRNA gene sequences could be used for the detection of* Salmonella spp. *and those designed from the toxin genes of* S. aureus *or* E. coli *cells could be used for the detection of these pathogenic bacterial cells. On the part of the molecular typing studies for Staphylococcal enterotoxin A (SEA)* S. aureus *strains isolated in Taiwan and USA, we found that although SEA S. aureus strains from geographically far distant locations showed considerable genetic diversity, strains of certain PFGE pattern might be the predominant or the most disseminated strains.*

INTRODUCTION

Pathogenic bacteria, such as *Salmonella* spp., pathogenic *Escherichia coli, Yersinia enterocolitica, Staphylococcus aureus*, and recently, *Listeria monocytogenes* are important because they often cause food poisoning incidents and human disease. For some of these bacteria, such as *Salmonella*, pathogenic *E. coli.*, *L. monocytogens* and *S. aureus*, detection of the cells or the toxin released is important for food safety or is required for food inspection. The conventional microbiological methods for detection of these bacteria, however, usually include multiple subculture and biotype or serotype identification steps and, thus, are laborious and time-consuming. For example, 5-7 days and 4-8 days may be required for *Salmonella* and *S. aureus* detection, respectively (Food and Drug Administration 1995; Wolocott 1991). For some pathogenic bacteria, such as enterotoxigenic *E. coli* (ETEC), the detection of its toxigenicity using a bioassay method is complicated and laborious. Therefore, in the past years, rapid methods for detection of these specific bacteria have been intensively studied and some of these methods have been commercialized. These methods include improved rapid biochemical tests and various types of immunoassays, such as fluorescent antibody techniques, reverse phase latex agglutination (RPLA) method, radioimmunoassays (RIA), or enzyme-linked immunosorbent assay (ELISA) (Cox *et al.* 1987, Wolocott 1991).

Recently, two rapid methods using bacteria-specific or toxin specific DNA or oligonucleotide fragments have been developed for the detection of pathogenic bacteria in food samples. These methods are the DNA-DNA hybridization method and the polymerase chain reaction (PCR) method. These methods have been used in detection of various bacteria spp. and their toxin genes. So far, many reports regarding the design and use of the DNA probes and PCR primers for the detection of pathogenic bacteria have been documented. In this report, we will show several approaches to obtain the DNA probes or PCR primers which can be used for the specific detection of some food pathogens, or the enterotoxin or virulence genes of some pathogenic bacteria. For example, *Salmonella* specific DNA probes and PCR primers could be obtained by molecular cloning techniques and by comparison of the DNA sequences of bacterial 16S r RNA genes (Tsen *et al.* 1993, 1994; Lin and Tsen 1995a,b). Staphylococcal enterotoxin A, B, C, D and E specific DNA probes or PCR primers could be designed from the staphylococcal enterotoxin genes (Tsen *et al.* 1993, 1994). Heat-labile and heat-stable enterotoxins and Shiga-like toxin I and II genes specific PCR primers could be designed from these virulence genes and used for the detection of pathogenic *E. coli* cells (Tsen *et al.* 1996, 1997). Application of these DNA probes and PCR primers for food inspection was also successful (Tsen *et al.* 1993a,b, 1994a,b, 1995, 1996a, 1997; Lin and Tsen 1995a,b).

Since reports regarding the use of pulsed field gel electrophoresis (PFGE) techniques in subtyping of specific enterotoxigenic *S. aureus* strains isolated from food samples are limited, and also, such subtyping data may be useful for the epidemiological study and for the tracing of contamination source once an outbreak occurs, we therefore in this report also investigated the PFGE types for SEA *S. aureus* strains isolated in Taiwan and obtained from USA. Results indicated that, although SEA *S. aureus* strains from geographically far distant locations showed considerable genetic diversity, strains of certain PFGE pattern might be the most disseminated strains and could be found in local strains and strains from far distant areas, such as USA (Tsen *et al.* 1995, 1996b).

MATERIALS AND METHODS

Bacterial Strains

Salmonella isolates with various serogroups, *E. coli* strains with various virulence factors, such as enterotoxigenic *E. coli* (ETEC) (including heat labile toxin I, II, heat stable toxin (ST) I, II ETEC), Shiga-like toxin producing *E. coli* (including enterohemorrhagic *E. coli* (EHEC), enteropathogenic *E. coli* (EPEC) and enteroinvasive *E. coli* (EIEC), type A, B, C, D, E enterotoxins producing *S. aureus* strains are known and used. Other bacterial strains including strains of the family of *Enterobacteriaceae*, such as *E. coli*, *Klebsiella*, *Serratia*, *Citrobacter* and *Shigella* spp. etc were used in our study. These bacterial strains were obtained from the American Type Culture Collection

(ATCC), Rockville, MD. USA, the United States Department of Agriculture (USDA), Washington, D.C., USA and the Culture Collection and Research Center (CCRC), Hsin-Chu, Taiwan. Other strains used were laboratory isolates from foods or clinical sources. Some other strains were generous gifts from the Food Research Institute (FRI), University of Wisconsin, Madison, WI., USA, etc.

Media Used

Luria broth (LB), plate count agar (PCA), lactose-combined tetrathionate (CTET) broth, Gram negative broth (GN), Baird-Parker base (BP), Trypticase say agar (TSA), brain heart infusion (BHI) and MacConKey broth, etc., were used.

Methods

1. Molecular cloning of a *Salmonella* specific DNA fragment which could be used for *Salmonella* detection (Tsen *et al.* 1993a).
2. Sequence analysis of the 1.8 kb Hind III DNA fragment which is specific for *Salmonella* detection (Tsen *et al.* 1993a).
3. Designing of oligonucleotide probes and PCR primers for *Salmonella* detection (Tsen *et al.* 1993a, 1994a).
4. Use of *Salmonella* specific DNA probes and PCR primers for specific detection of *Salmonella* contaminated in food samples (Tsen *et al.* 1993a, 1994a).
5. Sequence analysis of the 16S rRNA genes of *Salmonella* spp. and some other enterobacteria (Lin and Tsen 1995a).
6. Design of 16S rDNA targeted oligonucleotide probes and PCR primers for *Salmonella* detection (Lin and Tsen 1995a,b).
7. Use of the gene sequence data available in Gene Bank/EMBL database to design the DNA probes and PCR primers for the specific detection of Staphylococcal enterotoxin A, B, C, D and E genes (Tsen *et al.* 1993b, 1994b).
8. Use of the gene sequence data available in Gene Bank/EMBL database for the designing of PCR primers which could be used for the specific detection of the genes coding for heat labile toxin I, II (LTI, LTII), heat stable toxin (ST) I, II of ETEC cells, Shiga-like toxin (SLT) I and II of EHEC cells (Tsen *et al.* 1996a, 1997).
9. Application of the DNA probes and PCR primers for the specific detection of virulent *E. coli* cells and enterotoxigenic *S. aureus* strains contaminated in various food samples (Tsen *et al.* 1993b, 1994b, 1996a, 1997).

Sequences and lengths of the PCR primers used for the above study were described in our reports (Tsen *et al.* 1993a,b, 1994a,b, 1995, 1996a, 1997; Lin and Tsen 1995a,b). Part of these sequences are shown in Table 1.

RESULTS AND DISCUSSION

Possible Use of a 1.8 kb DNA Fragment for the Specific Detection of *Salmonella* in Foods

The aim of this study was to find a specific DNA probe for the detection of Salmonella in foods. A 1.8 kb Hind III DNA fragment cloned from *S. typhimurium* was tested for its specificity by hybridization to *Salmonella* strains of different serotypes as well as to non-*Salmonella* bacteria. The ^{35}S-labeled Hind III DNA fragment hybridized with all of the common and uncommon *Salmonella* isolates but did not hybridize with other non-*Salmonella* isolates tested. Hybridization efficiencies of this 1.8kb DNA probe to *Salmonella* strains of different serotypes were nearly the same. When this probe was applied to the detection of *Salmonella* exogenously added to a variety of foods, bacterial flora naturally occurring in foods did not interfere with the assay. Thus, the hybridization specificity of this 1.8kb DNA probe was established.

TABLE 1.
PART OF THE PCR PRIMERS DEVELOPED FOR THE DETECTION OF FOOD PATHOGENS

Primer (5' →3')	Sequence	length (base no)
Salmonella spp.		
TS11	GTCACGGAAGAAGAGAAATCCGTACG	26
TS4	GCGGATCGTGCAACTGCGGTACGTA	25
TS5	GCGGATCGTGCAACTGCGGTACGTA	25
TS6	TTGTCAGGGTACTTAGCG	18
16S F 1	TGTTGTGGTTAATAACCGCA	20
16S III	CACAAATCCATCTCTGGA	18
E. coli		
LT I 1	GCTGACTCTAGACCCCCAG	19
LT I 2	TGTAACCATCCTCTGCCGGA	20
ST I 1	GGAGGTAAIATGAAIAAIIIAATITT	26
ST I 2	TTACAACAIAITTCACAGCAGTAA	24
ST II 1	CGTGTGAACATTATAGACAAATA	24
ST II 2	ACCATTATTTGGGCGCCAAG	21
LT51[b]	CCGGTATTACAGGGGTCTGA	20
LT31	GTGCATGATGAATCCAGGGT	20
S. aureus enterotoxin		
A1	AAAGTGCCGATCAATTTATGGCTA	24
A2	GTAATTAACCGAAGGTTCTGTAGA	24
D1	GCAGATAAAAATCCAATAATAGGA	24
D2	ATCTAAAGAAACTTCTTTTTGTAC	24
E1	TTACAAAGAAATGCTTTAAGC	21
E2	TAAACCAAATTTTCCGTG	18

DNA Sequence of a *Salmonella*-Specific DNA Fragment and the Use of Oligonucleotide Probes for *Salmonella* Detection

Hybridization specificity of a 1.8 kb Hind III DNA fragment isolated from S. *typhimurium* by a molecular cloning technique was confirmed by colony hybridization with 327 *Salmonella* isolates of various serotypes and 56 non-*Salmonella* isolates including *Enterobacteriaceae* closely related to *Salmonella,* such as *E. coli, Klebsiella, Citrobacter* and *Shigella*. It was found that this 1.8 kb DNA fragment was highly specific for all the *Salmonella* isolates tested. The DNA sequence of this 1.8 kb DNA fragment was then determined by the dideoxynucleotide chain termination method. According to this DNA sequence, six oligonucleotide fragments ranging from 17- to 26- mer were then chemically synthesized and tested for their hybridization specificities. Results showed that three of the six oligonucleotide fragments are highly specific for all 327 *Salmonella* strains tested and can be used as probes for the specific detection of *Salmonella* in foods or other samples.

Possible Use of a Polymerase Chain Reaction Method for Specific Detection of *Salmonella* in Beef

A rapid and sensitive polymerase chain reaction (PCR) method for the detection of *Salmonella* isolates with different serotypes is described. Based on the DNA sequence of a cloned 1.8 kb Hind III DNA fragment which could hybridize with all the *Salmonella* isolates tested but not with any of the non-*Salmonella* isolates including *Enterobacteriaceae* closely related to *Salmonella*, oligonucleotide fragments ranging from 18- to 26- mer were synthesized and tested for their possible use as PCR primers. Results showed that three oligonucleotides, called TS11, TS4 and TS5 could be used in pairs of TS11/TS4 and TS11/TS5. The molecular weight of the PCR product amplified with *Salmonella* DNA was 1179 bp for primers TS11/TS4 and 375 bp for primers TS11/TS5. Primer TS5 could also be used as a checking probe to identify the PCR product amplified from primers TS11/TS4. An example of the PCR results is shown in Fig. 1. TS6 is a checking probe located between TS11 and TS5. Study of the detection sensitivity showed that DNA from N $\times$ 10^0 or N $\times$ 10^1 cells of *Salmonella* could be detected unambiguously either with primers TS11/TS5 or with primers TS11/TS4. When these PCR primers were used for the detection of salmonellae in beef, N $\times$ 10^0 to N $\times$ 10^1 cells per gram of beef could be detected and the endogenously contaminated microflora in the food sample did not interfere with the detection.

Development and Evaluation of Two Novel Oligonucleotide Probes Based on 16S rRNA Sequence for the Identification of *Salmonella* in Foods

DNA sequence in the V3 to V6 region of the 16S rRNA gene of *S. enteritidis* was determined. By comparison of this sequence with those of *E. coli* and *Proteus vulgaris* obtained from GenBank/EMBL database, three oligonucleotides termed as 16S I, 16S II and 16S III were synthesized. Hybridization of these oligonucleotides with 325 *Salmonella* isolates and some non-*Salmonella* isolates including the *Salmonella* closely related species of the family of *Enterobacteriaceae* showed that 16S II could not be used as a *Salmonella* specific-probe. 16S I and 16S III hybridized with all the *Salmonella* isolates tested, the former also hybridizing with *Citrobacter* spp. and the latter hybridizing with *Klebsiella pneumoniae* as well as *Serratia marcescens*. Since enrichment of the target cells in food samples was usually required prior to the DNA hybridization assay, the interference from these non-*Salmonella* isolates could be prevented by enrichment by culturing in lactose-combined tetrathionate (CTET) broth followed by

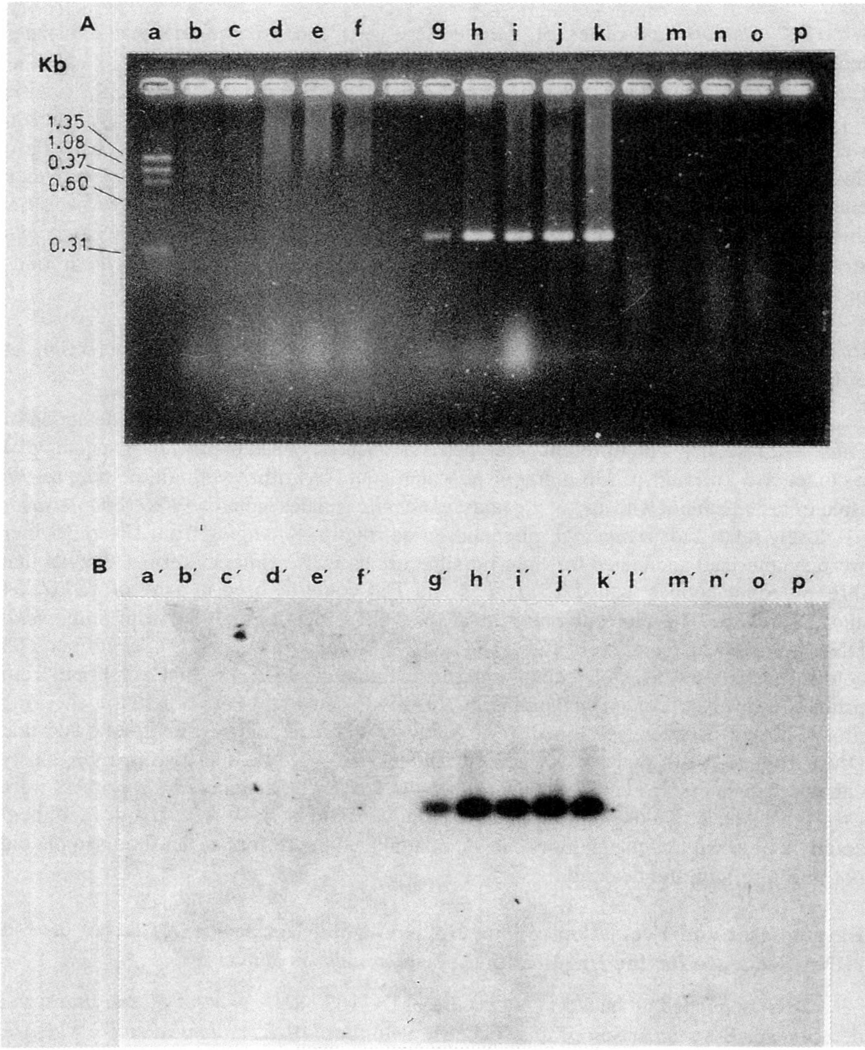

FIG. 1. AGAROSE GEL ELECTROPHORESIS OF THE PCR PRODUCTS AMPLIFIED WITH PRIMERS TS11/TS5 (A) AND SOUTHERN BLOT HYBRIDIZATION OF THE PCR PRODUCTS WITH ^{32}P-LABELED OLIGONUCLEOTIDE TS6 (B).

Lane a represents $\phi\chi$ 174 DNA digested with *Hae* III and lanes b→}p represent the PCR products amplified from *Salmonella* and non-*Salmonella* DNAs. Lanes b'→p' show the hybridization results for the PCR products from lanes b→p. Lanes b-f for PCR products amplified with DNAs from *Acinetobacter calcoaceticus*, *Citrobacter freundii*, *C. amalonaticus*, *C. diversus*, *C. Koseri*; lanes g-k, for PCR products amplified from *Salmonella berta*, *S. haardt*, *S. derby*, *S. bousso*, *S. muenchen*; lanes l-p: for PCR products amplified from *E. coli*, *Shigella flexneri*, *Klebsiella pneumoniae*, *Enterobacter aerogenes* and *E. carotovora*.

Gram-negative (GN) broth at 37°C and/or 43°C. Such a culture step could inhibit the growth of *Klebsiella* spp., *Ser. marcescens* and/or *Citrobacter* spp. and allow the specific detection of *Salmonella*.

Use of Two 16S DNA Targeted Oligonucleotides as PCR Primers for the Specific Detection of *Salmonella* in Foods

A 16S DNA targeted polymerase chain reaction (PCR) method specific for the detection of *Salmonella* isolates with various serotypes was developed. The primers used for such a PCR method were 16SF1 and 16SFIII. 16SF1 is the reverse and complementary strand of 16SI which has been shown to be able to hybridize with *Salmonella* and *Citrobacter* spp. 16III on the other hand, is able to hybridize with *Klebsiella* and *Serratia* spp. in addition to *Salmonella*. Although 16SF1 and 16SIII were not specific to *Salmonella* only, when they were used as PCR primers, only the *Salmonella* isolates could be specifically detected. The interference from *Citrobacter, Klebsiella* and *Serratia* spp. could be prevented. None of the other non-*Salmonella* isolates including strains of the family of *Enterobacteriaceae* closely related to *Salmonella* generated the false-positive reaction. When this PCR system was used for the detection of *Salmonella* cells artificially contaminated in food samples, results obtained were satisfactory. A detection limit of N $\times 10^0$ cells per assay could be obtained.

Novel Oligonucleotide Probes for Identification of Enterotoxigenic *Staphylococcus aureus*

Based on the DNA sequences coded for *Staphylococcus aureus* enterotoxins (SE) A, B, C, D and E, oligonucleotides unique to each enterotoxin gene were synthesized and used as probes for the identification of types A, B, C, D and E enterotoxigenic *S. aureus*. Probes A1, C1, D1 and E1 encode amino acid 124 (Lys) to 131 (Leu) of SEA, 52 (Asn) to 59 (Lys) of SEC, 26 (Ala) to 33 (Gly) of SED and 15 (Leu) to 21 (Ser) of SEE, respectively. Probes A2, B2, C2 and E2 are the complementary sequences for genes encoding amino acid 189 (Ser) to 196 (Tyr) of SEA, amino acid 232 (Val) to 239 (Lys) of SEB, amino acid 122 (His) to 129 (Glu) of SEC and amino acid 161 (His) to 166 (Leu) of SEE, respectively. The hybridization specificities for these oligonucleotide probes were confirmed by colony hybridization with standard isolates of enterotoxigenic *S. aureus* and some other bacterial strains. Despite the high degree of homology among these *S. aureus* enterotoxin genes, each probe allows specific identification with total discrimination from other types of enterotoxin genes. DNA from non-enterotoxigenic *S. aureus* or from non-*S. aureus* isolates does not interfere with the hybridization result. In addition, probes designed for SEE gene detection allow discrimination of SEE strains that, when assayed with a staphylococcal enterotoxin A, B, C, D detection kit by reversed passive latex agglutination (SET-RPLA), would be grouped together with enterotoxin A producing strains. When these oligonucleotide probes were used for a survey of enterotoxigenic types of *S. aureus* isolated from frozen foods, the results showed that SEA, SEB and SEAB were the major enterotoxigenic types.

Use of the Polymerase Chain Reaction for Specific Detection of Type A, D and E Enterotoxigenic *Staphylococcus aureus* in Foods

By comparison with the DNA sequences coding for *S. aureus* enterotoxins (ents) A, B, C, D and E, oligonucleotides unique to the entA, entD and entE genes were synthesized and used as polymerase chain reaction (PCR) primers for the specific detection of type A, D or E enterotoxigenic *S. aureus*. The relative molecular weights of the PCR products amplified with these primers were 210, 333 and 456 bp, respectively. Despite the high relatedness among these *S. aureus* enterotoxin genes, each primer pair allows specific detection with total discrimination from other types of enterotoxigenic *S. aureus*. DNA from non-enterotoxigenic *S. aureus* or from non-*S. aureus* would not interfere with the PCR results either. Primers designed for entE detection allow the discrimination of entE strains that, when assayed by a serological method, might be classified as entA-producing strains. Study of the detection sensitivity showed that by using these primers, DNA from 10^0 cells of enterotoxigenic *S. aureus* could be detected unambiguously. When these oligonucleotide primers were used for the detection of *S. aureus* in foods, 10^0 to 10^1 cells per gram of food could be detected and the naturally contaminated microflora in the food sample did not interfere with the detection.

Use of Novel Polymerase Chain Reaction Primers for the Specific Detection of Heat-Labile Toxin I, and Heat-Stable Toxin I and II Enterotoxigenic *Escherichia coli* in Milk

Enterotoxigenic *E. coli* (ETEC) strains which produce heat-labile and/or heat-stable toxins (LT and ST) have been some of the most important microorganisms causing food- and waterborne diseases. Rapid and sensitive methods for the specific detection of enterotoxigenic *E. coli* are thus important. Although *quite* a few polymerase chain reaction (PCR) primers have been developed for the specific detection of ETEC genes coding for LT I, ST Ia, and ST Ib, only a few primers have been designed for the detection of ST II and ST Ia, together with ST Ib ETEC. By gene-sequence comparison and serial PCR assay studies, we were able to develop novel PCR primers specific for the detection of LT1 and ST Ia as well as ST Ib and STII enterotoxin-coding genes of *E. coli* cells. An example of the multiplex PCR detection of LT I and ST II genes of *E. coli* cells is shown in Fig. 2. The DNA sequences of these PCR primers are different from those reported by other laboratories. Studies on the detection sensitivities of these PCR primers showed that when cell lysate rather than the total DNA obtained by the phenol-chloroform-isoamyl alcohol extraction method was used for PCR, a lower detection limit, i.e., 10^1 or 10^2 CFU target cells per assay could be obtained. When such a cell-lysis method was used for the PCR detection of ETEC cells in a variety of milk samples, such as whole, <2% fat, skim, and raw milk samples, it was found that if target cells in these milk samples were precultured in MacConKey broth for 8 h prior to cell lysis, as few as 10^0 cells per g of whole, <2% fat, or skim milk samples, and 10^2 cells per g of raw milk sample could be detected.

Plasmid Profiles and Pulsed-Field Gel Electrophoresis for Type A Enterotoxigenic *Staphylococcus aureus* Isolated from Foods

Reports regarding the use of plasmid profile and pulsed field gel electrophoresis

(PFGE) in subtyping of specific enterotoxigenic *S. aureus* isolated from food samples are limited. We isolated 176 strains of *S. aureus* from food samples and showed that 64 of these strains are enterotoxigenic as determined by staphylococcal enterotoxin A, B, C, D detection kit by reversed passive latex agglutination (SET-RPLA) method. Of these 64 enterotoxigenic strains, 45 by SET-RPLA or 44 by polymerase chain reaction (PCR) were identified to be staphylococcal enterotoxin A (SEA) producing strains. All these 64 enterotoxigenic strains could be grouped into three patterns of antibiogram when their antibiotic susceptibilities to penicillin G, oxacillin, vancomycin and methicillin were investigated. Strains resistant to penicillin G, but susceptible to the other three antibiotics were of the major pattern since 50 of the 64 enterotoxigenic strains tested showed such pattern of antibiotic susceptibility. Plasmid deoxyribonucleic acid (DNA) analysis for the 45 SEA strains showed that four types of plasmid profiles could be obtained. When chromosomal DNA of these SEA strains were digested with SmaI and subjected to the PFGE analysis, a total of eight genome types were observed. In addition, 28 of these 45 SEA strains tested could be grouped into one specific type of these eight genome types. Results shown in this report may be useful for the epidemiological study and for the tracing of contamination source when a food poisoning outbreak occurs.

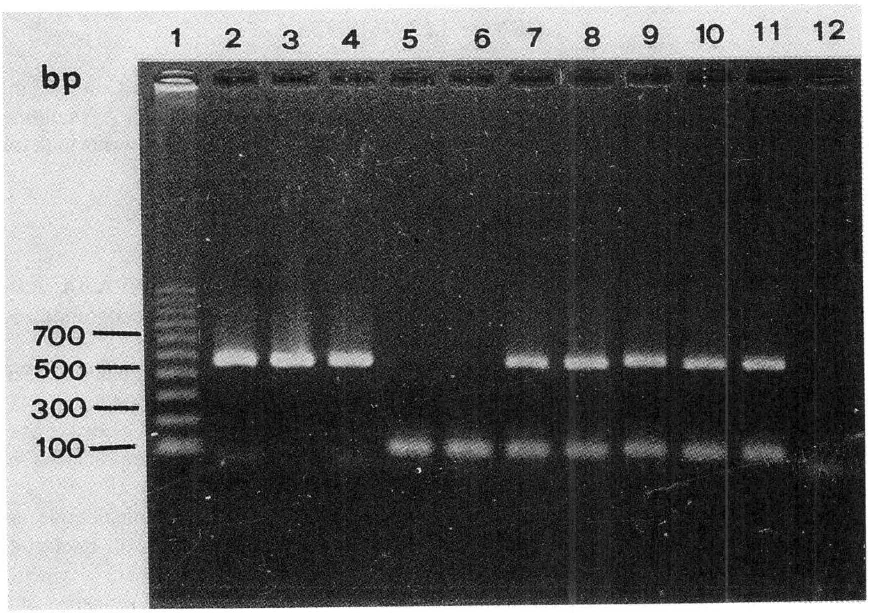

FIG. 2. DETECTION OF LT I AND/OR ST II GENES OF ENTEROTOXIGENIC *ESCHERICHIA COLI* STRAINS USING MULTIPLEX PCR SYSTEM

The PCR primers used were LT I 1/LT I 2 and ST II 1/ST II 2. Lane: 100 bp DNA ladder; lane 2-12 represent PCR products amplified from cell lysates of ETEC strains of ATCC 43886 (LT I h) (lane 2); ATCC 35401 (LT I h + ST I h) (lane 3; ATCC 43886 (LT I)/ATCC 31618 (ST I) (lane 4); UM 4247 (ST II) (lane 5); UM 4247/ATCC 31618 (ST I a) (lane 6); ATCC 43886/UM 4247 (lane 7); ATCC 35401/UM 4247 (lane 8); ATCC 43886/ATCC 31618/UM 4247 (lane 9); PT 18 (LT I + ST II) (lane 10); PT 18/ATCC 31618 (lane 11) and ATCC 31618 (lane 12). For each assay, the bacteria numbers used were 10^6 CFU.

Comparison of Type A Enterotoxigenic *Staphylococcus aureus* Strains Isolated from Geographically Far Distant Locations by Pulsed Field Gel Electrophoresis

Staphylococcal enterotoxin A (SEA) is one of the major staphylococcal enterotoxins which may cause food-borne outbreaks. In order to investigate the difference in genomic types and to elucidate the most disseminated strains for enterotoxin A-producing strains of *S. aureus,* a total of 60 SEA *S. aureus* strains isolated from food and clinical samples in Taiwan and 30 SEA *S. aureus* strains obtained from geographically far distant locations were compared for their pulsed field gel electrophoresis (PFGE) patterns. The rare cutting endonuclease SmaI generated 10 distinct genome patterns for the 60 local SEA isolates and 15 and eight genome patterns, respectively, for the 20 and 10 SEA strains originally isolated from the USA and other countries. The local isolates are less diverse in genome patterns as compared to the USA isolates. Of all these PFGE patterns, a certain pattern, such as pattern 3, is shared by the food and clinical isolates and the local and foreign isolates. Thus, although SEA *S. aureus* strains from geographically far distant locations showed considerable genetic diversity, PFGE pattern 3 strain might be one of the most disseminated strains.

ACKNOWLEDGMENTS

The author thanks the National Science Council, the Agriculture Council, the Department of Health, Taipei, Taiwan and the United States Department of Agriculture, USA for support of the research grants used in this study. The author also wants to thank all his students who participated in these researches.

REFERENCES

COX, N.A., FUNG, Y.C., BAILEY, J.S., HARTMAN, P.A. and VASAVADA, P.C. 1987. Miniaturized kits, immunoassays and DNA hybridization for recognition and identification of food borne bacteria. Dairy Food Sanit. *7*, 628–631.

FOOD and DRUG ADMINISTRATION. 1995. Bacteria Analytical Manual, 8th Ed. Association of Analytical Chemists. Arlington, Va. USA.

LIN, C.K. and TSEN, H.Y. 1995a. Development and evaluation of two novel oligonucleotide probes based on 16S rRNA sequence for the identification of *Salmonella* in foods. J. Appl. Bacteriol. *78*, 507–520.

LIN, C.K. and TSEN, H.Y. 1995b. Use of two 16S rRNA targeted oligonucleotides as PCR primers for the specific detection of *Salmonella* in foods. J. Appl. Bacteriol. *80*, 659–666.

TSEN, H.Y., WANG, S.J., ROE, B.A. and GREEN, S.S. 1993a. DNA sequence of a *Salmonella* specific DNA fragment and the use of oligonucleotide probe for *Salmonella* detection. Appl. Microbiol. Biotechnol. *35*, 339.

TSEN, H.Y., YANG, R.Y. and HUANG, F.Y. 1993b. Novel oligonucleotide probes for isolation and identification of enterotoxigenic *S. aureus*, J. Ferment. Bioengin. *76*, 7–13.

TSEN, H.Y., LIOU, J.W. and LIN, C.K. 1994a. Possible use of a PCR method for specific detection of *Salmonella* in foods. J. Ferment. Bioengin. *77*, 132–143.

TSEN, H.Y., LIOU, J.W. and HU, H.H. 1994b. A colorimetric microtiter plate sandwich DNA hybridization system for the detection of *Salmonella* in foods. J. Ferment. Bioengin. *78*, 12–18.

TSEN, H.Y., YU, G.K. and LIN, I.T. 1995. Plasmid profiles and pulsed field gel electrophoresis for type A enterotoxigenic *S. aureus* isolated from foods. J. Food Protect. *58*, 147–153.

TSEN, H.Y., CHI, W.R. and LIN, C.K. 1996a. Use of novel PCR primers for the specific detection of heat labile toxin I, and heat stable toxin I and II enterotoxigenic *E. coli* in milk. J. Food Protect. *59*, 795–802.

TSEN, H.Y., YU, G.K. and HU, H.H. 1996b. Comparison of type A enterotoxigenic *S. aureus* isolated from geographically distant locations by pulsed field gel electrophoresis. J. Appl. Bacteriol. *82*, 485–493.

TSEN, H.Y., JIAN, L.Z. and CHI, W.R. 1997. Use of a multiplex PCR system for the simultaneous detection of heat labile toxin I and heat stable toxin II genes of ETEC in skim milk and porcine stool. J. Food Protect. (in press).

WOLOCOTT, M.J. 1991. DNA based rapid methods for the detection of food-borne pathogens. J. Food Protect. *54*, 387–401.

PARADOX OF FOOD SAFETY: MICROBIAL HAZARDS

MARY Y. WANG

California Department of Health Services
Sacramento, CA

and

B.S. LUH

University of California
Davis, CA

ABSTRACT

The paradox of food safety has caused consumer concerns and they are demanding more positive assurance of safety, i.e., foods free of microbial hazards. In years past, chemicals and pesticide residues were high profile food safety concerns but today, they are microbes (such as emerging pathogens, E. coli O157:H7, Salmonella enteritidis, *and* Vibrio vulnificus*). This presentation will help the readers to become more familiar with the investigation of foodborne illness outbreaks, including surveillance data and epidemiologic findings on emerging pathogens linked to the outbreaks. Discussion will highlight the dilemma of regulatory infrastructure and prevention controls for resolutions of health emergencies and other safety problems in foods. Lastly, suggestions for proactive responses that the food industry can take in today's changing market and how academia can help to ensure food safety.*

INTRODUCTION

Food safety and health is one of the important subjects emphasized by all public health agencies in the United States; agencies include the state and local health departments and the federal government, the Food and Drug Administration (FDA), the Center for Disease Control and Prevention (CDC), and the U.S. Department of Agriculture (USDA). Today's food safety issues, microbiological or chemical, are complex and new approaches are necessary to meet consumer demands in a changing marketplace. The potential threat of chemicals and environmental substances contaminating the food supply is still a concern to the consumer. However, the most serious food safety problem in the U.S. today is arguably foodborne disease of microbial origin. The Council for Agricultural Science and Technology (CAST) reported in 1994 that each year there are an estimated 6.5 to 33 million cases of foodborne diseases. USDA (1996) reports that the cost of human illness are estimated to be \$9.3-\$12.9 billion annually and \$2.9-\$6.7 billion are attributed to foodborne bacteria. Of the foodborne disease outbreaks where etiology was determined between 1987-1992, CDC (1996) reports that 79% of outbreaks (90% of the cases) were due to bacterial agents. Chemical agents caused 14%, parasites caused 2% and viruses caused 4% of outbreaks.

During the past few decades, several foodborne pathogens have emerged where there are limited knowledge about their role in food safety. In addition, new ways of doing things have caused many changes in the dietary patterns of consumers, such as increased use of new processing technology for extended shelf-life with added choices of convenient foods, increasing numbers of susceptible individuals and the aging population, and lastly, a constant demand for a global world supply. Microorganisms, although only a small percentage of which are pathogenic, are ubiquitous in the environment and often contaminate raw agricultural food products, including many foods of animal origin. Also, humans may introduce pathogens into foods during production, processing, distribution and preparation. Every person involved in the food chain must recognize the need for vigilance in controlling microbiological hazards because foodborne disease is largely preventable.

Some of the more recent publications on foodborne diseases, food microbiology, food virology, and general food safety have been published by APHA (1995), CAST (1994), CDC (1994, 1996), Hackney *et al.* (1996), Hedberg and Osterholm (1993), Hui *et al.* (1994), and USDA (1995, 1996). Other references on the subject have also been published by Knabel (1995), Ray (1996), and in FDA's Food Code (1997a). This report covers the recent food safety issues on microbial hazards, with emphasis on three pathogens (*E. coli* O157:H7, *Salmonella enteritidis*, and *Vibrio vulnificus*).

FOODBORNE DISEASE INVESTIGATION AND SURVEILLANCE

Surveillance of foodborne disease outbreaks began over a century ago and the early surveillance data have led to many important public health rules to reduce foodborne diseases. Todd (1994) illustrated a structure that a team effort among federal, state and local health departments and laboratories is necessary to form the foundation for a surveillance system. An effective surveillance would require prompt investigation of any reported foodborne disease outbreak and a well coordinated effort at all levels. In addition, all investigations must be conducted in a thorough and timely manner to prevent any spread of the disease. The procedures for investigating foodborne disease outbreaks are described by Morse *et al.* (1994) and IAMFES (1988). Once the etiologic agent, a food vehicle responsible, and a source of contamination are identified, intervention and controls are implemented to prevent future outbreaks (CDC 1994).

In California, the local health departments are required to report foodborne disease outbreaks to the California Department of Health Services (CDHS) in which the surveillance data are used at both the state and national level to monitor trends in foodborne disease outbreaks. CDHS received a total of 63 foodborne disease outbreaks (1,219 total cases) reports in 1995. As illustrated in Fig. 1, 39% had a confirmed etiology, 32% had a suspected etiology, and 27% had an unknown etiology. Of the confirmed etiology (25 outbreaks, 679 cases), 24 outbreaks were due to bacterial agents and one outbreak (97 cases) was due to a viral agent (Norwalk virus). Figure 2 shows the etiologic agents responsible for the outbreaks: *Salmonella enteriditis* caused 10 outbreaks (161 cases); other *Salmonella* serotypes caused 7 outbreaks (142 cases); *Shigella* caused 2 outbreaks (32 cases); *Clostridium botulinum* caused 2 outbreaks (2 cases); *E. coli* O157:H7 caused one outbreak (5 cases); *Clostridium perfringens* caused one outbreak (100 cases); and *Staphylococcus aureus* caused one outbreak (140 cases).

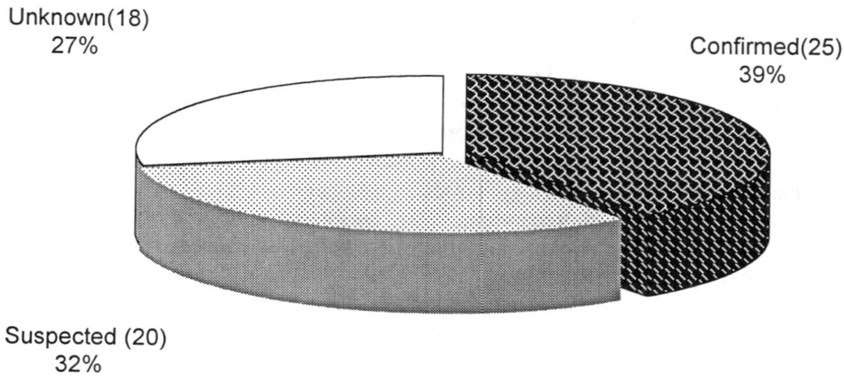

FIG. 1. CALIFORNIA FOODBORNE OUTBREAKS - 1995
N = 63 Outbreaks
Source: California Department of Health Services, Division of Communicable Disease Control, Surveillance and Statistics Section

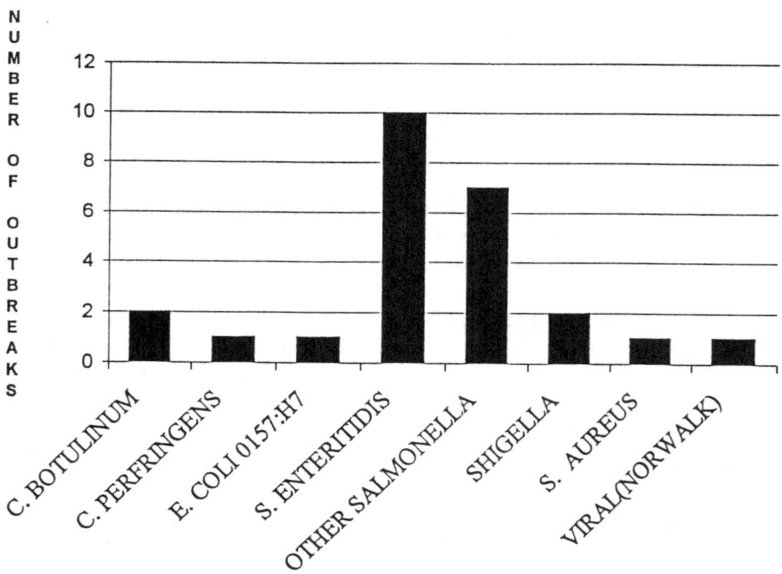

FIG. 2. CALIFORNIA FOODBORNE OUTBREAKS - 1995 BY CONFIRMED ETIOLOGY
N = 25 Outbreaks
Source: California Department of Health Services, Division of Communicable Disease Control, Surveillance and Statistics Section

To monitor national trends in foodborne diseases, CDC recently set up five FoodNet active surveillance sites in the United States (California, Connecticut, Georgia, Minnesota and Oregon); in 1996, of the 7,259 laboratory-confirmed cases, 33 resulted in death. The seven pathogens and their incidence of causing disease in the monitoring project are: *Campylobacter* (45%), *Salmonella* (29.5%), *Shigella* (17.2%), *E. coli* O157:H7 (5.3%), *Yersinia* (1.9%), *Listeria* (0.9%) and *Vibrio* (0.2%). Also in 1996, CDC identified five clusters of foodborne disease: salmonellosis in Oregon linked to alfalfa sprouts; *E. coli* O157:H7 infections in Connecticut and Illinois associated with lettuce, *E. coli* O157:H7 infections in Connecticut linked to unpasteurized apple cider, and *E. coli* O157:H7 infections in a daycare center in Minnesota; and Yersiniosis in Georgia linked to chitterlings.

EMERGING FOODBORNE PATHOGENS

Recent foodborne disease outbreaks in the United States have caused concerns in food safety because of several emerging pathogens and unusual vehicles of transmission. The following is a brief discussion of three emerging foodborne pathogens.

Escherichia coli O157:H7

Escherichia coli (E. coli) bacteria normally live in the intestines of humans and animals. Although most strains of this bacteria are harmless, several are known to produce toxins that can cause diarrheal illnesses. One particular *E. coli* strain called O157:H7 can cause severe bloody diarrhea and kidney failure (Hemolytic Uremic Syndrome or HUS) in young children (MacDonald and Osterholm 1993). The first foodborne disease outbreak linked to ground beef occurred in 1982, but it was not until the 1993 outbreak associated with a fast-food restaurant that *E. coli* O157:H7 infection was recognized as an emerging cause of foodborne disease (CDC 1993). There are an estimated 10,000 to 20,000 cases occurring in the United States each year and most cases have been associated with eating undercooked, contaminated ground beef. However, person-to-person contact in child care centers and nursing homes is also an important mode of transmission. Infection can also occur during swimming in or drinking contaminated water.

When cooking ground beef, the *E. coli* O157:H7 bacteria, if present, can be destroyed by heating to 155°F (FDA 1997a). However, in 1996 several *E. coli* O157:H7 outbreaks implicated plant foods that previously have not been considered to be potentially hazardous. These are ready-to-eat foods, such as fresh unpasteurized apple juice and chopped lettuce (CDC 1997a,b). Therefore, additional control measures must be considered for foods that may be contaminated with low levels of *E. coli* O157:H7 bacteria. The food industries recognize the potential problem with this pathogen, and are working with the regulatory agencies to develop and establish preventive measures throughout the food chain. Currently, farmers, growers, processors and distributors are implementing comprehensive Quality Assurance programs based on Good Manufacturing Practices (GMP) regulations and the Hazard Analysis and Critical Control Point (HACCP) system to ensure finished product quality and safety.

Salmonella enteritidis

Salmonellosis is the most commonly reported cause of foodborne disease in the United States. Salmonella food poisoning has the potential to affect any person exposed to it, and the disease can be life threatening to the susceptible populations, the elderly, the young and those who are immunocompromised. *Salmonella enteritidis* infections became a public health problem in the United States in the early 1980s, and is an important public health problem in many countries today. Shell eggs have been the most commonly implicated food item in *Salmonella enteritidis* outbreaks because the organism can be present inside a perfectly normal appearing egg (St. Louis *et al.* 1988). Eggs, meat, poultry, milk and other foods are safe when handled properly. Shell eggs are safe when stored in the refrigerator, individually and thoroughly cooked and promptly consumed after cooking. Consumers should be advised to keep eggs refrigerated to prevent bacteria in the eggs, if present, from growing. Cooking will destroy the bacteria present; however, if contaminated egg is eaten raw or undercooked then there is a potential risk of salmonellosis.

Salmonella enteritidis is the common serotype responsible for a large number of sporadic cases of salmonellosis reported in California, as well as in the United States. In September 1994, a major multistate outbreak of *Salmonella enteritidis* infection occurred, in which a nationally distributed brand of ice-cream was implicated (Hennessy *et al.* 1996). The product was recalled and further epidemiologic and microbiological investigations were conducted. Apparently, the ice cream mixes were transported from one processing facility to another in a tanker truck that previously hauled liquid raw eggs. As a result, the FDA and the USDA jointly promulgated a proposed regulation for transporting and storing potentially hazardous foods requiring a HACCP-type system for temperature monitoring (*Federal Register* 1996).

Vibrio vulnificus

Molluscan shellfish (oysters, clams and mussels) have long been known to be associated with marine pathogens and biotoxins. Illnesses associated with consumption have been attributed to Hepatitis A virus, Norwalk virus, and bacterial agents such as *Salmonella* spp. and *Vibrio* spp. (Rippey 1994). Today eating raw shellfish is relatively common and oyster bars are doing a brisk business across the United States. Very few consumers are aware that eating raw bivalve mollusks can pose a significant health risk, especially to those with compromised immune systems.

Individuals with underlying diseases are at greatest risk for septicemia (blood poisoning) with *Vibrio vulnificus*, a dangerous bacterium naturally occurring in the marine environment. Generally, the bacteria are transmitted either through consumption of raw shellfish or wound exposure to seawater. *Vibrio vulnificus* and raw molluscan shellfish consumption present a challenge to public health and the scientific community because of the severity of illness it causes. It may be mild illnesses for healthy individuals but deadly to highly susceptible individuals.

Presently, virtually all known foodborne *Vibrio vulnificus* cases where the sources of shellfish were known have involved the consumption of raw oysters harvested from the Gulf Coast states during the warmer months. There may have been cases where sources of oysters were not determined. California has its share of *Vibrio vulnificus* cases that are associated with raw shellfish consumption. In March 1991, CDHS adopted regulations requiring warning to be posted at retail food facilities where certain raw oysters are sold. To date (from 1983 to 1996), of the total number of 41 cases reported in California, 32 cases were associated with the consumption of raw oysters.

PROACTIVE RESPONSES

Currently there is a significant shortage of scientific knowledge on foodborne pathogens, and proactive control measures are needed to deal with today's changing market. The following areas need more academic research: (1) determine the exact microbial causes of human disease via the foodborne route; (2) identify sources of contamination and transmission to food vehicle; (3) study the elements affecting pathogen's survival and growth in foods; (4) research on the infective dose to human, especially for those who are more susceptible; (5) survey the ecology of the pathogen and its interaction with the food environment, both in raw food (plant or animal sources) and in processed food; and (6) develop scientific data for predictive modeling of the characteristics of foodborne pathogens. In addition, a critical need in food safety research is the development of rapid and reliable diagnostic methods to detect pathogens in foods. Bio-engineered testing kits, such as those employing Enzyme-Linked Immunosorbent Assays (ELISA) based on monoclonal antibody technology, are currently being developed which may be adopted as official methods in the future.

Academia, industry and government must work closely together to fill the gap to ensure consumers that the food supply is safe. The National Advisory Committee on Microbiological Criteria for Foods (NACMCF) endorses HACCP as an effective and rational means of assuring food safety from harvest to consumption and preventing problems from occurring. Many of the HACCP principles are already in place in the FDA-regulated low-acid canned foods, and have been incorporated into the FDA's Food Code since 1993. The Food Code serves as a model legislation for state agencies that inspect restaurants and retail food establishments in the United States. Recently, HACCP-based inspection and microbial pathogen monitoring are incorporated into the USDA Food Safety and Inspection Services meat and poultry inspection programs. The FDA also promulgated HACCP regulations for inspection of fish and seafood products. Several other segments of the food industry, such as the lettuce and apple juice producers, have developed HACCP training for their growers and processors as part of their voluntary Quality Assurance programs.

NATIONAL FOOD SAFETY INITIATIVE

The challenge of food safety is fully discussed in the recently published National Food Safety Initiative in which a federal interagency strategy is being developed to prevent future foodborne diseases (FDA 1997b). The important approaches to the National Food Safety Initiative are: (1) *Surveillance*. To increase from 5 to 8 sentinel sites in the Active Foodborne Disease Surveillance Program; electronically linking the sites with the federal agencies to speed detection and response to outbreaks; creating a national electronic network for bacterial "fingerprinting". (2) *Inspection*. Optimizing FDA's food inspection program by employing HACCP; enhancing federal/state partnerships to facilitate the rapid transfer of inspection results. (3) *Risk assessment*. Filling food safety information gaps by establishing a risk assessment consortium;

developing dose-response assessment models and better techniques for assessing microbial and chemical risks. (4) *Bioscience Research*. Coordinating research efforts to develop needed detection methods, drug therapies, pathogen prevention made up of industry, consumer, state and local food protection agencies to develop and share information on strategies and safe handling tools. (5) *Education*. Launching a focused educational campaign aimed at changing unsafe handling by food workers. Convening a national food safety education made up of industry, consumer, state and local food protection agencies to develop and share information on food safety. (6) *Outbreak Coordination*. Establish a foodborne response group made up of federal and state representatives to coordinate the investigations into and communications on significant outbreaks of foodborne diseases.

REFERENCES

APHA. 1995. Control of communicable diseases manual. Benenson, A.S. (ed). An official report of the American Public Health Association. 16th Ed.

CAST. 1994. Foodborne pathogens: risks and consequences. Council for Agricultural Science and Technology. Task Force Report No. 122.

CDC. 1993. Update: multistate outbreak of *Escherichia coli* O157:H7 infections from hamburgers -- Western United States 1992-93. MMWR *42*, 258–263.

CDC. 1994. Addressing emerging infectious disease threats: A prevention strategy for the United States. Centers for Disease Control and Prevention, U.S. Department of Health & Human Services, Atlanta, Georgia.

CDC. 1996. Surveillance for Foodborne-Disease Outbreaks -- United States, 1988-1992. Center for Disease Control and Prevention *Surveillance Summaries*, October 25, 1996; 45 (No.SS-5).

CDC. 1997a. Outbreaks of *E.coli* O157:H7 and Cryptosporidium associated with drinking unpasteurized apple cider - Connecticut and New York. MMWR *46*, 4–8.

CDC. 1997b. Foodborne diseases active surveillance network -- 1996. MMWR *46*, 258–261.

CDHS. 1996. Foodborne disease outbreak summary reports -- California 1995 surveillance data. California Department of Health Services, Division of Communicable Disease Control, Surveillance and Statistics Section.

CDHS. 1991. Raw oyster warning and tag and labeling requirements. Title 17, California Code of Regulations. Section 13675.

FEDERAL REGISTER. 1996. Transportation and storage requirements for potentially hazardous foods. Food Safety and Inspection Service, USDA; FDA, DHHS. November 22, 1996. Washington D.C. *61*, 59372–59382.

FDA. 1997a. Food Code. Recommendations of the United States Department of Health and Human Services, Public Health Service, Food and Drug Administration. Washington D.C.

FDA. 1997b. Food safety from farm to table: a national food safety initiative, report to the President, May 1997. U.S. Dept. of Health & Human Services, U.S. Dept. of Agriculture, and the U.S. Environmental Protection Agency. [Internet access: http://www.fda.gov]

HACKNEY, C., PEIRSON, M.D. and BANWART, G. 1996. Basic Food Microbiology, 3rd Ed., Chapman Hall, New York.

HEDBERG, C.W. and OSTERHOLM, M.J. 1993. Outbreaks of foodborne and waterborne viral gastroenteritis. Clin. Microbiol. Rev. *6*, 199–210.

HENNESSY, T.W., HEDBERG, C.W., SLUTSKER, L., WHITE, K.E., BESSER-WIEK, J.M., MOEN, M.E., FIELDMAN, J., COLEMAN, W.W., EDMONSON, L.M., MACDONALD, K.L. and OSTERHOLM, M.T. 1996. A national outbreak of *Salmonella enteritidis* infections from ice-cream. New England J. Med. *334*, 1281–1286.

HUI, Y.H., GORHAM, J.R., MURRELL, K.D. and CLIVER, D.O. 1994. Foodborne disease handbook - diseases caused by bacteria, Volume 1. Marcel Dekker, Inc., New York, Basel, Hong Kong.

IAMFES. 1988. Procedures to investigate foodborne illness. International Association of Milk, Food and Environmental Sanitarians, Inc. 4th Ed. - 1987 (Revised & Updated-1988), Des Moines, Iowa.

KNABEL, S.J. 1995. Foodborne illness, role of home food handling practices. Food Technol. *49*, 119–130.

MACDONALD, K.L. and OSTERHOLM, M.T. 1993. The emergence of *Escherichia coli* O157:H7 infection in the United States. The changing epidemiology of foodborne disease. JAMA. *269*, 2264–2266.

MORSE, D.L., BIRKHEAD, G.S. and GUZEWICH, J.J. 1994. Investigating foodborne disease. *In* Foodborne Disease Handbook, Vol. 1. Diseases Caused by Bacteria. Y.H. Hui, J.R. Gorham, K.D. Murrell and D.O. Cliver (eds.). Marcel Dekker, Inc., New York, Basel, Hong Kong.

RAY, B. 1996. Fundamental Food Microbiology. CRC Press, Boca Raton, New York, London, Tokyo.

RIPPEY, S.R. 1994. Infectious diseases associated with molluscan shellfish consumption. Clin. Microbiol. Rev. *7*, 419–425.

ST. LOUIS, M.E., MORSE, D.L., POTTER, M.E., DEMELFI, T.M., GUZEWICH, J.J., TAUXE, R.V. BLAKE, P.A. and the *Salmonella enteritidis* Working Group. 1988. The emergence of grade A eggs as a major source of *Salmonella enteritidis* infections. JAMA. *259*, 2103–2107.

TODD, E.C.D. 1994. Surveillance of foodborne disease. *In* Foodborne Disease Handbook, Vol. 1. Diseases Caused by Bacteria. Y.H. Hui, J.R. Gorham, K.D. Murrell and D.O. Cliver (eds.). Marcel Dekker, Inc., New York, Basel, Hong Kong.

USDA. 1995. Tracking foodborne pathogens from farm to table: data needs to evaluate control options. T. Roberts, H. Jensen, and L. Unnevehr (eds.) U.S. Department of Agriculture, Economic Research Service, Food and Consumer Economics Division. Misc. publ. no. 1532.

USDA. 1996. Bacterial foodborne disease: medical costs and productivity losses. Economic Research Service, USDA. Agriculture economic report no. 741.

CONSUMER FOOD SAFETY CONCERNS: ACCEPTANCE OF NEW TECHNOLOGIES THAT ENHANCE FOOD SAFETY

CHRISTINE M. BRUHN

University of California, Davis
One Shields Ave.
Davis, CA 95616-8598

ABSTRACT

Microbiological safety has been United States consumers' most frequently volunteered food safety concern for several years, and in the last few years the percentage of people expressing concern has increased. Concern about pesticides, antibiotics or hormones used in animal production, and additives or preservatives used in processing have gradually decreased over the past eight years.

Consumer concern about microbiological safety could enhance receptivity to newer technologies which enhance microbiological safety, such as food irradiation, laser or high pressure treatment. Educational programs on new technologies must begin with consumer benefits. Enhanced microbiological safety, even though it is an invisible benefit, can be potent. While some consumers will maintain a cautious stance toward an unfamiliar technology, many will try a new product if the benefits seem real and other safety and quality concerns are addressed.

Attitude studies have demonstrated that when given science-based information, from 60% to 90% of consumers prefer the advantages irradiation processing provides. Experience with food irradiation indicates food processed by this technology is accepted and even receives a premium in the marketplace.

INTRODUCTION

Consumers demand food with an increasingly high level of safety. They expect protection from natural substances and hazards added by human intervention. Although some prefer to trust in "natural" or traditional processes, many seek protection through modern science and technology.

When United States consumers are given the opportunity to volunteer the greatest food safety threat, they mention microbiological hazards and spoilage most frequently. The percentage of consumers who specifically mention this hazard increased from 29% in 1990 to 69% in 1997 (Abt Associates 1997). This high rating contrasts to only 10% volunteering pesticide residues and 6% stating chemicals. When specifically asked, 82% identified bacteria as a serious health risk in 1997, significantly more than those classifying pesticide residues, 66%; product tampering, 65%; antibiotic or hormone residues, 43%; nitrites or food additives, 28% as a serious health risk.

Consumer perception as to who should be primarily responsible to ensure that product safety has shifted. In 1988 almost half of the consumers accepted personal responsibility for safety with 45% replying "yourself as an individual" (Opinion Research

1990). Government was identified by 29% and consumer groups by 15%. By 1997, only 29% cited personal responsibility, government responsibility slipped to 20% and consumer groups to 6% (Abt Associates 1997). In contrast, an increased percentage of consumers are placing responsibility on manufacturers and food processors, with 7% citing this group in 1988 and 23% in 1997. Additionally, an increasing percentage of consumers expect supermarkets to take primary responsibility. Only 3% identified supermarkets in 1988 compared to 20% in 1997.

Many manufacturers and retailers have responded to these increased expectations with increased emphasis on employee training and adoption of safe manufacturing practices such as the Hazard Analysis Critical Control Point method. Processors can also utilize newer technologies such as food irradiation that increase the microbiological safety of raw ingredients. Retailers may feature products processed by safety-enhancing technology.

Food irradiation can significantly increase the safety of raw meat or poultry by destroying microbiological pathogens (Thayer *et al.* 1996). In this process, food is exposed to high levels of energy from radioactive isotopes such as cobalt or from X ray machines. The effect of this treatment varies by the amount of energy used. A high dose sterilizes spices and substitutes for the fumigant, ethylene oxide. Pathogens in raw poultry and meat can be reduced by as much as 99.9% by a lower "pasteurization" dose of radiation. Grain and produce can be disinfected by still lower doses, and natural decay of some fruit and vegetables can be retarded. Irradiation is an effective quarantine treatment for the Mediterranean fruit fly and other pests and can substitute for these pest control uses of methyl bromide.

Irradiation is a cold treatment. The food maintains an unprocessed, fresh-like character. The safety of irradiation is endorsed by the World Health Organization, the American Medical Association, United States Food and Drug Association, the American Dietetic Association, the American Veterinary Medical Association, the Institute of Food Technologists, and various health and safety authorities in over 30 countries.

In the United States, irradiation is approved for spices to decontaminate and disinfest insects, destruction of pathogens in poultry, control *Trichinella spiralis* in pork, delay maturation of fruits and vegetables, and disinfest wheat or fruits (Thayer *et al.* 1996). A petition to approve the irradiation of fresh and frozen red meat is pending.

Introduction of irradiated foods into the marketplace has been slow, due in part to uncertainty of consumer acceptance. Some activist groups claim consumers will reject irradiated food; others state that irradiation is unnecessary. This paper will review recent attitude surveys and market response to irradiated food and will identify information of greatest consumer interest.

CONSUMER CONCERNS

Since the process of asking about an area will cause some to express concern, responses to a specific processing method or ingredient are more accurately interpreted by comparing change over time, or contrasting attitudes toward one area with those of another within the same sample. This comparison indicates irradiation is considered a serious risk by fewer people than other areas and the percentage viewing irradiation as risky is decreasing. The Food Marketing Institute annual attitude surveys indicates 33% classified irradiation as a serious health risk comparable to 43% classifying antibiotics and hormone residues and 28% classifying nitrites, and 21% classifying additives as serious risks (Abt Associates 1997). Since the late 1980's, 10% fewer considered irradiation a serious risk; 8% believe irradiation and 7% believe additives do not pose a risk. A relative ranking of food processing methods surveyed by the Gallup Organization found that irradiation, food preservatives, and use of chlorination generated a similar concern rating (Gallup *et al.* 1993).

A study among Georgia consumers (n=446) found concerns for pesticides, animal drug residues, growth hormones, food additives, and bacteria were significantly higher than concern for food irradiation (Resurreccion *et al.* 1995). Concern ratings for irradiation and naturally occurring toxins was comparable. More persons believed irradiation was "no problem," (20%); than other potential food safety issues such as food additives, (11%); growth hormones (8%); animal drugs (7%); and pesticides (7%).

EFFECTS OF EDUCATION

When asked about irradiation, people have questions about product safety, nutritional quality, potential harm to employees, and potential danger from living near an irradiation facility. Consumer studies consistently demonstrate that when provided with science-based information, a high percentage of consumers prefer irradiated foods (Bruhn 1995).

The effect of information and product samples on consumer attitudes was documented in a Purdue University study (Pohlman *et al.* 1994). Initially, about half of the sample of 178 residents were willing to buy irradiated foods. After viewing an eight minute video tape, *The Future of Food Preservation, Food Irradiation,* subjects knowledge and willingness to buy irradiated food increased to 90%. Willingness to buy increased to 99% among those who both saw the video tape and sampled irradiated strawberries.

This video tape has been evaluated among other audiences. *The Future of Food Preservation, Food Irradiation* video tape and other educational pieces were shown to military personal (Schutz 1994). In follow-up interviews, the percentage of soldiers who expressed major concern in the control group (received no educational intervention) decreased from 33 to 29% and those expressing no concern increased from 8 to 27%. This change may have resulted from repeat exposure to the concept of irradiation. Among those soldiers viewing the video tape, 17% expressed major concern and 38% no concern about irradiated food. Those soldiers likely to select irradiated food in the military dining commons increased from 21 to 61% after viewing the video tape. Over 80% indicated they were likely to choose irradiated field rations.

A USDA funded project in California and Indiana used the video tape to evaluate the impact of a brief educational program on community leaders attitudes and knowledge of food irradiation (Bruhn and Mason 1996). After a brief introduction, *The Future of Food Preservation, Food Irradiation* was shown, followed by a question and answer period and summary of the effect of irradiation on food. Consumers gained knowledge of specific food irradiation facts and their interest in purchasing irradiated foods increased. After participating in this program, consumer concern about the safety of irradiated foods decreased from 19% to 11%. Confidence in the safety of irradiated food increased with those likely or very likely to try irradiated food increasing from 57 to

83%. There was no difference in attitudes or knowledge between California and Indiana consumers.

People do not always do what they say. A University of Georgia shopping simulation test showed a significant increase in the proportion of consumers purchasing irradiated ground beef after exposure to an educational program on the benefits of food irradiation. After receiving information, 71% selected irradiated beef, including half of those who were uncertain and 62% of those originally stating they would not purchase irradiated food (Gallup *et al.* 1993).

MARKET EXPERIENCES

Irradiation offers significant consumer advantages in food safety, quality, and convenience. Actual marketing experience in several parts of the United States demonstrates that consumers will purchase irradiated conventional and tropical fruit and poultry. Persons opposed to scientific and technological innovations find irradiation unacceptable; they have been estimated as 5-10% of the population (Brand Group 1986).

Consumer response to labeled irradiated food has been positive. Irradiated mangoes sold well in Florida in 1986. In March 1987, irradiated Hawaiian papayas available as a one day trial at two markets in Southern California outsold the identically priced non irradiated counterpart by greater than ten to one (Bruhn and Noel 1987). Irradiated apples marketed in Missouri were favorably received (Terry and Tabor 1990). A record amount of irradiated strawberries were sold in Florida in 1992 (Marcotte 1992). Thereafter, numerous irradiated produce items have been marketed in the Chicago area (Pszczola 1992). Since the Fall of 1995, tropical fruit from Hawaii has been sold at Carrot Top (Chicago) and several Midwest markets in collaboration with a study to determine quarantine treatment. From 1995 through October, 1996, eleven shipments of fruit consisting of papaya (10,020 pounds), atemoya (7,302 pounds), rambutan (1,168 pounds), lychee (3,080 pounds), starfruit (2,264 pounds), banana (380 pounds), Chinese taro (30 pounds), and oranges (200 pounds) were shipped to Isomedix plant near Chicago for irradiation between 0.25 Kg (Kilogrey) and 1.0 Kg (Wong 1996). In late 1996 fruit was also marketed in ethnic markets in San Francisco and Los Angeles. Fruit was well received by consumers; however, one Midwest retailer withdrew due to threats from an activist organization. By 1997, 100,000 pounds of irradiated Hawaiian tropical fruit has been sold on the mainland (Wong 1997).

The market response to irradiated poultry was tested in Kansas. In 1995 labeled irradiated poultry captured 60% of the market share when priced 10% less than store brand, 39% when priced equally, and 30% when priced 10% higher (Anonymous 1995b). In 1996 market share increased to 63% when the irradiated product was priced 10% less than the store brand, 47% when priced equally, and 18 and 17% when priced 10 or 20% higher (Fox 1996). The irradiated product sold better in the more up-scale store, capturing 73% of the market when priced 10% lower, 58% when priced equally, and 31 and 30% when priced 10 or 20% higher. This is consistent with other attitude surveys and marketplace data that indicate irradiation is more accepted in up-scale markets.

Chicken irradiated to destroy bacterial contamination is being used for employee and patient food service in some Florida healthcare facilities (Anonymous 1995a). Lawyers have noted that there are greater risks for a food company to not use irradiation than to use it (Robeck 1996). Irradiated chicken is also being used in a restaurant chain in Florida. The executive chef indicates he chose irradiated food for the greater safety. At the Institute of Food Technologists annual meeting, Chef Scott Dickerson said irradiated poultry is, "the cheapest peace of mind I could imagine" (Dickerson 1997).

Through focus group studies consumers indicate the most important information about irradiation is the process' long term record of safety, endorsement by health authorities, maintenance of food flavor and nutritive value and protection from bacteria which could lead to illness (Gallup *et al.* 1993).

CONCLUSIONS

Consumer research and market experience indicates many consumers are ready to purchase safety-enhanced irradiated food. When consumers are provided additional information on the benefits of irradiation, the percentage of consumers ready to purchase irradiated food increases. The food processing and retail industry can meet consumer demand for safety-enhanced products by offering irradiated products. Given the opportunity, consumers will buy high quality, safety-enhanced irradiated food.

REFERENCES

ABT ASSOCIATES INC. 1997. Trends in the United States, Consumer attitudes and the supermarket, 1996. Food Marketing Institute, Washington, DC.

ANONYMOUS. 1995a. Florida hospitals make irradiated chicken buy. Food Service Director *8*(2), 1.

ANONYMOUS. 1995b. The irradiation option. Food Safety Consortium *5*(3), 1–5.

BRAND GROUP. 1986. Irradiated seafood product. A position paper for the seafood industry. Final report. Chicago, IL.

BRUHN, C.M. 1995. Consumer attitudes and market response to irradiated food. J. Food Protection *58*(2), 175–181.

BRUHN, C.M. and MASON, A. 1996. Science and Society: A public information program on food innovations. Final Report USDA FY 1994 Special Projects, Project no 94–EFSQ–1–4141. U.S. Department of Agriculture, Washington, D.C.

BRUHN, C.M. and NOEL, J.W. 1987. Consumer in–store response to irradiated papayas. Food Technol. *41*(9), 83–85.

DICKERSON, S. 1997. Food irradiation and HACCP. 1997 Institute of Food Technologists annual meeting, Orlando, Florida.

FOX, J.A. 1996. Personal communication. Department of Agricultural Economics, Kansas State University, Manhattan, Kansas.

GALLUP ORGANIZATION, ABT Associates, Center for Food Safety and Quality Enhancement, University of Georgia. 1993. Consumer awareness, knowledge and acceptance of food irradiation. American Meat Institute Foundation, Arlington, Virginia.

MARCOTTE, M. 1992. Irradiated strawberries enter the US market. Food Technol. *46*(5), 80.

OPINION RESEARCH. 1990. Trends. Consumer attitudes and the super–market. Food Marketing Institute, Washington, D.C.

POHLMAN, A.J., WOOD, O.B. and MASON, A.C. 1994. Influence of audiovisuals and food samples on consumer acceptance of food irradiation. Food Technol. *48*(12), 46–49.

PSZCZOLA, D.E. 1992. Irradiated produce reaches midwest market. Food Technol. *46*(5), 89–92.

RESURRECCION, A.V.A., GALVEZ, F.C.F., FLETCHER, S.M. and MISRA, S.K. 1995. Consumer attitudes toward irradiated food: Results of a new study. J. Food Protect. *58*(2), 193–196.

ROBECK, M.R. 1996. Product liability issues related to food irradiation. Food Technol. *50*(2), 78–82.

TERRY, D.E. and TABOR, R.L. 1990. Consumers' perceptions and willingness to pay for food irradiation. Proceedings of the Second International Conference on Research in the Consumer Interest, August 1990.

THAYER, D.W., JOSEPHSON, E.S., BRYNJOLFSSON, G. and GIDDINGS, G. 1996. Radiation Pasteurization of Food. Council for Agricultural Science and Technology. *7*, 1–10.

WONG, L. 1996. Personal communications. Plant Industry Administrator, Department of Agriculture, State of Hawaii, Honolulu, Hawaii.

WONG, L. 1997. Personal communications. Plant Industry Administrator, Department of Agriculture, State of Hawaii, Honolulu, Hawaii.

CONSUMER PREFERENCE GROUPS — MEASUREMENT, IMPLICATIONS, AND CHALLENGES

JOEL L. SIDEL, HERBERT STONE, HEATHER THOMAS
and HOWARD G. SCHUTZ

Tragon Corporation
365 Convention Way
Redwood City, CA 94063

ABSTRACT

In most all markets, whether they be new or mature, consumers are free to choose among a variety of food products that are competitively priced and often technologically similar. Advertising, pricing, shelf location, and packaging influence initial trial, and sensory acceptance influences repeat purchase. Competition for a consumer's loyalty and food expenditure requires that manufacturers accurately anticipate consumer wants and needs, and rapidly develop and market those products. Critical to accurately anticipating consumer wants and needs is knowing "who is the current or potential consumer for the product", "how best to measure consumer preference", "are consumers homogeneous in their preferences", and "what sensory characteristics drive acceptance." Answers to the latter two questions impact the number and type of products to develop, the sensory delivery for those products, and how best to market those products.

New approaches to using sensory evaluation, and the application of multivariate statistical techniques provide important information and insights about consumer preferences and the heterogeneity of those preferences. Preference group research answers why a product in a sensory test is liked by some consumers and disliked by others, and what formulation is most likely to satisfy these different preferences. Obtaining this information is possible through the application of contemporary sensory evaluation practices, testing large and diverse product sets, and identifying properly qualified consumers. Cluster analysis and preference mapping identify different preference groups in the population, and sensory analysis identifies sensory characteristics that differentiate the preference groups. This presentation provides examples from our preference group research, and focuses on how the information was developed and the implications of those results for more successful product development efforts. The importance of integrating this information with the advertising, pricing, and related marketing issues also will be considered.

INTRODUCTION

In most markets, whether they are new or mature, consumers have many choices among the products available. These products are competitively priced and often technologically very similar. Advertising, pricing, shelf location, and packaging attract and influence initial trial, while sensory acceptance influences repeat purchase. Historically, companies have responded to increased competition and other changes in the marketplace by introducing new brands as well as developing less costly products. At times both of these approaches will compete with each other to the point that consumer perceived quality will be compromised. Companies usually take this approach primarily because they underestimate consumer knowledge of the products available to them in the marketplace or apply standardized techniques to contemporary problems. Competition for a consumer's loyalty and that portion of their food expenditure, requires that manufacturers accurately anticipate consumer wants and needs, and rapidly develop and market those products. Critical to accurately anticipating consumer wants and needs is knowing the answers to a series of questions: who is the current or potential consumer for that product, how best to measure preference, are preferences changing, are consumers homogeneous in their preferences, and what sensory characteristics drive preference. Answers, especially to the latter two questions impact the number and type of products that could be developed, the key sensory characteristics for those products, and how best to market them.

With this brief overview of the marketplace, it is encouraging to note that there are systems in place that allow us to answer many of these questions and provide products that better meet consumer expectations.

New approaches to using sensory evaluation, and the application of multivariate statistical techniques provide important information and insights about consumer preferences, the heterogeneity of those preferences and the sensory characteristics that drive those differences. Preference group research answers why a product in a sensory test is liked by some consumers and disliked by others, and what formulation is most likely to satisfy these different preferences. Obtaining this information is possible through the application of contemporary sensory evaluation practices, testing sufficiently large and diverse product sets, and identifying properly qualified consumers. Cluster analysis and preference mapping provide a means for identifying different preference groups in the population, and sensory analysis identifies the characteristics that differentiate these groups.

In this discussion we describe the means by which such preference behavior can be identified and characterized along with the implications for developing and marketing new and improved products.

MEASUREMENT

No sensory acceptance test finds that all consumers prefer the same product or have the same rank order for a group of products, a result which by itself is not surprising. For the most part these differences represent the individual preferences of those consumers, and to a lesser extent consumer insensitivity and judgment error. While it would seem that such differences represent brand loyalty and related factors, such a view would be overly simplistic. These preference differences represent a more complex challenge. Can one formulate a product that will please more consumers, especially those with different preferences and thus increase market share and profitability? Is more than one product necessary to satisfy the expectations of these consumers? Contemporary consumer research provides insights and answers to these questions which are described here.

Products

A simple two product test is very useful for identifying preference differences but it is not very helpful in establishing a relationship among sensory, analytical and preference measures or accounting for preference differences. Such relationships are best developed from multiproduct tests. Typically 15 or more products selected to represent a broad range of sensory, analytical, and preference differences are tested. The focus is on the range of variables represented by the different products, rather than the individual products. A limited amount of product similarity is desirable for estimating statistical reliability; however, too many can limit finding preference groups in that product category. Product sets typically include important competitive and experimental products, and may include products from other markets; e.g., those marketed in other countries. The latter are selected to fill sensory gaps not covered by the other products.

Consumers

A minimum of about 120 is typically recommended for finding reliable preference groups. This number can be increased to accommodate quota groups representing demographic and user groups of interest. For example, a reliable cell size for three age groups (minimum of 50 each) in each of two cities would require 300 consumers. Studies that include multiple cities and countries easily can exceed 500 consumers. The actual number of consumers tested should reflect the experience of the researcher, taking into account the extent of product variability, the precision of the measuring system, and the specific recruiting criteria. Some companies may have established minimum numbers that are acceptable. In any case, using fewer than about 75 responses for a group of potential interest can impact the usefulness of any subsequent models that are developed. Consumer qualification typically focuses on brands purchased, frequency of purchase, and specific user demographics. The importance of recruiting qualified consumers cannot be emphasized enough. The key to this component of the process is reflected in the subsequent product opportunities that are identified. General population groups are rarely used because they include too many market segments of little interest to the manufacturer.

Scorecard

The consumer scorecard we use consists of a 9-point hedonic question for overall opinion; however, other reliable acceptance measures may be used. Additional usage and attitude questions may be included, depending on the test objective.

Test Procedure

Typically, each consumer evaluates all the products, which requires their participation for as few as 2 to as many as 5 consecutive days. Consumers evaluate a set of four to six products following a monadic sequential presentation order, with a 1 to 3 min rest interval between evaluations. Following a 10 to 20 min rest break, a second set of four to six products are evaluated. This procedure is continued on subsequent days until all products are evaluated. The procedure assures that all consumers experience the full sensory context embodied in the entire product set. Although incomplete block designs can be used, they introduce risk by providing consumers with different sensory contexts.

Data Analysis

A variety of univariate and multivariate analyses are used for this research. Analysis of variance and multiple range tests identify significant product differences, and cluster analysis is used to identify different consumer preference groups. The analysis of variance and multiple range tests are reasonably uncomplicated statistical techniques, requiring little or no intervention by the analyst, whereas cluster analysis requires more from the analyst. Various numbers of clusters are examined, with different "seeds" and "stricts". The analyst decides if there are clusters, when the clusters are stable, and if they provide useful information. Not all analysts are equally skilled at extracting maximal information from cluster analysis. Some analysts may require as few as three to four cluster analyses to develop the skills necessary for accurate clustering, others may require substantially more training. SAS FASTCLUS (SAS Institute Inc. 1990) was used to derive the following results.

RESULTS

The results described herein were obtained from a larger optimization effort considering several product categories. They typically reveal that consumers are not homogeneous in their product preferences.

Product - Flavored Light Alcohol Beverage

This particular product category has very broad appeal and in one sense, it is a market that can be easily entered. It also means that it is difficult to encourage the consumer to sample your product from among the many available, and, once sampled, convince that consumer to continue to use your brand. Knowledge about consumer preferences and the sensory characteristics that have the most influence become very important, especially if those consumers exhibit different preferences. This particular test was fielded in an Asian country; however, the results are not unique to that location.

Two-hundred consumers, qualified as likers and users of products in this beverage category, were recruited to a central location test site. An array of 12 competitive and experimental products were evaluated on three consecutive days. A trained QDA® panel also evaluated the products. Of specific interest to this discussion are the cluster analysis and the preference-attribute correlations. A three cluster solution was obtained from the consumer preference scores. There were 69 consumers each in clusters 1 and 2, and 57 consumers in cluster 3. The preference ratings for the three clusters are provided in Fig. 1, along with the correlation of preference scores for the three groups. Groups 1 and 2 had high negative correlations (r = -0.72) with one another. The four best liked products for Group 1 were the four least liked by Group 2, and the least liked product for Group 1 was among the best liked by Group 2. Group 3 had a low correlation with the two other groups (r = -0.03 and r = -0.25, respectively).

The individual sensory attributes listed in Table 1 correlated well (r = ±0.50 and higher) with the preference scores for the different cluster groups. Ten of them had values that exceeded ± 0.76. Group 1 preferred products that had a clear appearance and were low in color; i.e., more pale and not dark, and were low in intensity for most taste and aftertaste attributes except for fruit and sweet flavor. The direction for many of the preferred attributes for Group 2 was opposite to that for Group 1. Group 2 preferred products that were high in color; i.e., brighter, had a less clear appearance, and also were strong for most taste and aftertaste attributes, except for sour, fruit, and, sweet taste. Group 3 preferences were not easily defined; these consumers preferred products

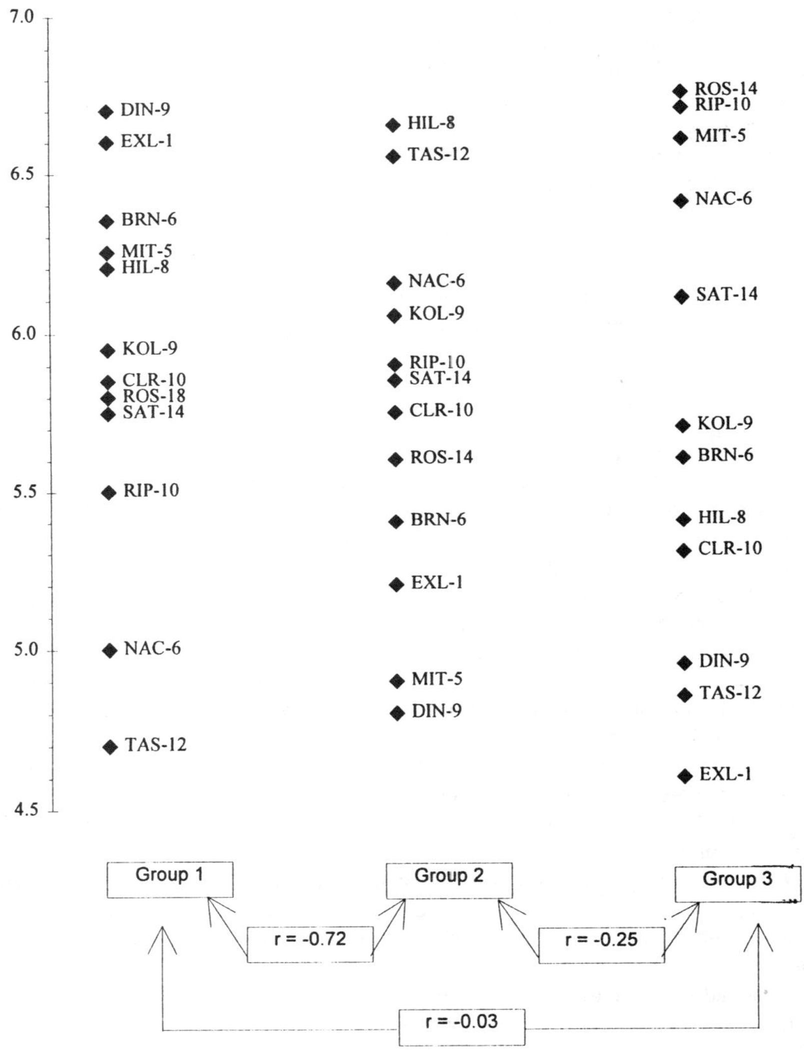

FIG. 1. CLUSTER GROUP ACCEPTANCE MEANS FOR FLAVORED LIGHT ALCOHOL BEVERAGE

TABLE 1.
SENSORY ATTRIBUTES MOST HIGHLY CORRELATED WITH CONSUMER PREFERENCES FOR A FLAVORED LIGHT ALCOHOL BEVERAGE

Attribute	Group 1 (N = 69) "Low Strength"	Group 2 (N = 69) "High Strength"	Group 3 (N = 57) "Diverse"
Color	- - -	+ + +	0
Clarity	+ + +	- - -	0
Brightness	0	0	+ +
Sweet Aroma	0	- -	- -
Overall Taste	- - -	+ ++	0
Bitter Taste	- - -	+ + +	0
Harsh Taste	- - -	+ + +	0
Sour Taste	- -	0	0
Sweet Taste	+ +	- - -	0
Fruit Taste	+ +	- - -	0
Alcohol Taste	- - -	+ +	0
Burnt Taste	- - -	+ +	0
Lingering Aftertaste	- - -	+ + +	0

Correlation Code	Negative	Positive
.00 to .25	0	0
.26 to .50	-	+
.51 to .75	- -	+ +
.76 to .99	- - -	+ + +

that were bright and sparkling (represented by Groups 1 and 2). The results suggest that further clustering may be possible, that these consumers liked many products or had not reached a definite choice. The preference map shown in Fig. 2 integrates the cluster, preference, and driver attribute information. Diverse preferences may explain why some categories readily support products representing a broad range of sensory differences.

DISCUSSION

Information about consumer preference groups, their likes and dislikes, and the attributes important to them allow food manufacturers to make informed decisions about which sensory characteristics will improve acceptance. Companies need to use different development strategies, depending on the types of cluster groups in the category. For opposite cluster types (e.g., high strength vs. low strength) the manufacturer may want to optimize for the two product styles. A diverse cluster preferring sweet, fruity, and value added characteristics offer opportunities for many alternative products that are optimized for one or more of those characteristics. Alternatively, a compromise strategy is possible for the manufacturer interested in offering only one product for a category.

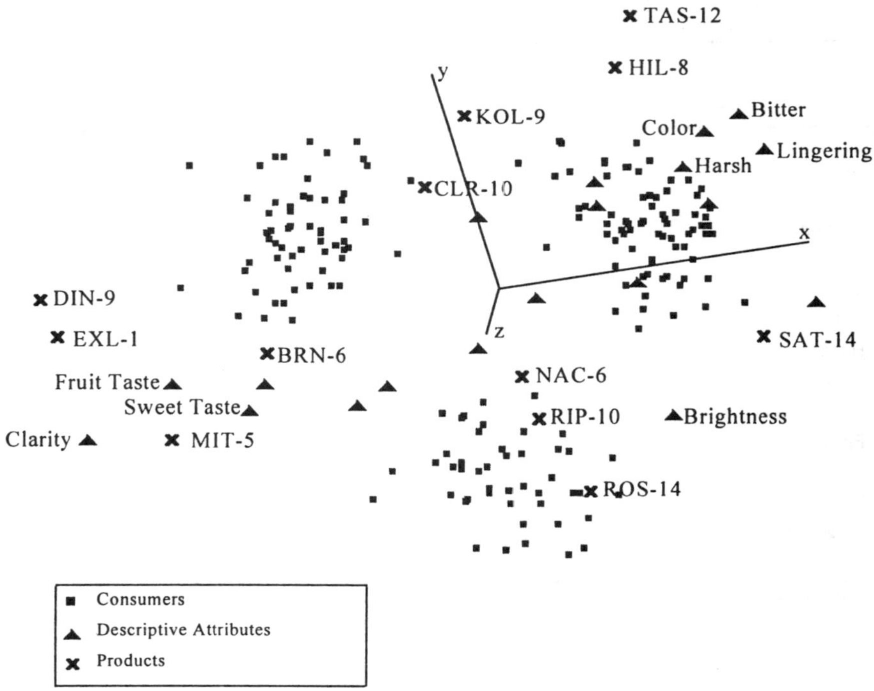

FIG. 2. PREFERENCE MAP FOR FLAVORED LIGHT ALCOHOL BEVERAGE

Once the likes and dislikes of the diverse groups are understood, product development can focus on optimizing attributes that are liked and minimizing disliked attributes. For example, if one cluster prefers a buttery characteristic and is neutral to sweet, and another cluster prefers sweet and is neutral to buttery, it is reasonable to develop a product appealing to both groups that is sweet and buttery. A compromise strategy is most likely to succeed in product categories that do not contain significant numbers of consumers with opposite style preferences.

THE MARKETING CHALLENGE

This discussion focused on the successful use of a technology for determining the presence of consumer preference groups, and for identifying product characteristics that appeal most to those groups. Preference information has significant value to product development, but a well liked product is no guarantee of market success. More information is needed about the consumers in the preference groups, and the estimated sizes of the groups to develop a successful marketing strategy (assuming the business plan can accommodate it).

Consumer Cluster Profile

Traditional consumer profiles are specified in demographic terms, such as age, sex, and income. For the majority of our preference group research, there is little or no correlation between traditional demographics and membership in a specific cluster group. Other variables are needed to describe and classify members of a cluster group. We customarily include a large array of lifestyle, usage, and behavioral questions in cluster research. Once stable clusters are identified, discriminant analysis of those responses is used along with the demographic information to develop a behavioral profile of those consumers. The resulting discriminant function usually will correctly classify 75 to 90% or more of the cluster group members. This questionnaire provides a comprehensive profile of the consumer that can be subsequently used to screen for consumers that belong to a specific cluster group.

Cluster Group Size and Product Volume Projection

It also is necessary to assess the stability of a cluster and, for volume projections, to determine the relative size of that cluster in the population of concept acceptors and potential purchasers. This is more easily determined when clustering is a regular part of a category tracking system. Otherwise, cluster size reliability estimates have to be done during follow-up product development tests. The percentage of each cluster of the total consumer group can give a first estimate of their relative size in the population.

Cluster groups are of interest to food manufacturers only to the degree that those consumers represent a viable business opportunity. Potential market size depends on many factors including the number of consumers that prefer a product's sensory characteristics and marketing's success at persuading those consumers to try the product. Cluster information is important for selecting and testing with the appropriate consumer, and for assessing what information most likely will result in product trial. As illustrated below, consumers may not know what it is they like about a product.

In subsequent research on the clusters reported in this study we found that not all cluster groups are aware, or will believe, that they prefer products they scored best when not branded. When asked which brands and attributes they prefer for this category, Cluster 1 consumers in the light alcohol study describe attributes and products more closely associated with Cluster 2 preferences than with their own. The preferred product imagery for Cluster 1 consumers communicates a strong flavor experience while the preferred product delivers a less strong flavor experience. Accurate volume predictions will account for the combination of imagery and sensory experience most desired by the consumer.

CONCLUSION

Results from the sensory testing paradigm described in this research offers evidence that consumer preference for foods is diverse rather than homogeneous, and that preference groups are not readily defined by traditional demographic segmentation. There are recurring preference patterns observed across the different consumer groups, and they cover a broad range of products, regions, and cultures. Future research will need to focus on how behavioral factors such as lifestyle and attitudes shape sensory experiences, and how those factors interact with physiological factors to shape consumer preference. The sensory measurement tools and statistical analysis methods for determining the presence of cluster groups is available. They provide business opportunities as well as raise important issues about the value of aggregate data. Consumer preference groups are found for the majority of food categories. Successful business strategies will fully exploit how best to use this powerful consumer information.

REFERENCES

ANONYMOUS. 1989. SAS/STAT® User's Guide, Version 6, 4th Edn., Volume 1, SAS Institute Inc., Cary, NC. pp. 823–849.

GREENHOFF, K. and MACFIE, H.J.H. 1994. Preference mapping in practice. *In* Measurement of Food Preferences, (H.J.H. MacFie and D.M.H. Thompson, eds.), Blackie, Academic and Professional, pp. 137–166.

PANGBORN, R. 1981. Individuality in responses to sensory stimuli. *In*: Criteria of Food Acceptance. How Man Chooses What He Eats. (J. Solms and R.L. Hall, eds.) Forster Verlag AG, Zurich.

SCHUTZ, H.G., DAMRELL, J.K. and LOCKE, B.H. 1972. Predicting hedonic ratings of raw carrot texture by sensory analysis. J. Texture Studies *3*, 227–232

SIDEL, J.L., STONE, H. and THOMAS, H.A. 1994. Hitting the target: Sensory and product optimization. Cereal Foods World *39*, 826–830.

STONE, H. and SIDEL, J.L. 1981. Quantitative descriptive analysis in optimization of consumer acceptance. Presented at: Eastern Food Science and Technology Conference on *Strategies of Food Product Development*. IFT, Lancaster, PA. Unpublished.

STONE, H. and SIDEL, J.L. 1993. Sensory Evaluation Practices, 2nd edn. Academic Press, San Diego, CA.

NEUROBIOLOGY AND PSYCHOPHYSICS OF ORAL IRRITATION

E. CARSTENS

Section of Neurobiology, Physiology & Behavior
University of California, Davis
Davis, CA 95616

ABSTRACT

A variety of naturally-occurring chemicals such as capsaicin in red chili, or nicotine in tobacco, irritate mucous membranes. To study trigeminal mechanisms of oral irritation, we have used both psychophysical methods in humans, and electrophysiological methods in anesthetized animals, to investigate sensations and responses of trigeminal neurons elicited by application of a variety of irritant chemicals to the oral cavity.

In the psychophysical studies, subjects used a visual analog scale to rate the intensity of irritant sensations elicited by repeated application of capsaicin (0.5-5 ppm) or nicotine (0.1%) to one side of the dorsal tongue. The magnitude of irritation increased with repeated capsaicin (sensitization), but decreased with repeated nicotine. After a rest period, the side pretreated with capsaicin was less sensitive to further capsaicin or nicotine, while the side pretreated with nicotine was less sensitive to nicotine but not capsaicin, indicating an asymmetric cross-desensitization effect. The cholinergic antagonist, mecamylamine, reduced irritation from nicotine but not capsaicin, indicating involvement of peripheral neuronal nicotinic receptors in nicotine-evoked irritation. We are also examining interactions among other irritant chemicals such as NaCl and citric acid.

Electrophysiology experiments were conducted using thiopental-anesthetized rats. Nearly all neurons recorded in the superficial layers of the dorsomedial trigeminal subnucleus caudalis responded to epilingual application of at least one irritant chemical, and many neurons responded to all nine chemicals tested (histamine, nicotine, capsaicin, piperine, mustard oil, serotonin, acidified phosphate buffer, NaCl and ethanol). The neuronal population responded to 75% of tested chemicals. The response incidence was independent of the order of chemicals tested, except for capsaicin which desensitized subsequent responses. Onset and duration of averaged responses were longest for capsaicin, piperine and mustard oil. Responses significantly increased in a dose-related manner for histamine (9×10^{-1} to 1×10^{-4} M), nicotine (6×10^{-1} to 1×10^{-4} M), NaCl (0.5-5 M), ethanol (15-50%), and pH 4-1. Successive responses to repeated application decreased significantly for nicotine, NaCl, serotonin, capsaicin and piperine. Spontaneous firing increased significantly 5-10 min after capsaicin, consistent with its prolonged irritant sensation. Responses to histamine and nicotine were pharmacologically antagonized, indicating the involvement of separate receptor mechanisms

These data support the idea of a common chemical sense ("chemesthesis"), whereby different irritant chemicals activate a common population of trigeminal sensory neurons, presumably via independent peripheral transduction mechanisms.

INTRODUCTION

Irritation is a commonly used but poorly defined term for an unpleasant sensation, soreness or inflammation that is not necessarily painful. Upon exposure to the skin or mucous membranes, chemicals in a variety of consumer products evoke an irritant sensation yet are nonetheless sought after. Examples are capsaicin from red chili peppers, piperine in black pepper, nicotine in tobacco, and ethanol in drinks and cosmetics. Chemically-evoked irritation is often reported to have qualities of warmth, burning, pricking, stinging, tingling and/or numbness (e.g., Cliff and Heymann 1992). Presently it is uncertain whether qualitative differences in irritation evoked by various chemicals can be reliably discriminated, or if there is a unitary "common chemical sense" (Parker 1912). Furthermore, there is incomplete information regarding the sensory receptors innervating mucous membranes that convey irritation, and very little information regarding the processing of irritation by the central nervous system. The major aims of this paper are to discuss recent psychophysical studies on the oral sensory effects and interactions of irritant chemicals, and to review the underlying neural mechanisms of irritation emphasizing studies from our laboratory on the trigeminal system.

PSYCHOPHYSICAL STUDIES OF ORAL IRRITATION

A variety of chemicals elicit oral and cutaneous irritation or pain (reviewed in Green *et al.* 1990; Green and Lawless 1991), including capsaicin (Green 1989, 1991; Karrer and Bartoshuk 1991), piperine (Lawless and Stevens 1990), nicotine (Jarvik and Assil 1988), NaCl (Green and Gelhard 1989), citric acid (Gilmore and Green 1993), zingerone (Green 1993; Prescott and Stevenson 1996a,b), menthol (Cliff and Green 1994, 1996; Gwartney and Heymann 1995), methyl salicylate (Green and Flammer 1989), camphor (Green 1990), ethanol (Green 1988), cinnamic aldehyde (Green 1991) and CO_2 (Yau and McDaniel 1990, 1991; Green 1992). Sensations from some of these irritants (capsaicin, NaCl, citric acid, cinnamic aldehyde, menthol) are cross-desensitized by capsaicin (Green 1991; Geppetti *et al.* 1993; Gilmore and Green 1993; Cliff and Green 1996; Green 1996), suggesting that the irritation is triggered by activating a common population of capsaicin-sensitive sensory nerve fibers.

The best-studied chemical irritant is capsaicin, which elicits an intraoral burning sensation that increases in magnitude across trials of sequential stimulation at short intervals (sensitization), with a marked decrease in sensory magnitude (self-desensitization) when re-applied after a 5-15 min waiting period (Green 1989, 1991; Karrer and Bartoshuk 1991). Interestingly, when capsaicin is recurrently applied following self-desensitization, the magnitude of irritation increases again suggesting that capsaicin's irritant action overcomes the self-desensitization (Green 1996).

We were interested in testing if nicotine, the irritant in tobacco smoke, has sensory effects like those of capsaicin (Dessirier *et al.* 1997). Using a sequential stimulation paradigm similar to that of Green (1989), we verified the sensitizing effect of capsaicin (Fig. 1). In contrast, nicotine evoked irritation that decreased in magnitude across trials (Fig. 1). A similar decline in sequential ratings of oral irritation was recently reported for menthol (Cliff and Green 1994, 1996) and zingerone (Prescott and Stevenson 1996b), while sensitization occurs with sequential application of 0.8 M NaCl (Green and Gelhart

1989). Conceivably, sensitization and desensitization may reflect different mechanisms by which irritants excite chemosensitive nociceptors.

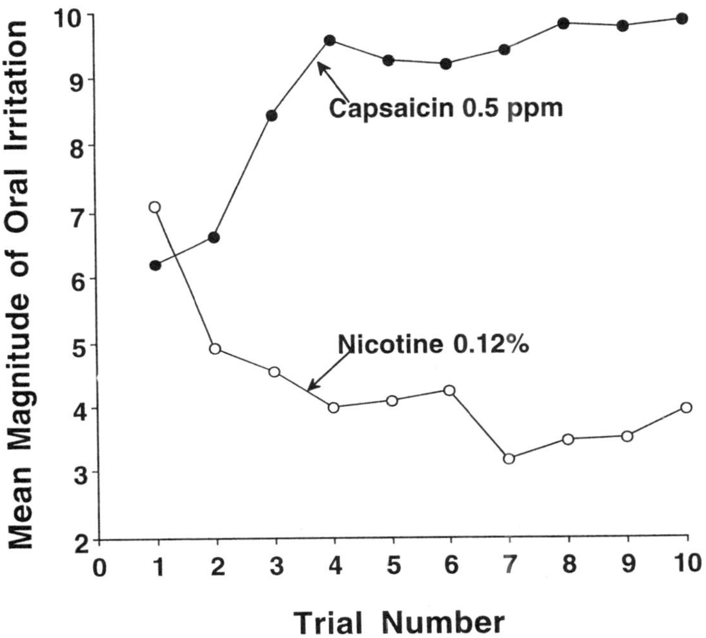

FIG. 1. DIFFERENTIAL RESPONSES TO REPEATED APPLICATION OF NICOTINE VS. CAPSAICIN

Graph plots mean ratings of the intensity of irritation for each of 10 sequential applications of 0.12% nicotine or 0.5 ppm capsaicin, applied by filter paper in 35 μl volumes. Subjects rated irritation using a visual analog scale with endpoints "no sensation" and "most intense irritation imaginable". Ratings were taken 25 sec following chemical application. See Dessirier *et al.* 1997, for details. Reproduced with permission of Oxford University Press.

We also developed a 2-alternative forced-choice paradigm to test for cross-desensitization by sequentially stimulating one side of the tongue with capsaicin or nicotine, and after a rest period applying one or the other chemical bilaterally and asking subjects to choose which side of the tongue gave rise to a stronger sensation. We observed self-desensitization for both capsaicin and nicotine, and a non-reciprocal cross-desensitization of capsaicin to nicotine but not vice versa. The nicotinic antagonist, mecamylamine, prevents irritation from nicotine (Jarvik and Assil 1988) but not capsaicin (J.-M. Dessirier, M. O'Mahony and E. Carstens, unpublished observations). These results suggest that capsaicin and nicotine may both act on a common population of intraoral chemosensitive nociceptors that express both capsaicin ("vanilloid") receptors and neuronal nicotinic cholinergic receptors in the terminal membrane. This idea receives support from recent electrophysiological studies showing that a subset of trigeminal ganglion neurons is depolarized by both chemicals (Liu and Simon 1996a). The ability of capsaicin to cross-desensitize to nicotine and other irritants may involve its binding to the capsaicin receptor (Szallasi 1994) to open cation channels, allowing an influx of Ca^{2+} to initiate intracellular events leading to a generalized decrease in the excitability of the nociceptor membrane (Cholewinski *et al.* 1993; Chard *et al.* 1995; Liu and Simon 1996b). The self-desensitization observed psychophysically with nicotine might reflect a direct pharmacological desensitization of the neuronal nicotinic receptors (Ochoa *et al.* 1990), which would not cross-desensitize to other non-cholinergic irritants.

NEUROBIOLOGY OF ORAL IRRITATION

Overview of Trigeminal System

Chemical irritants in the oral cavity excite chemosensitive polymodal nociceptors whose free endings are located in the mucosal epithelium and lamina propria (Holland 1984). Primary afferent fibers of nociceptors travel in the lingual nerve, via the mandibular division of the trigeminal nerve, to terminate in brain stem trigeminal subnuclei caudalis, interpolaris and oralis (Torvik 1956; Hamilton and Norgren 1984; reviewed in Norgren 1984; Schults 1992). Nociceptive inputs terminate largely in nucleus caudalis, where they synapse onto second-order neurons which represent the face and oral cavity in a somatotopically organized manner (e.g., Kruger and Michel 1962; Darian-Smith *et al.* 1963; Nord 1968; Rowe and Sessle 1972; Mosso and Kruger 1973; Yokota 1975; Price *et al.* 1976; Dostrovsky and Hellon 1978; Yokota and Nishikawa 1977, 1980; Hu *et al.* 1981; Amano *et al.* 1986; Hu 1990; Anton *et al.* 1992; Strassman and Vos 1993; Bereiter *et al.* 1994; McHaffie *et al.* 1994; Coimbra and Coimbra 1994; Mineta *et al.* 1995; reviewed in Schults 1992). Neurons in the interstitial (paratrigeminal) nucleus, like those in caudalis, are also somatotopically arranged and respond to noxious stimuli (see Schults 1992). A population of neurons in subnucleus oralis also responds to noxious facial stimuli (Dallel *et al.* 1990; Raboisson *et al.* 1991). Nociceptive neurons in caudalis, oralis and paratrigeminal nuclei are thus well suited to transmit information on oro-facial pain.

Lingual Nociceptors

Electrophysiological studies have shown that single lingual nerve afferents respond to chemical stimuli including various salts, menthol, ethanol, CO_2, nicotine, organic acids, and less frequently capsaicin (Hellekant 1965; Kawamura and Adachi 1967; Okuni 1978; Sostman and Simon 1991; Komai and Bryant 1993; Wang *et al.* 1993; Lundy and Contreras 1994; Brand and Bryant 1994; Bryant and Moore 1995). Lingual C-fiber afferents may exhibit a degree of chemoselectivity, since most responded to different salt solutions but few of them responded to nicotine and none to capsaicin (Wang *et al.* 1993). Recent patch-clamp studies have shown that a subset of trigeminal ganglion neurons are depolarized by both capsaicin and nicotine (Liu and Simon 1996a; see above), by capsaicin and acid (Garcia-Hirschfeld *et al.* 1995), and by capsaicin, piperine and zingerone in a manner that is blocked by the capsaicin antagonist, capsazepine (Liu and Simon 1996c). Thus, some trigeminal receptors appear capable of responding to multiple irritant chemicals.

Trigeminal Nucleus Caudalis

The chemical sensitivity of central trigeminal neurons will reflect that of the synaptic inputs they receive from lingual afferent fibers. There are relatively few studies of central trigeminal neuronal responses to irritant chemicals in general (Mosso and Kruger 1973; Amano *et al.* 1986; Raboisson *et al.* 1991, 1995; Hu *et al.* 1992; Peppel and Anton 1993; Yu *et al.* 1993; Meng *et al.* 1997), and none on irritant chemical stimulation of the lingual epithelium. We therefore initiated anatomical and electrophysiological studies to address whether individual trigeminal neurons can respond to different classes of irritants applied to the tongue.

Anatomical c-Fos Studies. To determine the location within the trigeminal complex of neurons that are activated by irritants on the tongue, we employed the method of c-fos immunohistochemistry (Carstens *et al.* 1995). This method capitalizes on the observation that central neurons that are directly excited by noxious stimuli express the nuclear immediate-early gene, c-fos (Zimmermann and Herdegen 1994). Epilingual application of nicotine, capsaicin, piperine or histamine each produced a similar distribution of c-fos-immunoreactive cell nuclei in the superficial layers of the dorsomedial trigeminal nucleus caudalis bilaterally (Fig. 2), as well as in other brain stem areas including the area postrema, nucleus of the solitary tract, and paratrigeminal nuclei. The dorsomedial caudalis area is particularly interesting since the tongue is represented here, making this area a likely relay in the trigeminal pathway for irritation from the tongue.

Electrophysiological Studies. A drawback of the c-fos method is that it provides a "snapshot" in time of the distribution of all neurons activated by one particular chemical stimulus, but cannot determine if one and the same neuron is activated by different chemicals, or if there are separate populations of "chemospecific" neurons grouped near one another with each responding only to one chemical. For this reason, we performed electrophysiological experiments to determine if single neurons in this region of trigeminal caudalis can respond to application of a spectrum of irritant chemicals applied to the dorsal surface of the tongue (Carstens *et al.* 1997).

Extracellular recordings were made from single neurons located in the superficial layers of dorsomedial caudalis of barbiturate-anesthetized rats. All neurons responded to mechanical and noxious thermal ($>48°C$) stimulation of the ipsilateral tongue, as well as to application of one or more of a panel of irritant chemicals (histamine, nicotine, capsaicin, piperine, mustard oil, serotonin (5-HT), acidified phosphate buffer at pH 6 to 1, NaCl and ethanol). A typical example is shown in Fig. 3. Each row shows peristimulus-time histograms (PSTHs) of responses to a given chemical. The bottom row shows, from left to right, responses to physical stimuli, piperine and carbonated water. Most importantly, this neuron gave responses of similar magnitude to each chemical tested (middle column of PSTHs). Responses increased in a dose-related manner (1st 3 PSTHs in rows 1-7). Successive responses to repeated applications of 5-HT, nicotine, capsaicin and mustard oil decreased markedly across trials (rows 1, 4, 7 and 8), while successive responses to the other chemicals decreased less or not at all. The neuron's

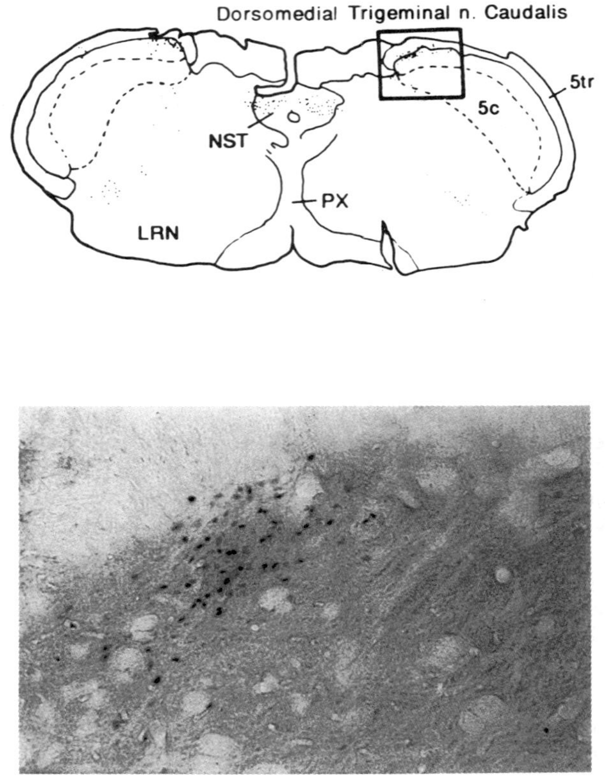

FIG. 2. DISTRIBUTION OF C-FOS-IMMUNOREACTIVE NEURONS IN DORSOMEDIAL TRIGEMINAL NUCLEUS CAUDALIS

Top drawing is a cross-section through the rat caudal brainstem. Dashes indicate loci of cell nuclei immunopositive for c-fos 2 hr following epilingual application of 0.5% nicotine. The box indicates the region that is shown in the photomicrograph below of immunopositive nuclei (black) in dorsomedial caudalis. A similar distribution of immunoreactivity was also seen after epilingual application of other irritants (capsaicin, piperine, histamine). See Carstens *et al.* 1995, for experimental details. Abbreviations: 5c, trigeminal nucleus caudalis; 5tr, spinal tract of trigeminal nerve; LRN, lateral reticular nucleus; NST, nucleus of the solitary tract; PX, pyramidal decussation.

receptive field was on the ipsilateral anterior tongue and chin (Fig. 2, inset figurine), and the recording site was in dorsomedial caudalis (lower right drawing in Fig. 2). This neuron is representative of the population of 32 neurons, which responded to 75% of all tested chemicals (up to 10 per neuron). Responses significantly increased in a dose-related manner for histamine ($9x10^{-1}$ to 10^{-4} M), nicotine ($6x10^{-1}$ to 10^{-4} M), NaCl (0.5-5 M), ethanol (15 to 50%), and acid at pHs 4 to 1 (Fig. 3). Successive responses to

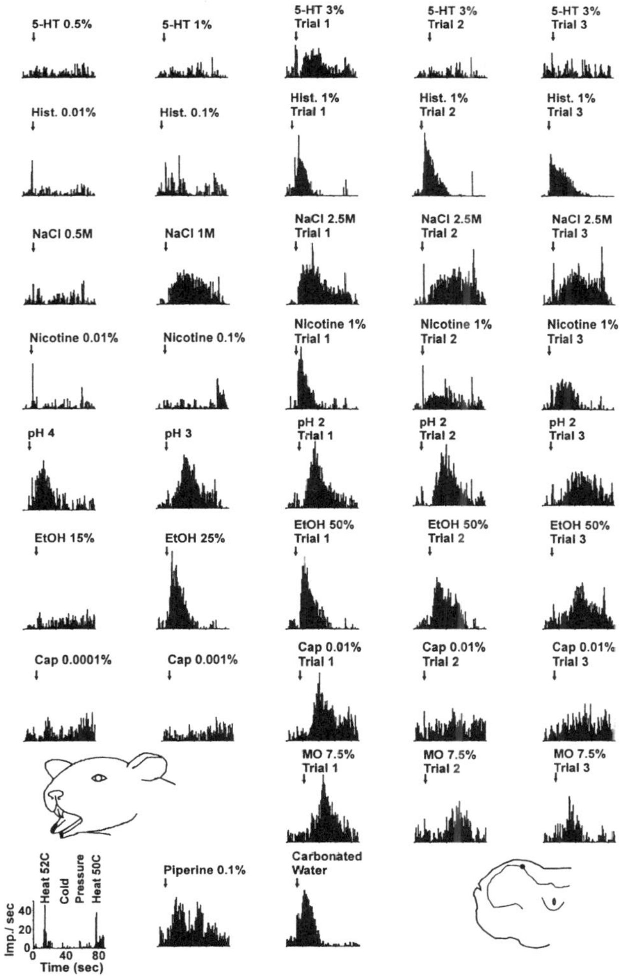

FIG. 3. EXAMPLE OF RESPONSES OF INDIVIDUAL TRIGEMINAL NEURON TO DIFFERENT CHEMICALS

Each row of peristimulus-time histograms (PSTHs; bin width: 1 sec) shows responses to application of one chemical. Stimuli (0.1 ml) were delivered topically to the dorsal tongue and left on for 60 sec, followed by rinse with 0.9% saline. The first 7 rows show, from left to right, responses to increasing doses (1st 3 PSTHs) and to repeated application at one dose (last 3 PSTHs). Row 8 shows responses to repeated mustard oil (MO), and the bottom row shows responses to physical stimuli (left PSTH), piperine (middle PSTH) and carbonated water (right PSTH). Abbreviations: Hist = histamine; pH = acidified phosphate buffer at indicated pH value; EtOH = ethanol (50%), cap = capsaicin; MO = mustard oil. Lower left inset drawing shows receptive field (solid) on ipsilateral tongue and chin. Lower right inset shows recording site (dot) on drawing of brain stem section.

repeated application decreased significantly for nicotine, NaCl, 5-HT, capsaicin and piperine. Responses to histamine and nicotine were selectively reduced by ceterizine (H1 antagonist) and mecamylamine, respectively, indicating that distinct receptor mechanisms mediate responses to these two irritants. An interesting observation was that neurons' spontaneous firing rates (in the absence of stimulation) significantly increased 5-10 min following an initial suprathreshold application of capsaicin, commensurate with its prolonged irritant sensation in the mouth. Furthermore, the firing rate waxed and waned similar to variations in perceived intensity of capsaicin irritation. Finally, following capsaicin the neurons were usually unresponsive to subsequent application of irritant chemicals, indicative of cross-desensitization.

The results indicate that individual nociceptive trigeminal neurons are typically activated by many different irritant chemicals. The data therefore support the notion of a common chemesthetic sense, since different types of irritant chemicals evoke a similar discharge in a population of trigeminal neurons. Nonetheless, it is conceivable that humans have at least a crude ability to discriminate among different irritants. For example, discrimination between irritation from acids and salts might be aided by concomitant gustatory (sour or salty) sensations, although the way the central nervous system integrates taste and trigeminal information for flavor discrimination is not known. The tasteless chemicals capsaicin and piperine are reported to elicit qualitatively different sensations of stinging, biting and piercing vs. itching (Lawless and Stevens 1990). Histamine evokes a "pungent burning" or horseradish -like sensation (Heubner 1925) or pricking sensation (author's unpublished observation) that appears to be subjectively distinct from the burning sensation elicited by capsaicin on the tongue. A potential means of discrimination might be that individual trigeminal neurons respond preferentially at a higher frequency to one chemical, while responding at a lower frequency to other irritant chemicals. The nervous system could discriminate between different irritants by comparing inputs from a population of such preferentially-responsive neurons (across-fiber population coding), analogous to neural mechanisms proposed for taste coding (e.g., Norgren 1984; Scott and Plata-Salaman 1991). It is also possible that chemospecific trigeminal neurons exist, so that discrimination is accomplished using both a specificity code and across-fiber comparison. More studies are needed to determine if there are sub-populations of trigeminal neurons with degrees of chemoselectivity, in addition to those that respond indicriminately to a wide variety of irritant chemicals.

ACKNOWLEDGMENTS

The studies reported in this paper were supported by a grant from the California Tobacco Disease-Related Research Program, #4IT-0087 and by a Fulbright senior research award.

REFERENCES

AMANO, N., HU, J.W. and SESSLE, B.J. 1986. Responses of neurons in feline trigeminal subnucleus caudalis (medullary dorsal horn) to cutaneous, intraoral and muscle afferent stimuli. J. Neurophysiol. *55*, 227–243.

ANTON, F., HERDEGEN, T., PEPPEL, P. and LEAH, J.D. 1992. C-Fos-like immunoreactivity in rat brainstem neurons following noxious chemical stimulation of the nasal mucosa. Neurosci. *41*, 629–641.

BEREITER, D.A., HATHAWAY, C.B. and BENETTI, A.P. 1994. Caudal portions of the spinal trigeminal complex are necessary for autonomic responses and display Fos-like immunoreactivity after corneal stimulation in the cat. Brain Res. *657*, 73–82.

BRAND, J.G. and BRYANT, B.P. 1994. Receptor mechanisms for flavour stimuli. Food Qual. Pref. *5*, 31–40.

BRYANT, B.P. and MOORE, P.A. 1995. Factors affecting the sensitivity of the lingual trigeminal nerve to acids. Am. J. Physiol. *268*, R58–0R65.

CARSTENS, E., KUENZLER, N. and HANDWERKER, H.O. 1997. Activation of neurons in superficial layers of dorsomedial trigeminal subnucleus caudalis by application of a wide spectrum of irritant chemicals to the rat tongue. Submitted.

CARSTENS, E., SAXE, I. and RALPH, R. 1995. Brainstem neurons expressing c-fos immunoreactivity following irritant chemical stimulation of the rat's tongue. Neurosci. *69*, 939–953.

CHARD, P.S., BLEAKMAN, D., SAVIDGE, J.R. and MILLER, R.J. 1995. Capsaicin-induced neurotoxicity in cultured dorsal root ganglion neurons: involvement of calcium-activated proteases. Neurosci. *65*, 1099–1108.

CHOLEWINSKI, A., BURGESS, G.M. and BEVAN, S. 1993. The role of calcium in capsaicin-induced desensitization in rat cultured dorsal root ganglion neurons. Neurosci. *55*, 1015–1023.

CLIFF, M.A. and GREEN, B.G. 1994. Sensory irritation and coolness produced by menthol: evidence for selective desensitization of irritation. Physiol. Behav. *56*, 1021–1029.

CLIFF, M.A. and GREEN, B.G. 1996. Sensitization and desensitization to capsaicin and menthol in the oral cavity - interactions and individual differences. Physiol. Behav. *59*, 487-494.

CLIFF, M. and HEYMANN, H. 1992. Descriptive analysis of oral pungency. J. Sens. Stud. *7*, 279–290.

COIMBRA, F. and COIMBRA, A. 1994. Dental noxious input reaches the subnucleus caudalis of the trigeminal complex in the rat, as shown by c-fos expression upon thermal or mechanical stimulation. Neurosci. Lett. *173*, 201–204.

DALLEL, R., RABOISSON, P., WODA, A. and SESSLE, B.J. 1990. Properties of nociceptive and non-nociceptive neurons in trigeminal subnucleus oralis of the rat. Brain Res. *521*, 95–106.

DARIAN-SMITH, I., PROCTOR, R. and RYAN, R.D. 1963. A single-neurone investigation of somatotopic organization within the cat's trigeminal brain-stem nuclei. J. Physiol. *168*, 147–157.

DESSIRIER, J.-M., O'MAHONY, M. and CARSTENS, E. 1997. Oral irritant effects of nicotine: psychophysical evidence for decreased sensation following repeated application and lack of cross-desensitization to capsaicin. Chem. Sens. (in press).

DOSTROVSKY, J.O. and HELLON, R.F. 1978. The representation of facial temperature in the caudal trigeminal nucleus of the cat. J. Physiol. *277*, 29–47.

GARCIA-HIRSCHFELD, J., LOOPEZ-BRIONES, L.G., BELMONTE, C. and VALDEOLMILLOS, M. 1995. Intracellular free calcium responses to protons and capsaicin in cultured trigeminal neurons. Neurosci. *67*, 235–243.

GEPPETTI, P., TRAMONTANA, M., DELBIANCO, E. and FUSCO, B.M. 1993. Capsaicin desensitization to the human nasal mucosa selectively reduces pain evoked by citric acid. Brit. J. Clin. Pharmacol. *35*, 178–183.

GILMORE, M.M. and GREEN, B.G. 1993. Sensory irritation and taste produced by NaCl and citric acid - effects of capsaicin desensitization. Chem. Sens. *18*, 257–272.

GREEN, B.G. 1988. Spatial and temporal factors in the perception of ethanol irritation on the tongue. Percept. Psychophys. *44*, 108–116.

GREEN, B.G. 1989. Capsaicin sensitization and desensitization on the tongue produced by brief exposures to a low concentration. Neurosci. Lett. *107*, 173–178.

GREEN, B.G. 1990. Sensory characteristics of camphor. J. Invest. Dermatol. 94, 662–666.

GREEN, B.G. 1991. Capsaicin cross-desensitization on the tongue: psychophysical evidence that oral chemical irritation is mediated by more than one sensory pathway. Chem. Sens. *16*, 675–689.

GREEN, B.G. 1992. The effects of temperature and concentration on the perceived intensity and quality of carbonation. Chem. Sens. *17*, 435–450.

GREEN, B.G. 1996. Rapid recovery from capsaicin desensitization during recurrent stimulation. Pain *68*, 245–253.

GREEN, B.G. and FLAMMER, L.J. 1989. Methyl salicylate as a cutaneous stimulus: a psychophysical analysis. Somatosens. Mot. Res. *6*, 253–274.

GREEN, B.G. and GELHARD, B. 1989. Salt as an oral irritant. Chem. Sens. *14*, 259–271.

GREEN, B.G. and LAWLESS, H.T. 1991. The psychophysics of somatosensory chemoreception in the nose and mouth. *In* Smell and Taste in Health and Disease, Getchell, T.V., Doty, R.L., Bartoshuk, L.M. and Snow, J.B. (eds.), Raven, New York, pp. 235–253.

GREEN, B.G., MASON, J.R. and KARE, M.R. 1990. Chemical Senses, Vol. 2, Irritation. Dekker, New York.

GWARTNEY, E. and HEYMANN, H. 1995. The temporal perception of menthol. J. Sens. Stud. *10*, 393–400.

HAMILTON, R.B. and NORGREN, R. 1984. Central projections of gustatory nerves in the rat. J. Comp. Neurol. *222*, 560–577.

HELLEKANT, G. 1965. The effect of ethyl alcohol on non-gustatory receptors of the tongue. Acta Physiol. Scand. *65*, 243–250.

HEUBNER, W. 1925. Zur Pharmakologie der Reizstoffe. Arch Exp. Path. Pharmak. *107*, 129–154.

HOLLAND, G.R. 1984. Innervation of oral mucosa and sensory perception. *In* The Structure and Function of Oral Mucosa, Meyer, J., Squier, C.A. and Gerson, S.J. (eds.), Pergamon, New York, pp. 195–217.

HU, J.W. 1990. Response properties of nociceptive and non-nociceptive neurons in the rat's trigeminal subnucleus caudalis (medullary dorsal horn) related to cutaneous and deep craniofacial afferent stimulation and modulation by diffuse noxious inhibitory controls. Pain *41*, 331–345.

HU, J.W., DOSTROVSKY, J.O. and SESSLE, B.J. 1981. Functional properties of neurons in cat trigeminal subnucleus caudalis (medullary dorsal horn). I. Responses to oral-facial noxious and nonnoxious stimuli and projections to thalamus and subnucleus oralis. J. Neurophysiol. *45*, 173–192.

HU, J.W., SESSLE, B.J., RABOISSON, P., DALLEL, R. and WODA, A. 1992. Stimulation of craniofacial muscle afferents induces prolonged facilitatory effects in trigeminal nociceptive brain-stem neurones. Pain *48*, 53–60.

JARVIK, M.E. and ASSIL, K.M. 1988. Mecamylamine blocks the burning sensation of nicotine on the tongue. Chem. Sens. *13*, 213–217.

KARRER, T. and BARTOSHUK, L. 1991. Capsaicin desensitization and recovery on the human tongue. Physiol. Behav. *49*, 757–764.

KAWAMURA, Y. and ADACHI, A. 1967. Electrophysiological analysis of taste effectiveness of soda water and CO_2 gas. *In* Olfaction and Taste II, Hayashi, T. (ed.) Pergamon, NY, pp. 431–437.

KOMAI, M. and BRYANT, B.P. 1993. Acetazolamide specifically inhibits lingual trigeminal nerve responses to carbon dioxide. Brain Res. *612*, 122–129.

KRUGER, L. and MICHEL, F. 1962. A single neuron analysis of buccal cavity representation in the sensory trigeminal complex of the cat. Arch. Oral Biol. *7*, 491–503.

LAWLESS, H.T. and STEVENS, D.A. 1990. Differences between and interactions of oral irritants: neurophysiological and perceptual implications. *In* Chemical Senses, Vol. 2, Irritation, Green, B.G., Mason, J.R. and Kare, M.R. (eds.), Dekker, New York, pp. 197–211.

LIU, L. and SIMON, S.A. 1996a. Capsaicin and nicotine both activate a subset of rat trigeminal ganglion neurons. Am. J. Physiol. Cell Physiol. *39*, C1807-C1814.

LIU, L. and SIMON, S.A. 1996b. Capsaicin-induced currents with distinct desensitization and Ca^{2+} dependence in rat trigeminal ganglion neurons. J. Neurophysiol. *75*, 1503–1514.

LIU, L. and SIMON, S.A. 1996c. Similarities and differences in the currents activated by capsaicin, piperine, and zingerone in rat trigeminal ganglion cells. J. Neurophysiol. *76*, 1858–1869.

MCHAFFIE, J.G., LARSON, M.A. and STEIN, B.E. 1994. Response properties of nociceptive and low-threshold neurons in rat trigeminal pars caudalis. J. Comp. Neurol. *347*, 409–425.

MENG, I.D., HU, J.W., BENETTI, A.P. and BEREITER, D.A. 1997. Encoding of corneal input in two distinct regions of the spinal trigeminal nucleus in the rat: cutaneous receptive field properties, responses to thermal and chemical stimulation, modulation by diffuse noxious inhibitory controls, and projections to the parabrachial area. J. Neurophysiol. *77*, 43–56.

MINETA, Y., EISENBERG, E. and STRASSMAN, A.M. 1995. Distribution of fos-like immunoreactivity in the caudal medullary reticular formation following noxious facial stimulation in the rat. Exp. Brain Res. *107*, 34–38.

MOSSO, J.A. and KRUGER, L. 1973. Receptor categories represented in spinal trigeminal nucleus caudalis. J. Neurophysiol. *36*, 472–488.

NORD, S.G. 1968. Receptor field characteristics of single cells in the rat spinal trigeminal complex. Exp. Neurol. *21*, 236–243.

NORGREN, R. 1984. Central neural mechanisms of taste. *In* Handbook of Physiology. Section 1. The Nervous System, Vol. III, *Sensory Processes*, Part 2, (Geiger, S.R. ed., Darian Smith I., Vol. ed.), Am. Physiol Soc., Bethesea, pp. 1087–1128.

OCHOA, E.L.M., LI, L. and MCNAMEE, M.G. 1990. Desensitization of central cholinergic mechanisms and neuroadaptation to nicotine. Mol. Neurobiol. *4*, 251–287.

OKUNI, Y. 1978. Response of lingual nerve fibres of the rat to pungent spices and irritants in pungent spices. Shika Gakuho *78*, 325–339.

PARKER, G.H. 1912. The relation of smell, taste and the common chemical sense in vertebrates. J. Acad. Natl. Sci. Ser. 2, *15*, 221–234.

PEPPEL, P. and ANTON, F. 1993. Responses of rat medullary dorsal horn neurons following intranasal noxious chemical stimulation: effects of stimulus intensity, duration and interstimulus interval. J. Neurophysiol. *70*, 2260–2275.

PRESCOTT, J. and STEVENSON, R.J. 1996a. Psychophysical responses to single and multiple presentations of the oral irritant zingerone: relationship to frequency of chili consumption. Physiol. Behav. *60*, 617–624.

PRESCOTT, J. and STEVENSON, R.J. 1996b. Desensitization to oral zingerone irritation: effects of stimulus parameters. Physiol. Behav. *60*, 1473–1480.

PRICE, D.D., DUBNER, R. and HU, J.W. 1976. Trigeminothalamic neurons in nucleus caudalis responsive to tactile, thermal and nociceptive stimulation of monkey's face. J. Neurophysiol. *39*, 936–953.

RABOISSON, P., BOURDIOL, P., DALLELL, R., CLAVELOU, P. and WODA, A. 1991. Responses of trigeminal subnucleus oralis nociceptive neurones to subcutaneous formalin in the rat. Neurosci. Lett. *125*, 179–182.

RABOISSON, P., DALLELL, R., BOURDIOL, P., CLAVELOU, P., SESSLE, B.J. and WODA, A. 1995. Effects of subcutaneous formalin on the activity of trigeminal brain stem nociceptive neurones in the rat. J. Neurophysiol. *73*, 496–505.

ROWE, M.J. and SESSLE, B.J. 1972. Responses of trigeminal ganglion and brain stem neurones in the cat to mechanical and thermal stimulation of the face. Brain Res. *42*, 367–384.

SCHULTS, R.C. 1992. Nociceptive neural organization in the trigeminal nuclei. *In* The Initial Processing of Pain and Its Descending Control: Spinal and Trigeminal Systems, Light, A.R. (ed.), Karger, New York, pp. 178–202.

SCOTT, T.R. and PLATA-SALAMAN, R. 1991. Coding of taste quality. *In* Smell and Taste in Health and Disease, Getchell, T.L. (ed.), Raven, New York, pp. 345–368.

SESSLE, B.J., HU, J.W., DUBNER, R. and LUCIER, G.E. 1981. Functional properties of neurons in cat trigeminal subnucleus caudalis (medullary dorsal horn). II. Modulation of responses to noxious and non noxious stimuli by periaqueductal gray, nucleus raphe magnus, cerebral cortex, and afferent influences, and effect of naloxone. J. Neurophysiol. *45*, 193–207.

SOSTMAN, A.L. and SIMON, S.A. 1991. Trigeminal nerve responses in the rat elicited by chemical stimulation of the tongue. Arch. Oral Biol. *36*, 95–102.

STRASSMAN, A.M. and VOS, B.P. 1993. Somatotopic and laminar organization of Fos-like immunoreactivity in the medullary and upper cervical dorsal horn induced by noxious facial stimulation in the rat. J. Comp. Neurol. *331*, 495–516.

SZALLASI, A. 1994. The vanilloid (capsaicin) receptor: receptor types and species differences. Gen. Pharmacol. *25*, 223–243.

TORVIK, A. 1956. Afferent connections to the sensory trigeminal nuclei, the nucleus of the solitary tract, and adjacent structures. J. Comp. Neurol. *106*, 51–141.

WANG, Y., ERICKSON, R.P. and SIMON, S.A. 1993. Selectivity of lingual nerve fibers to chemical stimuli. J. Gen. Physiol. *101*, 843–866.

YAU, N.J.N. and MCDANIEL, M.R. 1990. The power function of carbonation. J. Sens. Stud. *5*, 117–128.

YAU, N.J.N. and MCDANIEL, M.R. 1991. The effect of temperature on carbonation perception. Chem. Sens. *16*, 337–348.

YOKOTA, T. 1975. Excitation of units in marginal rim of trigeminal subnucleus caudalis elicited by tooth pulp stimulation. Brain Res. *95*, 154–158.

YOKOTA, T. and NISHIKAWA, N. 1977. Somatotopic organisation of trigeminal neurons within caudal medulla oblongata. *In* Pain and the Trigeminal Region, Anderson, D.J. and Matthews, B. (eds.), Amsterdam: Elsevier, pp. 243–257.

YU, X.-M., SESSLE, B.J. and HU, J.W. 1993. Differential effects of cutaneous and deep application of inflammatory irritant on mechanoreceptive field properties of trigeminal brain stem nociceptive neurons. J. Neurophysiol. *70*, 1704–1707.

ZIMMERMANN, M. and HERDEGEN, T. 1994. Control of gene transcription by Jun and Fos proteins in the nervous system: beneficial or harmful molecular mechanisms of neuronal response to noxious stimulation? Am. Pain Soc. J. *3*, 33–48.

DATA COLLECTION AND ANALYSIS METHODS FOR CONSUMER TESTING

JEAN-XAVIER GUINARD

Department of Food Science and Technology
University of California, Davis
Davis, CA 95616

ABSTRACT

Understanding consumer behavior and knowing which product attributes drive consumer acceptance are key to successful development and marketing of new products. Sensory properties are critical determinants of consumer acceptance. The food industry and academia have developed various methods to measure consumer acceptance, and to relate it to instrumental (physical and chemical) and sensory (descriptive) measures of sensory properties.

The first task of the consumer scientist is to select a test design and protocol, and a consumer population. Applications, advantages and limitations of laboratory tests (which may use company employees or preferably externally-recruited consumers), central location tests (e.g., mall intercept), and home-use tests, are outlined. Experimental design issues (e.g., number of consumers, number of samples, first-order and carry-over effects, complete vs. incomplete designs) are also addressed. Measures of consumer acceptance include (1) degree of liking of the product overall, and/or of specific product attributes, usually on a 9-point hedonic scale, (2) preference measures (paired-preference or preference ranking), or (3) purchase intent. We propose that additional measures of consumer purchase (do consumers actually buy the product?) and consumption behavior (do consumers actually eat or drink the product?) be carried out as well.

Statistical methods which examine individual consumer responses and/or relate them to analytical variables have recently been introduced (e.g., internal and external preference mapping, multiple factor analysis). These methods use various linear and non-linear models and various criteria for goodness of fit of each consumer to the models. They provide a more thorough picture of consumer preferences than traditional methods which only relate averaged acceptance ratings (across a population of consumers) to analytical variables.

INTRODUCTION

The primary purpose of consumer or affective tests is to assess the personal response (acceptance, degree of liking, preference, purchase intent,...) by current or potential consumers of a product, a product concept, or specific product characteristics. Consumer tests are a necessary complement to analytical tests (e.g., instrumental and sensory measurements of sensory properties), which they typically follow in the sequence of tests. They are used mainly by manufacturers of consumer goods, but also by providers of services (hospitals, banks), and even the US Army, where many tests were first developed, and continue to be (Cardello 1994; Meiselman 1994). Applications of consumer testing are many, including product maintenance, product improvement/optimization, development of new products, and assessment of market potential. To conduct a consumer test, a group of individuals is selected from a sample of some larger population for whom the product (or service) is intended. That sample is typically drawn from so-called 'users and likers' of the product. The source of consumers may be employees (not recommended, except for preliminary tests), local residents, or the general population. Three types of formats and settings may be used (e.g., laboratory tests, central location tests, and home-use tests) depending on the purpose and type of consumer test being carried out. The applications, advantages and drawbacks of these alternatives are shown in Table 1.

TABLE 1.
APPLICATIONS, ADVANTAGES AND LIMITATIONS OF LABORATORY TESTS, CENTRAL LOCATION TESTS, AND HOME-USE TESTS

	Laboratory Tests
Applications	Product maintenance, improvement/optimization and/or development (with specially-recruited consumers). Preliminary tests in the product development process (with employees).
Advantages	Product preparation and presentation can be carefully controlled and procedural biases can be minimized. A large number of samples may be tested (over several sessions if necessary).
Limitations	Laboratory conditions are different from actual conditions of use.
	Central Location Tests
Applications	Product maintenance, improvement/optimization and/or development.
Advantages	Many consumers may be recruited. The product is tested by the end-users. Test conditions are controlled by the experimenter. High return of responses.
Limitations	The number of questions or tasks in the ballot may be limited. Test conditions may not be ideal (interferences from the environment).
	Home-Use Tests
Applications	Product maintenance, improvement/optimization and/or development.
Advantages	The product is prepared and tested under natural conditions of use. Information may be based on repeated use of the product. Experimental designs can be fully utilized. More information may be collected because more time is available for completion of the scoresheet.
Limitations	Time consuming (1 to 4 weeks to complete). The number of consumers tested may be limited. Low return of responses. Few samples can be tested not to upset the natural use situation. No control by the experimenter over the preparation and/or use of the product.

METHODS USED IN CONSUMER TESTS

The various methods that may be used to collect consumer responses are shown in Table 2. Focus groups are a primarily qualitative tool for testing the acceptability of a product or concept (the latter proves useful in the early stages of product development). The most widely used scale in consumer testing is the 9-point hedonic scale (Peryam and Pilgrim 1957), a bipolar scale from 1 = dislike extremely to 9 = like extremely, with 5 = neither like nor dislike. Variations of that scale include 7-point scales with faces showing different levels of sadness or happiness, and words such as 'yummy' or 'yacky', or 'super good' and 'super bad', which are suited for testing children (Kimmel *et al.* 1994).

TABLE 2.
METHODS TYPICALLY USED FOR CONSUMER TESTING

Focus groups	(Casey and Krueger 1994)
Scales & Questionnaires	9-point hedonic scale (Peryam and Pilgrim 1957)
	Hedonic line scales (Pangborn *et al.* 1989)
	Hedonic magnitude estimation scales (Moskowitz and Sidel 1971; Pearce *et al.* 1986)
	Semantic ratio scale (Schutz and Cardello 1997)
	Facial hedonic scale (Kimmel *et al.* 1994)
	"Just-right" scales (Meilgaard *et al.* 1991)
	Attribute diagnostics questionnaire (Meilgaard *et al.* 1991)
	Appropriateness scale (Schutz 1988)
	5-point purchase intent scale (Meilgaard *et al.* 1991)
	Purchase probability scale (Solheim and Lawless 1996)
Preference tests	Paired-preference test (see Roessler *et al.* (1978) for data analysis)
	Preference ranking (see Basker (1988) for data analysis)
Signal detection	R-index (Cliff *et al.* 1997; Chauhan and O'Mahony 1993; Vié *et al.* 1991)

With attribute diagnostic questionnaires, the consumer is expected to rate not only overall liking of the product, but also liking for specific sensory attributes. This can be valuable additional information for the manufacturer. In a study of the contribution of attribute liking to overall liking across six food categories, Moskowitz and Krieger (1995) found taste/flavor was the most important contributor to overall liking, followed by texture and appearance. They found a variety of different patterns, however, across the consumers tested. We recently carried out a consumer test on 24 lager beers with 170 consumers divided in 6 categories according to age (individuals in their 20s, 30s or 40s) and gender (men or women). Table 3 shows Pearson's correlation coefficients between liking for specific attributes and overall degree of liking in the 6 categories of consumers. Hedonic ratings for all attributes were significant predictors of overall liking. For all categories except women in their 20s, degree of liking of taste was the best predictor of overall degree of liking (Table 3), consistent with the results of Moskowitz and Krieger (1995).

TABLE 3.
PEARSON'S CORRELATION COEFFICIENTS BETWEEN OVERALL DEGREE OF LIKING AND ATTRIBUTE LIKING RATINGS FOR 24 LAGER BEERS BY 170 CONSUMERS CLASSIFIED ACCORDING TO AGE AND GENDER
All coefficients are significant at $p<0.001$.

Attributes	Consumer category					
	Men, 20s	Men, 30s	Men, 40s	Women, 20s	Women, 30s	Women, 40s
Appearance	0.924	0.890	0.840	0.932	0.822	0.738
Carbonation	0.853	0.817	0.747	0.925	0.819	0.670
Aroma	0.919	0.893	0.898	0.948	0.825	0.879
Taste	0.976	0.979	0.941	0.962	0.977	0.974
Body	0.971	0.952	0.913	0.969	0.917	0.875
Aftertaste	0.941	0.918	0.867	0.901	0.880	0.907

"Just right" scales are used to assess whether the consumer feels specific attributes are too weak, too strong or just right. Preference tests (e.g., paired-preference or preference ranking) may be more powerful than scaling methods in terms of discriminating among samples. They offer the advantage of being relatively easy tasks for consumers. They can only be used, however, with a limited number of samples (ranking more than 5 samples can be complex).

Signal detection theory is being applied more and more to consumer testing, and R-index measures of preference or liking can be derived from various difference test, scaling and ranking protocols.

PROBLEMS AND ISSUES IN CONSUMER TESTING

How Many Consumers Should Be Tested?

The issue of the number of consumers required for a typical consumer test is not addressed sufficiently in the sensory evaluation literature. Whereas most sensory scientists are satisfied to use what is considered a 'typical' number of judges for a given test (e.g., 30 for a paired-preference test, and 100 for hedonic or purchase intent scaling), there are statistical means to determine what an appropriate number of consumers should be for a given application. These means are collectively known as 'power analysis' (Fleiss 1986). It requires estimates of the variance and of within-subject correlations for the measurement to be carried out in the sensory test (e.g., hedonic or purchase intent scaling), as shown in the following example.

Let us pretend we want to measure the sensory acceptability of 5 prototypes on a 9-point hedonic scale. From previous consumer studies, we can assume a variance estimate

(Mean Square Error or MSE) of 2.5 and a within-subject correlation (ρ) of 0.6. These estimates are very conservative. They assume a large dispersion of hedonic responses among consumers (e.g., high variance) and a low internal consistency of hedonic ratings among consumers (e.g., low within-subject correlation). More typical estimates may be closer to 2.0 and 0.75, respectively. Let us assume as well that a difference of 0.7 on the 9-point hedonic scale between the mean ratings of two prototypes would be statistically significant. To achieve a power ($1 - \beta$) of 90%, with a two-tailed α of 0.05, we would need to sample 35 consumers. To achieve powers of 95 or 99%, we would need to sample 45 or 65 consumers, respectively. How do these numbers change with estimates of 2.0 for MSE and 0.75 for ρ? Powers of 90, 95 and 99% would be achieved with 20, 25 and 35 consumers, respectively. These numbers clearly suggest samples of 100-300 consumers might be an overkill.

Moskowitz (1997) examined sample size from the viewpoint of psychophysical scaling: what is the necessary sample size at which the average rating stabilizes? His empirical data suggest that sample sizes of 40-50 consumers generate stable averages, and that beyond 80 consumers the average is not particularly affected by sample size. In a response to Moskowitz's paper, McEwan (1997) rightfully asks "if two groups of 50 consumers from the same consumer segment are used, how confident will one be of obtaining the same mean value?". We carried out a study of the effects of sugar and acid on the acceptability of frozen yogurt (Guinard *et al.* 1994), which offers a partial answer to that question. It shows a remarkable level of consistency among responses from three groups of about 50 consumers (Fig. 1). The same mean hedonic ratings and the same regressions relating degree of liking to acid concentration were found for the three groups!

This is undoubtedly because the homogeneity of the sample of consumers is just as important as the number of consumers in the sample. It should be a homogeneous population of users and likers of the product, i.e., the target population for that product. In our frozen yogurt study, the three groups tested were college students (from the same university). The concept of population homogeneity is expressed in the variance and within-subject correlation estimates required for the power analysis calculations. A less homogeneous population would require higher variance estimates and possibly lower within-subject correlation estimates, and in turn higher numbers of consumers for achieving adequate power.

Which Experimental Design Should be Used?

Sensory scientists should be aware of the advantages and limitations of fully- vs. partially-randomized designs and of complete vs. incomplete designs. The so-called first order effect is an important bias to consider in consumer testing. The sample tasted first in a series typically receives a higher acceptability or hedonic rating than the other samples. We experienced this phenomenon first hand in our study of consumer liking for lager beers. Table 4 shows the mean hedonic ratings obtained by the beers according to their position in the design (tasted first vs. second vs. third...) for two tasting conditions (blind vs. informed, i.e., with knowledge of brand and price). We found that the beer tasted first received a significantly higher hedonic rating than the beers tasted second through eighth ($p<0.05$). Carry over effects (the effects of a given sample on the next sample) can also be significant in consumer testing.

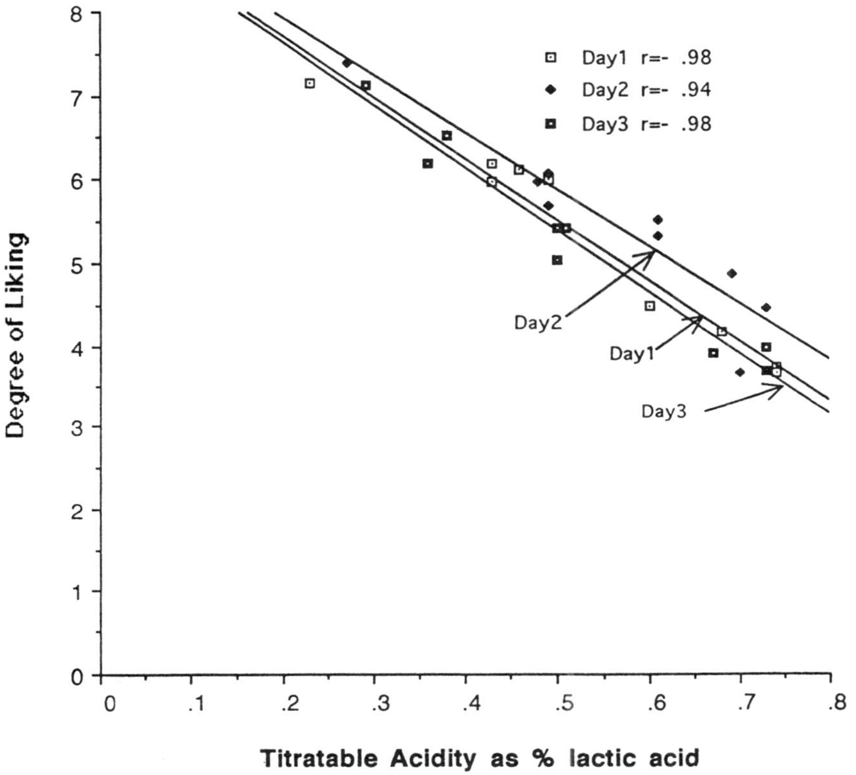

FIG. 1. DEGREE OF LIKING OF FROZEN YOGURT VERSUS TITRATABLE ACIDITY FOR 3 POPULATIONS OF COLLEGE STUDENT CONSUMERS (Day 1, n = 40; Day 2, n = 47; Day 3, n = 54).

TABLE 4.
MEAN HEDONIC RATING ON A 9-POINT HEDONIC SCALE VS. ORDER OF PRESENTATION WITHIN A SESSION (FIRST THROUGH EIGHTH) IN A CONSUMER TEST OF 24 LAGER BEERS WITH 170 CONSUMERS, IN TWO TASTING CONDITIONS (BLIND VS. INFORMED, E.G., WITH KNOWLEDGE OF BRAND AND PRICE)

	Order of presentation in the session							
	1st	2nd	3rd	4th	5th	6th	7th	8th
Condition 1	5.93	5.30	5.47	5.77	5.65	5.49	5.53	5.40
Condition 2	5.79	5.60	5.45	5.58	5.45	5.51	5.62	5.63

First-order and carry-over effects can be avoided by using a fully randomized design in which each sample is presented in each position the same number of times and each sample appears before and after each of the other samples the same number of times as well. Such designs are known as MOLS (Mutually Orthogonal Latin Squares) and detailed examples are found in Wakeling and MacFie (1995). Needless to say, a preset number of consumers is required to use a MOLS design. For example, a multiple of 72 would be required for testing the acceptability of 9 samples with a complete design.

The issue of whether each consumer should taste all the samples (complete design), or whether he/she should only taste a subset (incomplete design) often comes up because of logistical, psychophysical and statistical considerations. Indeed, it might be unrealistic to have a consumer evaluate 6 hot dog samples for a number of parameters at a sitting during a mall intercept because (1) the time availability of the consumer is limited, (2) the logistics of serving 6 hot samples at a time are complex, and (3) fatigue, context and carry-over effects will bias the outcome of the test. In such instances incomplete designs may be used. They may place a significant burden on the quality of the data analysis, however (see section on data analysis below).

What Else is Needed? Monitoring Consumer Behavior During Purchase and Consumption

The question as to whether sensory consumer tests as described in the previous section are good predictors of actual consumer purchase and consumption behavior remains. Indeed, many factors besides sensory properties may influence consumer behavior (Meiselman 1994, 1996; McEwan and Thompson 1988). Does a high rating on a 9-point hedonic scale imply that the consumer will actually buy the product, use it, and buy it again? Ultimately, the latter is the information the manufacturer is after. Very few studies have attempted to answer that question. Meiselman's (1994) solution to this problem is a seven-phase testing sequence which he used for developing food products for U.S. Army soldiers: I. consumer marketing; II. individual item sensory testing; III. consumer meal testing — laboratory; IV. consumer meal testing — field; V. prototype testing; VI. extended ration use validation; and VII. quality control testing.

Large collaborative studies are needed to examine the value of sensory hedonic ratings for predicting consumer purchase and consumption behavior. If hedonic ratings are not necessarily good predictors, consumer testing must then go beyond sensory tests and include measures of first and repeated purchase (e.g., supermarket intercepts), and consumption (e.g., cafeteria/restaurant/home plate wastes, food frequency questionnaires, consumption journals, etc...) (Guinard *et al.* 1996).

STATISTICAL ANALYSIS OF CONSUMER DATA, AND OF THEIR RELATION WITH ANALYTICAL (INSTRUMENTAL AND/OR DESCRIPTIVE) DATA

The statistical methods used to analyze the results of consumer tests are just as important as the methods used to collect the data. Table 5 summarizes the various methods used for consumer data analysis. The first order of business is to determine whether there are significant differences in preference, liking, or purchase intent among the samples tested. This is typically done by applying two-tailed binomial statistics in the case of paired-preference or preference ranking data, and by applying analysis of variance in the case of hedonic or purchase intent ratings (O'Mahony 1986). The latter also examines variability among consumers. Multiple mean comparison tests are then used to compare individual means for the samples or the consumers.

TABLE 5.
STATISTICAL METHODS USED FOR THE ANALYSIS OF CONSUMER DATA.

ANALYZING DATA FROM CONSUMER TESTS
Binomial statistics (for paired-preference test data — Roessler *et al.* 1978)
Multiple sum of ranks comparisons (for ranking data — Basker 1988)
R-index (may be calculated with paired-preference, ranking or hedonic scaling data — Vié *et al.* 1991)
Analysis of variance (O'Mahony 1986)
Multiple mean comparisons (Fisher's Least Significant Difference, Duncan's Multiple Range Test,... — O'Mahony 1986)
Internal Preference Mapping (Greenhoff and MacFie 1994; McEwan 1996)
RELATING CONSUMER DATA TO ANALYTICAL DATA
Pearson's correlation coefficient (O'Mahony 1986)
Simple linear regression (O'Mahony 1986)
Polynomial regression (Guinard *et al.* 1997)
Response Surface Methodology (Giovanni 1983)
Multiple Regression (Schutz 1983)
Repertory Grid Method (Gains 1994)
Partial Least Square regression (Martens and Martens 1996)
External Preference Mapping (Schlich 1995)
Multiple Factor Analysis (Belin *et al.* 1996)

Several of the methods listed in Table 5 actually evaluate the relationships between consumer and analytical (instrumental and/or descriptive) data. The critical difference among those methods is whether they examine these relationships for the consumer population as a whole, or for each consumer individually. We find that both types of analyses should be carried out when an attempt is made to find predictors of consumer acceptance among analytical variables. The principles, applications, advantages and limitations of preference mapping — a relatively new set of multivariate techniques for analyzing consumer preferences — are discussed in the next section.

Preference Mapping Techniques

There are two kinds of preference mapping procedures, e.g., internal and external. Internal preference mapping is a principal component analysis (PCA) of the matrix of hedonic ratings across consumers (the variables) and products (the observations). The PCA should be carried out on the covariance matrix to allow for differences in the strength of the consumer preferences to be expressed. Results are presented in the form of a biplot (PC 2 vs. PC 1) in which consumers or products may be viewed. By comparing the distribution of the consumers and of the products, the analyst can figure out which product is liked best by the majority of consumers. Knowledge of the sensory characteristics of the products in turn allows the analyst to determine which sensory attributes are likely to drive acceptance for the various clusters of consumers in the biplot. Because of the dimensions of the matrix that is being analyzed, the biplot of the first two principal components may only account for a fairly limited amount of the variance in the data. The analyst is encouraged to examine consumer loadings on other principal components. This clearly is the main limitation of internal preference mapping.

External preference mapping (Schlich 1995) regresses individual consumer preferences onto the first two principal components of the covariance matrix of descriptive (or other analytical) ratings across products. Again, the covariance matrix should be used rather than the correlation matrix to allow for an accurate representation of the importance of each of the descriptive attributes (e.g., a longer vector means the attribute discriminated among the products). When a PCA is performed on a correlation matrix, the length of the attribute vectors cannot necessarily be taken as an accurate representation of their importance (ability to discriminate among the products). When different types of variables (sensory, instrumental,...) are used in a PCA, however, a correlation matrix must be used because it normalizes the data before analysis. To assess the value of an external preference map, it is important to consider (1) what proportion of the variance is accounted for by the first two dimensions (just like for any other PCA), and (2) what proportion of the consumers are fitted by the various models (not an issue with internal preference mapping, which fits all the consumers in the biplot). Details about the different models used to regress the hedonic ratings onto the first 2 PCs are found in Schlich (1995). These models are the vectorial, circular, elliptical (with maximum or saddle point) and quadratic models. The equation relating DOL (Y) for a consumer to PC 1 (X_1) and PC2 (X_2) may therefore range from a simple, linear one, e.g., $Y = a + b X_1 + c X_2$ to a complex, second-order one with quadratic and cross-product effects, e.g., $Y = a + b X_1 + c X_2 + d X_1^2 + e X_2^2 + f X_1X_2$.

The best model for a given consumer also has to fit the data for that consumer (as per the significance level of the regression equation) or else that consumer is excluded from the external preference map. So far, the percentage of consumers who could be fitted by one of the models has been the main limitation of external preference mapping. Indeed, if only 50% of the consumers are represented in the preference map biplot, the technique may not be that useful to product developers and marketers. This problem is apparent in the actual examples used by Schlich (1995). In our consumer test of lager beers, over 75% of the consumers were fitted by the external preference mapping models at the required minimum level of significance ($p = 0.25$ for wrongly not simplifying the model, and $p = 0.25$ for wrongly selecting a consumer). This improvement over previous studies can probably be credited to the high number of samples (24) on which the relationships were based. It is also worth noting that all the models were used in fitting these consumers onto the map. For some consumers a vectorial model gave the best fit, and for others the elliptical model with saddle point did.

The challenge of external preference mapping (and one point of criticism) is the interpretation of the results, since preferences are expressed as a function of two principal components, not simple analytical variables (sensory attributes or instrumental measures) as in the Regression Method by Schutz (1983). It remains that once a dense area of consumer preferences has been identified, one can then characterize an ideal product based on its position on the first two PCs (at the heart of that 'hot' preference area), develop the profile of sensory attributes that correspond to that position on the PCA, and then formulate the product accordingly. This multistep approach is rendered feasible by the fact that food manufacturers nowadays understand quite well the relation between ingredients/processes and sensory properties and are reasonably able to formulate a product with a specific set of sensory attributes.

Another requirement of most multivariate methods used to relate consumer data to analytical data is a large number of products on which to base these relationships. As mentioned above, however, it might not be feasible to have the consumer taste many samples. In such a case, incomplete designs may be used. The power and the validity of preference mapping techniques may be reduced, however, when only a limited subset of the products are tasted by the consumer (Schlich *et al.* 1996).

Example

The use of three statistical methods for analyzing consumer data is illustrated in Fig. 2. Hedonic ratings by a population of 144 young adult consumers for 9 ice cream samples varying in sugar and fat according to a 3^2 factorial design were analyzed by analysis of variance (means hedonic ratings are shown with Fisher's LSD in Fig. 2a), response surface methodology (the response surface relating degree of liking to sugar and fat levels is shown in Fig. 2b), and by internal preference mapping (both consumers and ice cream samples are shown in Fig. 2c). This example is meant to illustrate the need for both kinds of statistical approaches — those which focus on the population's (or sub-populations') average, and those which examine each consumer individually.

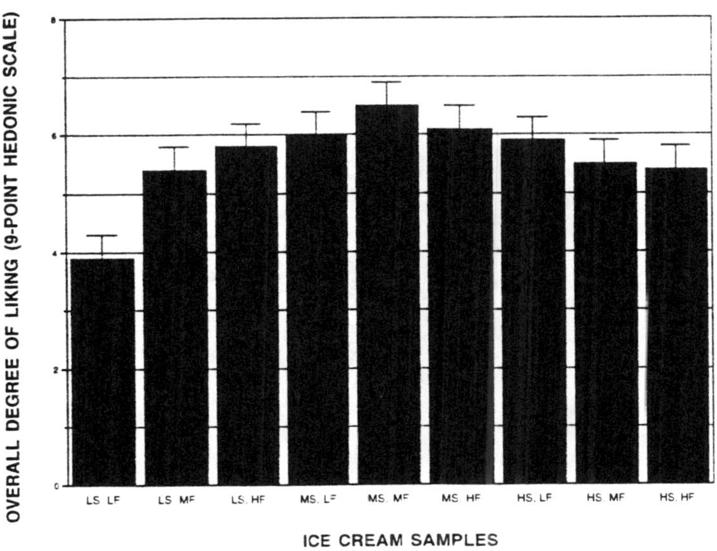

FIG. 2. CONTRAST BETWEEN STATISTICAL ANALYSES OF HEDONIC RATINGS FOR 9 ICE CREAM SAMPLES VARYING IN SUGAR (8, 13, OR 18% W/W) AND FAT (10, 14, OR 18% W/W) BY 144 YOUNG ADULT CONSUMERS.

a. Mean hedonic ratings with Fisher's LSD at $p<0.05$

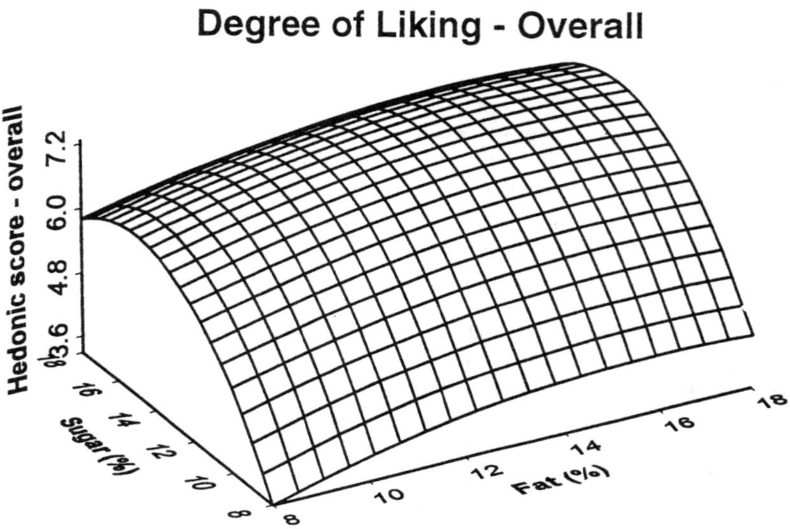

FIG. 2. b. Response surface relating mean degree of liking to sugar and fat concentrations;

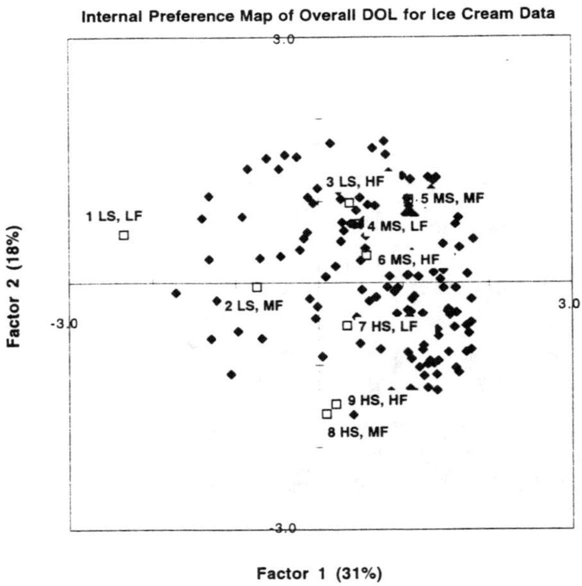

FIG. 2. c. Internal preference map showing both the samples and the consumers (L=low, M=medium, H=high; S=sugar, F=fat)

REFERENCES

BASKER, D. 1988. Critical values of differences among rank sums for multiple comparisons. Food Technol. *42*, 79–84.

BELIN, E., PAGES, J. HOSSENLOPP, J. and PALAGOS, B. 1996. Mise en relation de données consommateurs et de données sensorielles par différentes approches multidimentionnelles. Presented at the Third Sensometrics Meeting, June 19–21, Nantes, France.

CARDELLO, A. V. 1994. Consumer expectations and their role in food acceptance. *In* Measurement of Food Preferences, H.J.H. MacFie and D.M.H. Thomson (eds.). Blackie Academic & Professional, London. pp. 253–297.

CASEY, M. A. and KRUEGER, R. A. 1994. Focus group interviewing. *In* Measurement of Food Preferences, H.J.H. MacFie and D.M.H. Thomson (eds.). Blackie Academic & Professional, London. pp. 77–96.

CHAUHAN, J. and O'MAHONY, M. 1993. Use of a signal detection ranking analysis to measure preferences for commercial and 'health modified' cakes. J. Sens. Studies *8*, 69–75.

CLIFF, M.A., KING, M.C., SCAMAN, C. and EDWARDS, B.J. 1997. Evaluation of R-indices for preference testing of apple juices. Food Qual. Pref. *8*, 241–246.

FLEISS, J.L. 1986. The Design and Analysis of Clinical Experiments. John Wiley and Sons, New York.

GAINS, N. 1994. The repertory grid method. *In* Measurement of Food Preferences, H.J.H. MacFie and D.M.H. Thomson (eds.). Blackie Academic & Professional, London. pp. 51–76.

GIOVANNI, M. 1983. Response surface methodology and product optimization. Food Technol. *37*(11), 41–45, 83.

GREENHOFF, K. and MACFIE, H.J.H. 1994. Preference mapping in practice. *In* Measurement of Food Preferences, H.J.H. MacFie and D.M.H. Thomson (eds.). Blackie Academic & Professional, London. pp. 137–166.

GUINARD, J.-X., LITTLE, C., MARTY, C. and PALCHAK, T. 1994. Effect of sugar and acid on the acceptability of frozen yogurt to a student population. J. Dairy Sci. *77*, 1232–1238.

GUINARD, J.-X., ZOUMAS-MORSE, C., DIETZ, J., GOLDBERG, S., HOLZ, M., HECK, B. and AMOROS, A. 1996. Does consumption of beer, alcohol and bitter substances affect perception of bitterness? Physiol. Behav. *59*, 625–631.

GUINARD, J.-X., ZOUMAS-MORSE, C., MORI, L., UOTANI, B., PANYAM, D. and KILARA, A. 1997. Sugar and fat effects on sensory properties of ice cream. J. Food Sci. (In press).

KIMMEL, S., SIGMAN-GRANT, M.J. and GUINARD, J.-X. 1994. Sensory testing with young children. Food Technol. *48*(3), 92–99.

MARTENS, H. and MARTENS, M. 1996. Trends in PLS regression of relevance to sensometrics. Presented at the Third Sensometrics Meeting, June 19-21, Nantes, France.

McEWAN, J. A. 1996. Preference mapping for product optimization. *In* Multivariate Analysis of Data in Sensory Science, T. Naes and E. Risvik (eds.), Elsevier, Amsterdam. pp. 71–102.

McEWAN, J.A. 1997. Reply to: Base size in product testing: a psychophysical viewpoint and analysis. Food Qual. Pref. *8*, 257–258.

McEWAN, J.A. and THOMSON, D.M.H. 1988. A behavioural interpretation of food acceptability. Food Qual. Pref. *1*, 3–10.

MEILGAARD, M., CIVILLE, G.V. and CARR, B.T. 1991. Sensory Evaluation Techniques. CRC Press, Boca Raton, FL.

MEISELMAN, H. 1994. A measurement scheme for developing institutional products. *In* Measurement of Food Preferences, H.J.H. MacFie and D.M.H. Thomson (eds.). Blackie Academic & Professional, London. pp. 1–24.

MEISELMAN, H. 1996. Context in sensory testing. Presented at ECRO XII, August 25-31, Zurich, Switzerland.

MOSKOWITZ, H. 1997. Base size in product testing: a psychophysical viewpoint and analysis. Food Qual. Pref. *8*, 247–255.

MOSKOWITZ, H.R. and SIDEL, J.L. 1971. Magnitude and hedonic scales of food acceptability. J. Food Sci. *36*, 677–680.

MOSKOWITZ, H.R. and KRIEGER, B. 1995. The contribution of sensory liking to overall liking: an analysis of six food categories. Food Qual. Pref. *6*, 83–90.

O'MAHONY, M. 1986. Sensory Evaluation of Food. Statistical Methods and Procedures. Marcel Dekker, Inc., New York. 487 pp.

PANGBORN, R. M., GUINARD, J.-X. and MEISELMAN, H.L. 1989. Evaluation of bitterness of caffeine in hot chocolate drink by category, graphic and ratio scaling. J. Sens. Studies *4*, 31–53.

PERYAM, D.R. and PILGRIM, F.J. 1957. Hedonic scale method of measuring food preferences. Food Technol. *11*(9), Suppl. 9–14.

PEARCE, J.H., KORTH, B. and WARREN, C.B. 1986. Evaluation of three scaling methods for hedonics. J. Sens. Studies *1*, 27–46.

ROESSLER, E.B., PANGBORN, R.M., SIDEL, J.L. and STONE, H. 1978. Expanded statistical tables for estimating significance in paired-preference, paired-difference, duo-trio and triangle tests. J. Food Sci. *43*, 940–944.

SCHLICH, P. 1995. Preference mapping: relating consumer preferences to sensory and instrumental measurements. *In* Bioflavour '95. Analysis/Precursor Studies/Biotechnology. P. Etiévant and P. Schreier (eds.), INRA Editions, Versailles.

SCHLICH, P., CALLIER, P. and DEGOUD, S. 1996. The dark side of preference mapping. Presented at the Third Sensometrics Meeting, June 19-21, Nantes, France.

SCHUTZ, H. 1983. Multiple regression approach to product optimization. Food Technol. *37*(11), 46–48, 62.

SCHUTZ, H. G. 1988. Beyond preference: appropriateness as a measure of contextual evaluation of food. *In* Food Acceptability. D. M. H. Thomson (ed.), Elsevier Applied Science, London, pp. 115–134.

SCHUTZ, H. G. and CARDELLO, A. V. 1997. Development of a semantic ratio scale for assessing food liking/disliking. Presented at the 6th Food Choice Conference, June 25–27, Uppsala, Sweden.

SOLHEIM, R. and LAWLESS, H.T. 1996. Consumer purchase probability affected by attitude towards low-fat foods, liking, private body consciousness and information on fat and price. Food Qual. Pref. *7*, 137–143.

VIE, A., GULLI, D. and O'MAHONY, M. 1991. Alternative hedonic measures. J. Food Sci. *56*, 1–5, 46.

WAKELING, I.N. and MACFIE, H.J.H. 1995. Designing consumer trials balanced for first and higher orders of carry-over effect when only a subset of k samples from t may be tested. Food Qual. Pref. *6*, 299–308.

SENSORY PROPERTIES OF FRUITS AND VEGETABLES

DIANE M. BARRETT, ELBA CUBERO, IRENE LUNA-GUZMAN, CHARLENE WEE and JEAN XAVIER GUINARD

Department of Food Science and Technology
University of California, Davis

ABSTRACT

Fruits and vegetables offer the consumer unique color, flavor and texture attributes; however, control of processing conditions is required for optimization of sensory quality. Three studies in our laboratory illustrate correlations between instrumental and sensory evaluation of fruit and vegetable products.

Three varieties of corn and 2 varieties of broccoli were blanched for various times, frozen and stored for 9 months at 0°F. Instrumental and sensory analyses found significant differences between varieties in both commodities in terms of texture, flavor, aroma and color. Short blanch treatments eliminated undesirable sensory qualities and improved texture and sweetness while longer blanch treatments had an undesirable effect on color.

Textural integrity of fresh cut cantaloupe was improved in a second study by dipping pieces in solutions of calcium salts. Descriptive sensory panel measurements indicated that calcium lactate dips produced a sweeter, firmer product while calcium chloride dips resulted in a bitter, less firm product.

In a third study, three varieties of diced tomatoes were processed using aseptic, hot fill and cold fill processes and then evaluated for textural integrity using instrumental and sensory analyses. There were significant differences between both varieties and thermal processes, with the aseptically processed tomatoes being the most firm by both instrumental and sensory measures.

INTRODUCTION

Processing technologies targeted to preservation of fruit and vegetable products must maintain the unique color, flavor and texture attributes expected by consumers. Whatever preservation method is utilized, it must be designed to optimize sensory properties of the final product. Recent studies in our laboratory have focused on measurement and correlation of the instrumental and sensory properties of processed fruits and vegetables. Three separate studies focusing on the following will be cited: 1) blanched, frozen and stored vegetable quality; 2) fresh-cut cantaloupe texture; and 3) effects of different processing techniques on the textural attributes of diced tomatoes.

MATERIALS AND METHODS

Blanched, Frozen and Stored Vegetable Study

Three corn and two broccoli varieties were blanched for varying times and evaluated for residual lipoxygenase, peroxidase and cystine lyase activity. Samples stored

9 mo (0°C) were analyzed for content of flavor volatiles, free fatty acids, sugars, color, texture and sensory properties (flavor, aroma and texture). Methodology for all analyses is described in Barrett *et al.* (In preparation, 1997), but brief mention of methods will be made below.

Corn lipoxygenase (LPO) and peroxidase (POD) and broccoli POD were analyzed by the methods of Theerakulkait *et al.* (1995). Broccoli POD was measured according to the method of Chen *et al.* (1986), and broccoli cystine lyase (CL) was evaluated using the method of Friedemann and Haugen (1943). Flavor volatiles were measured by headspace analysis, utilizing cryofocusing prior to injection into a gas chromatograph (GC) with a DB-WAX (J&W Scientific, Folsom, CA) open tubular fused silica column and a flame ionization detector.

Free fatty acids were analyzed by mixing the sample with sulfuric acid and anhydrous sodium sulfate, sonicating, mixing with hexane and centrifuging to separate the aqueous and organic layers. Formic acid in diisopropyl ether was added and fatty acids were measured by GC. Sugars were evaluated by mixing the sample with isopropyl alcohol, diluting with deioinized water and analyzing by high performance liquid chromatography (HPLC). Color was analyzed using a Minolta CR-200 colorimeter and L*, a*, b* and hue angle measurements were taken. Texture analysis was carried out using the Kramer shear cell on a TA.XT2 Texture Analyzer (Texture Technologies Corp., Scarsdale, NY) and the test was run at 1 mm/sec and 90% strain.

A sensory panel of ten judges (6 women and 4 men) was selected for corn and broccoli descriptive analyses. A modified version of the Quantitative Descriptive Analysis (DA) method (Stone and Sidel 1993) was used to evaluate the sensory properties of the corn and broccoli samples. A 10-point numerical scale was used and all samples were evaluated in duplicate. Individual descriptors were generated for all sensory characteristics, and definitions (including mode of evaluation) and reference standards were developed for the final list of attributes. Panelists were trained in four separate sessions and then evaluated actual samples. Results were analyzed using Analysis of Variance (ANOVA) and Principal Component Analysis (PCA).

Textural Integrity of Fresh-Cut Cantaloupe

Fresh-cut cantaloupe melon pieces were treated with calcium salts and evaluated for sensory quality and for instrumental firmness following the method of Luna-Guzman *et al.* (1997, submitted). A paired-comparison test was used first to determine whether differences in bitterness and firmness of treated samples could be detected by consumers. Descriptive analysis was also carried out using 6 trained panelists. Aroma, flavor and texture descriptors were generated and panelists were trained in 5 sessions. Three additional sessions were required for sample analysis. Results were evaluated using ANOVA.

Processing Effects on Textural Attributes of Diced Tomatoes

Three varieties of tomatoes (Halley 3155, Heinz 8892 and Heinz 9382) were obtained from 2 different growing regions and processed using three different methods (aseptic, hot fill and cold fill). Diced tomato products were evaluated using three different instrumental methods with the TA.XT2 Texture Analyzer, e.g. Kramer shear, back extrusion and texture profile analysis (TPA). Descriptive analysis was carried out by 14 trained judges for 12 texture and 3 taste attributes. The effects of variety and processing method were assessed by ANOVA and PCA.

RESULTS AND DISCUSSION

Blanched, Frozen and Stored Vegetable Study

There were significant differences among the 3 corn varieties evaluated and they also behaved differently as a function of blanching time (Table 1). Corn peroxidase inactivation in all 3 varieties required an 8 min blanch while lipoxygenase inactivation required a 6 min blanch in sweet corn varieties A and B and a 4 min blanch in supersweet variety C. Reducing blanch time is desirable from a sensory standpoint, because longer blanch treatments generally reduce firmness and fresh corn attributes and increase cooked flavors. Analytical data showed that sucrose content increased with blanch times up to 4 min, and then was relatively constant.

TABLE 1.
MEANS FOR ENZYME ACTIVITY, COLOR AND FIRMNESS OF THREE BLANCHED CORN-ON-THE-COB VARIETIES (AVERAGED RESULTS)

Analysis	0 min	2 min	4 min	6 min	8 min
Hexanal (ppb)	0.38 a	0.28 b	0.29 b	0.32 ab	0.3 ab
Lipoxygenase	3.37 a	1.17 b	0.25 c	0 c	0 c
Peroxidase	8.44 a	6.26 b	1.90 c	0.73 cd	0 d
Chroma	38.84 b	50 a	48.61 a	50 a	49.42 a
L * Value	67.8 a	64.4 b	64.57 b	63.27 b	63.68 b
Hue	88.5 c	90.4 b	90.5 b	90.2 b	92 a
Firmness	129.1 b	163 ab	184 a	199 a	171 ab

Within a row, means sharing same subscripts are not significantly different

Supersweet corn variety C not only required the shortest blanch, but also was the most sweet, highest in overall flavor, cooked flavor and firmness and had the least number of undesirable sensory attributes after 9 mo of storage (Fig. 1). Variety B was found to be more yellow-orange in color, the most juicy with the least cooked in terms of flavor (Fig. 2). In addition, a husky aftertaste was retained in all blanch times with this variety and the grainy flavor increased with blanching. Sweet corn variety B had the greatest number of undesirable attributes, as compared to varieties A and C (Fig. 2 vs Fig. 1 and 3).

Sensory analysis indicated that variety A was the most starchy, least sweet, least juicy and had less cooked flavor and overall flavor intensity at any blanching time (Fig. 3). Rancid and moldy flavor and aroma were still detectable in the stored sweet corn varieties A and B which received a 4 min blanch, but not in supersweet variety C. A 6 min blanch may be required to eliminate these undesirable attributes in some corn varieties, but in this study undesirable attributes were eliminated from the supersweet variety C in just 4 min. Instrumental texture analysis of the means of the three varieties found that firmness increased with blanching up to 6 min, and then declined.

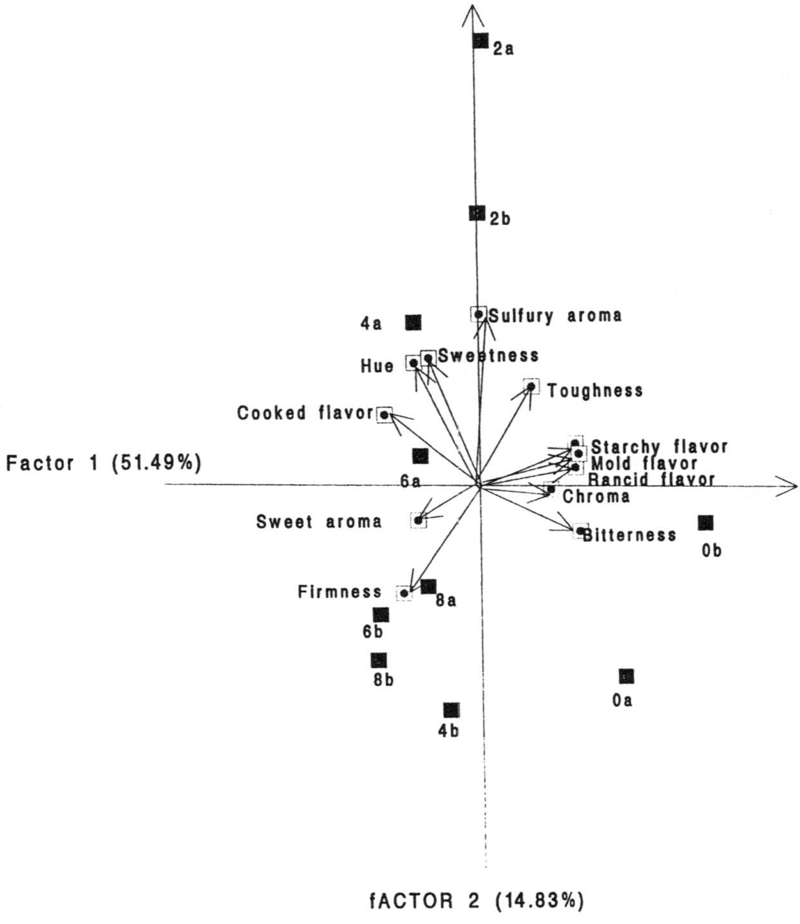

FIG. 1. PCA OF SENSORY ANALYSIS OF CORN VARIETY C

The two broccoli varieties responded to blanching time increases in a similar fashion, which resulted primarily in textural changes (Fig. 4 and 5). Broccoli became less firm, fibrous, crunchy and more juicy as blanching time increased. The instrumental texture data indicated that broccoli firmness increased with blanching up to 90 to 135 sec and then decreased. Blanched samples had a sulfury aroma and flavor, seaweedy aroma and flavor and smoked aroma and flavor but there was no significant difference among blanch times. Because bitterness increased with blanch time in variety A (Fig. 4) and textural attributes were less desirable as blanching increased (Fig. 4 and 5), there is incentive to maintain blanch times at 90 sec from a sensory standpoint. Complete inactivation of broccoli enzymes also required a 90 sec blanch. Dimethyl sulfide concentration was found to increase significantly between 90 and 135 sec, which presents another argument for maintaining broccoli blanch times at 90 sec to avoid off-aroma production.

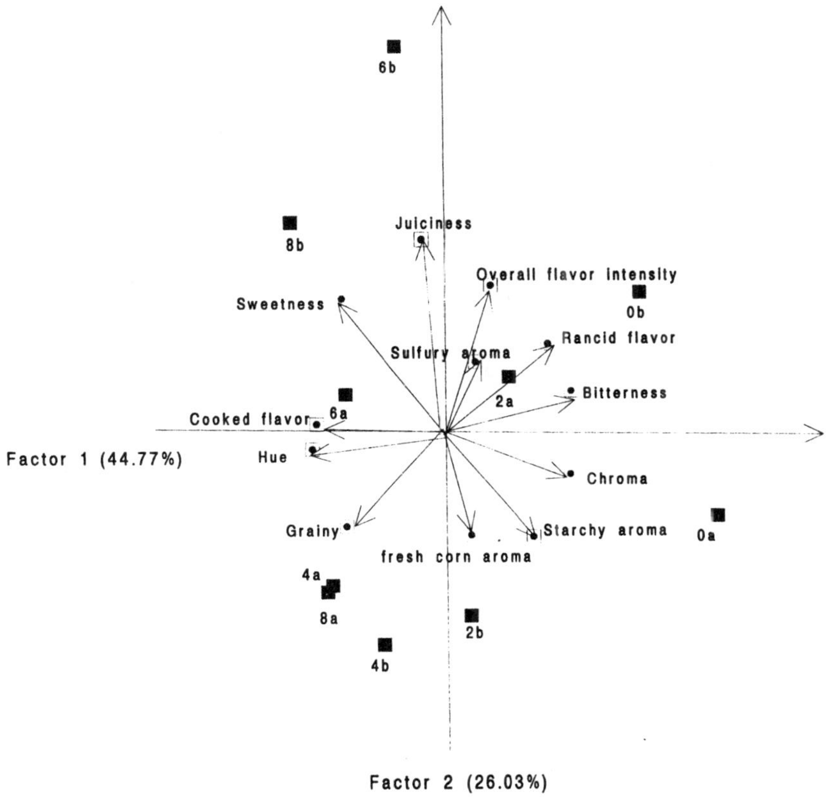

FIG. 2. PCA OF SENSORY ANALYSIS OF CORN VARIETY B

In general, both broccoli and corn color were positively affected by short blanch treatments, and longer blanch times resulted in undesirable effects on color. Blanch times for both corn and broccoli may be significantly reduced from current industry practices. Results from instrumental and sensory analyses were in fairly good agreement, and suggest that it may be possible to predict sensory quality using instrumental measurements.

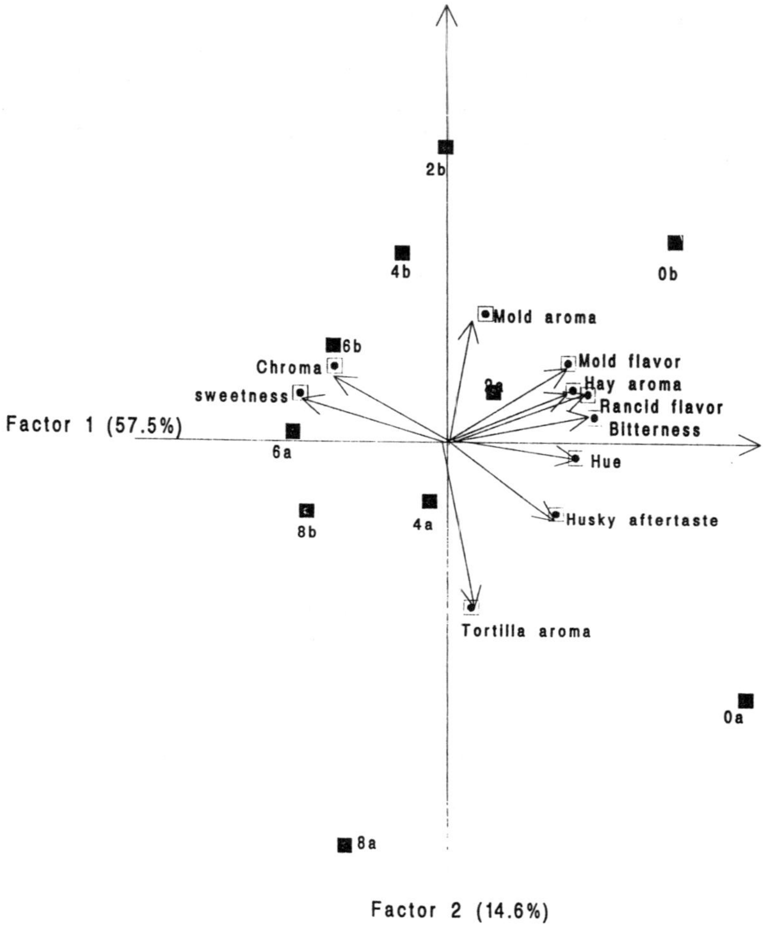

FIG. 3. PCA OF SENSORY ANALYSIS OF CORN VARIETY A

Textural Integrity of Fresh-Cut Cantaloupe

Both calcium salts used in this study imparted an improvement in texture (Fig. 6; Table 2); however, calcium lactate appeared to be significantly better than $CaCl_2$ in maintaining firmness throughout a 12 day storage period. Paired comparison tests showed that samples treated with as little as 1% $CaCl_2$ were perceived as having a significantly different taste and firmness than water treated samples. The trained panel developed 6 attributes to describe fresh-cut cantaloupe quality: melon flavor, sweetness, bitterness,

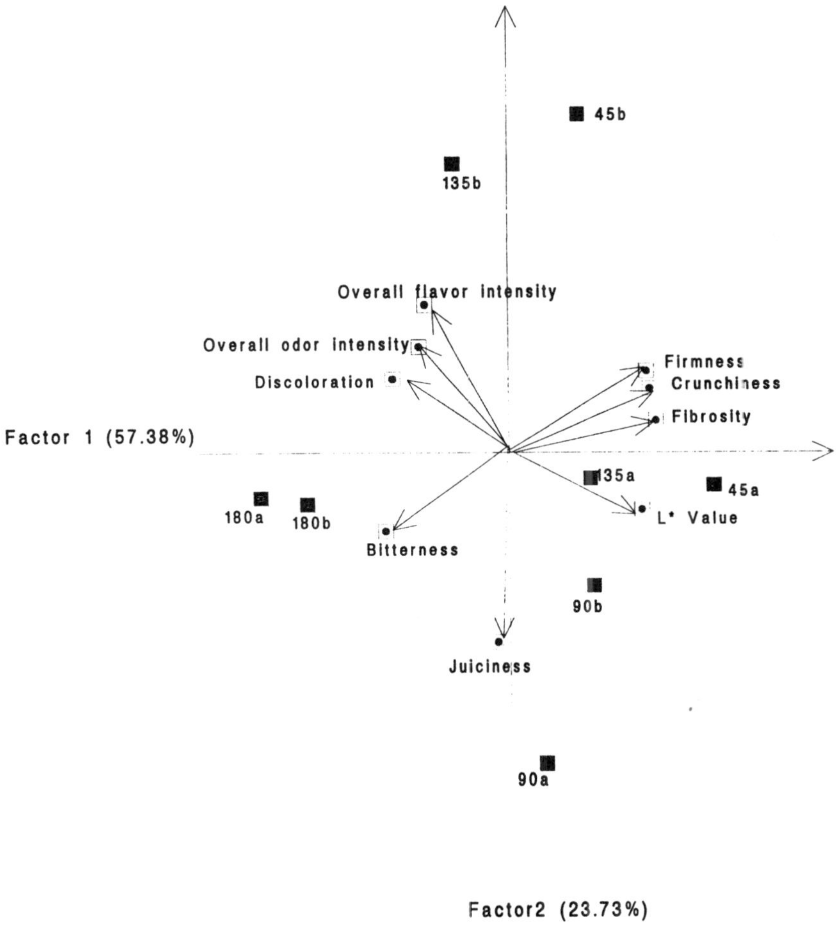

FIG. 4. PCA OF SENSORY ANALYSIS OF BROCCOLI VARIETY A

hardness (front teeth), crunchiness (molars) and moisture content. All of the calcium-treated samples were greater in hardness than just cut samples, but the samples treated with 2.5% calcium lactate were the most hard (Table 2). There were no significant differences found in sweetness; however, $CaCl_2$ treated samples were significantly more bitter than any other treatment. There was no significant bitterness detected in either calcium lactate or just cut samples. In this study, instrumental and sensory measures of firmness were very well correlated.

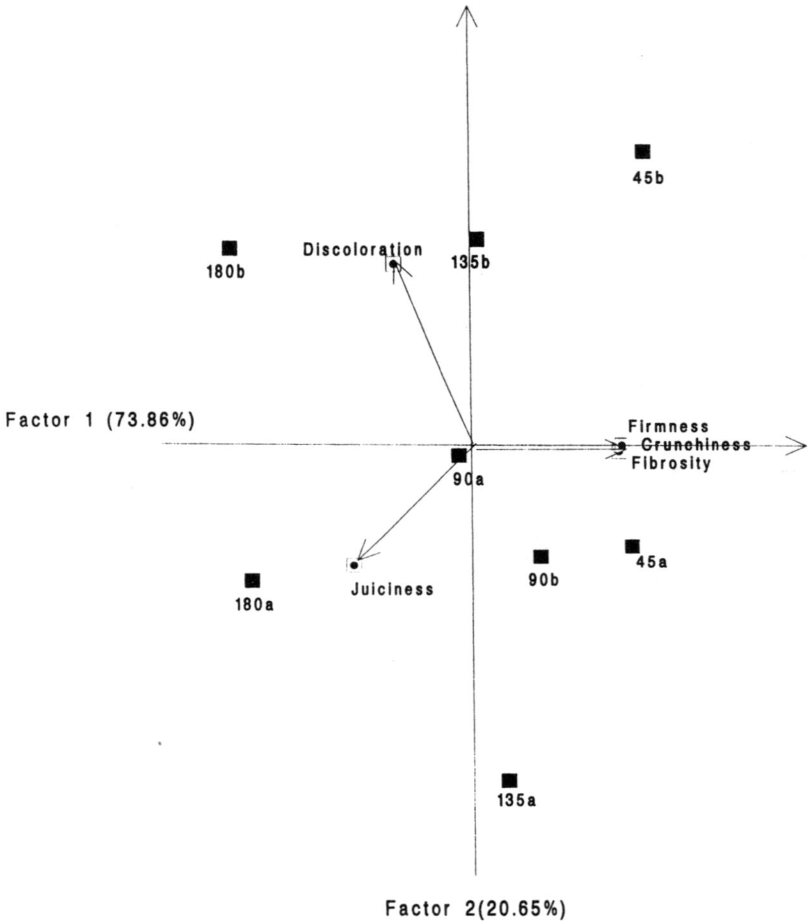

FIG. 5. PCA FOR SENSORY DATA FOR BROCCOLI VARIETY B

Processing Effects on Textural Attributes of Diced Tomatoes

Significant differences were determined between both tomato varieties and processing methods by both instrumental and sensory measurements. Sensory firmness differed significantly among processing treatments ($p < 0.001$), with the aseptic and hot fill methods yielding firmer tomatoes than the cold fill method (Fig. 7). Sensory firmness did not differ, however, between varieties. Sensory firmness was significantly correlated with instrumental firmness as determined by the back extrusion method ($r = 0.74$; $p < 0.001$), but the Kramer shear method was not as well correlated.

TABLE 2.
TABLE OF DESCRIPTIVE ANALYSIS OF FRESH-CUT CANTALOUPE

TREATMENT	Melon Flavor	Sweetness	Bitterness	Hardness	Crunchiness	Moisture Content
Just Cut	4.61 [ab]	4.18 [a]	2.64 [b]	3.41 [c]	4.36 [b]	5.95 [ab]
1% $CaCl_2$	3.18 [b]	3.74 [a]	4.78 [a]	5.14 [b]	5.04 [ab]	6.36 [a]
2.5% $CaCl_2$	4.23 [ab]	4.36 [a]	5.76 [a]	4.78 [b]	5.85 [a]	4.82 [bc]
1% $CaLactate_2$	5.63 [a]	3.89 [a]	2.74 [b]	4.73 [b]	4.96 [ab]	4.55 [c]
2.5% $CaLactate_2$	4.71 [b]	4.05 [a]	3.37 [b]	6.05 [a]	5.73 [a]	4.51 [c]

Significant differences were found among treatments for firmness (aseptic = hot fill > cold fill), chunkiness (aseptic > hot fill > cold fill), crunchiness (cold fill > aseptic = hot fill), fibrosity (hot fill = cold fill > aseptic), juiciness (hot fill = cold fill > aseptic), seediness (hot fill > cold fill = aseptic), mushiness (hot fill > cold fill = aseptic), sliminess (cold fill = aseptic > hot fill), rubberiness (cold fill = aseptic > hot fill), graininess (hot fill > aseptic = cold fill), acidity (aseptic > hot fill > cold fill) and saltiness (hot fill > aseptic > cold fill).

Variability between variety replicates was high for the aseptic and cold fill methods. PCA of the sensory data alone clearly separates the samples on the basis of processing method, with cold fill samples being more fibrous, grainy, mushy, seedy, juicy and salty, and aseptic samples being more firm, chunky and crunchy (Fig. 7). Hot filled products were in the central portion of the PCA diagram and had more neutral texture values. These results indicate that the aseptic method of processing is preferable.

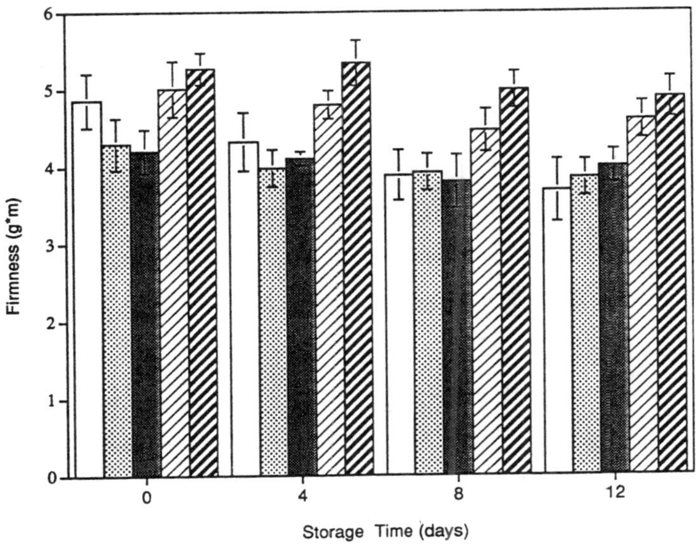

FIG. 6. EFFECT OF STORAGE TIME ON FIRMNESS OF FRESH-CUT CANTALOUPE TREATED IN VARIOUS WAYS

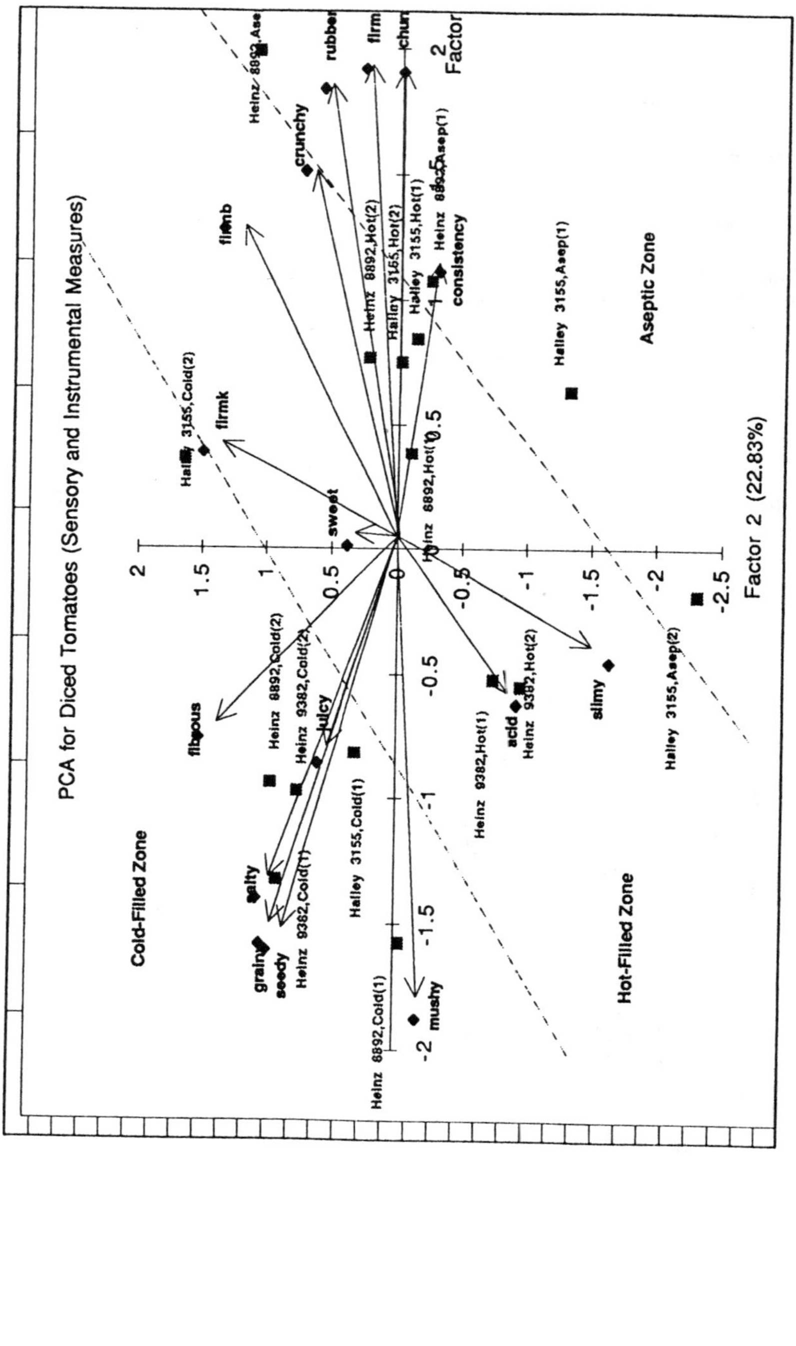

FIG. 7. PCA FOR DICED TOMATOES (SENSORY AND INSTRUMENTAL MEASURES)

CONCLUSIONS

Instrumental and sensory methods were good indicators of textural attributes in all the studies cited. The blanched, frozen and stored vegetable study also showed that instrumental and sensory evaluation of color and flavor attributes were closely related. In many instances, therefore, instrumental measurements of fruit and vegetable quality correlate well with and therefore may be used to predict sensory responses.

REFERENCES

BARRETT, D.M., CUBERO, E., GARCIA, E.L., RUSSELL, G.F., RAMIREZ, E., SHIRAZI, A. and GUINARD, J.X. 1997. Instrumental and sensory evaluation of steam blanched, frozen and stored corn and broccoli. (In preparation)

CHEN, A.O., LIM, M.H., PANGBORN, R.M. and WHITAKER, J.R. 1986. Unpublished data. U. of California, Davis, CA.

FRIEDEMANN, T.E. and HAUGEN, G.E. 1943. The determination of keto acids in blood and urine. J. Biol. Chem. *147*, 415–442.

LUNA-GUZMAN, I., BARRETT, D.M. and CANTWELL, M. 1997. Fresh-cut cantaloupe: Physiological responses and firmness variability with $CaCl_2$ and calcium lactate dips. Submitted to Postharvest Biology and Technology.

STONE, H. and SIDEL, J.L. 1993. Sensory Evaluation Practices. 2nd ed. Academic Press, Inc. New York, NY. 338p.

THEERAKULKAIT, C., BARRETT, D.M. and MCDANIEL, M.R. 1995. Sweet corn germ enzymes affect odor formation. J. Food Sci. *60*(5), 1034–1040.

EFFECT OF PROCESSING ON TEXTURE AND SENSORY QUALITY OF FROZEN PRECOOKED RICE

M.T. YAN and B.S. LUH

Department of Food Science and Technology
University of California
Davis, CA 95616

ABSTRACT

*Rice (*Oryza sativa L.*) is one of the important economic crops grown in California. This paper studies the effect of several processing variables on chemical, physical, and sensory quality of frozen pre-cooked Calrose rice. The variables include the Water/Rice ratio, freezing methods and storage temperature on sensory quality of the products. Results indicate that Calrose rice soaked in water at 25°C for 30 minutes will reach a moisture content of 30-31%. Rice cooked at a W/R ratio of 1.25 had a more desirable texture after cooking. Addition of soy oil and surfactant helps to improve grain separation and flavor acceptability of the product. Storage of the precooked products at 25, 12, 0, -12 and -25°C resulted in marked differences in texture and retrogradation of the starch. Changes are more pronounced at lower storage temperatures. Precooked rice frozen in the blast, plate and room freezer showed differences in shear press values and sensory quality.*

INTRODUCTION

Rice (*Oryza sativa* L.) is one of the most economically important crops grown in California. LaBell (1994) reported that per capita consumption of rice in the United States has increased from 6.4 kg in 1980 to 10.0 kg in 1990.

Research work on frozen cooked rice has been published by Boggs *et al.* (1951). The effect of parboiling and freezing on quality of Spanish rice varieties has been reported by Olalquiaga *et al.* (1986). General aspects of rice utilization have been published by Luh (1991). Recent progress in frozen food technology was reviewed by Mallet (1993), and manufacturing of frozen prepared meals by Shaevel (1993).

The important factors in developing new rice varieties are grain quality and yield. Webb (1991) made an excellent review on rice quality and grades. This paper reports on the effects of several processing variables on chemical, physical and sensory quality of frozen precooked Calrose rice.

MATERIALS AND METHODS

Rice. Two hundred forty pounds of Calrose medium grain rice were purchased from the California Rice Growers Association, West Sacramento, California. The rice was packed in 2-lb. plastic bags (12 bags in each cardboard box) and stored at 2°C upon receipt.

Washing. From each sample, 200 g of Calrose rice were washed in a home style strainer with running tap water for 10 s to remove free starch and extraneous materials.

Soaking. The washed rice sample was transferred to a beaker and soaked in distilled water at room temperature (25°C) for 15, 30, 45 and 60 min. The moisture content of the drained samples soaked for different time intervals was determined. The average of three replicates is reported. Soaking the rice in excess of water on moisture absorption at 35, 45 and 55°C was also studied.

Water/Rice Ratio. In each batch, 200 g of milled Calrose rice were soaked in distilled water for 30 min at 25°C. The amounts of distilled water used in cooking were 150, 200, 250, 300 and 350 ml, respectively. The average of three trials was used in each treatment. The frozen precooked rice samples were packaged in Scotchpack 16" Mylar-Polyethylene boil-in-the-bag pouches and tested for quality at various time intervals after processing.

Effect of Soy Oil/Surfactant in the Cooking Water

Two hundred twenty mL of the following solutions were used to cook 200 g of Calrose rice.

Soy oil/surfactant solutions. Soy oil with Tween 60 as surfactant were prepared [Tween 60 is polyoxyethylene sorbitan monostearate, a non-ionic emulsifier (ICI America, Inc.)]. Three oil emulsions were prepared: 5% oil with 0.5% Tween 60; 10% oil with 0.5% Tween 60; and 5% oil in water. Tween 60 was weighed and dissolved in water and warmed to 65-70°C.

Rice Cooking. Rice samples for texture and sensory studies were cooked in a Hitachi (RD-5901) electrical automatic rice cooker. The rice was cooked 12 min at the water/rice ratios described in the previous section. The cooked rice was allowed to stand for 10 min before removing the lid. The Hitachi rice cooker has a capacity for nine cups of cooked rice. The main heater functions at 550 Watts, and the warmer at 45 Watts.

Packaging. The cooked rice was cooled to room temperature and packed into Scotchpack 16" Mylar-Polyethylene boil-in-the-bag, and sealed with an electric sealer. It is important to minimize the air content of the head space before sealing. Unless otherwise mentioned, the cooked and packaged samples were stored at -23°C (-10°F) in a walk-in freezer room.

Freezing and Storage. To study the effect of storage temperature on quality, the packaged, cooked samples were stored at 25°, 12°, 0°, -12° and -18°C, respectively. Precautions were taken to avoid microbial growth on samples stored at 25, 12, and 0°C by the use of 0.5% potassium sorbate and 25 ppm sodium hypochlorite on a w/w basis.

Effect of Freezing Process. The packaged and cooked rice samples were frozen in a Conrad blast freezer (Barber Colman Co., Rockford, IL) at -40°C, a Freeze-Cel plate contact freezer (Dole Refrigerating Products Co. Ltd., Lewisburg, Oakville, Ont., Canada) at -20°C, and a walk-in freezer room at -18°C, respectively. The frozen and packaged products were stored at -18°C after the freezing process, and tested for quality at 0, 1, 5 and 10 days after freezing.

Starch Degradation Test

Iodine Adsorption. One mL of the sample containing 2% gelatinized starch and 10 mL of phosphate buffer at pH 7 were mixed. Five mL of the mixture were centrifuged at 12,000 × g for 15 min at 3°C. One mL of the centrifugate was mixed with 10 mL of iodine solution (0.01% I_2 and 0.02% KI in water). The optical density of the solution was read at 590 nm with a Bausch and Lomb Spectronic 20. The test measures the amount of iodine taken up by the amylose component.

Moisture Content. The milled rice was ground to pass a 20-mesh screen. Two g of the rice powder were weighed into a tared aluminum weighing dish. The dishes were dried in a vacuum oven at 70°C for five h, transferred into a desiccator, and cooled to room temperature. The dishes were weighed again on an analytical balance. The average of four readings was recorded. Similar conditions were used for determining the moisture content of cooked rice samples by the vacuum-oven drying method.

Texture. A Lee-Kramer shear press equipped with an electronic recording attachment was used for texture evaluation of the cooked rice. The frozen rice samples were thawed and allowed to reach room temperature (23-25°C) before testing. Fifty g of rice were weighed into a cylindrical cell (5.25 inner diameter × 4.3 cm height). A plunger consisting of 25 small cylindrical rods (0.4 cm diameter and 6.2 cm in length) was used to penetrate the rice sample. The plunger was adjusted to move downward at a rate of 42 s per stroke. A 500 lb gauge ring and a 0-100 attenuation were used. The area under the time-force curve was measured in square inches with a Hruden planimeter. The results are expressed as apparent work in ft-lbs. by multiplying the area in square inches by the factor 6.25. Four determinations were made for each sample; the average is reported.

Cohesiveness. Cohesiveness (stickiness) of the cooked rice was measured objectively in a cohesive meter made in our machine shop. It consists of a plastic plate (20.2 × 19.7 × 2.5 cm). Two cylindrical aluminum cylindrical dishes were hung, one on the left and one on the right side of a pulley with a chain. Twenty g of cooked rice were weighed onto the plastic plate just above the left side aluminum dish (A), and a weight of 1,500 g was placed on top of it for 15 s. The weights were then removed from dish A, and lead shots were slowly added to the aluminum dish (B) on the right side which was also connected to the pulley. The added lead shot were weighed and recorded as weight required to detach the aluminum dish A. The average of 15 readings was recorded. Cohesiveness may be defined as the work required to lift the aluminum dish (4.8 cm diameter × 4 cm deep) from the rice pressed for 15 s with 1,500 g of weight.

Sensory Evaluation. Sensory characteristics of the freshly cooked and various frozen samples were tested by a trained panel of 15 members, using a partially balanced block design (Pangborn 1984). The panel members rated the samples for aroma, cohesiveness, tenderness and flavor on a 1-10 scale as follows: 9-10, excellent; 7-8, good; 5-6, fair; 3-4, poor; and 1-2, very poor.

Frozen and stored rice was heated in the sealed plastic bag in a boiling water bath for 12 min and served simultaneously with fresh cooked rice for sensory comparisons.

RESULTS AND DISCUSSION

Effect of Time and Temperature on Water Absorption

The effect of soaking time on the rate of hydration of Calrose rice was studied. The grains were soaked in an excess of distilled water at 25°C for various time intervals. The moisture content of the soaked samples increased with time during the first 30 min. An equilibrium moisture level of 30-31% was reached in 30 + min. Further soaking resulted in no significant increase in moisture content of the rice (Fig. 1).

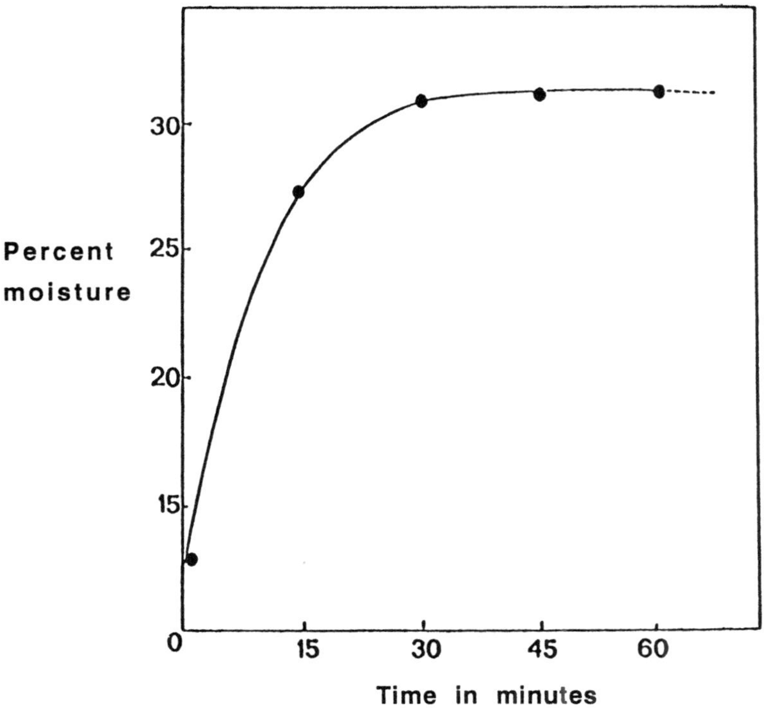

FIG. 1. RATE OF HYDRATION OF CALROSE RICE AT 25°C

The penetration of moisture through soaking assured no hard center in the cooked rice, a phenomenon that may occur when cooking is done manually. Failure to yield a cooked rice of satisfactory texture results from improper W/R ratio. Long grain rice (*0. indica*) may need a W/R ratio of 1.8 to 2.0 for satisfactory texture after cooking.

Effect of W/R Ratio on Texture

Results on the effect of water/rice (W/R) ratio on texture of the cooked rice is presented in Fig. 2. The sample with lower W/R ratio (0.75) gave a cooked product of firmer texture than those with higher ones. The sample prepared with highest W/R ratio of 1.75 (350 ml water/200 gm rice) resulted in a cooked product of very soft texture. All

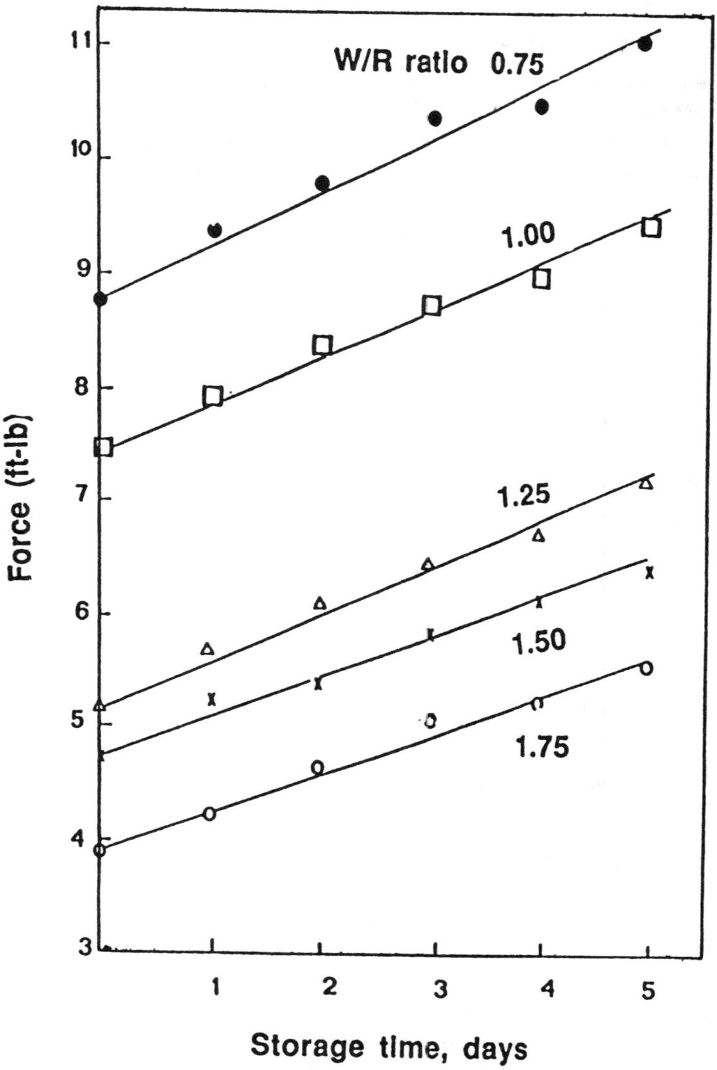

FIG. 2. EFFECT OF WATER/RICE RATIO ON TEXTURE OF COOKED CALROSE RICE (25°C)

the samples showed an increase in firmness during storage at 25°C. Since starch is the major component of rice, this phenomenon may be explained by the retrogradation of the gelatinized starch after the rice is cooked. Rice starch is composed of a branched fraction (amylopectin) and a linear fraction (amylose). The major linkage is alpha-1,4-D-glucopyranoside, but amylopectin contains, in addition, the alpha-1,6-D-glucopyranoside linkage at branch points. The degree of branching of amylopectin is 4-5%, a mean chain length of 20 to 28 anhydroglucose units has been determined by peroxidation. Amylopectin is the major fraction of rice starch. The amylose content of non-waxy milled rice is classified by Webb (1991) as follows: long grain, 21-23%; medium grain, 15-20%; and short grain, 15-20%. The amylose/amylopectin ratio is the most important factor determining the texture and eating quality of cooked rice. Table 1 lists the physicochemical characteristics of long, medium and short grain rice.

TABLE 1.
PHYSICOCHEMICAL (QUALITY) CHARACTERISTICS OF CONVENTIONAL COOKING AND PROCESSING LONG-, MEDIUM-, AND SHORT-GRAIN RICE TYPES

Milled Rice Characteristics	Conventional Cooking and Processing Type		
	Long	Medium	Short
Apparent amylose content, %	21-23	15-20	15-20
Alkali spreading value, average	3-5	5.5-7	5.5-7
Gelatinization temperature[a] °C	69-72	64-68	64-68
Gelatinization temperature type	Intermediate	Low	Low
Protein (N × 5.95), %	6-8	6-8	6-8
Amylographic paste viscosity, BU[b]			
Peak	650-850	700-900	700-900
Hot	350-400	350-400	350-400
Cool	650-850	650-800	650-800
Breakdown	300-400	350-450	350-450
Setback	-150- +150	-250- -50	-250- -50

[a]Amylographic gelatinization temperature.
[b]Bu = Brabender Units.
Source: Based on measurements of fully developed mature grains of conventional varieties within each grain type. Results of tests conducted at the Regional Rice Quality Laboratory, Beaumont, TX; adapted in part from Webb (1991).

Starch retrogradation involves the realignment and association of the starch chains, commonly thought to be amylose in dilute solution with formation of some crystalline structure. The latter can be determined by the increase in the crystalline X-ray diffraction pattern during retrogradation. Amylose is known to retrograde rapidly, particularly in dilute dilutions. Amylopectin retrogrades more slowly in starch systems where water availability is limited (Matsukura *et al.* 1983). They proposed a structure for retrograded starch where amylose-amylose, amylose-amylopectin and amylopectin-amylopectin associations occur. The medium grain rice (*O. japonia*) used in this study is well liked by many consumers in Oriental countries. The percentage of rice produced in the United States may vary from year to year, depending on the market demand. The long-grain rice (*O. indica*) usually accounts for 6% of the total production; medium-grain, 30%; and short-grain, the remainder (Childs 1989).

Cohesiveness. Effect of W/R ratio on cohesiveness of cooked rice is presented in Table 2. Measurements were conducted on cooked samples stored at 25°, 12°, and 0°C for one to five days. Preliminary studies indicated that rice samples stored at -12°C and -25°C which do not stick to the plate of the device is attributable to changes in W/R relationship. Results obtained here indicated some discrepancy of the results reported by Ozaki (1973) on changes of adhesiveness of cooked rice during storage and thawing. The cooked, frozen rice stored at -12° and -25°C and then thawed did not stick to the plate of the cohesiveness tester. It appears that water in the cooked rice became detached from the rice gel upon freezing and thawing. The resulting thawed rice did not return to its original cohesiveness.

Starch is an important constituent of rice, representing more than two-thirds of its dry weight. Starch in medium grain rice gelatinizes at 68-78°C. During cooking, in the presence of sufficient water, the starch granules swell. The amylopectin and amylose molecules also become hydrated, and the viscosity of the cooked rice increases. During granule swelling, some amylose diffuses from the granule and results in increase in viscosity. Much of the initially available water is adbsorbed to the starch granules during gelatinization, leaving a reduced quantity of unbound water to accommodate the solubilized starch, thereby causing the increase in viscosity.

Mitsuda and Nakajima (1977) immersed polished rice in 0.5% acetic acid for 10 min and then cooked the rice in the same acidified solution. The cooked rice was made into discs and kept in air-tight film bags at 30°C for 15 days. These discs had good retention of textural characteristics even after the longer storage period. Discs prepared by adding a small amount of 4.2% acetic acid to the cooked product exhibited better textural properties after storage. These treatments reportedly inhibit browning and retrogradation of the starch as well as growth of lactic acid bacteria and fungi. In Japan, the summer is hot and humid, and the smell, taste and appearance of cooked rice quickly turn bad due to drying, browning and the growth of bacteria and fungus. The present experiments confirm the work of Mitsuda and Nakajima (1977) that the texture of cooked rice became firmer while the cohesiveness of the cooked rice decreased during storage.

Sensory Evaluation. The effect of W/R ratio on the sensory quality of frozen rice is presented in Table 3. The samples were stored at -25°C, thawed and tested together with a freshly cooked sample at the end of 1, 3, and 6 months. Panel scores showed preference for the rice with a W/R ratio of 1.25, in cohesiveness and tenderness. The average aroma and flavor scores were highest in the sample with W/R ratio of 1.5.

The cohesiveness scores of the cooked rice decreased as the W/R ratio increased (Table 3, column 1). Storage of the samples at -25°C resulted in a slight decrease in aroma and flavor scores. The effect of storage at -25°C for 6 months on the sensory

TABLE 2.
EFFECT OF WATER/RICE (W/R) RATIO ON COHESIVENESS OF PRECOOKED CALROSE RICE DURING STORAGE

	Weight of lead shots (gm)[a]																	
Water to rice ratio	at 25°C Storage Time (days)						at 12°C Storage Time (days)						at 0°C Storage Time (days)					
w/r	0	1	2	3	4	5	0	1	2	3	4	5	0	1	2	3	4	5
0.75	174±3	163±4	161±5	158±4	140±6	-	-	151±9	143±8	135±5	128±6	115±5	-	132±7	116±10	111±9	104±8	100±1
1.00	183±2	177±3	166±6	165±9	144±7	-	-	162±6	151±7	144±8	130±5	122±5	-	135±5	118±7	115±8	109±9	106±1
1.25	197±4	135±4	174±4	170±6	156±8	-	-	167±5	159±9	150±12	146±8	135±3	-	142±8	130±6	123±10	114±9	110±9
1.50	204±4	192±4	183±5	189±5	180±7	-	-	179±4	162±6	160±5	143±9	141±6	-	148±9	121±7	119±11	123±10	141±8
1.75	226±3	220±2	208±3	194±5	188±6	-	-	181±3	171±5	158±7	150±7	149±2	-	157±6	136±9	138±7	132±7	129±6

[a]The average of 15 measurements were recorded.

TABLE 3.
EFFECT OF WATER/RICE (W/R) RATIO AND STORAGE ON SENSORY QUALITY OF FROZEN CALROSE RICE

Water to rice ratio	Cohesiveness Storage time (months)				Aroma Storage time (months)				Flavor Storage time (months)				Tenderness Storage time (months)			
(w/r)	0(fresh)	1	3	6	0	1	3	6	0	1	3	6	0	1	3	6
0.75	8.53	9.30	9.26	9.30	5.30	5.24	5.15	5.10	6.27	6.30	6.25	6.22	6.75	5.70	5.63	5.60
1.00	8.12	8.27	8.30	8.42	5.41	5.30	5.35	5.27	6.35	6.20	6.31	6.25	7.58	7.40	7.58	7.43
1.25	8.20	8.25	8.28	8.24	8.05	7.64	7.52	7.45	8.43	8.15	8.05	8.05	9.50	9.55	9.47	9.60
1.50	5.45	5.30	5.60	5.62	9.32	8.85	8.80	8.85	9.64	9.20	9.31	9.25	5.36	5.40	5.42	5.45
1.75	3.80	5.03	5.25	5.30	9.04	8.70	8.75	8.64	8.32	8.31	8.25	8.20	4.40	4.35	4.48	4.45
L.S.D. (P=.05)	0.40	0.53	0.49	0.70	0.48	0.65	0.67	0.38	0.56	0.72	0.52	0.44	0.76	0.74	0.53	0.62

[a]The panel score was based on a 1-10 scale: Excellent, 9-10; Good, 7-8; Fair, 5-6; Poor, 3-4; and Very Poor, 1-2.

quality of the products is presented. The samples cooked with W/R ratio of 1.25 to 1.50 were scored high in the frozen product. The least significant difference (L.S.D.) of the sensory scores are presented in Table 3. It appears that the cohesiveness and tenderness scores of the samples decreased rapidly when the W/R ratio was at 1.5, and even more at 1.75. Thus, the W/R ratio is a very important factor influencing the sensory quality of cooked rice.

Effect of Freezing Methods on Starch Degradation of Precooked Rice

Effect of freezing methods on texture (shear-press values) and starch retrogradation of the rice samples during storage at -18°C for different time intervals are presented in Table 4. The sample frozen in the room freezer (-25°C) and the plate contact freezer (-20°C) yielded higher shear-press values than samples frozen in the blast freezer (-40°C) indicating an increase in hardening in the slower freezing process. Among the three methods, the blast freezer method resulted in a more rapid cooling than the other two methods. The phenomenon may be explained in terms of ice-crystal formation. Slower freezing rates result in formation of larger ice crystals, faster rate of freezing results in formation of smaller ice crystals. Smaller ice crystals have less effect on the structure of the original material. Amolopectin is known to be slower in rate of retrogradation than amylose. After thawing, samples frozen in the blast freezer yielded a softer and more tender rice which coincides with the results on sensory evaluation by the panel members. Results from iodine adsorption corresponded to the shear-press tests. Freezing precooked rice caused rapid starch retrogradation which affects the physical and sensory quality of

TABLE 4.
EFFECT OF FREEZING METHODS AND FREEZING STORAGE ON TEXTURE (SHEAR PRESS VALUE) AND STARCH RETROGRADATION OF PRECOOKED CALROSE RICE STORED AT -18.3°C

	Storage time in days					
	1	3	5	7	9	Reheat H
A. Texture (shear press value in ft-lb)						
Blast freezer (-40°C)	6.16	7.03	8.35	9.46	10.20	5.26
Plate freezer (-20°C)	6.24	7.35	8.96	10.21	10.88	5.84
Room freezer (-25°C)	6.49	8.76	10.48	10.87	11.01	5.92
Freshly cooked - 5.75						
B. Retrogradation index by I_2 absorption method						
Blast	49.1	50.2	50.8	54.8	57.6	
Plate	52.2	54.3	57.5	61.2	65.3	
Room	53.3	59.4	67.2	71.9	75.3	

the rice. Throughout the present study, retrogradation of the gelatinized Calrose rice starch varied with different treatments. The bases of the differences are relative solubility and crystallinity of the gelatinized starch. Upon cooling in a dilute starch solution, the amylose molecules realign themselves by hydrogen bonding into an insoluble precipitate. In concentrated starch solutions, realignment is rapid and disordered. Association of the starch molecules occurs at limited locations and water is entrapped at the interstices.

Effect of Soy Oil/Surfactant

Experiments were carried out to study the effect of soy oil and Tween 60 surfactant in the cooking water followed by storage of the cooked rice at 0°C on texture of the cooked rice. Table 4 indicates firming of texture during frozen-storage. Addition of soy oil/surfactant to the cooking water reduced adhesiveness and resulted in good kernel separation. This is due to the compatibility of hydrophilic components of the surfactant with the hydrophilic surface of the rice; the kernels do not stick together. As the oil-surfactant forms a continuous film on the surface of rice kernel, the oily material becomes oriented on the outer portion of the coating with the hydrophobic-hydrophilic structure of the emulsion and acts as a bridge or bond between the oil and rice surface. Application of the oil emulsion did not significantly affect the rate or extent of retrogradation of the starch material, but it did improve the flavor acceptance of the product. In general, addition of oils to foods increase the flavor acceptance of the products by providing lubrication during the mastication process. The taste buds are activated by the presence of the oil film.

CONCLUSIONS

Medium grain Calrose rice (*Oryza sativa L, japonica*) has been very popular in the Asiatic countries as a staple food. This work demonstrates the importance of the W/R ratio in influencing the sensory quality of the cooked products. Addition of soy oil and Tween 60 as a surfactant improved grain separation and flavor acceptance of the cooked and frozen products. Important factors influencing the quality of frozen rice were the W/R ratio, and soaking condition before cooking. Marked difference in physical, chemical and sensory quality of the frozen rice was observed as related to freezing methods and storage temperature.

REFERENCES

BHATTACHARYA, K.R., SOWBHOGYA, C.M. and SWAMY, Y.M. 1982. Quality profiles of rice. A tentative scheme for classification. J. Text. Studies *47*:564.

BOGGS, M.M., SINNOTT, C.E., VASAK, O.K. and KESTER, E.R. 1951. Frozen cooked rice. Food Technol. *5*, 530.

CHILDS, N.W. 1989. U.S. Rice Distribution Patterns. U.S. Dept. Agric., ERS, Statistical Bull. 776, Washington, D.C.

FELLERS, D.A., MOSSMAN, A.P. and SUZUKI, H. 1983. Rice stickiness II. Application of an Instron method to make some varietal comparisons and study modification of milled rice by hot air treatment and other methods. Cereal Chem. *60*, 292.

JULIANO, B.O. *et al.* 1984. International cooperative test on texture of cooked rice. J. Text. Studies *15*, 357–376.

KUMAR, B.M., UPADHYAY, J.K. and BHATTACHARYA, K.R. 1976. Objective tests for stickiness of cooked rice. J. Text. Studies *7*, 271–278.

LaBELL, F. 1994. Faster cooking rice with integrity. Prepared Foods *163*(2), 65.

LUH, B.S. 1991. Canning, freezing and freeze-drying. *In*: Rice Utilization, Vol. II, second Ed., Chap. 7, pp. 147–175. Edited by B.S. Luh. An Avi Book, published by Van Nostrand Reinhold, New York.

LUH, B.S. 1991. Rice Utilization, Vol. II, Second Edition. An Avi Book, Van Nostrand, Reinhold, New York.

MALLETT, C.P. 1993. Frozen Food Technology. Blackie Academic & Professional. An Imprint of Chapman and Hall, London.

MATSUKURA, U., MATSUNAGA, A. and KAINUMA, K. 1983. Structural studies on retrograded normal and waxy corn starches. J. Japan Soc. Starch Sci. (Denpun Kagaka) *30*, 106–113.

MITSUDA, H. and NAKAJIMA, K. 1977. Storage of cooked rice. J. Food Sci. *42*, 1439–1443.

OLALQUIAGA, R., GUINARD, J-X. and SINGH, R.P. 1986. Effect of parboiling and freezing on quality of three Spanish rice varieties. J. Food Process. Preserv. *10*(3), 189.

OZAKI, N. 1973. Retrogradation of cooked rice (Part 2): Change of adhesiveness of cooked rice. J. Jap. Soc. Food Nutrit. *26*, 289.

PANGBORN, R.M. 1984. Sensory analysis as an analytical laboratory tool in food research. *In*: Modern Methods of Food Analysis (Edited by K.K. Stewart and J.R. Whitaker), p. 265, Avi Publishing Co., Westport, CT.

PERSSON, P.O. and LONDAHL, G. 1993. Freezing Technology. Edited by C.P. Mallett, Chap. 2, pp. 20–58. Blackie Academic & Professional. An Imprint of Chapman and Hall, London.

RICHARDSON, T. and FINLEY, J.W. 1985. Chemical Changes in Food During Processing. Avi Publishing Co., Inc., Westport, CT.

SHAEVEL, M.L. 1993. Manufacturing of frozen prepared meals. *In*: Frozen Food Technology, edited by C.P. Mallett, Chap. 10, pp. 270–302. Blackie Academic & Professional, An Imprint of Chapman and Hall, London.

STONE, H., SIDEL, J.L. and BLOOMQUIST, J. 1980. Quantitative descriptive analysis. Cereal Foods World *25*, 642.

WEBB, B.D. 1991. Rice quality and grades. *In*: Rice Utilization, Vol. II, Second edition, Chap. 5, pp. 89–119. Edited by B.S. Luh, Van Nostrand Reinhold, New York.

ENHANCING THE BIOSYNTHESIS OF ENDOGENOUS METHIONINE-RICH PROTEINS (MRP) TO IMPROVE THE PROTEIN QUALITY OF LEGUMES VIA GENETIC ENGINEERING

ALFREDO F. GALVEZ, M. JAMELA REVILLEZA, BENITO O. DE LUMEN and DEANNE C. KRENZ

Division of Nutritional Sciences and Toxicology
University of California
Berkeley, CA 94720-3104

ABSTRACT

The full nutritional potential of legume protein is limited by the relative deficiency of sulfur amino acids. A strategy we use is to increase the biosynthesis of non-abundant, endogenous methionine-rich protein (MRP) we identified in soybean seed. A cDNA (designated as Gm2S-1) encoding a novel MRP isolated from soybean cotyledon, the first ever cloned from a legume, has been isolated and characterized. The Gm2S-1 cDNA codes for a pre-proprotein that contains a signal peptide and a hydrophilic precursor protein that undergoes post-translational processing to generate a 43 amino acid small subunit (SSU), a 77 amino acid large subunit (LSU) and a 17 amino acid linker polypeptide. The LSU is a cotyledon-specific 8 kDa MRP containing 7.8% methionine and is also rich in lysine (13.0%) and cysteine (7.8%) with the precursor protein having balanced amounts of the other essential amino acids. Homology comparisons with other 2S albumins show that the encoded Gm2S-1 protein sequence is unique, and represents a new subclass which shares structural features with other albumins such as proteolytic cleavage sites and conserved locations of cysteine residues. The Gm2S-1 gene is an ideal candidate for overexpression to improve the nutritional quality of soybean and other legumes not only because of its high methionine content but also because of its high content of lysine which is commonly the first limiting essential amino acid in legume-cereal mixtures.

NUTRITIONAL RATIONALE AND GOALS

Methionine is the first limiting essential amino acid in legumes because the major storage proteins in legumes, the globulins, contain low amounts of this amino acid. Cysteine, although not an essential amino acid, is included with methionine because it has a sparing effect on methionine when added to the diet. This relative deficiency of legumes in sulfur amino acids, combined with its high lysine content, makes legumes nutritionally complementary with cereals which are first limiting in lysine and relatively high in methionine. Consequently, the overall protein quality of cereal-legume mixtures is better than that of either protein source alone.

Supplementation of legumes with free methionine improves their value in supporting animal growth and increases the efficiency of utilization of dietary protein (Bressani and Elias 1968). In the feeds of poultry and swine where soybean is the main protein source, methionine is used as a supplement. Little practical use of supplementation in human diets has been made despite clinical studies with humans demonstrating its effectiveness.

The rapid accumulation of knowledge about gene expression and regulation in plants has led to development of strategies to improve the nutritional quality of plant proteins through genetic engineering. The strategies for legume proteins have been discussed in a recent review and the reader is referred to this (de Lumen and Uchimiya 1997). Briefly, these are:

(a) introduction of methionine residues into major seed storage proteins;
(b) transfer of heterologous genes encoding MRP from other species;
(c) manipulation of key enzymes in biosynthetic pathways of essential amino acids;
(d) increasing the level of endogenous, non-abundant MRP in the target legume.

What would be the nutritional target of genetic engineering to enhance the protein quality of legumes? The sulfur amino acid requirements of humans and animals vary with age, with infants requiring the most (42 mg/g) and adults the least and growing pigs requiring more (48 mg/g) than human infants (FAO 1985). It is recommended that the essential amino acid requirement pattern of 2-5 year old children (25 mg/g) be used to evaluate protein quality for all ages, except those for infants (FAO 1985). Accordingly, the methionine + cysteine content of legumes has to be increased to approximately 25 mg/g protein to meet the requirements for humans except infants, to 42 mg/g protein for human infants and to 48 mg/g protein for swine. The digestibility of legume protein, which varies from 72-98%, also has to be considered. Taking soybean as an example, its average methionine + cysteine content of 22 mg/g protein (Liener 1978) has to be increased by 14% (for humans), by 91% (for infants) and by 118% (for swine). The average contents would have to be higher when protein digestibility is taken into consideration and for other beans whose methionine + cysteine contents are generally lower than those of soybean. In any case, animal feeding trials need to be carried out to establish the actual nutritional value of transgenic seeds.

ENHANCING THE BIOSYNTHESIS OF ENDOGENOUS METHIONINE-RICH PROTEINS

The strategy we have chosen in our laboratory to improve the nutritional quality of soybean protein is to enhance the biosynthesis of non-abundant, endogenous MRP. This could have the following advantages: (a) increasing the level of an endogenous protein is unlikely to be deleterious to the seed; (b) as a homologous protein, the MRP is expected to be processed and transported correctly and is less subject to proteolytic degradation; (c) the gene encoding MRP, as a homologous gene, could lead to a more stable integration into the host genome; (d) the finding that the transgenic Brazil nut MRP in soybean is allergenic to humans (Nordlee *et al.* 1996), adds significance to the search for non-allergenic MRP. Although it remains to be proven, the soybean MRP that we have isolated might have the additional advantage of non-allergenicity since it belongs to a MW class which has not been shown to be allergenic.

Our laboratory established that the MRPs are localized in the albumin (water soluble) fraction of soybean protein using a method based on the specific alkylation of the thioether moiety in methionine with [1-^{14}C]-iodoacetic acid (de Lumen and Kho 1987;

Kho and de Lumen 1988). Resolution of total protein by 2D-SDS PAGE identified a 10.8 kDa protein that has 12.1% methionine and although the N-terminus was sequenced, the insufficiency of MRP resulted in some ambiguity of the sequence (George and de Lumen 1991). Enrichment of the albumin fraction for the low molecular weight components by heparin affinity chromatography followed by 2D-SDS PAGE revealed three 8 kDa MRPs with different pI (Revilleza *et al.* 1996). The N-terminus of the most abundant and most acidic of the three MRPs, previously called 2D-1, was sequenced and the encoding cDNA, now termed Gm2S-1, has been cloned and characterized (Galvez *et al.* 1997). This is the first MRP cDNA ever cloned from a legume and is distinct from the cDNA coding for a cysteine-rich but methionine-poor albumin cloned from pea (Higgins *et al.* 1986).

Features of the Gm2S-1 DNA and Protein

The Gm2S-1 cDNA containing the open reading frame of the full length protein is found within the 1.5 kb EcoRI-BamHI fragment near the 3' end of a 2.5 kb clone (Fig. 1), isolated from a library prepared from midmaturation mRNA of soybean seed. Because of the chimeric nature of the 2.5 kb cDNA clone, the transcription initiation site of the Gm2S-1 coding region was not resolved although the ATG start site was present. Using a modified cRACE protocol (Maruyama *et al.* 1995), the transcription initiation site was established and is located 17 bp away from the ATG translation start site.

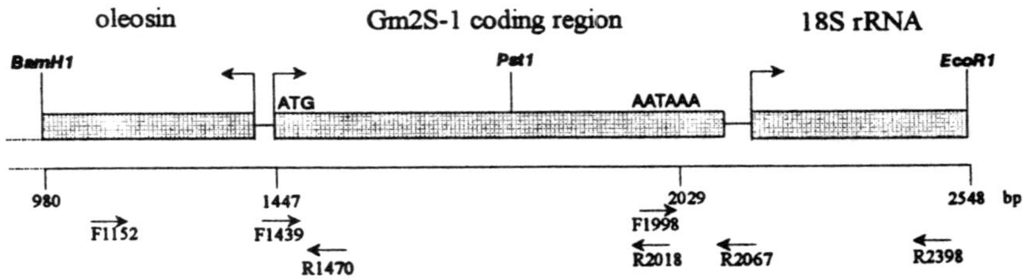

FIG. 1. DIAGRAM OF THE 1.5 KB *BAMH1-ECOR1* FRAGMENT CONTAINING THE COMPLETE CODING AND 3' UNTRANSLATED REGIONS OF GM2S-1 CDNA

The fragment is found at the 3' end of the chimeric 2.5 kb cDNA clone that was isolated from a mid-maturation cDNA library. The 1.5 kb fragment also contains a 326 bp cDNA fragment of 18S rRNA and a 628 bp fragment of a soybean oleosin gene that flank the Gm2S-1 cDNA at the 3' and 5' end, respectively. The primers used to obtain the complete DNA sequence and to generate the Gm2S-1 specific amplified product are shown as directional arrows from 5' to 3' below the diagram.

The Gm2S-1 cDNA encodes a 158-amino acid protein. The first 21 amino acids corresponds to a signal peptide sequence which is characteristically hydrophobic while the rest of the molecule is hydrophilic (Fig. 2). A search revealed that the next 43 amino

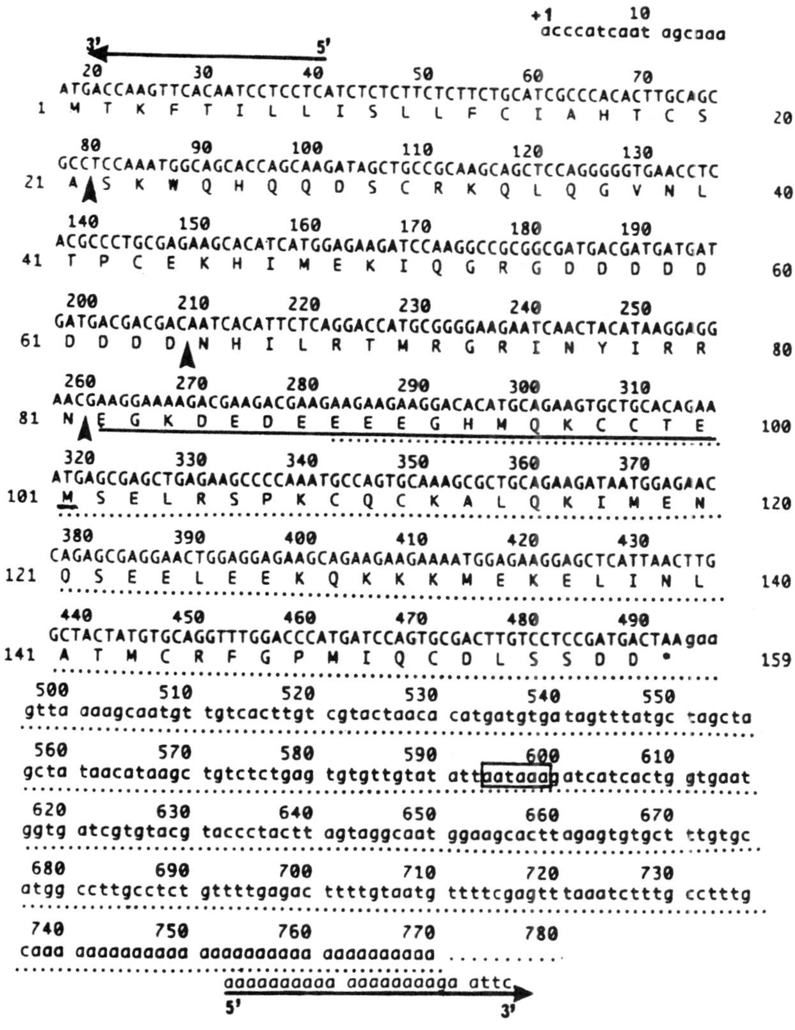

FIG. 2. COMPLETE DNA SEQUENCE AND ENCODED TRANSLATION PRODUCT OF THE GM2S-1 CDNA CLONE

Lower case letters denote the untranslated region of the cDNA while the coding region is in upper case letters. Arrows indicate the proteolytic cleavage sites of the precursor protein. The boxed DNA sequence shows the putative polyadenylation signal. Solid line shows the location of the 20 amino acid N-terminal sequence obtained from the microsequencing of the purified 8 kDa MRP (Revilleza *et al.* 1996), which differed from the encoded protein only by the substitution of alanine with cysteine at residue 17. Dotted line indicates the location and sequence of the PCR product that was generated from RACE and used as a probe to isolate the 2.5 kb cDNA clone from a mid-maturation soybean cotyledon cDNA library. Line arrows indicate the location of the oligo(dA)18-*EcoR1* and the Gm2S-1 specific primer used in cRACE to determine the transcription start site (+1).

acid segment (SSU) has 100% homology with an aspartic acid-rich peptide isolated from dried mature soybean seed (Odani *et al.* 1987). Post-translational processing should therefore include cleavage sites after 21-alanine and 64-aspartic acid to release the SSU. Based on the N-terminal sequence of the Gm2S-1 protein (Revilleza *et al.* 1996), there is a putative proteolytic cleavage site between 81-asparagine and 82-glutamic acid giving rise to a 77 amino acid polypeptide that corresponds to the mature 8 kDa Gm2S-1 protein (LSU) and a 17 amino acid linker peptide between the SSU and the LSU.

Figure 3 shows the hydrophobicity profile of the complete Gm2S-1 protein. Except for the 21 amino acid N-terminus that comprises the hydrophobic signal peptide, the pro-Gm2S-1 protein is mainly hydrophilic. The proteolytic cleavage sites corresponding to the asparagine residues at positions 65 and 81 are located at the most hydrophilic regions of the Gm2S-1 precursor protein.

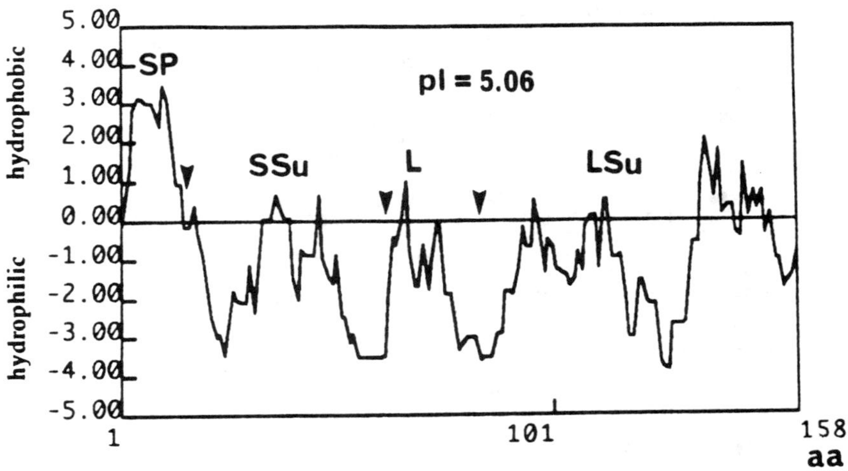

FIG. 3. HYDROPHOBICITY PLOT OF THE GM2S-1 PRECURSOR PROTEIN AS DETERMINED USING THE KYTE-DOOLITTLE ALGORITHM (1982) IN THE MACDNASIS SEQUENCE ANALYSIS PROGRAM

Arrows indicate the location of the putative proteolytic cleavage sites that produce the hydrophobic 21 amino acid signal peptide (SP) and the mainly hydrophilic propeptide. Note that the two proteolytic sites in the precursor propeptide that separates the small subunit (SSU), linker (L) and the large subunit (LSU) is located in the most hydrophilic region of the protein.

Multiple sequence alignment analysis with other 2S albumins (Fig. 4) showed that, like Gm2S-1, the albumins from Brazil nut, *Arabidopsis* and *Brassica napus* all contain a 21-22 amino acid signal peptide and undergo two proteolytic cleavages to generate mature heterodimeric proteins. Except for the identity of the SSU with the previously reported soybean aspartic acid-rich peptide, the rest of Gm2S-1 protein shows no

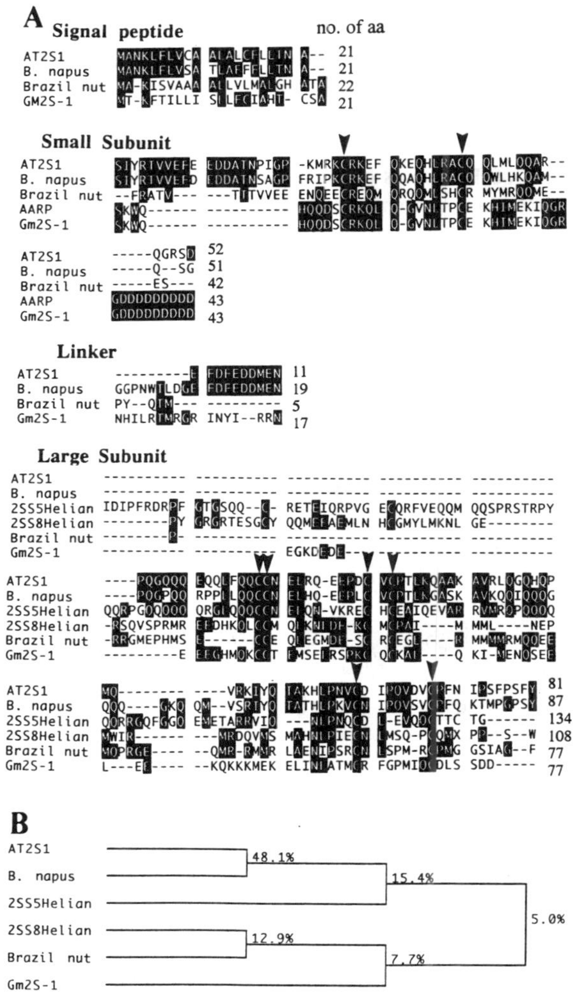

FIG. 4. SEQUENCE HOMOLOGY COMPARISON OF COMPONENT POLYPEPTIDES AMONG THE DIFFERENT 2S ALBUMINS UPON PROTEOLYTIC CLEAVAGE OF PRECURSOR PROTEINS

A: Multiple sequence alignments were done using the Higgins-Sharp algorithm (1988) in the MacDNASIS sequence analysis software (Hitachi). Shaded regions indicate 2 or more sequence match upon alignment. The signal peptide, SSU and linker polypeptides were compared among the dimeric 2S albumins from *Arabidopsis* (AT2S1), *Brassica napus* (*B. napus*), Brazil nut and Gm2S-1 including the aspartic acid-rich polypeptide that has a 100% sequence homology to the small subunit of Gm2S-1. Comparisons among the LSU included the monomeric 2S albumins from sunflower (2SS5Helian and 2SS8Helian). Arrows indicate the location of the conserved cysteine residues in the small and large subunits. B: Phylogenetic tree showing sequence homology among the LSU sequences as determined from the Higgins and Sharp (1988) pairwise sequence similarity algorithm in the MacDNASIS sequence analysis program (Hitachi).

significant homology with the other 2S albumins. However, the locations of cysteine residues in both SSU and LSU are conserved among the different plant species, indicating that the Gm2S-1 is related to other members of the 2S albumin family in secondary and tertiary structure rather than sequence homology.

Using a PCR fragment that contains the Gm2S-1 coding region as a probe, a transcript of about 700 bp size is detected as early as 3 weeks after flowering which persists up to 7 weeks but is completely absent in the mature seed. Maximal expression is observed at 5-6 weeks after flowering (Fig 5). The 700 bp Gm2S-1 transcript is present only in the cotyledon (5 weeks after flowering) and not in any other tissue (pod, leaf, root, and stem).

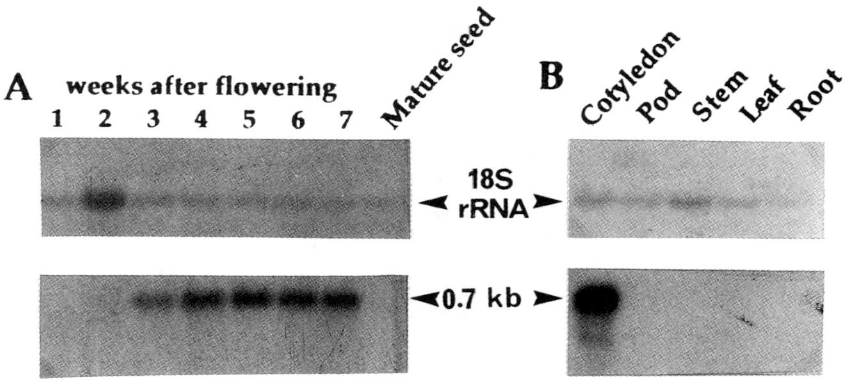

FIG. 5. NORTHERN ANALYSIS SHOWING TEMPORAL (A) AND SEED-SPECIFIC (B) EXPRESSION OF THE GM2S-1 CDNA

Approximately 20 μg of total RNAs isolated from developing soybean seeds and from other plant tissues was electrophoresed in a 1.5% denaturing agarose gel, and transferred to Hybond-N membrane by capillary transfer. The Northern blots were probed with a ^{32}P-labeled PCR fragment containing the full-length Gm2S-1 coding region and a 326 bp PCR fragment of the 18S rRNA cDNA that was used as an internal control to show equal loading of total RNA in each lane.

To compare the levels of Gm2S-1 mRNA and the 8 kDa Gm2S-1 protein at different stages of seed development, the low molecular weight-enriched albumin fraction of seed proteins isolated at different times after flowering, were resolved in 1D-SDS PAGE and tagged for methionine residues with [1-^{14}C]-iodoacetate. Detectable levels of the 8 kDa MRP fraction are seen at 5 weeks after flowering and maintained up to maturity (Fig. 6). The appearance of the maximal level of Gm2S-1 mRNA at 5 weeks after flowering coincides with the initial detection of the 8 kDa MRP fraction. The 8 kDa MRP fraction, as noted earlier, constitutes three differently charged proteins in 2D-SDS PAGE, in which Gm2S-1 is the most abundant and acidic (Revilleza *et al.* 1996).

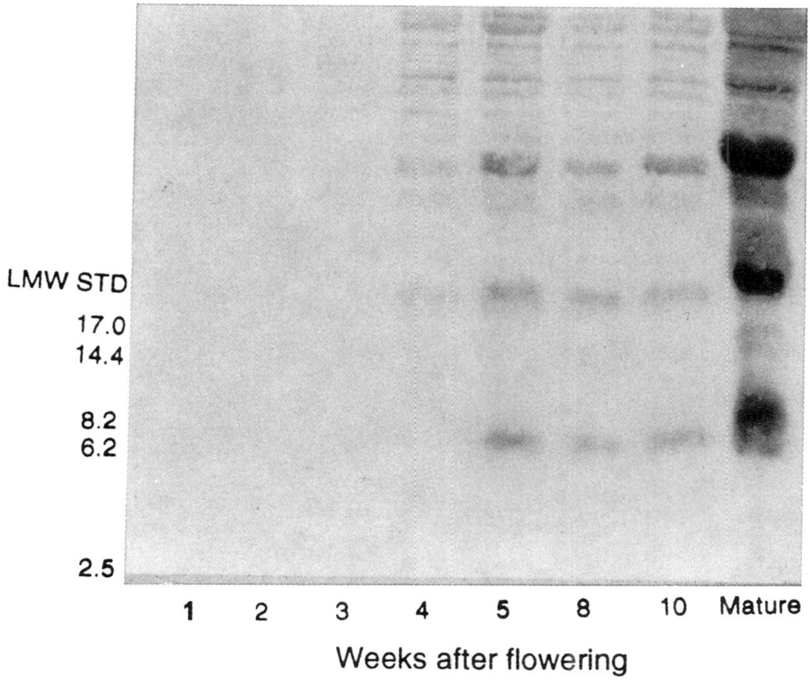

FIG. 6. AUTORADIOGRAPH OF LOW MOLECULAR WEIGHT ALBUMIN FRACTION WITH LABELED METHIONINE RESIDUES AT DIFFERENT STAGES OF SOYBEAN SEED DEVELOPMENT

One-dimensional SDS-PAGE was carried out on the low molecular weight-enriched albumin fraction isolated from developing cotyledons. The proteins were electroblotted onto Immobilon membrane (Millipore) and the methionine-containing albumins detected in the membrane by specific alkylation of the thioether moiety with [1-^{14}C]-iodoacetate.

Multiple DNA restriction fragments hybridized to the Gm2S-1 PCR probe in *HindIII*, *Eco RV*, *Pvu II*, *NcoI* and *XbaI* digests of soybean genomic DNA (Fig. 7). The Gm2S-1 cDNA, like the *Arabidopsis* 2S albumin multi-gene family (Krebbers *et al.* 1988), may not contain any introns. If this were true, the multiple fragments suggest the presence of at least two copies of the Gm2S-1 gene in the soybean haploid genome.

Amino Acid Composition of Gm2S-1 and other MRPs

The essential amino acid composition of the soybean 8 kDa MRP is compared with other MRPs whose cDNA have been cloned (Table 1). The Brazil nut MRP has been used in a number of plant species by several laboratories to increase the methionine content in seeds, resulting in varying levels of enhancement (Altenbach *et al.* 1989, 1992; de Clerq *et al.* 1990; Guerche *et al.* 1990; Saalbach *et al.* 1994). The most successful of these attempts led to an accumulation of Brazil nut MRP at levels of up to

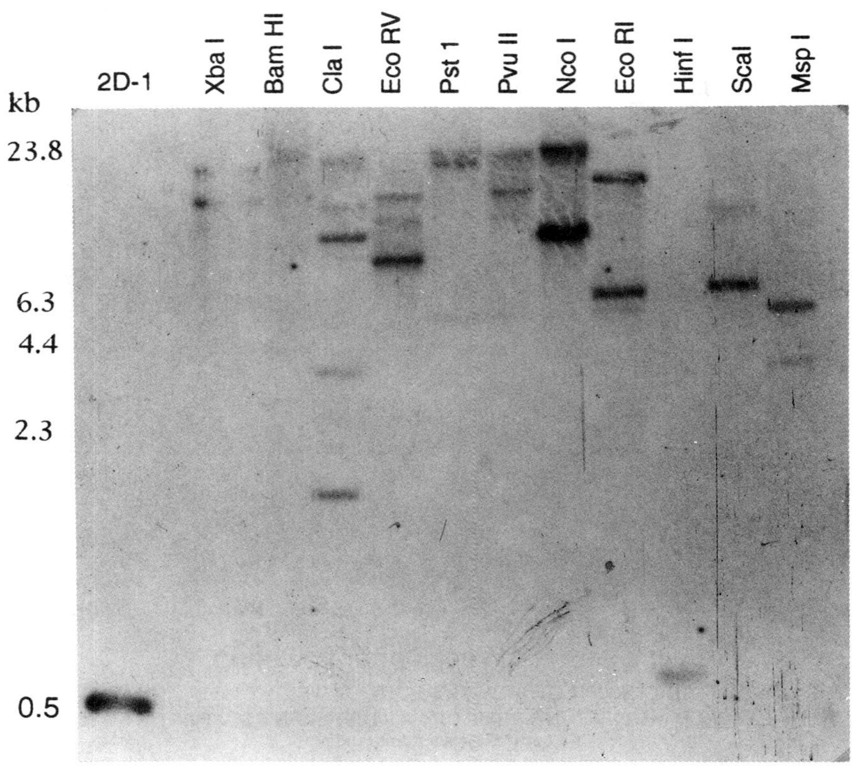

FIGURE 7. SOUTHERN ANALYSIS OF SOYBEAN GENOMIC DNA USING GM2S-1 PCR AMPLIFIED FRAGMENT AS PROBE

Eleven restriction enzymes were used to cut 10 μg of soybean genomic DNA and the resulting restriction fragments were separated on a 1% Tris-acetate agarose gel before transferring onto Genescreen Plus membrane (Dupont/NEN). Southern blots were prehybridized then hybridized with the ^{32}P-labeled Gm2S-1 PCR fragment.

8% of the total protein, equivalent to a 26% gain in methionine (Townsend *et al.* 1992; Nordlee *et al.* 1994). However, the heterologous Brazil nut MRP in transgenic soybean has been found to be allergenic (Nordlee *et al.* 1996). Soybean is a known source of allergens, although it is widely used for human foods (Shibasaki *et al.* 1980; Herian *et al.* 1990; Taylor 1992). Several allergens from soybean protein with subunit molecular weights from 14 to 60 kDa have been identified (Herian *et al.* 1990). Earlier studies in Japan have found allergenic activities in the major soy protein components, the 11 S-, 7S- and 2S-globulin fractions (Shibasaki *et al.* 1980). However, it should be noted from these studies that the low MW albumin fraction from which the Gm2S-18 kDa mature protein was isolated has not been shown to be allergenic. Nevertheless, the issue of Gm2S-1 protein allergenicity still remains to be resolved. Although the Gm2S-1 protein is endogenous to soybean, it is important to test it for allergenicity if it is to be used to enhance the nutritional quality of soybean for human consumption.

TABLE 1.
ESSENTIAL AMINO ACID COMPOSITION OF METHIONINE-RICH PROTEINS[a]

Amino acid	Corn 10 kDa	Corn 15 kDa	Rice 10 kDa	Brazil nut 12 kDa	Sunflower 10 kDa	Soybean 8 kDa
Met	22.5	11.3	20.0	18.8	15.5	7.8
1/2 cys	3.9	4.4	10.0	7.9	7.8	7.8
Lys	0.0	0.0	0.9	0.0	3.9	13.0
Trp	0.0	0.0	0.0	0.0	1.0	0.0
Thr	3.9	2.5	6.4	0.0	0.0	2.6
Ile	2.3	0.6	1.8	1.0	2.9	3.9
Leu	11.6	10.0	6.4	5.0	8.7	7.8
Phe	3.9	0.0	2.7	0.0	0.0	1.3
Val	3.9	2.5	1.8	0.0	1.9	0.0
His	2.3	0.0	0.9	2.0	2.9	1.3

[a] Values, % of total protein, are deduced from sequences of cloned cDNAs (Altenbach and Simpson 1990; Galvez *et al.* 1997).

In legume-cereal mixtures, lysine is commonly the first limiting essential amino acid. The 8 kDa Gm2S-1 protein contains 13% lysine in contrast with no lysine for all the other MRPs except that of sunflower and rice. This presents an advantage of using Gm2S-1 for overexpression to increase methionine and lysine as well. It is also interesting to note that at least one of the following essential amino acids is also lacking in some of the MRPs including Gm2S-1: tryptophan, threonine, phenylalanine and valine. If the enhanced synthesis of the MRP happens at the expense of other storage proteins, an imbalance of other essential amino acids could occur. However, this remains to be established through amino acid analysis of transgenic seeds and animal feeding studies.

FUTURE EXPERIMENTS

Since the 8 kDa soybean MRP is estimated to make up about 0.5% of the total extractable protein in soybean seed, we calculated that it has to be increased approximately 14-fold over wild type to increase the sulfur amino acid content of soybean to 25 mg/g, the requirement for 2-5 year old children (FAO 1985). It has been demonstrated that modifications in the CaMV 35S constitutive promoter resulted in seed-specific enhanced expression as high as 25- to 40-fold over wild type in tobacco seeds when a segment of the α'-subunit of β-conglycinin (soybean protein) promoter is inserted into the CaMV 35S promoter (Chen *et al.* 1988). A similar construct will be made by putting the cDNA encoding the signal peptide, the 17-amino acid polypeptide linker and the 8 kDa MRP (*signal peptide-polypeptide linker-8 kDa MRP*) downstream from the modified CaMV 35S promoter in which the β-conglycinin subunit has been inserted in the 5' to 3' orientation at the -90 position (courtesy of Dr. Roger Beachy). The NOS polyadenylation control region will be at the 3' end. If needed, we can add another copy of the modified CaMV 35S to further enhance the expression (Kay *et al.* 1987). Increasing the number of methionine residues in the 8 kDa protein would reduce the fold-increase of overexpression needed to achieve the nutritionally significant increase in sulfur amino acid mentioned above. The region between the 4th and 5th cysteine residues and towards the carboxyl end from the 6th cysteine residue are likely sites for addition of methionine residues since they have variable lengths among the different 2S albumins (Galvez *et al.* 1996). Methionine residues could be inserted in these regions. For example, addition of four additional methionine residues (two between the 4th and 5th cysteine and two after the 6th cysteine) will increase the methionine content of the 8 kDa protein to about 13.0% from 7.8%, and would reduce the required fold-increase from 14-fold to about 9-fold. The constructed gene expression cassettes will be cloned into the pGEM3Zf(+) vector (Promega, Madison, WI) for use in transient gene expression assay (Cho *et al.* 1995). To hasten the screening of the promoter constructs in soybean embryogenic tissue system, a gene expression cassette using the GUS reporter gene in place of the *signal peptide-polypeptide linker-8 kDa SRP* cDNA will also be made for visual quantitation of expression levels. Once the highest expressing constructs are selected, stable transformation will be carried out in collaboration with the Center for Soybean Tissue Culture and Genetic Engineering, University of Kentucky, which develops and refines transformation techniques for soybean.

ACKNOWLEDGMENTS

Supported in part by USDA NRICGP Grant # 94-02167 and the U.S. Soybean Board. We thank Dr. Robert Goldberg for the cDNA library, Merrill Shum, Cindy Kang, Abigail Jung, Ann Chou and Gyu Kim for laboratory assistance and Jing-jie Liu and Bill Odegard for helpful discussions.

REFERENCES

ALTENBACH, S.B., KUO, C.C., STARACI, L.C., PEARSON, K.W., WAINWRIGHT, C., GEORGESCU, A. and TOWNSEND, J. 1992. Accumulation of a Brazil nut albumin in the seeds of transgenic canola results in enhanced levels of seed protein methionine. Plant MoL. Biol. *18*, 235–245.

ALTENBACH, S.B., PEARSON, K.W., MEEKER, G., STARACI, L.C. and SUN, S.S.M. 1989. Enhancement of the methionine content of seed proteins by the expression of a chimeric gene encoding a methionine-rich protein in transgenic plants. Plant Mol. BioL. *13*, 513–522.

ALTENBACH, S.B. and SIMPSON, R.B. 1990. Manipulation of methionine-rich protein genes in plant seeds. TIBTECH *8*, 156–160.

BRESSANI, R. and ELIAS, L.G. 1968. Processed vegetable protein mixtures for human consumption in developing countries. Adv. Food Res. 16, 1–103.

CHEN, Z.L., PAN, N.S. and BEACHY, R.N. 1988. A DNA sequence element that confers seed-specific enhancement to a constitutive promoter. EMBO J. *7*, 297-302.

CHO, M.J., WILHOLM, J.M. and VODKIN, L.A. 1995. Cassettes for seed-specific expression tested in transformed embryogenic cultures of soybean. Plant Mol. Biol. Rep. *13*, 255–269.

DE CLERQ, A., VANDEWIELE, M., VAN DAMME, J., GUERCHE, P., VAN MONTAGU, M., VANDEKERCHOVE, J. and KREBBERS, E. 1990. Stable accumulation of modified 2S albumin seed storage proteins with higher methionine contents in transgenic plants. Plant Physiol. *94*, 970–979.

DE LUMEN, B.O. and UCHIMIYA, H. 1997. Molecular strategies to enhance the nutritional quality of legume protein: an update. AgBiotech News and Information *9*, 53N–58N.

DE LUMEN, B.O. and KHO, C.J. 1987. Identification of methionine containing proteins and quantitation of their methionine contents. J. Agric. Food Chem. *35*, 688–691.

FAO/WHO/UNU. 1985. Energy and protein requirements. WHO Tech.Rep. Ser. No.724. WHO Geneva, Switzerland.

GALVEZ, A.F., REVILLEZA, J.M. and DE LUMEN, B.O. 1997. A novel methionine-rich protein from soybean (*Glycme max*) seed: Cloning and characterization of encoding cDNA. (submitted).

GEORGE, A.A. and DE LUMEN, B.O. 1991. A novel methionine-rich protein in soybean: Identification, amino acid composition and N-terminus sequence. J. Agric. Food Chem. *39*, 224–227.

GUERCHE, P., DE ALMEIDA, E.R.P., SCHWARZTEIN, M.A., GANDER, E., KREBBERS, E. and PELLETIER, G. 1990. Expression of the 2S albumin from *Bertholletia excelsa* in *Brassica napus*. Mol. Gen. Genet. *221*, 306–314.

HERIAN, A.M., TAYLOR, S.L. and BUSH, R.K. 1990. Identification of soybean allergens by immunoblotting with sera from soy-allergic adults. Int. Arch. Allergy Appl. Immunol. *92* 193–198.

HIGGINS, T.J.V., CHANDLER, P.M., RANDALL, P.J., SPENCER, D.G., BEACH, L.R., BLAGROVE, R.J., KORTT, A.A. and INGLIS, A.S. 1986. Gene structure, protein structure, and regulation of the synthesis of a sulfur-rich protein in pea seeds. J. Biol. Chem. *261*, 11124-11130.

HIGGINS, D.G. and SHARP, P.M. 1988. CLUSTAL: a package for performing multiple sequence alignment on a microcomputer. Gene *73*, 237–244.

KAY, R., CHAN, A., DALY, M. and McPHERSON, J. 1987. Duplication of a CaMV 35S promoter sequence creates a strong enhancer for plant genes. Science *236*, 1299–1302.

KHO, C.J. and DE LUMEN, B.O. 1988. Identification and isolation of methionine - cysteine rich protein fraction in soybean seed. Plant Foods Human Nutr. *38*, 287–296.

KYTE, J. and DOOLITTLE, R.F. 1982. A simple method for displaying the hydropathic character of a protein. J. Biol. Chem. *157*, 105–132.

LIENER, I.E. 1978. Nutritional value of food protein products. *In* Soybeans: Chemistry and Technology, Vol. 1 Proteins. Smith, A.K. and Circle, S.J., eds. AVI Publishing, Westport, CT, pp. 203–277.

MARUYAMA, I.N., RAKOW, T.L. and MARUYAMA, H.I. 1995. cRACE: a simple method for identification of the 5's end of mRNAs. Nucl. Acids Res. *23*, 3796–3797.

NORDLEE, J.A., TAYLOR, S.L., TOWNSEND, J.A., THOMAS, L.A. and BUSH, R.K. 1996. Identification of a Brazil nut allergen in transgenic soybeans. New Engl. J. Med. *334*, 688–692.

NORDLEE, J.A., TAYLOR, S.L., TOWNSEND, J.A., THOMAS, L.A. and TOWNSEND, R. 1994. Investigations of the allergenicity of Brazil nut 2S seed storage protein in transgenic soybean. OECD Workshop on Evaluation of New Foods, Oriel College Oxford, UK.

ODANI, S., KOIDE T. and ONO, T. 1987. Amino acid sequence of a soybean (*Glycine max*) seed polypeptide having a poly (L-aspartic acid) structure. J. Biol. Chem. *262*, 10502–10505.

REVILLEZA, J.M., GALVEZ, A.F. and DE LUMEN, B.O. 1996. An 8 kDa methionine-rich protein from soybean (*Glycine max*) cotyledon: Identification, purification and N-terminal sequence. J. Agric. Food Chem. *44*, 2930–2935.

SAALBACH, I., PICKARDT, T., MACHEMEHL, F., SAALBACH, G., SCHIEDER, O. and MUNTZ, K. 1994. A chimeric gene encoding the methionine-rich 2S albumin of the Brazil nut (*Bertholetha excelsa* H.B.K.) is stably expressed and inherited in transgenic grain legumes. Mol. Gen. Genet. *242*, 226–236.

SHIBASAKI, M., SUSUKI, S., TAJIMA, S., NEMOTO, H. and KURUOME, T. 1980. Allergenicity of major component proteins of soybean. Int. Arch. Allergy Appl. Immun. *61*, 441–448.

TOWNSEND, J.A., THOMAS, L.A., KULSEK, E.S., DAYWALT, M.J., WINTER, K.R.K. and ALTENBACH, S.B. 1992. Improving the quality of seed proteins in soybean. Proceedings 4th Biennial Conf. Mol. Cell. Biol. Soybean. July 27-29, 1992. Iowa State University, Ames IA. p. 4.

GENES DIFFERENTIALLY EXPRESSED DURING FRUIT BODY DEVELOPMENT OF SHIITAKE MUSHROOM *LENTINULA EDODES*

G.S.W. LEUNG, M. ZHANG, W.J. XIE and H.S. KWAN

Department of Biology
The Chinese University of Hong Kong
Shatin, N.T., HONG KONG

ABSTRACT

We aim to improve Shiitake mushroom strains by first understanding the molecular mechanisms of fruit body development. Arbitrarily primed PCR fingerprinting of RNA (RAP) generates fingerprints that can be used to identify differentially expressed genes among RNA populations. We have used RAP to analyze RNAs prepared from four stages of Lentinula edodes *development — vegetative mycelium, primodium, young fruiting body and mature fruiting body. About one hundred putative differentially expressed RAP fragments were isolated, cloned and sequenced, from more than a thousand bands screened. Homology searches of these clones with databases identified clones that share high sequence similarity with known genes including those involved in cell cycle control, signal transduction, DNA binding, and intracellular molecule targeting.*

The levels of RNAs corresponding to the cloned and sequenced RAP products have been analyzed by both dot-blot hybridization using total cDNA as probes and by Northern hybridization using the cloned DNA as probes. The differential expression of these genes could be used to infer the importance of cell cycle control and signal transduction in the development of fruit body of the Shiitake mushroom.

INTRODUCTION

The fruiting process is the most important and conspicuous developmental process in the life cycle of the basidiomycetous mushrooms. Studies of the fruit body (basidiocarp) development of *Lentinula edodes* (syn. *Lentinus edodes*, common name: Shiitake, Xianggu, the black mushroom), the second most cultivated edible mushroom (Chang 1987), has been considered important for the prospect of improving its cultivation.

Fruit body development has been studied more extensively in three basidiomycetous mushrooms, *Coprinus cinereus, Schizophyllum commune,* and *L. edodes*. The physiology of fruiting has been quite well documented. Fruiting is initiated by environmental factors such as light, temperature, humidity, nutrition and air (Wessels 1994). Some chemical substances such as cyclic AMP can also induce fruiting in *C. cinereus* (Swamy *et al.* 1985) and may be an intracellular effector for fruiting of *L. edodes* (Hori *et al.* 1991). The molecular aspects of fruiting in response to these stimuli, however, have not been extensively studied.

Three genes abundantly expressed during fruit body formation of *L. edodes* have been cloned and sequenced. They are *priA* (Kajiwara *et al.* 1992), *priB* (Endo *et al.* 1994) and *mfbA* (Shishido 1992). PriA contains zinc-finger-like and zinc-cluster-like motifs and PriB contains zinc cluster and leucine zipper motifs. MfbA contains a cell surface attachment-promoting amino acid sequence. Their roles in fruit body development are also uncertain.

We have used the approach of RNA-AP-PCR (RAP, differential display) (Welsh *et al.* 1992; Liang and Pardee 1992) to study the fruit body development of *L. edodes*.

MATERIALS AND METHODS

Mushroom Strain and RNA Extraction

The Dikaryotic strain L54 with fast growth rate and good fruiting ability was grown on artificial logs of saw dust. Mycelium, primodia and fruiting bodies were harvested. Total RNA was extracted from these samples by the SDS-phenol extraction procedure of Sokolovsky *et al.* (1990).

RNA Fingerprinting and Reamplification

The total RNA from each growth stage was fingerprinted using the RNA-AP-PCR method of Welsh *et al.* (1992). Complementary DNA (cDNA) was first synthesized from total RNAs at 37°C with MMLV reverse transcriptase and arbitrary primers. The cDNA was then amplified by PCR with low annealing temperatures (e.g. 35°C) for 35 cycles. The amplified DNA products were separated by agarose gel electrophoresis, stained with ethidium bromide, and visualized under UV illumination. Differential bands that appeared in some stages but not others were cut from the gel. Each of the cut piece of gel was placed in a tube of water and heated at 65°C to extract the DNA. A 5 μl fraction of the extraction was amplified in 50 μl of PCR reaction mixture using hot start PCR and the same primers that generated the fingerprint. Reamplified PCR products were analyzed by agarose gel electrophoresis. Those with the expected size were saved for further analyses.

Dot-blot Hybridization

Dot blot hybridization is a method for verifying the expression patterns of RNA fingerprints (Mou *et al.* 1994). cDNAs were generated by reverse transcription of the total RNAs of the four stages. Radioactive probes were prepared from 0.5 μg of cDNA using the Megaprime DNA labeling system (Amersham).

The reamplified PCR products were denatured and aliquots of 15 μl were dot-blotted on four Hybond-N+ nylon membranes (Amersham) and then fixed by baking at 120°C for 30 min. A fragment of rRNA was dot-blottted as the control to calibrate the variations in hybridization efficiency and overall probe radioactivity. The membranes were then hybridized with the cDNA probes. The radioactive signals were visualized by autoradiography with X-ray films. The dots of DNA were presumed to be in excess and thus the signal intensity would reflect the level of the RNA in the probes that hybridized with the DNA in the dot.

Cloning of Reamplified Fragments and Sequence Determination

The PCR-Script™ SK (+) cloning kit and *E. coli* XL-1Blue (Stratagene, La Jolla, CA) were used to clone the RAP products according to the manufacturer's protocol. After transformation, miniprep DNA was prepared from the transformants. Nucleotide sequences of the cloned RAP products were determined by dideoxy sequencing (Tabor and Richardson 1987) of double stranded DNA, using the sequencing kit and Perkin Elmer Applied Biosystem Genetic Analyzer B310 (PE ABI, Foster City, GA).

Search of Sequence Homology

Nucleotide sequences of these clones were compared with current databases using the BLAST (Altschul *et al.* 1990) on the www server of the National Center of Biotechnology Information (NCBI, National Library of Medicine, NIH).

RESULTS AND DISCUSSION

RNA-Arbitrarily-Primed PCR of RNA from Different Fruiting Stages of *L. edodes*

RNA fingerprints from the four developmental stages of Shiitake mushroom using arbitrarily chosen primers showed more than 100 bands (RAP-products) that appeared in some of the stages but not in other stages. These bands were considered to be differentially expressed and were cut out from the gel and reamplified. Examples of fingerprints are shown in Fig. 1. Reamplified differential bands were screened with dot-blot hybridization to show putative differential expression.

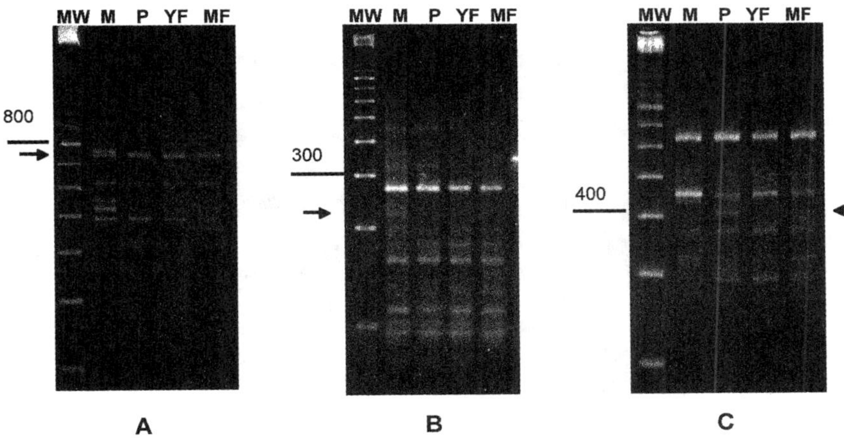

FIG. 1. RNA FINGERPRINTS OF *LENTINULA EDODES*. TOTAL RNA FROM THE FOUR DEVELOPMENTAL STAGES OF *LENTINULA EDODES* WERE FINGERPRINTED BY RAP-PCR WITH THE PROTOCOL AS LISTED IN MATERIAL AND METHODS USING 200 NG OF TOTAL RNA PER REACTION

The RAP products were resolved on a 3% Metaphorô agarose gel, ethidium bromide stained and visualized by UV illumination. Lane M, mycelium; lane P, primordium; lane YF, young fruiting body; lane MF, mature fruiting body. Size markers are the 100bp-ladder. Arrowheads indicate stage specific RAP-products. Primers used for the generation of RAP-PCR fingerprints were: (A) ARCAUP2; (B) LEPRIBLP1 and LERASUP1`; (C) LEPRIALP1.

Dot-blot Hybridization

Dot-blot hybridization was used as a secondary screening step for differentially expressed RAP-products. After hybridization and autoradiography, the X-ray films were scanned to quantify the intensities of the dots (Examples are given in Table 1). RAP-products that showed different dot intensities between any two of the four membranes were considered to be confirmed as differentially expressed in at least one stage (Fig. 2). These RAP-products were selected for cloning and sequence analysis.

TABLE 1.
RELATIVE SIGNAL LEVEL OF MRNA DETERMINED BY DOT HYBRIDIZATION

Clone	Gene	Relative intensity (-fold)			
		Vegetative mycelium	Primordium	Young fruit body	Mature fruit body
-	PriB	1	13.4	2.2	1.6
pMrG290a	Ubiquitin	1	5.2	1.6	0.5
pMrG500	MPP	1	41.0	8.0	2.7
pGD410	-	1	5.4	1.0	0.3
pE220	-	1	46.7	6.6	1.6
pGD480	-	1	17.7	23.0	1.4
pGD300	-	1	9.2	6.9	0.1
pMrG360	-	1	10.7	0.9	0.5

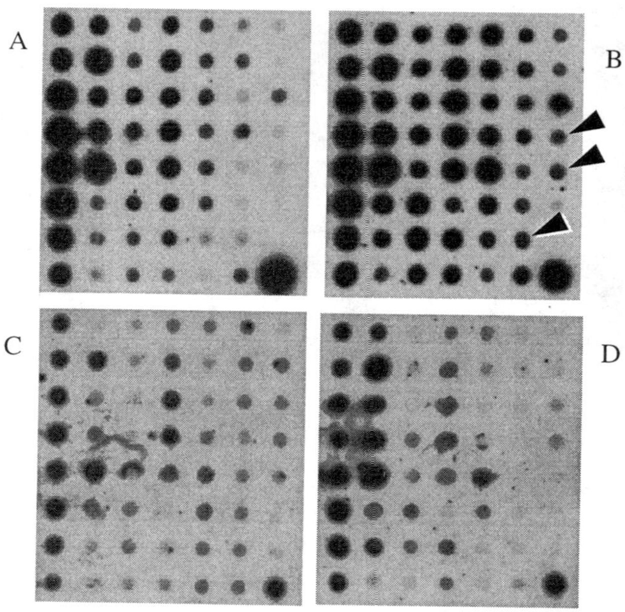

FIG. 2. DOT-BLOT HYBRIDIZATION. THE PROCEDURE IS DESCRIBED IN MATERIALS AND METHODS

The cDNA probes were synthesized from total RNA of (A) mycelium; (B) primordium; (C) young fruit body and (D) mature fruit body. The arrow heads indicate examples of differentially expressed rap products in the primodium stage.

Cloning, Sequencing and Identifying Fragments

The search of sequence homology with the NCBI link to all available DNA and protein databases using BLASTX showed the identities of some of the cloned gene fragments. Some of them are listed in Table 2. These genes mainly encode enzymes or proteins involved in signal transduction, cell cycle, intracellular molecule transport and metabolism. Genes involved in these cellular activities are: (a) signal transduction — mating factor A homolog, mitogen activated protein kinase (MAP kinase), byr2, and byr3; (b) cell cycle — cyclin B, CDC39, MAP kinase, and ubiquitin; (c) intracellular molecule transport — ubiquitin, mitochondrial processing peptidase beta subunit (MPP) and adaptin; (d) metabolism, H+-transporting ATPase, sugar transport protein, glycerol-3-phosphate dehydrogenase, and fructose 1,6 bisphosphatase.

TABLE 2.
A LIST OF RAP FRAGMENTS THAT WERE CLONED, SEQUENCED AND HOMOLOGY IDENTIFIED

Gene	Code	Primer(s)	Primer Sequences
18S rRNA	Au1000A	LEPRIAUP1	5′ CTACCCCCAACAAAGGAAATG 3′
α-Adaptin	Au500F	LEPRIAUP1	5′ CTACCCCCAACAAAGGAAATG 3′
byr2	GD300F	GalK-54	5′ TACGGTGGCGGAGCGCAGCA 3′
		DelC-23	5′ GTAAAACGACGGCCAGTACCAAG 3′
byr3 (cellular nucleic acid binding protein homolog)	C5-580P	C5	5′ CCGCACGCGCACGCAAGG 3′
CDC39	Au400P	LEPRIAUP1	5′ CTACCCCCAACAAAGGAAATG 3′
Cyclin B	Au500F	LEPRIAUP1	5′ CTACCCCCAACAAAGGAAATG 3′
Fructose 1,6 Bisphosphatase	BlRu250M	LEPRIBLP1	5′ GCGATCATGGATGAAAAGAACA3′
		LERASUP1	5′ GGCAAGTCACAGAACCTCATC 3′
Glycerol-3-phosphate dehydrogenase	MrG290P	M13RS-48	5′ AGCGGATAACAATTTCACACAGGA 3′
		GalK-54	5′ TACGGTGGCGGAGCGCAGCA 3′
H(+)-transporting ATPase	UpII770M	ARCAUP2	5′ TATGTCAACGAAGCGTAGTTTTAT 3′
Mating factor A homolog	GD480P	GalK-54	5′ TACGGTGGCGGAGCGCAGCA 3′
		DelC-23	5′ GTAAAACGACGGCCAGTACCAAG 3′
Mitochondrial Processing Peptidase β subunit	MrG500P	M13RS-48	5′ AGCGGATAACAATTTCACACAGGA 3′
		GalK-54	5′ TACGGTGGCGGAGCGCAGCA 3′
Mitogen-activated protein Kinase	C4-250P	C4	5′ CCACACGCGCACACGGGA 3′
Sugar transport	UpII700P	ARCAUP2	5′ TATGTCAACGAAGCGTAGTTTTAT 3′
Ubiquitin	MrG290P	M13RS-48	5′ AGCGGATAACAATTTCACACAGGA 3′
		GalK-54	5′ TACGGTGGCGGAGCGCAGCA 3′

CONCLUDING REMARKS

We have cloned and sequenced about sixty partial gene fragments (RAP clones). About twenty gene fragments from early developmental stages could be putatively identified by homology to known sequences in DNA sequence databases using BLAST. These genes belong mainly to three types — genes involved in signal transduction pathways, in DNA binding, and in intracellular molecule transport. These genes are of great interest for further studies because the isolation of these genes indicated the importance of signal transduction, transcriptional regulation, and intracellular molecule transport during early fruit body development. The signal transduction pathways are more closely related to developmental regulations and thus would be the first group of genes we wish to study.

ACKNOWLEDGEMENT

We thank Kwong-Kwok Wong, John Welsh, and Michael McCleland for introducing us to RAP-PCR and technical advices. M.Z. was supported by a post-doctoral fellowship of C.U.H.K. This study has been supported by Earmarked Grant for Research CUHK364/95M from Research Grants Council of UGC, Hong Kong to H.S.K.

REFERENCES

ALTSCHUL, S.F., GISH, W., MILLER, W., MYERS, E.W. and LIPMAN, D.J. 1990. Basic local alignment search tool. J. Mol. Biol. *215*, 403–410.

CHANG, S.T. 1987. World production of cultivated edible mushrooms in 1986. Mushroom J. Tropics *7,* 117–120.

ENO, H., KAJIWARA, S., TSUNOKA, O. and SHISHIDO, K. 1994. A novel cDNA, *priBc*, encoding a protein with a Zn(II)2Cys6 zinc cluster DNA-binding motif, derived from the basidiomycete *Lentinus edodes*. Gene *139,* 117–121.

HORI, K., KAJIWARA, S., SAITO, T., MIYAZAWA, H., KATAYOSE, Y. and SHISHIDO, K. 1991. Cloning, sequence analysis and transcriptional expression of a ras gene of the edible basidiomycete *Lentinus edodes*. Gene *105*, 91–96

KAJIWARA, S., YAMAOKA, K., HORI, K., MIYAZAWA, H., SAITO, T., KANNO, T. and SHISHIDO, K. 1992. Isolation and sequence of a developmentally regulated putative novel gene, *priA*, from the basidiomycete *Lentinus edodes*. Gene *114*, 173–178.

LIANG, P. and PARDEE, A. 1992. Differential display of eukaryotic messenger RNA by means of the polymerase chain reaction. Science *257,* 967–971.

MOU, L., MILLER, H., LI, J., WANG, E. and CHALIFOUR, L. 1994. Improvements to the differential display method for gene analysis. Biochem. Biophys. Res. Commun. *199,* 564–569.

SHISHIDO, K. 1992. Structure and function of the genes relating to the fruiting of *Lentinus edodes*. Proceed. The International Symposium on Recent Topics in Genetics, Physiology and Technology of the Basidiomycetes. Chiba, Japan. pp. 119–124.

SOKOLOVSKY, V., KALDENHOFF, R., RICCI, M. and RUSSO, V.E.A. 1990. Fast and reliable mini-prep RNA extraction from *Neurospora crassa.* Fungal Gen. Newsletters *37,* 41–43.

SWAMY, S., UNO, I. and ISHIKAWA, T. 1985. Regulation of cyclic AMP metabolism by incompatibility factors in *Corprinus cinereus*. J. Gen. Microbiol. *137,* 3211–3217

TABOR, S. and RICHARDSON, C.C. 1989. Selective inactivation of the exonuclease activity of bacteriopahge T7 DNA polymerase by *in vitro* mutagenesis. J. Biol. Chem. *264*, 6447–6458.

WELSH, J., CHADA, K., DALAL, S.S., CHENG, R., RALPH, D. and MCCLELLAND, M. 1992. Arbitrarily primed PCR fingerprinting of RNA. Nucl. Acids Res. *20,* 4965–4970.

WESSELS, J.G.H. 1994. Development of fruit bodies in homobasidiomycetes. The Mycota I, pp. 351–362. Springer-Verlag Berlin Heidelberg.

TRANSGENIC APPROACH TO IMPROVE PROTEIN, STARCH AND TASTE QUALITY OF FOOD PLANTS

SAMUEL S.M. SUN[1,2], MING-LI WANG[2], HELEN M. TU[2], WEI-NENG ZUO[2], LIWEN XIONG[2] and M.K. CHENG[1]

[1]Department of Biology
The Chinese University of Hong Kong
Shatin, NT, Hong Kong

[2]Department of Plant Molecular Physiology
University of Hawaii
Honolulu, Hawaii

ABSTRACT

Recent advances in plant biotechnology offer novel approaches for plant improvement. New and improved plant traits and products can be generated in transgenic plants through gene addition, subtraction, or pathway-redirection.

Using the gene addition approach, we demonstrated earlier that it is feasible to significantly enhance the content of essential methionine in transgenic seeds by the transfer and expression of a gene encoding the methionine-rich protein from Brazil nut. Using the same approach, a lysine-rich protein gene from winged bean is currently under study for protein quality improvement.

Mabinlin, a seed protein from mabinlang, has a sweet taste 400 times greater than sucrose. The gene for this sweet plant protein was cloned and transferred into potato and tobacco. Synthesis and correct cleavage of the precursor sweet protein was observed in the potato tubers and tobacco seeds.

Starch is the main component of taro corm, an important food crop. To genetically engineer the structure and functional property of taro starch, we had cloned and characterized the cDNAs encoding the small and large subunits of ADP-glucose pyrophosphorylase and the starch branching enzyme, and are studying the transgenic expression of these genes.

INTRODUCTION

Recent advances in plant molecular biology and biotechnology allow the isolation, transfer, and expression of specific genes in diverse target plant species. This genetic engineering could lead to: 1) creation of a new trait or plant product as a result of the added gene — gene addition; 2) partial or total removal of a target (undesirable) gene product — gene subtraction; and 3) change of the direction of a target pathway, resulting in modification in the amount or property of the pathway product — pathway redirection. These molecular approaches can be applied to improve the nutritional value of plant proteins, the taste quality of plant products, and the structure and functional property of starch.

ENHANCEMENT OF THE NUTRITIONAL QUALITY OF PROTEINS

Plant protein is a major source of dietary protein in the Asian Pacific regions. Though economic to produce, most plant proteins are nutritionally incomplete because of their deficiency in certain essential amino acids. For example, cereal proteins are low in lysine (Lys) and legume proteins are deficient in the sulfur amino acids, methionine (Met) and cysteine (Cys). Efforts to improve the essential amino acid balance in cereals and legumes through conventional breeding methods have met with little success.

We had earlier cloned a cDNA encoding a Met-rich 2S protein (18 mol% Met and 8 mol% Cys) in Brazil nut (BN2S) (Altenbach *et al.* 1987) and transferred and expressed it in transgenic tobacco seeds, demonstrating that it is feasible to enhance the Met content of the transgenic seeds by up to 30% through this approach (Altenbach *et al.* 1989). Similar enhancements were observed in transgenic rapeseed (Altenbach *et al.* 1992) and soybean (Townsend and Thomas 1994) using the same construct and approach. In an extension of this study, we were able to isolate Met-rich 2S proteins from seeds of paradise nut (PN2S) and cannonball (CB2S) of the Brazil nut family (Lecythidaceae) (Table 1; Zuo and Sun 1996) and observe expression levels of the paradise nut Met-rich 2S protein comparable to those of the BN2S in transgenic tobacco seeds (Zuo 1993). These Met-rich 2S proteins are thus promising candidates for protein quality improvement. It was shown recently, however, that the BN2S protein expressed in transgenic soybean causes allergenic reactions in some segments of the population (Nordlee *et al.* 1996). We are currently working to identify the allergenic determinant(s) of the BN2S protein.

TABLE 1.
AMINO ACID COMPOSITION OF PN2S, CB2S AND BN2S

Amino acid	PN2S mol%	CB2S mol%	BN2S mol%
Lys	2.8	0.3	1.6
His	1.9	1.7	1.9
Arg	10.6	15.5	12.1
Asx	4.9	2.8	4.4
Thr	3.3	-	0.5
Ser	6.4	6.3	5.6
Glx	23.3	27.4	23.1
Pro	7.7	8.1	6.5
Gly	7.2	4.7	7.5
Ala	4.2	1.8	1.8
Cys	4.3	4.5	9.7
Val	1.8	0.3	0.8
Met	14.0	19.9	16.1
Ile	1.1	0.2	0.7
Leu	5.7	5.6	5.7
Phe	0.9	0.8	0.4

To improve plant proteins that are deficient in essential lysine (Lys), we cloned a cDNA encoding an 18-kDa Lys-rich protein (LRP) from winged bean seeds (Sun *et al.* 1996). The LRP is currently used to construct chimeric genes under regulation of the seed-specific promoter of French bean phaseolin gene and to transform *Arabidopsis*. The enhancement effect of the LRP transgene on the Lys content of the transgenic *Arabidopsis* seeds will be analyzed.

IMPROVING THE TASTE QUALITY OF PLANT PRODUCTS

Humans and other animal species prefer, in general, substances that are sweet-tasting. However, excess sugar or calorie consumption is considered, at least partially, responsible for obesity and other health problems. Sweet plant proteins represent naturally-occurring low-calorie sweeteners and are potential candidates for genetically engineering plants for improved taste quality. We cloned and analyzed earlier the cDNAs encoding the isoforms of a sweet protein named mabinlin in the Chinese medicinal plant mabinlang (Sun *et al.* 1996). The mabinlin cDNA, under the regulation of the patatin, CaMV35S, and phaseolin promoters, respectively, was transferred into potato and tobacco. Results revealed that the sweet protein was expressed and properly processed in the potato tubers and tobacco seeds.

MANIPULATING THE STRUCTURE AND FUNCTIONAL PROPERTY OF TARO STARCH

Taro (*Colocasia esculenta*) is an important food plant of the South Pacific. It is a major staple for the people of Melanesia and Polynesia and a source of carbohydrates for the populations in South and Central America, Egypt, India, China and Japan. Taro corms contain 20% starch on a fresh weight basis and 70 to 80% on a dry weight basis. The granule size of taro starch is relatively small, less than 5 μm. Starch with a small granule size is considered a good filling agent for biodegradable plastics and cosmetics, and is suitable for use as a lipid substitute (Griffin and Wang 1983).

In order to genetically manipulate the amount, structure and functional property of the taro starch, we have cloned and characterized the cDNAs encoding 1) the ADP-glucose pyrophosphorylase (*Agp*, EC 2.7.7.27), which catalyzes the first step of starch biosynthesis, i.e. the formation of ADP-glucose, and is the rate limiting reaction in starch biosynthesis (Stark *et a*l. 1992), and 2) the starch branching enzyme (*Sbe*, EC 2.4.1.18), which catalyzes the synthesis of amylopectin, the branching polymer component of starch. The cDNA for the *Agp* large subunit is 2,083 bp in length, with a 174-bp 5′UTR, a 277-bp 3′ UTR, and a 1,631-bp ORF encoding a polypeptide of 543 amino acids in length and 59.9 kDa in molecular mass. The cDNA for the *Agp* small subunit is 1,955 bp in length, with a 95-bp 5′UTR, a 274-bp 3′ UTR, and a 1,596-bp ORF encoding a polypeptide of 531 amino acids and 57.6 kDa. Comparison of the two *Agp* subunit nucleotide sequences reveals a 61% identity at the NT level within the coding regions and 69% at the amino acid level, indicating that they are evolutionarily related. The cDNA for the *Sbe* is 3,087 bp in length with a 135-bp 5′ UTR, a 414-bp 3′ UTR, and a 2,538-bp ORF encoding a polypeptide of 845 amino acids and 95.7 kDa. Northern analysis shows that the transcripts of all these three genes are present only in the corms, not leaves, indicating that these genes probably represent the starch biosynthetic enzymes specific for sink tissue. We are currently preparing expression constructs for the transfer and expression of these genes in taro and other plants.

REFERENCES

ALTENBACH, S.B., PEARSON, K.W., LEUNG, F.W. and SUN, S.S.M. 1987. Cloning and sequence analysis of a cDNA encoding a Brazil nut protein exceptionally rich in methionine. Plant Mol. Biol. *8*, 239–250.

ALTENBACH, S.B., PEARSON, K.W., MEEKER, G., STARACI, L.C. and SUN, S.S.M. 1989. Enhancement of the methionine content of seed proteins by the expression of a chimeric gene encoding a methionine-rich protein in transgenic plants. Plant. Mol. Biol. *13*, 513-522.

ALTENBACH, S.B., KUO, C.C., PEARSON, K.W., WAINWRIGHT, C., GEORGESCU, A. and TOWNSEND, J. 1992. Accumulation of a Brazil nut albumin in seeds of transgenic canola results in enhanced levels of seed protein methionine. Plant Mol. Biol. *18*, 235–245.

GRIFFIN, G.J.L. and WANG, J.K. 1983. Industrial use. *In* Taro: A Review of *Colocasia esculenta* and its Potentials, J.K. Wang (ed.). University of Hawaii Press, Honolulu.

NORDLEE, J.A., TAYLOR, S.L., TOWNSEND, J.A., THOMAS, L.A. and BUSH, R.K. 1996. Identification of a Brazil-nut allergen in transgenic soybeans. New Engl. J. Med. *334*, 688-692.

STARK, D.M., TIMMERMAN, K.P., BARRY, G.F., PREISS, J. and KISHORE, G.M. 1992. Regulation of the amount of starch in plant tissue by ADP-glucose pyrophosphorylase. Science *258*, 287–292.

SUN, S.S.M., ZUO, W.N., TU, H.M. and XIONG L.W. 1996. Plant proteins: Engineering for improved quality. Ann. New York Acad. Sci. *792*, 37–42.

TOWNSEND, J.A. and THOMAS, L.A. 1994. Factors which influence the *Agrobacterium*-mediated transformation of soybean. J. Cell. Biochem. Suppl. *18A*, 78.

ZUO, W.N. 1993. Sulfur-rich 2S proteins in Lecythidaceae and their methionine-enriched forms in transgenic plants. Ph.D. dissertation, University of Hawaii.

ZUO, W.N. and SUN, S.S.M. 1996. Purification and characterization of the methionine-rich 2S seed proteins from the Brazil nut family (Lecythidaceae). J. Agric. Food Chem. *44*, 1206–1210.

EFFECT OF MICROBIAL TRANSGLUTAMINASE ENZYME ON KAMABOKO GEL FORMATION AND CROSS-LINKING REACTION OF MYOSIN HEAVY CHAINS

KOSAKU YASUNAGA[1], MASAKATSU YAMAZAWA[1], YOICHI ABE[2] and KEN-ICHI ARAI[2]

[1]National Research Institute of Fisheries Science of Japan
Fukuura 2-12-4, Kanazawa, Yokohama 236

[2]Rakuno Gakuen University
Ebetsu, Hokkaido 069, Japan

ABSTRACT

Frozen surimi of walleye pollack was ground with 3.0% NaCl in the presence and absence of 0.3% food additive containing transglutaminase (TGase). Each salt-ground meat was heated at 25° or 40°C for varied times (preheating gel) and this was followed by heating at 90°C for 30 min to produce kamaboko gel. Quality of the gel was evaluated from changes in the breaking strength (BS) and breaking strain (bs) as a function of the preheating time. The cross-linking profile of myosin heavy chains of each gel was also investigated.

The BS of kamaboko gels formed with the additive containing TGase increased at a much higher rate than the increase in bs of the same kamaboko gels. The cross-linking reaction of myosin heavy chains in the gel was markedly accelerated by the TGase, accumulating cross-linked products with larger molecular sizes. There was a good correlation between BS and spring constant (BS/bs) of the ordinary kamaboko gel products, formed from various grades of surimi, temperatures and durations of preheating, but not for the gels prepared with TGase. These results indicate that kamaboko gels prepared with TGase are harder and more heterogeneous in quality compared with the ordinary product.

INTRODUCTION

Transglutaminase (TGase) is widely distributed in nature. Ajinomoto Co. Inc. has succeeded in creating a method using bacteria for the mass production and commercialization of this enzyme and has proposed its applicability to a variety of food processes. This enzyme might improve the physical properties of various foods containing protein through the formation of covalent bonds between protein molecules.

The objective of this study is to examine the applicability of this enzyme to the gelation process of salt-ground meat from walleye pollack frozen surimi, which is an essential process in the production of kamaboko.

MATERIALS AND METHODS

Frozen surimi from walleye pollack was thawed and ground with 3.0 % NaCl (w/w) in the presence and absence of 0.3% food additive containing the microbial transglutaminase (w/w). The additive was composed of 1% transglutaminase, 75% calcium lactate, and 24% dextrin (Activa TG-K, Ajinomoto Co. Inc.) of which the enzyme activity was 100 units per gram. Although the principal component of the additive is Ca-lactate, the quality of kamaboko gel is not affected by this amount of lactate (Abe 1994). The temperature of the salt-ground meat was maintained at 8°C or below. The salt ground meat was stuffed into polyvinylidene tubes with a diameter of 30 mm and preheated at a set temperature in the range of 10 and 60°C for varied times (termed the preheating gel). The preheating gel was subsequently heated at 90°C for 20 min to produce kamaboko gel. The preheating and kamaboko gels were then sliced into 25 mm thickness and the breaking strength (g) together with the breaking strain (cm) were measured with a rheometer (Fudoh Co. Ltd., NRM2002J) using a spherical plunger of 5 mm in diameter.

Each 0.4 g of the gel was solubilized into 7.5 ml of 2% SDS-8 M urea-2% mercaptoethanol-20 mM Tris HCl (pH 8.0) on heating at 100°C for 2 min and followed by stirring at room temperature overnight. After centrifugation at 3,500 xg for 30 min, the amount of soluble protein in the supernatant was determined by the biuret method, and expressed as a relative value (%) using the value for each salt-ground meat before the preheating as 100%. Soluble protein (each 12 μg) was applied to SDS-PAGE using 5% polyacrylamide gels. The content of the protein component in the gels was determined according to the method of Numakura *et al.* (1989).

RESULTS AND DISCUSSION

In 1990, Numakura *et al.* reported that changes in gel properties and the cross-linking rate of myosin heavy chains of salt-ground meat from walleye pollack are dependent on the temperature and period of the preheating step. We also investigated the temperature and time dependent changes in breaking strength of kamaboko gel formed in the presence and absence of a food additive containing transglutaminase (TGase) as a function of preheating time. The results are shown in Fig. 1.

It was found that when the preheating was conducted at 30°C or below, the breaking strength of kamaboko gel formed with TGase was much higher than that of the gel without TGase. However, the breaking strain of the same gel with this enzyme was lower than that without TGase. On the other hand, when the preheating was conducted at 40°C or above, the breaking strength together with the breaking strain were both much higher than those without TGase.

Five lots of frozen surimi of different grades were also examined, and we found that there were also similar relative proportions between the breaking strength and breaking strain of kamaboko gel formed with and without TGase through preheating at 25°C and 40°C (Abe *et al.* 1996a). When the salt-ground meat with and without TGase was directly heated to 90°C, the breaking strength and breaking strain were both not affected by any further heating at 90°C. This may be caused by heat inactivation of the enzyme.

These results suggest that the forces between the myofibrillar proteins in the kamaboko gel, formed both in the presence and absence of TGase through preheating at

10-30°C and at 40-60°C, are evidently different from each other. Accordingly, the following study was conducted on the quality of the two types of kamaboko gels formed in the presence and absence of TGase through preheating at 25°C and at 40°C.

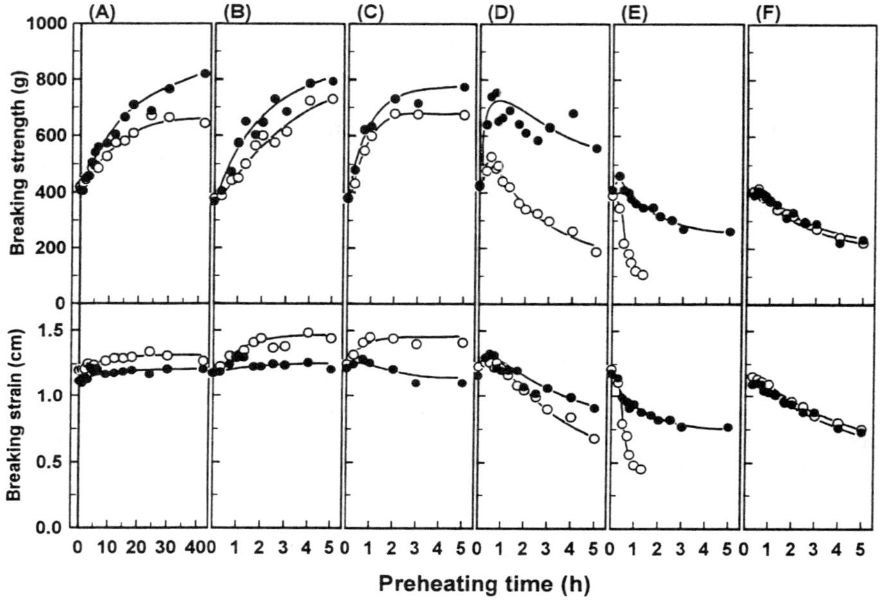

FIG. 1. CHANGES IN BREAKING STRENGTH AND BREAKING STRAIN OF KAMABOKO GEL FROM WALLEYE POLLACK FROZEN SURIMI AS A FUNCTION OF PREHEATING TIME AT VARIOUS TEMPERATURES
A, 10°C; B, 25°C; C, 30°C; D, 40°C; E, 60°C; F, 90°C.
○, without TGase; ●, with TGase.

The effect of TGase on changes in the breaking strength and breaking strain of both the preheating and kamaboko gels were then investigated as a function of the preheating time. The results are shown in Fig. 2. When preheated at 25°C (A), the breaking strength of the preheating gel without TGase was reinforced during a subsequent heating at 90°C for 30 min, whereas the breaking strain of the same gel declined with the 90°C heating. When mixed with TGase (B), the breaking strength of the preheating gel markedly increased and was reinforced further by a subsequent 90°C heating, whereas the breaking strain value of the same preheating gel remained almost constant during the same processes.

When preheated at 40°C, there were also the same increases in the breaking strength of kamaboko gel induced by TGase and by heating at 90°C, while the breaking strain remained at the same level.

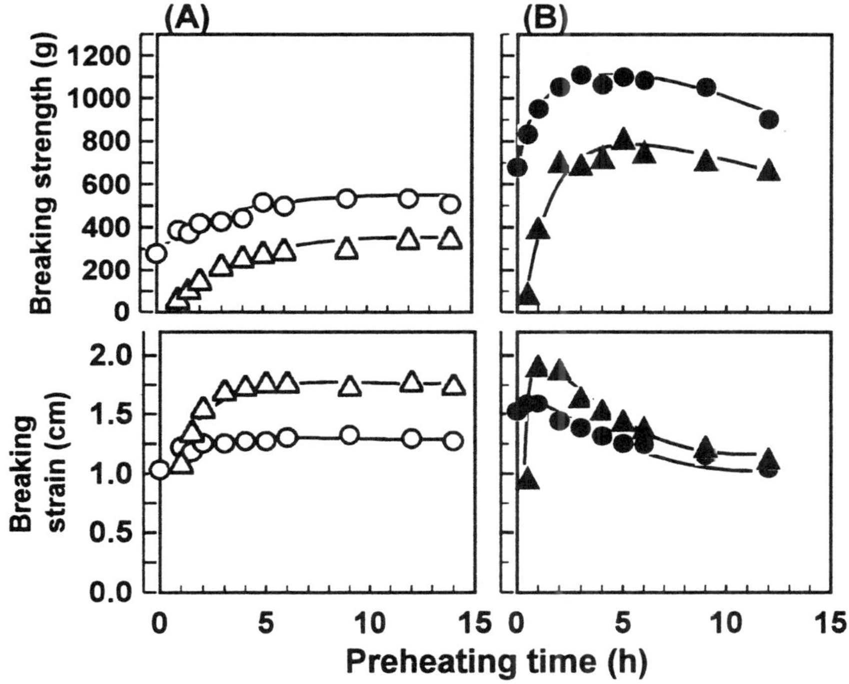

FIG. 2. CHANGES IN BREAKING STRENGTH AND BREAKING STRAIN OF PREHEATING AND KAMABOKO GELS WITH A FOOD ADDITIVE CONTAINING TRANSGLUTAMINASE FROM WALLEYE POLLACK FROZEN SURIMI AS A FUNCTION OF PREHEATING TIME AT 25°C.
A, without TGase; B, with TGase.
●, ○, kamaboko gel; ▲, Δ, preheating gel.

The preheating and kamaboko gels shown in Fig. 2 were solubilized into SDS-urea-mercaptoethanol mixtures. The soluble proteins were analyzed to determine their subunit composition by SDS-PAGE and densitometry. In Fig. 3, the solubility of the myofibrillar proteins in the preheating (b) and kamaboko (d) gels formed with (B) and without (A) TGase into the SDS-urea-mercaptoethanol medium is shown as a function of the preheating time at 25°C. The cross-linking profiles of myosin heavy chains (a,c) in the same preheating and kamaboko gels are also shown in this figure.

On gel formation without TGase, the cross-linking reaction of myosin heavy chains in the preheating gel was relatively slow. The decrease in the amount of myosin heavy chain accompanied by the accumulation of its cross-linked product (HCn1) and the cross-linking reaction in the preheating gel did not continue during the following 90°C heating. When mixed with TGase, the cross-linking reaction of myosin heavy chains in the preheating gel accelerated remarkably and its cross-linked products with larger molecular

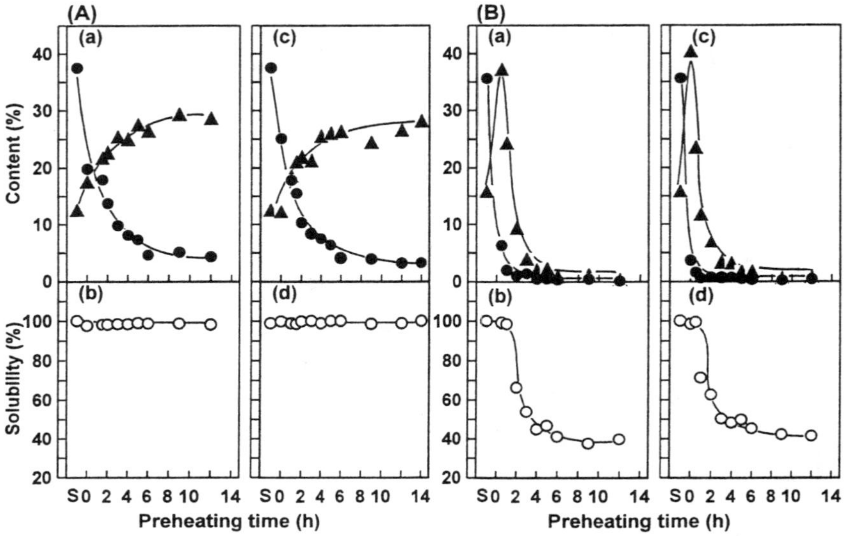

FIG. 3. CROSS-LINKING PROFILES OF MYOSIN HEAVY CHAINS IN PREHEATING AND KAMABOKO GELS FORMED WITH AND WITHOUT A FOOD ADDITIVE CONTAINING TRANSGLUTAMINASE AND SOLUBILITY OF MYOFIBRILLAR PROTEINS IN EACH GEL INTO SDS-UREA-MERCAPTOETHANOL MEDIUM AS A FUNCTION OF PREHEATING TIME AT 25°C

A, without TGase; B, with TGase.

a,c, cross-linking profiles of myosin heavy chains; b,d, solubility of myofibrillar proteins

●, Myosin heavy chain (HC); ▲, Cross-linked myosin heavy chains, migrating into 5% polyacrylamide gel (HCn1).

sizes accumulated (HCn2, HCn3). This reaction in the preheating gel with TGase also did not continue during subsequent heating at 90°C. In addition, the solubility of the myofibrillar proteins with SDS-urea-mercaptoethanol medium in the preheating and kamaboko gels formed with TGase decreased to a large degree with the progress of preheating time, while the gels without TGase were mostly soluble.

With the preheating at 40°C, essentially similar results as those at 25°C, showing that the changes in the breaking strength and breaking strain induced by addition of TGase and by 90°C heating proceeded separately with reaction rate of cross-linking of myosin heavy chains.

It is therefore evident that a marked reinforcement in the breaking strength of the preheating gel during heating at 90°C takes place essentially without the accompanying continuation of cross-linking of myosin heavy chains. When mixed with TGase, a more marked reinforcement of the breaking strength of the preheating gel occurred also without any continuation of the cross-linking reaction of myosin heavy chains.

Accordingly, as to the forces contributing to the changes in breaking strength and breaking strain of the preheating gel caused by the subsequent 90°C heating, we suggest that additional non-covalent type bonds between the myosin heavy chains and/or other myofibrillar proteins may form. In particular, there is a possibility that hydrophobic interactions among the protein molecules formed during heating at 90°C may largely contribute to the kamaboko gel formation.

Finally, we tried to characterize the quality of the kamaboko gel produced with TGase. The characterization of the kamaboko gel was made by calculating the value of breaking strength/breaking strain (termed the spring constant). In 1996, we reported that there was a positive correlation between the spring constant and the breaking strength of the kamaboko gel with a high correlation coefficient (Fig. 4A, Abe *et al.* 1996b). The correlation was not affected by the grades of the frozen surimi, temperatures or periods for preheating of the salt-ground meat. However, plots of the spring constant against the breaking strength of the kamaboko gel produced with TGase tended to deviate markedly with the progress of preheating time from the linear relation obtained for ordinary kamaboko gels (Fig. 4B).

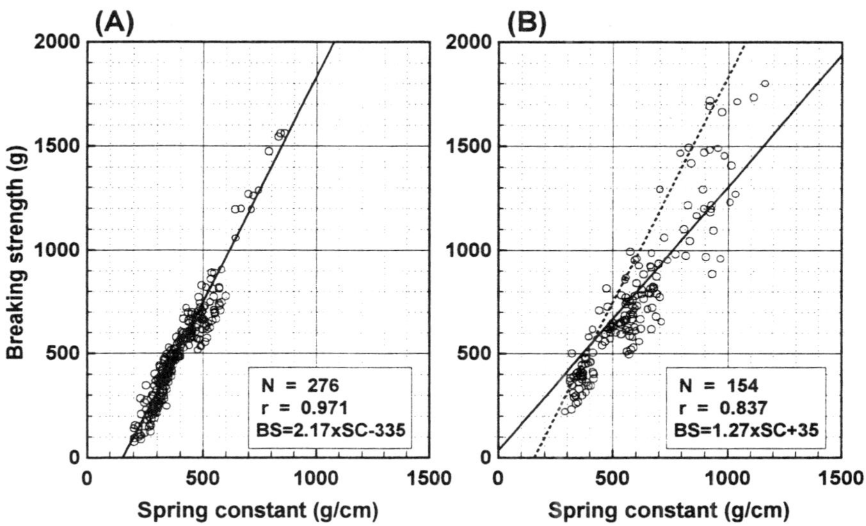

FIG. 4. RELATION BETWEEN SPRING CONSTANT AND BREAKING STRENGTH OF KAMABOKO GEL FROM WALLEYE POLLACK FROZEN SURIMI IN THE PRESENCE AND ABSENCE OF A FOOD ADDITIVE CONTAINING TRANSGLUTAMINASE

A, without TGase; B, with TGase. N, number of samples; r, coefficient of correlation; BS, breaking strength; SC, spring constant.

The spring constant was calculated as breaking strength/breaking strain. A regression line was calculated using the least squares methods.

Therefore, it is clear that the kamaboko gels produced with the aid of microbial transglutaminase are harder and more heterogeneous in quality, because the spring constant is poor relative to the breaking strength.

REFERENCES

ABE, Y. 1994. Quality of kamaboko gel prepared from walleye pollack surimi with an additive containing transglutaminase. Nippon Suisan Gakkaishi (Japan) *60*,381–387.

ABE, Y., YASUNAGA, K., KITAKAMI, S., MURAKAMI, Y., OTA, T. and ARAI, K. 1996a. Quality of kamaboko gels from walleye pollack frozen surimis of different grade on applying additive containing TGase. Nippon Suisan Gakkaishi (Japan) *62*,439–445.

ABE, Y., YASUNAGA, K., KITAKAMI, S., MURAKAMI, Y., OTA, T., MIHORI, T. and ARAI, K. 1996b. Characteristics of two-step heating gels from frozen surimi with a food additive containing TGase or a bovine plasma powder. Nippon Suisan Gakkaishi (Japan) *62*, 446–452.

NUMAKURA, T., MIZOGUCHI, R., KIMURA, I., TOYODA, K., FUJITA, T., SEKI, N. and ARAI, K. 1989. Changes in gel forming ability of myosin heavy chain of Alaska pollack surimi denatured by heat treatment. Nippon Suisan Gakkaishi (Japan) *55*,1083–1090.

NUMAKURA, T., KIMURA, I., TOYODA, K. and FUJITA, T. 1990. Temperature-dependent changes in gel strength and myosin heavy chain of salt-ground meat from walleye pollack during setting. Nippon Suisan Gakkaishi (Japan) *56*,2035–2043.

PHENOLICS: THEIR IMPACTS ON PROTEOLYTIC ACTIVITY

RASHDA ALI and SHAHINA NAZ

Department of Food Science and Technology
University of Karachi
Karachi-75270, Pakistan

ABSTRACT

The effect of some phenolic compounds on common proteases was studied. Proteases from different groups were selected and naturally-occurring phenolics from edible and inedible sources were reacted with substrates (caseins) under different conditions. The proteolytic activity was measured and reasons for effects on proteases or substrates were evaluated. The phenomenon of enhancement, inhibition or no effect on the overall enzymic activity were noted. The possible mechanism for the increase, decrease or no effect in the enzymic activity is discussed.

INTRODUCTION

It is often experienced that even goal-oriented research may divert its route to give birth to a completely new era for scientific investigations. One finds a similar story while reviewing the history of enzyme inhibitors which were accidentally discovered by protein chemists and enzymologists while exploring the key point/site of action of these biological catalysts. Chemical changes at the cellular level are governed greatly by endogenous or exogenous (in case of invasion) enzymes. Thus ripening of fruits may be delayed by inhibiting the various enzymes involved in hydrolysis, oxidation or browning of fruits (Spanos and Wrolstad 1994). In view of the mode of linkage, i.e. covalent or non covalent, enzyme inhibitors are classified as irreversible and reversible, respectively. It seems that enzyme inhibitors may also be classified as direct or indirect depending upon whether enzyme itself or its cofactor, prosthetic group, enzyme enhancer or substrate is involved in decreasing the enzyme activity. While discussing the mechanism of inhibition, numerous reasons may be given for limiting the enzymatic action such as presence of a substrate analog, conformational change in the enzyme, aggregation of the enzyme or the substrate, etc.

Phenolics, both as monomers or polymers, are known to minimize or to stop the enzymatic activity *in vivo* or *in vitro* food systems and thus are regarded as an effective tool for modification of flavor, texture, color or for preservation of food (Babic *et al.* 1993). The role of phenolic compounds in food systems, although still obscure, has been repeatedly observed in certain natural food processes [Mosel and Herrmann 1974]. Simple and complex phenolic acids, tannins, quinones, coumarins and flavonoids are the major groups of phenolic compounds widely distributed in food commodities ranging from 0.1-0.2 g/100 g in fresh fruits; the amount mostly decreases on storage (Friend and Rhodes 1981). Phenolics having other reactive groups such as acidic, aldehydic, methoxy, etc. show potential for complexation with other components present in food (Stohr and Herrmann 1975).

Ballentine (1992) has discussed the astringency in flavor of tea due to interactions of a variety of phenolics, especially tannins (condensed and hydrolyzable), within themselves and with other molecules such as proteins of mucous membrane lining of the mouth. The mouth-biting effect of most of the fruits is due to the phenolics and substituted phenolics (Hulme 1963, 1970). Phenolics, being charged particles, associate themselves with cations or metals, causing discoloration of the fruit tissues often observed during pulping, blanching and storage of fruits (Belitz and Grosch 1987). The tannin-protein complex (TPC) *in vitro* produces the turbidity, mouth feel and haze in hot or cold beverages. The presence of TPC is desirable in food commodities; however, free tannins in food are regarded as antinutrients in view of their interference with digestive enzymes; thus, they diversely affect biological, NPU and PER values of proteins (Salunke *et al.* 1982). Perhaps it correlates with the old belief that black tea is comparatively more harmful than white tea where tannins in tea have already formed complexes with milk proteins sparing biologically active or inactive proteins in the digestive gut of the animals for performing their natural functions.

The antimicrobial behavior of the phenolics is the basic cause of resistance in plants in view of their increased secretion and deposition against bacterial and fungal infections (Faith *et al.* 1992). The use of tannins as biocides in agriculture is increasing due to their effective role in controlling insects during growth in field and storage, so they have been named "biological pesticides" (Laks 1989). The role of phenolics as antioxidants in food has already been discussed by Pratt (1992). Protein protease-inhibitors found in plant and animals are now considered as possible therapeutic and cancer-chemopreventives (Le Guen and Birk 1993). In view of the antienzymic activity of the phenolic compounds they may prove to be equivalent to protein protease-inhibitor for controlling malignancy in animal tissues. Phenolics have also shown potential health benefits by interacting with metabolites in various ways (Ho *et al.* 1992) in spite of their definite antinutritional behavior in many food items as legumes.

The role of phenolics as enzyme inhibitors is less explored presently. Tannins, the major polyphenolics in nature, have long been known as antinutrients for their adverse actions on the digestive enzymes (Hagerman and Butler 1989). Jansman and co-workers (1993) reported the very interesting results on rats fed with high-tannin diet which produced hypertrophy of the parotid glands. However, a self-defensive mechanism was developed by immediate secretion of proline-rich-proteins (PRPs) in saliva which show high affinity for binding with tannins to decrease their effects. It has been observed that PRPs as salivary proteins are only produced during stress, indicating their involvement in a defense control system. All the digestive enzymes are not inhibited by tannins, especially the gastric enzymes, because of the unfavorable acidic pH for tannin-protein complexation. However, trypsin, α-amylase and lipase were inhibited in the chick jejunum (Longstaff and McNab 1991a; Yuste *et al.* 1992). Oh and Hoff (1986) found that the digestive proteases, such as trypsin, chymotrypsin and pepsin, are inhibited by tannins in grapes. Generally, the polyphenols from lucerne, sorghum grain and malt, and hull of faba bean are reported to minimize the activity of proteases (trypsin and pepsin), α-amylase, cellulose, lipase etc. (Milic *et al.* 1972; Daiber 1975; Griffiths and Jones 1977; Davis and Hoseney 1979).

The suppressed enzyme activity was regained by addition of polyvinylpyrrolidone illustrating the enzyme-tannin interaction as tannins were later released to restore enzyme action (Longstaff and McNab 1991a; Longstaff *et al.* 1993). Tannins are also known to enhance activity of lipase in rats (Horigom *et al.* 1988). The stimulation and inhibition of tryptic activity by tannins has been well demonstrated *in vitro* (Mole and Waterman 1985). Tannins react with many other enzymes as well, forming enzyme-tannin complexes (Villanueva *et al.* 1987).

The phenolic-protein interaction (Ali and Sayeed 1992, 1994, 1995), including that of tannins, is established through electrostatic, hydrogen, hydrophobic and covalent bonding. The mechanism of covalent linkage suggests the possibility of phenolics altering the bioactivity of sulfhydryl proteases as phenolics, on oxidation, develop potential charges to form a covalent linkage with either amide or the sulfhydryl group of the enzyme, thus inhibiting the activity of the sulfhydryl proteases. It is another reason for the antinutrient behavior of phenolic compounds in food (Haslan *et al.* 1992).

MATERIALS AND METHODS

All the chemicals used were of analytical grade supplied either by Merck or BDH. Double-distilled deionized water was used throughout the experiments.

Preparation of Enzyme-Quinone Phenolic Acids and Casein Solutions

Initially the stock solutions of the enzymes, trypsin and papain (0.1%) of varying pH were prepared by dissolving 0.1 g of the enzymes in 100 ml of acetic acid-acetate buffers (for pH 5.0, 5.5 and 6.0) and 100 ml of phosphate buffers (for pH 6.5, 7.0, 7.5 and 8.0) and then diluting the 1 ml of stock solution to 100 ml with corresponding buffer.

The stock solutions of the quinones, juglone and lawsone phenolic acids such as vanillic, caffeic and carminic acids (0.001-0.008%) were prepared by dissolving 0.1 g of the substance in 100 ml deionized water and then diluting 1, 2, 3, 4, 5, 6, 7 and 8 ml of the stock solution to 100 ml with deionized water. Solution of the 0.1% casein was prepared by dissolving 0.1 g casein in 100 ml of buffer (pH 7.5).

Preparation of (1:100) Enzyme-Substrate (Casein) Reactions

To ascertain the activity of the enzymes (trypsin and papain) and optimum range of the pH of the respective enzymes, 2 ml of 0.1% casein was mixed with 2 ml of the enzyme solution (0.001%) and 2 ml of the buffer (pH 5.0, 5.5, 6.0, 6.5, 7.0 and 8.0) in test tubes. The test tubes were incubated at a temperature of 37°C for 10 min. The unhydrolyzed protein was precipitated by adding 4 ml of 5% TCA solution. The absorbance of the hydrolyzed substrate was recorded on a UV-Visible spectrophotometer (Shimadzu model 160A) at 280 nm against a blank containing 2 ml of 0.1% casein, 2 ml of the corresponding buffer and 4 ml of TCA solution.

Preparation of Enzyme, Substrate, Quinone/Phenolic Acid (1:100:1) Solutions

To observe the change in enzyme activity, if any, due to interaction of the quinones (juglone, lawsone) and phenolic acids as vanillic, caffeic and carminic acids with enzyme and substrate, enzyme and substrate containing 2 ml casein and 2 ml enzyme was mixed with 2 ml of each of the quinones/phenolic acids and after 10 min, the reaction was stopped by addition of 5% TCA solution. The absorbance was recorded at 280 nm against blank sample containing 2 ml each of the casein, quinone/phenolic acids, TCA and the buffer.

Preparation of Enzyme, Substrate, Quinone/Phenolic Acids Reactions Varying the Ratios of Quinones

The enzyme and substrate solution (1:100) was mixed with the quinone in the ratio of enzyme, substrate, quinone (1:100:1), 1:100:2, 1:100:3, 1:100:4, 1:100:5, 1:100:6, 1:100:7 and 1:100:8 to evaluate the limits of the concentration of the quinone required to completely inhibit the enzyme activity. After 10 min the reactions were stopped by adding 4 ml of 5% TCA as above.

RESULTS AND DISCUSSION

The two enzymes trypsin and papain representing the serine protease and sulfhydryl groups of proteases, respectively, were treated with two classes of phenolics, i.e. quinone and phenolic acids to evaluate the effect of interaction between enzymes and polyphenols. Carminic acid is a quinone as well an acid and perhaps is more strong in inhibition in view of having both groups in the structure. The studies, although at a very premature stage, shows that quinones, i.e. juglone, lawsone and carminic acid, inhibit trypsin. Juglone at pH 5 had no effect on trypsin activity in spite of increasing the concentration of quinone; however, at pH 7.5 the juglone showed linear inhibition pattern with increasing concentration of quinone (Fig. 1 and 2). The 1:6 concentration of trypsin-juglone is optimal, after which the inhibition is not affected. The lawsone at pH 5 showed

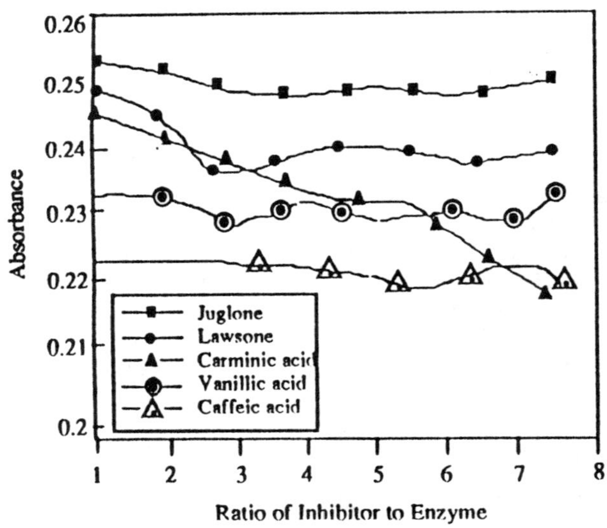

FIG. 1. EFFECT OF VARIOUS QUINONES ON ENZYMIC ACTIVITY OF TRYPSIN AT VARYING CONCENTRATION OF THE QUINONE AND AT A CONSTANT CONCENTRATION OF CASEIN AS SUBSTRATE AND AT A CONSTANT pH OF 5.0.

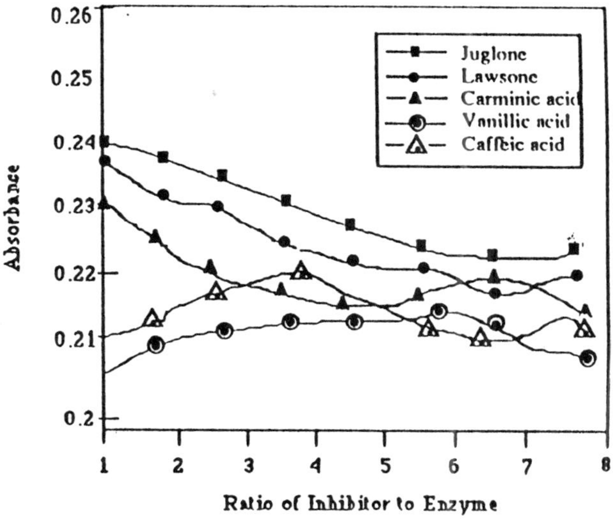

FIG. 2. EFFECT OF VARIOUS QUINONES ON ENZYMIC ACTIVITY OF TRYPSIN AT VARYING CONCENTRATION OF THE QUINONE AND AT A CONSTANT CONCENTRATION OF CASEIN AS SUBSTRATE AND AT A CONSTANT pH OF 7.5.

better inhibition effect at its low concentration at pH 5 and pH 7.5. Lawsone seems to be slightly more effective than juglone in controlling tryptic activity.

Out of the three phenolic acids, carminic, vanillic and caffeic, carminic acid is the most effective and more pronounced at low pH as expected from acids (Fig. 1 and 2). Vanillic and caffeic acids showed negligible effect at both pHs. It is too early to draw a conclusion; however looking at the structure it seems that the number of hydroxyl groups, presence of quinone and acidic groups increase the inhibitory activity.

Similarly, the -SH protease papain reacted with the quinones and phenoic acids producing interesting results for further investigations. Juglone was found to inhibit papain only at pH 5 while pH 8 was ineffective for inhibition (Fig. 3 and 4). Lawsone was more effective in its inhibition than juglone at both pH values. The vanillic and caffeic acids were almost ineffective in behavior towards papain at either pH. The most pronounced inhibition was exhibited by carminic acid against papain at pH 5 and 8. Carminic acid was also found to be the best inhibitor of trypsin among the five compounds tested.

Looking at the structure-function relationship, it looks obvious that carminic acid, containing all the three reactive groups (quinone, hydroxyl and carboxylic) is a better inhibitor than quinones consisting only of quinone and hydroxyl group or phenolic acids with hydroxyl and carboxylic acid groups.

Since the hydroxyl group is common in all three types of the inhibitors used, it seems that the increase in inhibitory effect of carminic acid is due to the presence of both quinone and carboxylic acid groups. However, more experimental work is required to be carried out using proposed inhibitors with similar structures as carminic acid for drawing a definite conclusion.

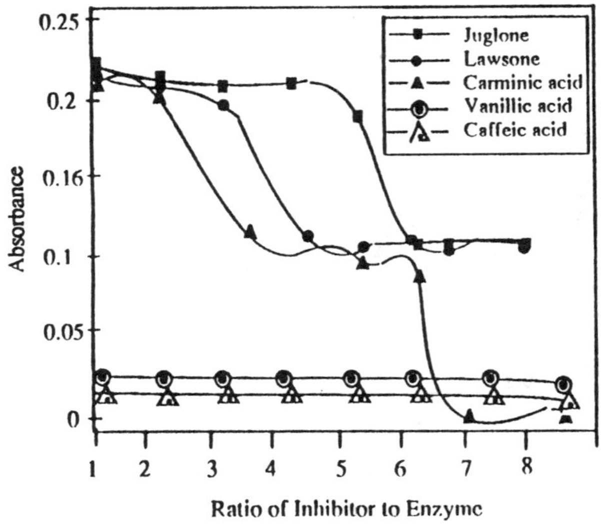

FIG. 3. EFFECT OF VARIOUS QUINONES ON ENZYMIC ACTIVITY OF PAPAIN AT VARYING CONCENTRATION OF THE QUINONE AND AT A CONSTANT CONCENTRATION OF CASEIN AS SUBSTRATE AND AT A CONSTANT pH OF 5.0

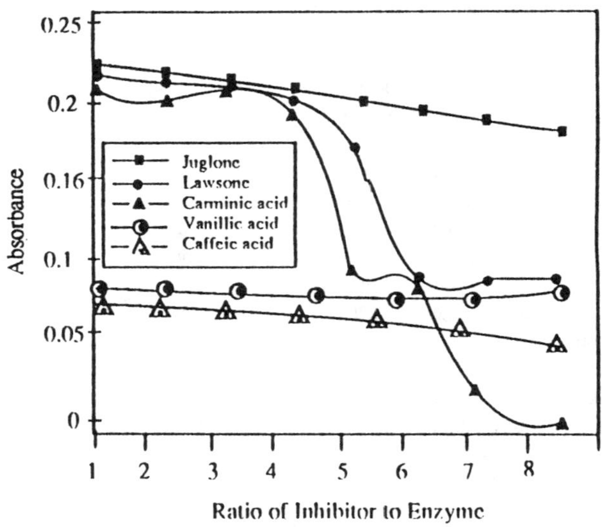

FIG. 4. EFFECT OF VARIOUS QUINONES ON ENZYMIC ACTIVITY OF PAPAIN AT VARYING CONCENTRATION OF THE QUINONE AND AT A CONSTANT CONCENTRATION OF CASEIN AS SUBSTRATE AND AT A CONSTANT pH OF 8.0.

Caffeic acid

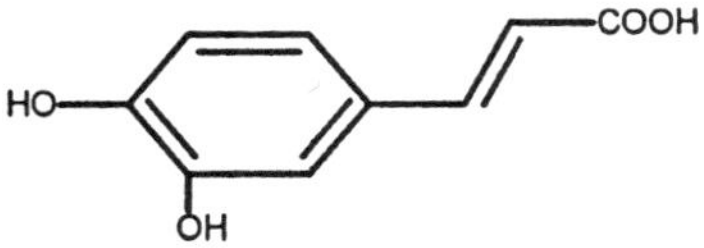

Juglone

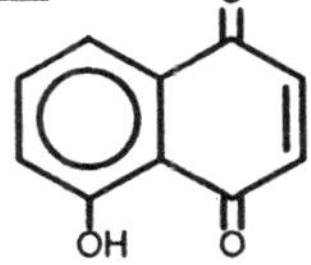

Vanillic acid

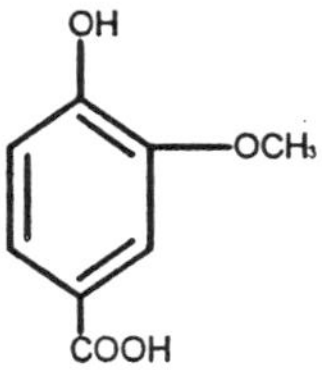

Lawsone

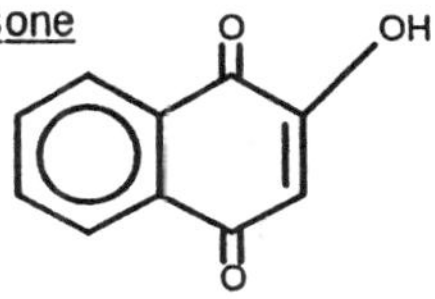

Carminic acid

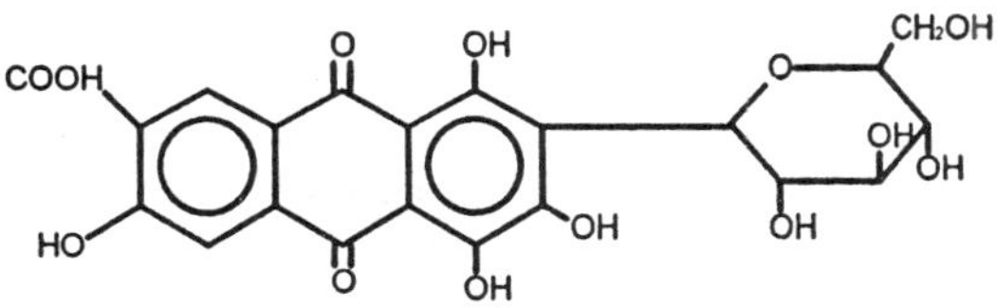

REFERENCES

ALI, R. and SAYEED, S.A. 1995. A sensitive novel staining agent for the resolved proteins on PAGE. Int. J. Pept. Protein Res. *45*, 97–99.

ALI, R. SAYEED, S.A., WHITAKER, J.R. and ATTA-UR-RAHMAN, 1994. Elucidation of structure and functional properties of anthocyanin bound protein from *Pumica granatus*. *19th IUPAC Symposium on the Chemistry of National Products*, Jan 16–20. Karachi, Pakistan.

ALI, R. and SAYEED, S.A. 1997. Lawsone: Phenolic of Henna and its potential use in protein-rich foods and staining. *In* Antinutrients and Phytochemicals in Food (F. Shahidi, ed.) ACS Symp. Ser. *662*, 223–244.

BABIC, I., AMIOT, M.J., NGUYEN, T.C. and AUBERT, S. 1993. Changes in phenolic content in fresh ready-to-use shredded carrots during storage. J. Food Sci. *58*, 351–356.

BALLENTINE, D.A. 1992. Manufacturing and chemistry of tea. *In* Phenolic Compounds in Food and Their Effects on Health. I. Analysis, Occurrence, and Chemistry. (C.T. Ho, C.Y. Lee and M.T. Haung, eds.) ACS Symp. Ser. *506*, 102–117.

BELITZ, H.-D. and GROSCH, W. 1987. Food Chemistry, 1st English Ed., Springer-Verlag, Heidelberg, pp. 592–602.

BUTLER, L.G. 1988. Effect of condensed tannins on animal nutrition. *In* Chemistry and Significance of Condensed Tannins. (R.W. Hemingway and J.J. Karchesy, eds.). Plenum Press, New York, pp. 343–396.

DAIBER, K.H. 1975. Enzyme inhibition by polyphenols of sorghum grain and malt. J. Sci. Food Agric. *26*, 1399–1411.

DAVIS, A.B. and HOSENEY, R.C. 1979. Grain sorghum condensed tannins. I. Isolation, estimation, and selective adsorption by starch. Cereal Chem. *56*, 310–314.

FAITH, N.G., YOUSEF, A.E. and LUCHANSKY, J.B. 1992. Inhibition of *Listeria monocytogenes* by liquid smoke and isoeugenol, a phenolic component found in smoke. J. Food Safety *12*, 263–314.

FRIEND, J. and RHODES, M.J.C. (eds.) 1981. Recent Advances in the Biochemistry of Fruits and Vegetables. Academic Press, London-New York.

GRIFFITHS, D.W. and JONES, D.I.H. 1997. Cellulase inhibition by tannins in the testa of field beans (*Vicia faba*). J. Sci. Food Agric. *28*, 983–989.

HAGERMAN, A.E. and BUTLER, L.G. 1989. Choosing appropriate methods and standards for assaying tannin. J. Chem. Ecol. *15*, 1795–1810.

HASLAN, E., LILLEY, T.H., WARMINSKI, E., LIO, H., CAI, Y., MARTIN, R., GAFFNEY, S.H., GOUDLING, P.N. and LUCK, G. 1992. Polyphenol complexation: A study in molecular recognition. *In* Phenolic Compounds in Food and Their Effects on Health. I. Analysis, Occurrence and Chemistry. (T. Ho, C.Y Lee and M.T. Huang, eds.), ACS Symp. Ser. *506*, 8–50.

HO, C.T., LEE, C.Y. and HUANG, M.T. (eds.) 1992. Phenolic Compounds in Food and Their Effects on Health.I. Analysis, Occurrence and Chemistry. ACS Symp Ser. *506*.

HORIGOME, T., KUMAR, R. and OKAMOTO, K.O. 1988. Effects of condensed tannins from leaves of fodder plants on digestive enzymes in vitro and in the intestines of rats. Br. J. Nutr. *60*, 275–285.

HULME, A.C. 1963. Biochemistry of fruits (Kretovich, V.L. and Pijanowski, E., eds). Proc. Intern. Congr. Biochem. 5th, Moscow, 1961, *8*, 43–153 (Publ. 1963).

HULME, A.C. (ed.) 1970. The Biochemistry of Fruits and Their Products. Vol. 1, Academic Press, London, New York.

JANSMAN, A.J.M., FROHLICH, A.A. and MARQUARDT, R.R. 1994. Production of proline-rich proteins by the parotid glands of rats fed diets containing tannins from faba beans (*Vicia faba L.*) J. Nutr. *124*, 249–258.

JANSMAN, A.J.M., VERSTEGEN, M.W.A. and HUISMAN, J. 1993. Effects of dietary inclusion of hulls of faba beans (*Vicia faba L.*) with a low and high content of condensed tannins on some physiological parameters in piglets. Anim. Feed Sci. Techn. *43*, 239–257.

LAKS, G. 1989 Condensed tannins as a source of novel biocides. *In* Chemistry and Significance of Condensed Tannins. Plenum Press, New York, NY pp. 330–377.

LE GUEN, M.P. and BIRK, Y. 1993. Protein protease inhibitors from legume seeds: nutritional effects, mode of action and structure-function relationship. Wageningen Press, The Netherlands, pp. 157–171.

LONGSTAFF, M. and MCNAB, J.M. 1991a. The inhibitory effects of hull polysaccharides and tannins of field beans (*Vicia faba L.*) on the digestion of amino acids, starch and lipid and on digestive enzyme activities in young chicks. Br. J. Nutr. *65*, 199–216.

LONGSTAFF, M. and MCNAB, J.M. 1991b. The effect of concentration on tannin-rich beans hulls (*Vicia faba L.*) on activities of lipase (EC 3.1.1.3) and α-amylase (EC 3.2.1.1) in digesta and pancreas and on the digestion of lipid and starch by young chicks. Br. J. Nutr. *66*, 139–147.

LONGSTAFF, M., FEUERNSTEIN, D., MCNAB, J.M. and MCCORQUODALE, C. 1993. The influence of proanthocyanidin-rich bean hulls and levels of dietary protein on energy metabolizability and nutrient digestibility by adult cockerels. Br. J. Nutr. *70*, 335–367.

MILIC, B.L., STOJANOVIC, S. and VUCUREVIC, N. 1972. Lucerne tannins. II. Isolation of tannins from lucerne, their nature and influence on the digestive enzymes in vitro. J. Sci. Food Agric. *23*, 1157–1162.

MOLE, S. and WATERMAN, P.G. 1985. Stimulatory effects of tannins and cholic acid on tryptic hydrolysis of proteins: Ecological implications. J. Chem. Ecol. *11*, 1323–1332.

MOSEL, H.D. and HERRMANN, K. Changes in catechins and hydroxycinnamic acid derivatives during development of apples and pears. J. Sci. Food Agric. *25*, 251–256.

OH, H.I. and HOFF, J.E. 1986. Effect of condensed grape tannins on the *in vitro* activity of digestive proteases and activation on their zymogens. J. Food Sci. *51*, 577–580.

PRATT, D.E. 1992. Natural antioxidant from plant material. *In* Phenolic Compounds in Food and Their Effects on Health. I. Analysis, Occurrence and Chemistry (C.T. Ho, C.Y. Lee and M.T. Huang, eds). ACS Symp. Ser *506*, 54–71.

SALUNKE, D.K., JADHAV, S.J., KADAM, S.S. and CHAVAN, J.K. 1982. Chemical, biochemical and biological significance of polyphenols in cereals and legumes. CRC Crit. Rev. Food Sci. Nutr. *17*, 227–305.

SPANOS, G.A. and WROLSTAD, R.E. 1994. Phenolics of apple, pear and white grape juices and their changes with processing and storage. – A review. J. Agric Food Chem. *40*, 1478–1487.

STOHR, H. and HERRMANN, K. 1975. Die phenolischen Inhaltsstoffe des Obstes. VI. Die phenolischen Inhaltsstoffe der Johannisberen, Starchelbeerne und Kulturheidelbeeren. Veranderungen der Phenolsauren und Catechine wahrend Wachstum und Reife von schwarzen Johannisbeern. Z. Lebensm. Unters. Forsch. *159*, 31–37.

VILLANUEVA, M.R., MARTINEZ, J.A. and LARRALDE, J. 1987. Intestinal disaccharidase and dipeptidase activities on growing rats fed on a raw field bean diet. J. Sci. Food Agric. *39*, 163–168.

YUSTE, P., LONGSTAFF, M. and MCCORQUODALE, C. 1992. The effect of proanthocyanidin-rich hulls and proanthocyanidin extracts from bean (*Vicia faba L.*) hulls on nutrient digestibility and digestive enzyme activities in young chicks. Br. J. Nutr. *67*, 57–65.

CHARACTERIZATION OF LIPASE AND ITS APPLICATION IN DEFATTING OF FISH

QIAO-QIN SHI, YI ZHENG, JIANZHONG HUANG and SONG-GANG WU

Biological Engineering College
Fujian Normal University
Fujian, Fuzhou, 350007
P.R. China

ABSTRACT

Enzymatic characteristics of a lipase from Penicillium expansum *PF868 were investigated and its application to fish defatting was tested. The optimum temperature and pH for the lipase were determined to be 36°C and pH 9.4, respectively, while the enzyme was found to be stable at temperatures lower than 35°C at pH 6.0-10.6. When applying the enzyme to mackerel fish processing, the fish were most efficiently defatted at 30-35°C at pH 9.0-9.4 at a concentration of 20 U/ml H_2O of the lipase (U = units).*

INTRODUCTION

Lipase can hydrolyze lipid into glycerol and fatty acids; it is used to produce fatty acids and to defat fish in processing (Fu and Gao 1992). We have successfully isolated a lipase from *Pencillium expansum* PF868 with activity of 10,000 U/g. In this work, its enzymatic properties were first studied, and its application in fish processing as a defatting agent was attempted.

MATERIALS AND METHODS

Lipase was produced by *Penicillium expansum* PF868 with a specific activity of 10,000 U/g. Olive oil (AR), bean oil and fish oil were purchased from grocery stores; mackerel fish were obtained from Ninbo Ocean Fishery Corporation in Ninbo (Zhejiang, China).

Determination of Lipase Activity

Lipase activity was determined according to the method of Shen (1974).

TLC of Oil and Hydrolyzed Oil by Lipase

Thin layer chromatography (TLC) of oil and hydrolysis were carried out according to the methods of Tao (1993), Gao (1992) and Chao (1995). The adsorption agent was silica gel G, the spread agent was ether: petroleum ether (boiling point from 60 to 90°C): acetic acid (70:30:1); and the displaying agent was iodine vapor.

GC Analysis

Fatty acids were analyzed by the method of Huang (1993).

Defatting Process of Mackerel Fish with Lipase

Commercial processed mackerel fish was produced by the following procedures: removal of head and tail from the fresh fish, slicing, defatting, flavoring, roasting and packing.

Defatting of mackerel fish was carried out in this study by suspending the fresh mackerel fish in water of pH 9.0 adjusted with Na_2CO_3 by 1 to 1 weight ratio, and incubated at 30 ± 2°C for 20 min and the water was agitated by gas.

Determination of Lipid

Lipid was determined by the method of Shen (1974).

RESULTS AND DISCUSSION

Enzyme Characteristics of the Lipase

The Optimum Temperature. Lipase activity was determined after its reaction mixture was incubated at various temperatures for 15 min. Effect of temperature on lipase activity is shown in Fig. 1. The maximum activity was observed at 36°C; the remaining activity of the lipase was more than 75% between 22-45°C, indicating a wide range of functional temperature. The decrease in activity at higher temperatures is a result of temperature effect on stability of the enzyme, while the increase in (rate) activity at the lower temperature is due to the effect of temperature on increasing the rate of conversion of substrate to product.

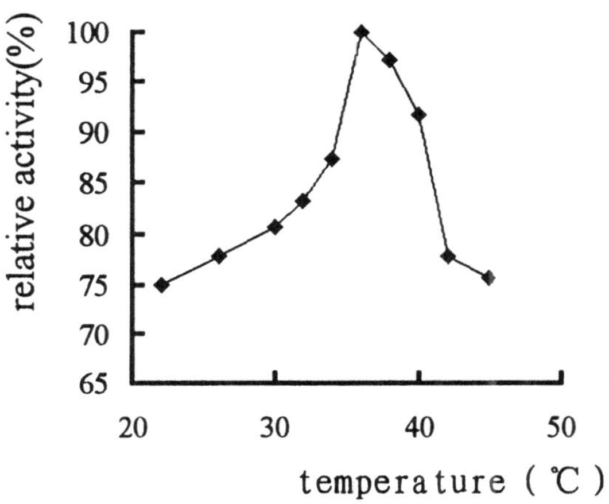

FIG. 1. OPTIMUM TEMPERATURE OF LIPASE

Heat Stability. Lipase solutions were incubated at various temperatures in the absence of substrate at a fixed time, and the remaining activity was determined. Effect of temperature on lipase activity is shown in Fig. 2. As is clear from the figure, lipase was stable at 30°C for 60 min and at 35°C for 30 min. The higher the incubation temperature, the higher the rate of activity loss.

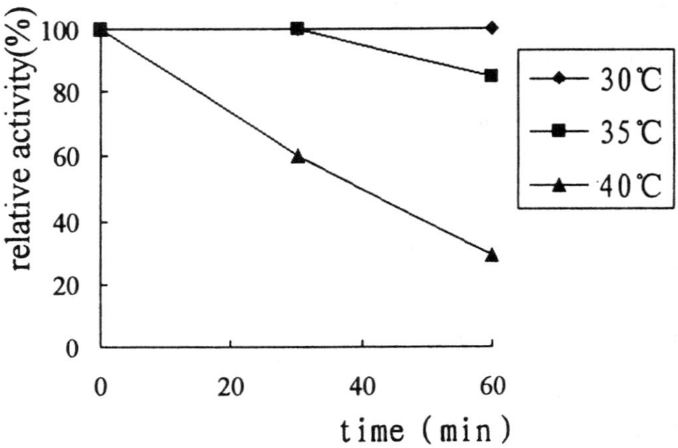

FIG. 2. EFFECT OF TEMPERATURE ON STABILITY OF LIPASE

Optimum pH. Lipase activity was determined in reaction mixtures at different pH; the results are shown in Fig. 3. The optimum pH for the lipase was 9.4; more than 60% of the activity remained between pH 7.0 and pH 10.6, indicating that the lipase may be an alkaline lipase.

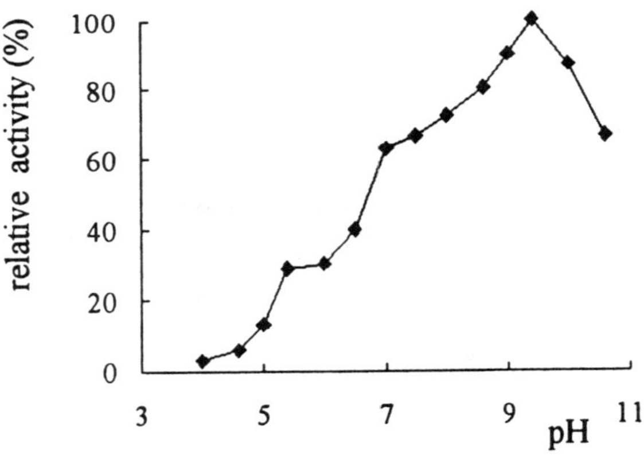

FIG. 3. OPTIMUM pH OF LIPASE

pH Stability. The lipase was incubated with buffer solutions of various pHs at 4 °C for 24 h, and the remaining lipase activity was determined as shown in Fig. 4. Full activity was retained between pH 7.0 and pH 10.6, and 90% activity remained at pH 6.0, suggesting that pH 6.0-10.6 is a suitable pH range for the lipase. When the pH was lower than 6.0, the enzyme was unstable. Therefore, an acid pH is not suitable for the lipase.

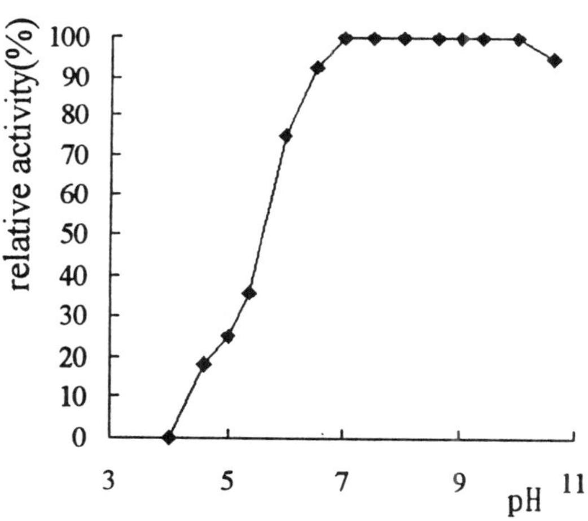

FIG. 4. EFFECT OF pH ON STABILITY OF LIPASE

Hydrolysis of Various Oils with the Lipase

Oils were hydrolyzed with the lipase in a 1:1 water/oil system with addition of the lipase at a concentration of 100 U/ml oil. The reaction mixtures were incubated at 32°C in a shaking bed rotating at 150 r/min for 36 h. The reaction mixture was sampled in the course of hydrolysis for determination of the total fatty acid value and hydrolysis rate. The ether extracts of each sample were separated by TLC (picture not shown), and the fatty acid section was collected and concentrated under vacuum, then analyzed by GC. The results are shown in Table 1.

As is shown in Table 1, the composition of the hydrolyzed fatty acid is almost in accord with the fatty acid content of the raw oil and the lipase exhibited a higher hydrolytic ability on lipids consisting of unsaturated fatty acids. When fish oil was hydrolyzed, C20:5 concentration in the total fatty acids increased from 24.2% to 46.0%, and C22:6 from 9.5% to 25.4%.

Defatting of Mackerel Fish with the Lipase

Optimum Temperature for Defatting. Fish were defatted with the lipase by the above-stated method with a lipase concentration of 20 U/ml at different temperatures. The mixture was sampled and the defatting rate determined.

TABLE 1.
COMPARISON OF THE FATTY ACID COMPOSITION OF OILS AND HYDROLYZED FREE FATTY ACIDS BY GC

sample	saturated fatty acid				unsaturated fatty acid					
	C12:0	C14:0	C16:0	C18:0	C16:1	C18:1	C18:2	C18:3	C20:5	C22:6
bean oil	/	12.2	3.9	/	23.0	53.4	7.4	/	/	
bean oil acid	22.8	14.9	8.9	/	/	19.3	32.0	1.8	/	
fish oil	/	5.7	9.0	1.6	6.2	16.3	5.1	19.5	24.2	9.5
fish oil acid	/	0.2	0.3	0.2	/	0.7	0.7	26.4	46.0	25.4
olive oil	/	/	0.7	3.5	1.9	76.1	7.5	0.3	/	/
olive oil acid	/	/	16.7	/	/	83.3	/	/	/	/

[1]not found

As is shown in Fig. 5, the optimum defatting temperature was 33°C. Even at room temperature (25-30°C), the lipase still exhibited high defatting ability. Therefore, relatively low temperatures at 28-33°C can be used for the defatting process, guaranteeing both a high defatting rate and fish meat of good quality.

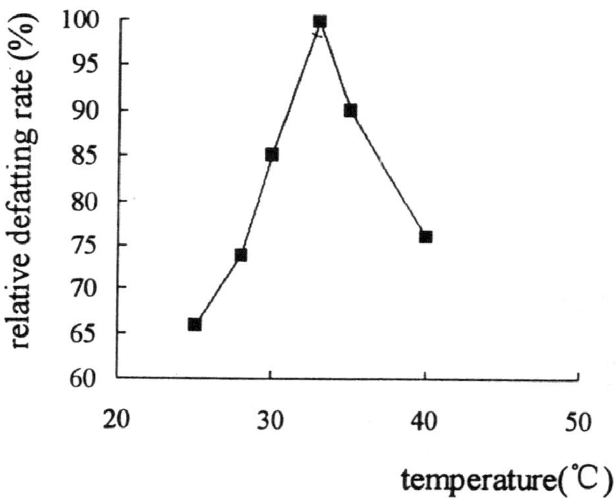

FIG. 5. OPTIMUM TEMPERATURE OF DEFATTING BY LIPASE

Optimum pH for Defatting. Fish defatting with the lipase was carried out by the above-stated methods at different initial pH adjusted with Na_2CO_3. The reaction mixture was sampled, and the defatting rate determined. Figure 6 shows that the optimum defatting pH was in the alkaline range. In the experiment, we adjusted the pH with small amounts of Na_2CO_3, which might enhance the defatting effect, and help with the removal of fatty acids since Na^+ binds to free fatty acids.

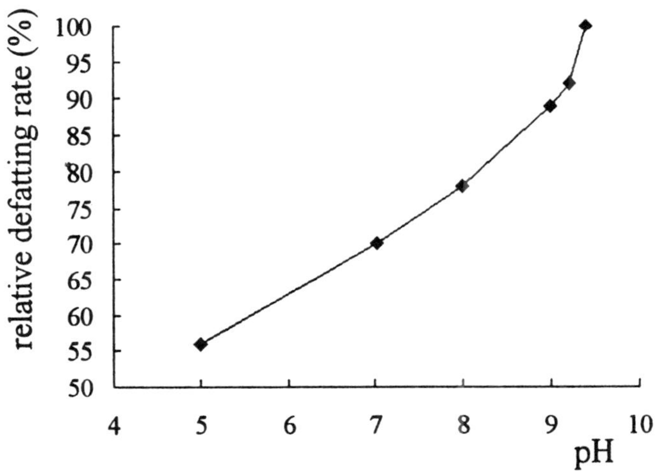

FIG. 6. OPTIMUM pH OF DEFATTING BY LIPASE

Optimum Lipase Concentration for Defatting. Fish defatting was carried out at different lipase concentrations, and the reaction mixture was sampled, and the lipid determined. The results are shown in Table 2.

TABLE 2.
EFFECT OF THE CONCENTRATION OF LIPASE ON DEFATTING OF FISH

number	lipase concentration (u/ml)	lipid content (%)	defatting rate (%)
1	10	14.2	24.9
2	20	11.8	37.6
3	40	8.9	52.9
4	60	9.1	51.9
5	4% Na_2CO_3	13.6	28.0
6	CK	18.9	/

As is shown in Table 2, the defatting effect at 20 U/ml lipase concentration was better than that by alkaline treatment. The lipase concentration was set to be 20 U/ml considering the cost of the lipase. Comparison of the quality of the products and semi-products defatted by enzymatic treatment and alkali treatment is shown in Table 3.

SUMMARY

The optimum temperature and pH of lipase from *Pencillium expansum* PF868 were 36°C, and pH 9.4, respectively. The enzyme was stable at temperatures lower than 35°C and in the pH range of 6.0-10.6. The lipase exhibited high activity in hydrolyzing fish oil, indicating that the lipase might be useful in the lipid industry, such as in fish processing.

TABLE 3.
COMPARISON OF THE PRODUCTS AND SEMI-PRODUCTS DEFATTED BY ENZYMATIC TREATMENT AND ALKALI TREATMENT

	alkali treatment	enzymatic treatment
semi-product (fish chip)	deep shade and greasy	light-color and ungreasy
product	uneasy to keep integrity deep shade, little acerbity with greasy surface keeping one month, taste unfavorably	easy to keep integrity light color, savory with ungreasy surface keeping one month, taste normally

The optimum conditions for fish chip defatting were 30-35°C and pH 9.0-9.4 at a lipase concentration of 20 U/ml H_2O.

REFERENCES

CHAO, S.G. 1995. The substrate specificity of lipase and its application potentiality. Prog. Biochem. Biophys. *22*(1), 9–13. (In Chinese)

FU, X. and GAO, K.Y. 1992. Hydrolysis of oils and fats catalyzed by lipase. Refined Petroleum Chem. Ind. *6*, 5–11. (in Chinese)

GAO, K.Y. 1992. Studies on hydrolysis of oils and fats catalyzed by 8901 lipase. Refined Petroleum Chem. Ind. *6*, 67–71. (In Chinese)

HUANG, W.K. 1993. The Detection and Analysis of Food. China Industry Press, Beijing. (In Chinese)

SHEN, Y.Q. 1974. Studies on lipase of *Eremothecium ashbyii* Du-32, Acta Microbiol. Sinica, *14* (1), 95–102. (in Chinese)

TAO, W.Q. 1993. Comparison of catalytic characteristics between lipase from different sources. J. Wuxi Institute of Light Industry *124* (2), 118–128. (In Chinese)

FLAVOR ESTER SYNTHESIS BY MICROBIAL LIPASES IN NON-AQUEOUS PHASE

XU YAN and CHANG KECHANG

School of Biotechnology
University of Light Industry
Wuxi 214036, P.R. China

ABSTRACT

The comparison of low molecular weight flavor ester synthesis in heptane, water, and solvent-free solution showed that higher molar conversion yields were obtained in non-aqueous phase due to shifting thermal equilibrium of the reaction for most of them tested. Suitable lipases for the synthesis reaction were screened, indicating that lipases from Mucor miehei, Candida rugosa, Pseudomonas sp *and porcine pancreas had higher yield with maximum yield of 93.5% conversion after 24 h obtained by* mucor miehei *lipase under 0.25 substrate concentration. The effect of chain length of carboxylic acids and alcohols on esterification exhibited that molar conversions were getting higher with the longer length of substrate chain under chain length of carboxylic acids ($C_2 \sim C_8$) and n-alcohols ($C_1 \sim C_8$). From the half-life period of esterification for different flavor ester production, it was observed that lipases were more stable in batch reaction with substrate chain length with longest one 981 h of half-life period.*

INTRODUCTION

With strong fruit flavor, low molecular weight esters are a large group of organic compounds used as flavors and fragrances. Extracted from plant materials, however, natural flavor esters are often scarce and expensive for commercial application in food, beverage, cosmetic and pharmaceutical industries which have great demands for them (Stofberg and Grundschober 1987). The use of biocatalysis for production of flavor esters has the potential for satisfying the increasing demands. Enzymatic esterification of flavor esters has the advantage of catalyzing reactions more specifically than chemical synthesis under mild condition and higher yield over microbiological production (Peter 1993; Kazlauskas 1993).

Triacylglycerohydrolases (EC 3.1.1.8) (or lipases) are the enzymes that have been used for the hydrolysis of acylglycerides in the oil industry and in recent years they have been researched to catalyze the reversible reaction: esterifying reaction in aqueous, non-aqueous and solvent-free phase (Bjorkling 1991; Welsh *et al.* 1990 and Xu *et al.* 1997). Higher capability for esterification and transesterification in non-aqueous phase increased lipase applications in organic synthesis. Enzymatic synthesis of aliphatic esters of longer chain substrates have shown their easy esterification due to their low polarity and good fit with the active site of lipase (Ota *et al.* 1990). Low molecular flavor esters synthesized from shorter chain substrates, however, have received considerably less attention comparably since substrates easily strip the essential water around enzymes to cause their deactivation (Chulalaksanaukul *et al.* 1990).

The objectives of our study were to (1) identify suitable lipase source with flavor ester synthesis; (2) choose appropriate media for enzymatic catalysis; (3) describe the effects of chain length of carboxylic acids ($C_2 \sim C_8$) and n-alcohols ($C_1 \sim C_8$) on the lipase mediated synthesis of low molecular flavor esters; and (4) investigate lipase's stability in esterification.

MATERIALS AND METHODS

Materials

Lipase preparations tested were *Mucor miehei* and *Aspergillus niger* from Novo Nordisk Industries Denmark; *Candida rugosa* (1) and porcine pancreas from Sigma Chemical Co; *Candida rugosa* (2), *Pseudomonas sp*, and *Mucor javanicus* from Amano Seiyaku Company; *Phycomyces nitens* from Takeda Yakuhin; *Candida sp* from Institute of Microbiology, Academia Sinica; *Candida lipolytica* from Synder Enzyme Company. Treated by 4A molecular sieve (Dalian catalyst plant) overnight for removal of water, all of the alcohol, carboxylic acid substrates, and heptane (analytically pure) were purchased from the Chemical Company of Shanghai, China.

Esterification Method

Flavor ester synthesis was conducted in 100 ml stoppered flasks with 15 ml heptane containing equal concentration of 0.25 M substrate and 0.1 g lipase. The mixture was incubated in batches, shaken at 150 rpm at a temperature of 30°C for 48 h.

Product Analysis Method

Aliquots of 100 μl reaction mixture were withdrawn and filtered by membrane periodically. Each sample was diluted in 5 ml heptane containing 0.1 ml of 10% n-heptane as an internal standard. Analysis was done by injecting a sample of 1 μl into a SP 3700 gas chromatograph (Beifen) equipped with a SE-30 fused silica capillary column (30 m × 0.25 mm i.d) and a hydrogen flame-ionization detector and SP 4290M Integrator (Spectra-Physics). Oven temperature by programmed temperature was held at 50°C for 3 min before being elevated to 150°C for 2 min at 10°C/min. Injector and detector temperature were set at 250°C. The carrier gas was nitrogen.

The molar conversion was defined as (molar of ethyl hexanate ÷ molar of initial hexanoic acid) × 100%.

The half life of lipase in batch was defined as the time when batch molar conversion decreased to the half of original conversion.

RESULTS AND DISCUSSION

Comparison of Flavor Ester Synthesis in Different Media

With the same molar substrates and amount of enzyme added, the comparison of seven flavor ester's synthesis catalyzed by MML (*Mucor miehei* lipase) in heptane, water, and solvent-free solution were conducted. The esters tested were synthesized from ethanol with different acyl donors: acetic acid, propionic acid, butyric acid, valeric acid, hexanoic acid, heptanoic acid, and octonoic acid. With a higher than 90% molar conversion yield, the data in Fig. 1 showed that lipase from *Mucor miehei* was more active in heptane than in water and a solvent-free solution. Even for some more difficultly synthesized esters, such as ethyl acetate and ethyl propionate, molar conversion yields in non-aqueous phase were 20% and higher than 40% respectively. The main reasons for the phenomenon were that a suitable solvent not only shifted the equilibrium of esterification reaction to give high yield but also did not distort the essential water layer that stabilized the lipase in microwater environment. Being more hydrophilic, the substrate seriously hampered the synthesis of the short chain ethyl esters (lower C_8) with consistently lower than 10% of molar conversion yield in water. So we did the esterification in solvent-free solution. With increasing carboxylic acid chain length, however, substrate conversion in solvent-free solution were getting higher with about 60% for ethyl heptanoate and octanoate.

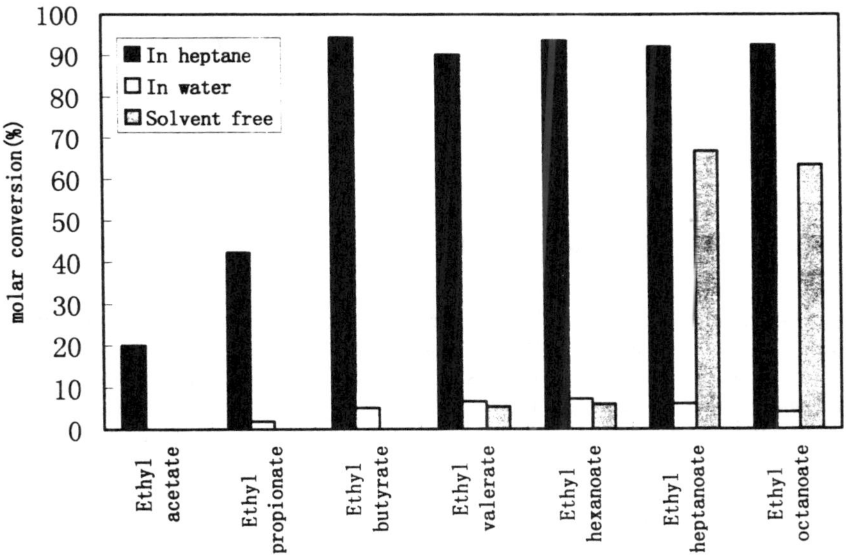

FIG. 1. COMPARISON OF FLAVOR ESTER SYNTHESIS BY MML IN HEPTANE, WATER, AND SOLVENT-FREE

Screening Trials of Suitable Lipases for Flavor Ester Synthesis

Under the same conditions, ethyl hexanoate esterification was used for screening suitable lipases. High 80% molar conversion yields were produced by MML, CRL-1, PPL, and PSL in all enzyme preparations tested (Table 1). The maximum yield was obtained by MML with 93.50% conversion yield in concentration of 33.66 g ethyl hexanoate per liter solvent. It was shown that substrate specificity of lipases varied considerably, depending on the enzyme, i.e, on the sources from which the lipases were produced. It is interesting to note that lipases from the same microbe *Candida rugosa* but from different suppliers had very different behavior in esterification.

TABLE 1.
ETHYL HEXANOATE ESTERIFICATION BY VARIOUS MICROBIAL LIPASES

Lipase source*	Degree of esterification (%)	Relative activity (%)
MML	93.50	100.00
CRL-1	86.25	92.25
PPL	89.02	95.21
CLL	32.56	34.82
CSL	61.20	65.45
PNL	18.19	19.45
MJL	16.00	17.11
ANL	8.50	9.09
PSL	87.06	93.11
CRL-2	30.23	32.33

* MML, *Mucor miehei* lipase
MJL, *Mucor javanicus* lipase
ANL, *Aspergillus niger* lipase
PSL, *Pseudomonas sp* lipase
CRL-2, *Candida rugosa* lipase
PNL, *Phycomces nitens* lipase
CRL-1, *Candida rugosa* lipase
PPL, Porcine pancreatic lipase
CLL, *Candida lipolytical* lipase
CSL, *Candidas* lipase

Effects of Chain Length of Carboxylic Acids and n-Alcohols on the Flavor Ester Synthesis

Effects of chain length of carboxylic acids and n-alcohols on molar conversion yield. In general, lipases exhibited a distinct specificity as regards the chain lengths of substrate acids and alcohols for synthesis in solvent phase. It was shown that the longer the chain length of acid and alcohol components were, the higher the degree of esterification achieved by MML (Fig. 2). It seemed that chain length of carboxylic acids had more influence on conversion yield than that of alcohols. The yields of acetate esters of various alcohol were almost identical with less than 30% molar conversion. Similar results have been reported by G. Langrad for different lipases as a result of inactivation of enzyme after the essential water was stripped.

Effects of chain length of carboxylic acids and n-alcohols on the stability of lipases in the flavor ester synthesis. The differences of the specificity of MML to substrate was observed not only in substrate conversion but also in their stability expressed by the half-life period of lipase in solvent phase (Table 2). The ethyl esters ($C_4 \sim C_8$ carboxylic acid) had longer half-life periods than ethyl acetate and ethyl propioatae.

We have shown in this study that microbial lipase catalyzed the flavor ester synthesis more actively in heptane than in water and solvent-free system. The lipases from different sources had different specificity to substrate acid and ethanol to give different conversion yields. The maximum production was obtained by lipase from *Mucor miehei* in synthesis of ethyl hexanoate. Most flavor esters tested were synthesized by MML in more than 90% conversion yield and with more than 900 h of half life. Lipase mediated synthesis of flavor esters has potentially industrial application in flavor and fragrant production because of higher conversion yield, stability of enzyme, and easy reuse of enzyme.

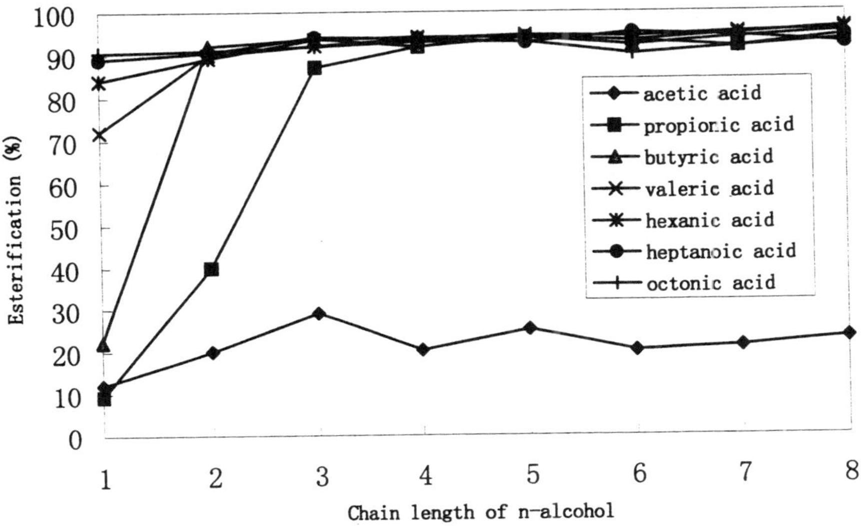

FIG. 2. EFFECT OF CHAIN LENGTH OF CARBOXYLIC ACID AND N-ALCOHOL ON THE DEGREE OF ESTERIFICATION

TABLE 2.
HALF LIFE PERIOD OF MML IN LOW MOLECULAR WEIGHT FLAVOR ESTER SYNTHESIS

Esters	Half life (hr)
Ethyl acetate	140
Ethyl propionate	275
Ethyl butyrate	975
Ethyl valerate	923
Ethyl hexanoate	981
Ethyl heptanoate	925
Ethyl octanoate	951

REFERENCES

BJORKLING, F., GODTFREDSEN, S.E. and KIRK, O. 1991. The future impact of industrial lipases. TIBTECH. *9*, 360–363.

CHULALAKSANAUKUL, W., CONDORET, S., DELORME, P. and WILLEMOT, R.M. 1990. Kinetic study of esterification by immobilized lipase in *n*-hexane. FEBS Letter *276*, 181–184.

KAZLAUSKAS, R.J. 1993. Biocatalysis-becoming more predictable and selective. TIBTECH. *11*, 439–440.

OTA, T., TAKANO, S. and HASEGAWA, T. 1990. Synthesis of C_{18}-fatty acid esters in organic solvent by lipase from *Candida cylindrecea*. *54*(6), 1571–1572.

PETER, J.C. 1993. The use of biotransformations for the production of flavours and fragrances. TIBTECH. *11*, 478–488.

STOFBERG, J. and GRUNDSCHOBER, F. 1987. Consumption ratio and food predominance of flavoring materials. Perfumer and Flavorist *24*, 27.

WELSH, F.W., WILLIAMS, R.E. and DAWSON, K.H. 1990. Lipase mediated synthesis of low molecular weight flavor esters. J. Food Sci. *55*, 1679–1682.

XU, Y. and ZHANG, K.C. 1997. Microbial lipase mediated synthesis of ethyl hexanoate for Chinese liquor in solvent phase. Chinese Alcoholic Beverage. *3*, 12–15.

XU, Y. and ZHANG, K.C. 1998. Flavor ester synthesis by microbial lipases in heptane phase. Chinese J. Biotechnol. Submitted.

STUDIES OF THE FERMENTATION PROPERTIES OF THE LIPID-PRODUCING MICROORGANISM — *MORTIERELLA ISABELINA* M-018

SONG-GANG WU, JIANZHONG HUANG, XIAO-LAN ZHOU, YAO-XIN LIN, BI-FENG XIE and QIAO-QIN SHI

Biological Engineering College
Fujian Normal University
Fujian, Fuzhou, 350007
P.R. China

ABSTRACT

The mutant M-018 from Mortierella isabelina, *capable of accumulating 79.2% lipids consisting of various polyunsaturated fatty acids, was successfully screened and cultured. The optimal culture conditions for mycelial growth were determined to be a medium containing glucose and yeast extract as major carbon and nitrogen sources, respectively, at a carbon to nitrogen ratio of 20/1 at 28°C. The optimal conditions for lipid production was a medium using glucose as carbon source and yeast extract as nitrogen source at carbon to nitrogen ratio of 60/1 at 25°C. Urea (0.3%) and* Zn^{2+} *(500 ppm) were found to give greatly increased lipid iodine values.*

INTRODUCTION

Lipid is an important nutritional component as well as a major material in industrial production. Lipid from microorganisms is apparently a new and interesting source of lipid. It can not only replenish the present inadequate lipid resource from animals and plants, and substitute for edible oil and industrial oil, but it is also a good source of lipids with high value, physiological function and special application. With elucidation of physiological function of polyunsaturated fatty acids (PUFAs), PUFAs producing microorganisms have become one of the major fields of great interest (Max *et al.* 1993; Shaw 1990; Kendrick and Ratledge 1990). Suzuki (1981) reported production of linoleic acid by *Mortierella* with a lipid content in mycelium up to 48-52%. We successfully screened and cultured a mutant *Mortierella isabelina* M-018 which could accumulate lipids up to 72.5-76.8% from soil. The optimal carbon and nitrogen sources and optimal culture conditions for the strain were investigated in this work in order to further improve lipid-producing capability of the strain.

MATERIALS AND METHODS

Microorganism, Media and Cultivation

The strain *Mortierella isabelina* M-018 used in this work was screened and cultured by this group and preserved in the strain center of our College. Medium A, used as seed cultural medium, consisted of 5% glucose, 0.5% urea, 0.1% KH_2PO_4, 0.2% $MgSO_4$, and 0.25% yeast extract. Medium B, used for lipid production, contained 10% glucose, 0.2% yeast extract and 0.5% $(NH_4)_2SO_4$. The strain was inoculated into a 250 ml shaking flask containing 50 ml of medium, and incubated at 28°C for 24 h with reciprocal shaking (200 strokes/min). Cultivation for lipid-production was carried out at 26°C for 72 h with reciprocal shaking (250 strokes/min).

Determination of Lipid Concentration

Lipid concentration was determined according to the method of Shimizu *et al.* (1989).

Determination of Iodine Value of Lipid

Lipid iodine value was determined by the method of Li *et al.* (1994).

Extraction and Determination of Fatty Acids

Fungal cells were harvested by suction filtration, washed with 50 ml of water and then dried at 100°C overnight. The dried cells were suspended in 5 ml of methylene chloride-10% methanolic HCl (1:1, v/v) for three h at 50 °C. As an internal standard, *n*-heptadecanoic acid (0.5 mg) usually was included in the methanolysis mixture. After extraction with 20 ml of *n*-hexane, followed by evaporation, the fatty acid methyl esters were dissolved in 0.05-0.1 ml of acetonitrile and then analyzed by gas liquid chromatography (GLC). The conditions for GLC were the same as those described previously (Yamada *et al.* 1989), except for the following modifications: glass column (3 mm × 2 m) packed with 5% Advans DS on 80/100 mesh Chromosorb W (Shimadzu, Kyoto); column temperature, 190°C; and injection port temperature of 240°C. Mycelial fatty acid composition values are reported in weight percent.

Determination of Mycelial Mass

Fungal growth was measured by determining the mycelial weight after drying at 100°C overnight.

RESULTS AND DISCUSSION

Analysis of Mycelium Fatty Acid Composition in *Mortierella isabelina* Mutant M-018

Results shown in Table 1 indicate that the lipid of mutant M-018 mycelium had a high content of polyunsaturated fatty acids including oleic acid, linolenic acid and γ-linolenic acid.

Effect of Carbon Sources on Mycelial Growth and Lipid Anabolism

The carbon source is used for energy by cells when they grow. Effects of different carbon sources on cell growth and lipid production were investigated. The tested carbon sources included glucose, maltose, lactose and so on. Results are shown in Table 2.

TABLE 1.
ANALYSIS OF MYCELIAL FATTY ACID COMPOSITION IN *MORTIERELLA ISABELINA* M-018

Kind of fatty acids	Content (%)
C14:0	1.1
C14:1	0.1
C16:0	23.1
C16:1	6.3
C18:0	1.3
C18:1	48.8
C18:2	10.9
C18:3	6.9
C20:0	0.5
C20:1	0.9
Others	0.1

TABLE 2.
THE EFFECT OF CARBON SOURCES ON THE MYCELIAL GROWTH AND LIPID ANABOLISM IN *M. ISABELINA* M-018

Carbon sources (10%)	Mycelial mass (g/l)	Lipid content (%)	Lipid iodine value
Glucose	31.2	66.4	83.4
Sugar	24.6	46.5	84.3
Starch	21.2	40.2	82.7
Maltose	29.3	52.5	88.5
Lactose	20.1	41.3	82.1
Dextrin	24.4	44.5	80.4

The results indicate that glucose was the best carbon source for mycelial growth and lipid anabolism of the strain M-018. It should be noted that several carbon sources had little effect on lipid iodine value.

Effect of Nitrogen Sources on the Mycelial Growth and Lipid Anabolism

Various organic and inorganic compounds and natural nutrients were tested by adding 0.3% of those materials to medium B in place of the yeast extract. Dry cells cultured in the different nitrogen source media were obtained. As shown in Table 3, different nitrogen sources had a large influence on the mycelial growth and lipid anabolism of strain M-018. $(NH_4)_2SO_4$, NH_4NO_3 and urea were suitable for growth of mycelium while peptone and beef extracts were good for lipid anabolism. Yeast extract was not only effective on growth but also enhanced lipid production. Urea increased lipid iodine value.

TABLE 3.
THE EFFECT OF NITROGEN SOURCES ON THE MYCELIAL GROWTH AND LIPID ANABOLISM IN *M. ISABELINA* M-018

Nitrogen sources (0.3%)	Mycelial mass (g/L)	Lipid content (%)	Lipid iodine value
Yeast extract	32.8	68.2	83.0
$(NH_4)_2SO_4$	32.4	57.4	79.2
KNO_3	22.5	58.9	77.9
NH_4NO_3	40.2	51.0	78.7
$NaNO_3$	28.2	58.5	79.4
$NH_4H_2PO_4$	34.5	54.2	78.6
NH_4Cl	22.5	60.1	87.4
Peptone	22.4	67.6	79.5
Beef extract	23.7	66.3	84.2
Urea	31.2	48.1	102.8

Influence of C/N on the Mycelial Growth and Lipid Anabolism

Mycelium cell growth required a large amount of nitrogen source while lipid anabolism required much less nitrogen. Figure 1 shows the influence of C/N on mycelial growth and lipid production. The optimal C/N for mycelial growth was 20/1, but for lipid production was 60/1.

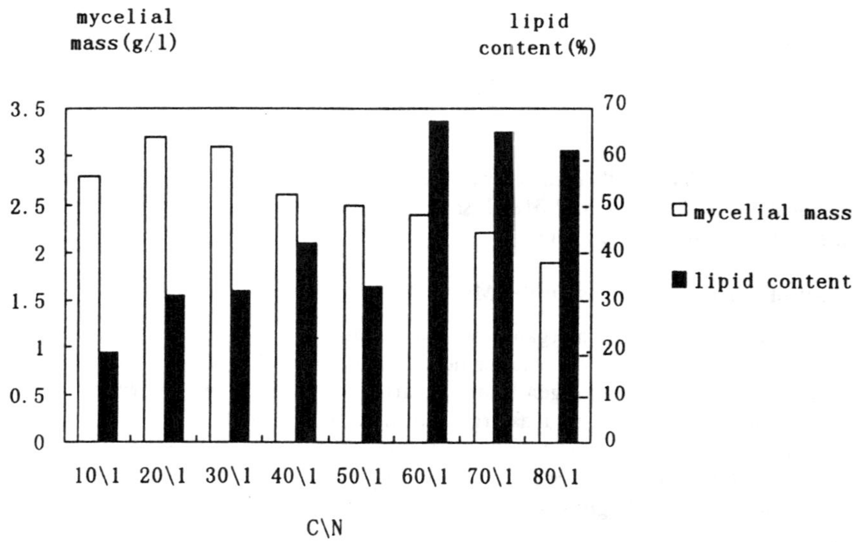

FIG. 1. EFFECT OF C/N ON MYCELIAL GROWTH AND LIPID ANABOLISM

Effect of Cultural Temperature on Mycelial Growth and Mycelial Lipid Anabolism

Figure 2 shows that the optimal temperature for mycelium growth was 25-30°C , different from the optimal temperature for lipid production. A large amount of lipid accumulated at 15-20°C. It also should be noted that lipid iodine values became higher with decrease of cultural temperature.

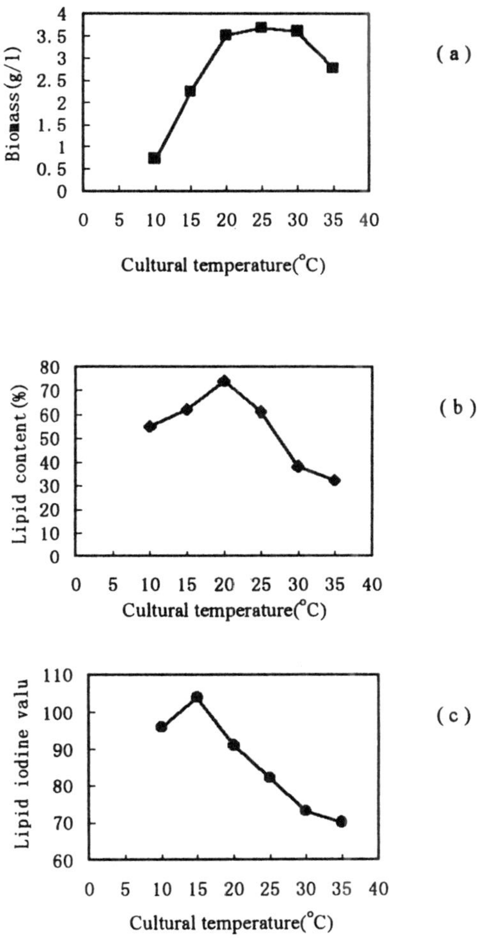

FIG.2 EFFECT OF CULTURAL TEMPERATURE ON MYCELIUM GROWTH AND LIPID ANABOLISM

(a) temperature on biomass; (b) temperature on lipid content; (c) temperature on lipid iodine value.

Effect of Sodium Citrate Concentration on Mycelial Growth and Lipid Anabolism

As shown in Table 4, cell weight per liter of cultural broth increased with the sodium citrate concentration. The amount of biomass reached 44 g/L of culture broth with 1.0% sodium citrate. Within 0.2-0.5% sodium citrate, lipid content in mycelium reached 66.3-67.4%. The concentration of sodium citrate was less influential on lipid iodine value.

TABLE 4.
EFFECT OF SODIUM CITRATE CONCENTRATION ON MYCELIAL GROWTH AND LIPID ANABOLISM

Concentration (%)	Mycelial mass (g/L)	Lipid content (%)	Lipid iodine value
0	0.9	51.4	79.5
0.1	24	58.3	80.3
0.2	32	67.4	82.6
0.5	38	66.4	80.1
0.75	41	57.2	79.4
10	44	56.1	79.8

Effect of Zn^{2+} on Mycelial Growth and Lipid Production

The mycelial lipid iodine value varied markedly depending on the addition of Zn^{2+} to the lipid-producing medium. Table 5 demonstrates the highest lipid iodine value of 108 in the present of 500 ppm Zn^{2+}, but iodine value was only 80.40 without Zn^{2+}; addition of Zn^{2+} to the medium had little effect on mycelium growth and lipid production.

TABLE 5.
EFFECT OF ZN^{2+} ON MYCELIAL GROWTH AND LIPID ANABOLISM

Concentration (ppm)	Mycelial mass (g/L)	Lipid content (%)	Lipid iodine value
0(contrast)	31.8	67.4	80.4
100	32.4	68.3	83
200	31.5	68.7	91
500	33.1	66.5	108
800	32.6	67.7	97
1000	31.6	68.0	95

REFERENCES

KENDRICK, A. and RATLEDGE, C. 1990. Microbial lipid technology: microbial formation of polyunsaturated fatty acids. Lipid Technol. *2*, 62–66.

LI, J.W., XIAO, N.G., YU, R.Y. and YUAN, M.X. 1994. Method for lipid iodine value assay. *In* Experimental Theory and Methods for Biochemistry. Beijing University Press, Beijing. pp. 139–141.

KENNEDY, M.J., READER, S.L. and DAVIES, R.J. 1993. Fatty acid production characteristics of fungi with particular emphasis on gamma linolenic acid production. Biotechnol. Bioengin. *42*, 625–634.

SHIMIZU, S., AKIMOTO, K., KAWASHIMA, H., SHINMEN, Y. and YAMADA, H. 1989. Production of dihomo-γ-linolenic acid by *mortierella alpina* IS-4. J. Am. Oil Chem. Soc. *66*, 237–241.

SHAW, R. 1965. The occurrence of gamma linolenic acid in fungi. Biochem. Biophys. Acta *98*, 230–237.

SUZUKI, O., YOKOCHI, T. and YAMASHINA, T. 1981. Studies on production of lipid in fungi II. Lipid composition of six species of mucorales in Zxgomyces. J. Jpn. Oil Chem. Soc. *30*, 863–868.

YAMADA, H., SHIMIZU, S., SHINMEN, Y., KAWASHIMA H. and AKIMOTO, K. 1989. Biotechnological processes for production of poly-unsaturated fatty acids. J. Dispersion Sci. Technol. *10*, 561–579.

SUBJECT INDEX